AF837282

Gene Therapy for Cancer

CANCER DRUG DISCOVERY AND DEVELOPMENT

BEVERLY A. TEICHER, SERIES EDITOR

Transforming Growth Factor-β in Cancer Therapy, Volume II: *Cancer Treatment and Therapy,* edited by *Sonia Jakowlew, 2007*

Transforming Growth Factor-β in Cancer Therapy, Volume 1: *Basic and Clinical Biology*, edited by *Sonia Jakowlew, 2007*

Microtubule Targets in Cancer Therapy, edited by *Antonio T. Fojo, 2007*

Cytokines in the Genesis and Treatment of Cancer, edited by *Michael A. Caligiuri, Michael T. Lotze, and Frances R. Balkwill, 2007*

Regional Cancer Therapy, edited by *Peter M. Schlag and Ulrike Stein, 2007*

Gene Therapy for Cancer, edited by *Kelly K. Hunt, Stephan A. Vorburger, and Stephen G. Swisher, 2007*

Deoxynucleoside Analogs in Cancer Therapy, edited by *Godefridus J. Peters,* 2006

Cancer Drug Resistance, edited by *Beverly A. Teicher,* 2006

Histone Deacetylases: *Transcriptional Regulation and Other Cellular Functions*, edited by *Eric Verdin,* 2006

Immunotherapy of Cancer, edited by *Mary L. Disis,* 2006

Biomarkers in Breast Cancer: *Molecular Diagnostics for Predicting and Monitoring Therapeutic Effect*, edited by *Giampietro Gasparini and Daniel F. Hayes,* 2006

Protein Tyrosine Kinases: *From Inhibitors to Useful Drugs*, edited by *Doriana Fabbro and Frank McCormick,* 2005

Bone Metastasis: *Experimental and Clinical Therapeutics*, edited by *Gurmit Singh and Shafaat A. Rabbani,* 2005

The Oncogenomics Handbook, edited by *William J. LaRochelle and Richard A. Shimkets,* 2005

Camptothecins in Cancer Therapy, edited by *Thomas G. Burke and Val R. Adams,* 2005

Combination Cancer Therapy: *Modulators and Potentiators,* edited by *Gary K. Schwartz,* 2005

Cancer Chemoprevention, Volume 2: *Strategies for Cancer Chemoprevention,* edited by *Gary J. Kelloff, Ernest T. Hawk, and Caroline C. Sigman,* 2005

Death Receptors in Cancer Therapy, edited by *Wafik S. El-Deiry,* 2005

Cancer Chemoprevention, Volume 1: *Promising Cancer Chemopreventive Agents,* edited by *Gary J. Kelloff, Ernest T. Hawk, and Caroline C. Sigman,* 2004

Proteasome Inhibitors in Cancer Therapy, edited by *Julian Adams,* 2004

Nucleic Acid Therapeutics in Cancer, edited by *Alan M. Gewirtz,* 2004

DNA Repair in Cancer Therapy, edited by *Lawrence C. Panasci and Moulay A. Alaoui-Jamali,* 2004

Hematopoietic Growth Factors in Oncology: *Basic Science and Clinical Therapeutics,* edited by *George Morstyn, MaryAnn Foote, and Graham J. Lieschke,* 2004

Handbook of Anticancer Pharmacokinetics and Pharmacodynamics, edited by *William D. Figg and Howard L. McLeod,* 2004

Anticancer Drug Development Guide: *Preclinical Screening, Clinical Trials, and Approval, Second Edition,* edited by *Beverly A. Teicher and Paul A. Andrews,* 2004

Handbook of Cancer Vaccines, edited by *Michael A. Morse, Timothy M. Clay, and Kim H. Lyerly,* 2004

Drug Delivery Systems in Cancer Therapy, edited by *Dennis M. Brown,* 2003

Oncogene-Directed Therapies, edited by *Janusz Rak,* 2003

Cell Cycle Inhibitors in Cancer Therapy: *Current Strategies,* edited by *Antonio Giordano and Kenneth J. Soprano,* 2003

Chemoradiation in Cancer Therapy, edited by *Hak Choy*, 2003

Gene Therapy for Cancer

Edited by

Kelly K. Hunt, MD

The University of Texas M. D. Anderson Cancer Center, Houston, TX

Stephan A. Vorburger, MD, MCR

Inselspital Bern, University of Bern, Bern, Switzerland

Stephen G. Swisher, MD

The University of Texas M. D. Anderson Cancer Center, Houston, TX

Humana Press
Totowa, New Jersey

999 Riverview Drive, Suite 208
Totowa, New Jersey 07512
www.humanapress.com

Cover design by Carlotta Craig
Cover illustration: Figure 3 from Chapter 17, "Nonviral Genetic Vaccines for Cancer," by Steven R. Little, Daniel G. Anderson, and Robert Langer
This publication is printed on acid-free paper. ∞
ANSI Z39.48-1984 (American National Standards Institute)
Permanence of Paper for Printed Library Materials

For additional copies, pricing for bulk purchases, and/or information about other Humana titles, contact Humana at the above address or at any of the following numbers: Tel.:973-256-1699; Fax: 973-256-8341; Email: orders@humanapr.com; or visit our Website: http://humanapress.com

Printed in the United States of America. 10 9 8 7 6 5 4 3 2 1

E-ISBN 1-59745-222-X 13-digit ISBN 978-1-58829-472-2
Library of Congress Cataloging-in-Publication Data
Gene therapy for cancer / edited by Kelly K. Hunt, Stephan A. Vorburger, Stephen G. Swisher.
p. ; cm. — (Cancer drug discovery and development)
Includes bibliographical references and index.
ISBN 1-58829-472-2 (alk. paper)
1. Cancer—Gene therapy. I. Hunt, Kelly K. II. Vorburger, Stephan A. III. Swisher, Stephen G. IV. Series.
[DNLM: 1. Neoplasms—genetics. 2. Neoplasms—therapy. 3. Gene Therapy—methods. QZ 266 G3253 2007]
RC271.G45G463 2007
616.99'40694—dc22 2006012653

Preface

The possibility of treating cancer, a disease defined by genetic defects, by introducing genes targeting these very alterations has led to an immense interest in gene therapy for cancer. Although incremental successes have been realized, enthusiasm for gene therapy has declined due to an increasing number of obstacles. These obstacles include vector systems that do not reach systemic metastases, therapeutic genes with redundant mechanisms allowing for cellular resistance, and toxicities in clinical trials leading to premature closure of these studies. Different tactics to overcome or circumvent these obstacles have catalyzed the development of a wide range of gene therapy approaches. Thus far, almost two-thirds of gene therapy trials have focused on cancer. This reflects the concept that gene therapy approaches for the treatment of cancer do not necessarily require long-term expression of the gene as is necessary for the treatment of primary genetic defects like hemophilia or juvenile diabetes. Unlike the treatment of genetic defects, where expression of the corrected gene needs to be strong, permanent and, sometimes regulated, tactics to treat tumors can be based on temporary and locally limited effects. In addition, cancer cells have different properties than normal cells and this allows for targeting gene therapy to specific cells, a major advantage over current antitumor therapies, which are also toxic to normal cells and tissues.

Gene Therapy for Cancer covers the current ideas and technology of gene therapy, as well as the demanding task of bringing it to and applying it in clinical trials. The book is divided into three major parts: (1) Vectors used in gene therapy against cancer, (2) targets and specific approaches for the therapy of cancer, and (3) clinical applications of cancer gene therapy.

The delivery of an antitumor gene, a toxic agent, or an immunostimulating drug selectively to tumor cells is one of the most crucial steps in achieving successful cancer gene therapy. We have dedicated a considerable portion of *Gene Therapy for Cancer* to a description of the various aspects of gene delivery including vehicles (vectors), their characteristics, and production methods.

Knowledge of the specific strategies and targets for the treatment of cancer has increased dramatically over the past decade. These range from methods that induce immediate cancer cell death through expression of genes that trigger the cell-death program or by reactivating pathways that render mutated cells susceptible to antitumor agents. Additional methods run the gamut from the correction of underlying defects at molecular levels to activation of the immune system or the tumor microenvironment. Understanding the basic underlying oncogenic changes allows for development of vectors engineered to exploit these gene mutations through selective spread of the vector in tumor cells with the specific changes. Background knowledge, technical details, and preclinical and clinical results are provided by specialists in each of these approaches.

Probably more so than in any other antitumor therapy, bringing gene therapy approaches to the clinic is a difficult task burdened by numerous regulations and limited by scarce funding opportunities. We have asked experts in clinical gene therapy trials to discuss the trials and tribulations of realizing advances in gene therapy at the preclinical level to the benefit of patients with cancer. The readers will gain significant insight into these difficulties and learn how to overcome the obstacles on the way from the laboratory to the bedside. Gene therapy approaches and results that have reached the stage of clinical testing are described by their principal investigators.

With *Gene Therapy for Cancer* we have sought to provide a comprehensive and in-depth view of currently available techniques for cancer gene therapy, including their limitations and the potential for future advances. This should prove to be a valuable resource for both researchers and clinicians in the field. With this approach we hope to provide an opportunity for clinicians and researchers to communicate their perspectives, allowing for increased collaboration and perhaps more rapid advances in this challenging field.

We would like to thank all the specialists who dedicated their valuable time to provide the most important and exciting advances in cancer gene therapy for this book. We are deeply grateful to our families for their continuous support, endless patience, and understanding.

Kelly K. Hunt, MD
Stephan A. Vorburger, MD
Stephen G. Swisher, MD

CONTENTS

CONTRIBUTORS

ROBERT J. AMATO • *Scott Department of Urology, Baylor College of Medicine, Houston, TX*

DANIEL G. ANDERSON • *Chemical Engineering Department, Massachusetts Institute of Technology, Cambridge, MA*

GUSTAVO AYALA • *Department of Pathology, Baylor College of Medicine, Houston, TX*

GLEN N. BARBER • *Department of Microbiology and Immunology, University of Miami School of Medicine, Miami, FL*

DAVID L. BARTLETT • *Division of Surgical Oncology, University of Pittsburgh, Pittsburgh, PA*

DORA BOCANGEL • *Introgen Therapeutics, Houston, TX*

E. BRIAN BUTLER • *Department of Radiology, Baylor College of Medicine, Houston, TX*

SUNIL CHADA • *Introgen Therapeutics, Houston, TX*

SRICHARAN CHALIKONDA • *Division of Surgical Oncology, University of Pittsburgh, Pittsburgh, PA*

DAVID T. CURIEL • *Gene Therapy Center, University of Alabama, Birmingham, AL*

BINGLIANG FANG • *Department of Thoracic and Cardiovascular Surgery–Research, The University of Texas M.D. Anderson Cancer Center, Houston, TX*

YUMAN FONG • *Department of Surgery, Memorial Sloan-Kettering Cancer Center, New York, NY*

JUAN FUEYO • *Department of Neuro-Oncology/Research, The University of Texas M. D. Anderson Cancer Center, Houston, TX*

TETSUO FUJITA • *Scott Department of Urology, Baylor College of Medicine, Houston, TX*

DAVID M. GERSHENSON • *Department of Gynecologic Oncology, The University of Texas M.D. Anderson Cancer Center, Houston, TX*

STANTON L. GERSON • *Division of Hematology-Oncology, Case Western Reserve University School of Medicine, Cleveland, OH*

ELIZABETH A. GRIMM • *Department of Experimental Therapuetics, The University of Texas M.D. Anderson Cancer Center, Houston, TX*

GABRIEL N. HORTOBAGYI • *Department of Breast Medical Oncology, The University of Texas M.D. Anderson Cancer Center, Houston, TX*

LEAF HUANG • *Center for Pharmacogenetics, Department of Pharmaceutical Science, University of Pittsburgh, Pittsburgh, PA*

MIEN-CHIE HUNG • *Department of Molecular & Cellular Oncology, The University of Texas M.D. Anderson Cancer Center, Houston, TX*

KELLY K. HUNT • *Department of Surgical Oncology, The University of Texas M.D. Anderson Cancer Center, Houston, TX*

SATOSHI INOUE • *Department of Thoracic and Cardiovascular Surgery, The University of Texas M. D. Anderson Cancer Center, Houston, TX*

WILLIAM R. JARNAGIN • *Hepatobiliary Service, Department of Surgery, Memorial Sloan-Kettering Cancer Center, New York, NY*

DOV KADMON • *Scott Department of Urology, Baylor College of Medicine, Houston, TX*

NORIYUKI KASAHARA • *Department of Medicine, UCLA Geffen School of Medicine, Macdonald Research Laboratories, Los Angeles, CA*

DAVID H. KIRN • *Department of Clinical Pharmacology, University of Oxford Medical School, Oxford, UK*

FREDERICK F. LANG • *Department of Neurosurgery, The University of Texas M. D. Anderson Cancer Center, Houston, TX*

ROBERT S. LANGER • *Chemical & Biomedical Engineering, Massachusetts Institute of Technology, Cambridge, MA*

PUI-YAN LEE • *Center for Pharmacogenetics, Department of Pharmaceutical Science, University of Pittsburgh, Pittsburgh, PA*

STEVEN K. LIBUTTI • *Surgery Branch, National Cancer Institute, Bethesda, MD*

STEVEN R. LITTLE • *Departments of Chemical Engineering and Bioengineering, University of Pittsburgh, Pittsburgh, PA*

TA-CHIANG LIU • *Molecular Neurosurgery Laboratory, Massachusetts General Hospital, Harvard Medical School, Boston, MA*

ROBERT M. LORENCE • *Wellstat Biologics Corporation, Gaithersburg, MD*

KENNETH LUNDSTROM • *BioXtal / Cancer Therapeutic Sciences, Switzerland*

RAYMOND E. MEYN, JR. • *Department of Experimental Radiation Oncology, The University of Texas M. D. Anderson Cancer Center, Houston, TX*

ABNER M. MHASHILKAR • *Introgen Therapeutics, Houston, TX*

BRIAN J. MILES • *Scott Department of Urology, Baylor College of Medicine, Houston, TX*

RIO MIYAHARA • *Department of Thoracic and Cardiovascular Surgery, The University of Texas M. D. Anderson Cancer Center, Houston, TX*

IAN J. MOHR • *Department of Microbiology, New York University School of Medicine, New York, NY*

ANUPAMA MUNSHI • *Department of Experimental Radiation Oncology, The University of Texas M. D. Anderson Cancer Center, Houston, TX*

KOJI NARUISHI • *Scott Department of Urology, Baylor College of Medicine, Houston, TX*

ABUJIANG PATAER • *Department of Thoracic and Cardiovascular Surgery, The University of Texas M.D. Anderson Cancer Center, Houston, TX*

ANDREW L. PECORA • *The Cancer Center, Hackensack University Medical Center, Hackensack, NJ*

RICHARD H. PIN • *Department of Surgery, Memorial Sloan-Kettering Cancer Center, New York, NY*

SELVARANGAN PONNAZHAGAN • *Department of Pathology, University of Alabama at Birmingham, Birmingham, AL*

RAJAGOPAL RAMESH • *Department of Thoracic and Cardiovascular Surgery–Research, The University of Texas M.D. Anderson Cancer Center, Houston, TX*

MAURA REINBLATT • *Department of Surgery, Memorial Sloan-Kettering Cancer Center, New York, NY*

JACK A. ROTH • *Department of Thoracic and Cardiovascular Surgery–Research, The University of Texas M.D. Anderson Cancer Center, Houston, TX*

JUSTIN C. ROTH • *Division of Hematology/Oncology, Case Western Reserve University, Cleveland, OH*

DMITRY M. SHAYAKHMETOV • *Division of Medical Genetics, Department of Medicine, University of Washington, Seattle, WA*

CHAO-ZHONG SONG • *Division of Medical Genetics, Department of Medicine, University of Washington, Seattle, WA*

RENATA STRIPECKE • *Department of Medicine, David Geffen School of Medicine, University of California (UCLA), Los Angeles, CA*

STEPHEN G. SWISHER • *Department of Thoracic and Cardiovascular Surgery, The University of Texas M. D. Anderson Cancer Center, Houston, TX*

ANITA T. TANDLE • *Surgery Branch, National Cancer Institute, Bethesda, MD*

BIN S. TEH • *Michael E. DeBakey Veterans Affairs Medical Center, Houston, TX*

TIMOTHY C. THOMPSON • *Scott Department of Urology, Baylor College of Medicine, Houston, TX*

TERRY L. TIMME • *Scott Department of Urology, Baylor College of Medicine, Houston, TX*

NAOTO T. UENO • *Department of Blood and Marrow Transplantation, The University of Texas M. D. Anderson Cancer Center, Houston, TX*

GIACOMO G. VECIL • *Department of Neurosurgery, The University of Texas M.D. Anderson Cancer Center, Houston, TX*

URS VON HOLZEN • *Department of Surgical Oncology, The University of Texas M. D. Anderson Cancer Center, Houston, TX*

STEPHAN A. VORBURGER • *Department of Visceral and Transplantation Surgery, Inselspital Bern, University of Bern, Bern, Switzerland*

HONGYU WANG • *Scott Department of Urology, Baylor College of Medicine, Houston, TX*

THOMAS M. WHEELER • *Department of Pathology, Baylor College of Medicine, Houston, TX*

JUDITH K. WOLF • *Department of Gynecologic Oncology, The University of Texas M. D. Anderson Cancer Center, Houston, TX*

MASATO YAMAMOTO • *Gene Therapy Center, University of Alabama, Birmingham, AL*

DUEN-HWA YAN • *Department of Molecular and Cellular Oncology, The University of Texas M. D. Anderson Cancer Center, Houston, TX*

LIDONG ZHANG • *Department of Thoracic and Cardiovascular Surgery, The University of Texas M. D. Anderson Cancer Center, Houston, TX*

I Vectors

1 Adenovector-Mediated Cancer Gene Therapy

Bingliang Fang, MD, PhD
and Jack A. Roth, MD

CONTENTS

Summary

Early-region (E1)-deleted, replication-defective adenovectors have been widely used in preclinical and clinical studies of cancer gene therapy. Recently, the use of conditional replicating or oncolytic adenovectors in cancer gene therapy or virotherapy has received much attention. Clinical trials with E1-deleted adenovectors and oncolytic adenovirus have shown that adenovector-mediated cancer gene therapy is well tolerated and can produce clinical responses in patients with advanced diseases. Moreover, numerous strategies to improve vector safety and therapeutic efficacy have been explored, including vector modification and the development of vector formulations to enhance transduction efficiency, to modulate tropism for vector targeting, to improve controlled or tissue-specific transgene expression, and to reduce vector-related toxicity. Yet, much has to be improved in this type of vector system to ensure its future success in clinical applications.

Key Words: Adenovirus; gene therapy; neoplasia; vector targeting; apoptosis; clinical trials.

1. INTRODUCTION

The use of adenoviruses as expression vectors in mammalian cells and in the development of recombinant vaccines dates back to the mid-1980s *(1–3)*. Their use as vectors in gene therapy was inspired by a report in 1990 that in vivo administration of an adenovirus expressing ornithine transcarbamylase corrected inherited defects of this enzyme in mice *(4)*. Since that time, numerous adenovectors expressing a variety of genes for in vivo gene transfer have been reported. Most of these adenovectors have been constructed by replacing the adenoviral early (E)1 region with an expression cassette

From: *Cancer Drug Discovery and Development: Gene Therapy for Cancer*
Edited by: K. K. Hunt, S. A. Vorburger, and S. G. Swisher © Humana Press Inc., Totowa, NJ

for the desired transgene. Because adenovectors are amenable to construction and purification to high titers and can efficiently transduce a variety of tissues in vivo *(5–10)*, they are today one of the most widely used vectors for in vivo gene delivery and gene therapy. They are the most frequently used vectors in clinical studies of cancer gene therapy *(11–15)* .

Numerous promising preclinical studies on adenovector-mediated cancer gene therapy have led to many phase I/II clinical trials of this vector. For example, published data from clinical trials of a p53 adenovirus and an oncolytic ONYX-015 adenovirus have shown that repeated administration of these adenoviral vectors is feasible and well tolerated. Repeated intratumoral administration of Ad-p53 results in continued transgene expression of the wild-type *p53* gene and can mediate clinical responses, including a pathologically complete response in a subset of patients with cancers resistant to chemotherapy or radiotherapy *(16–19)*. However, these studies also found that the effects of gene therapy alone were often limited. The favorable clinical responses were observed most often in patients whose treatment was combined with conventional therapies *(16–19)*. Other preclinical and clinical studies, however, have demonstrated that vector-related lethal toxicity can occur when a vector is administered systemically at a high dose *(20–22)*. Thus, it is clear that much still needs to be improved in adenovector-mediated cancer gene therapy to achieve maximal therapeutic efficacy and minimal toxicity.

2. BIOLOGICAL BASIS OF ADENOVIRUSES

The adenovirus was first isolated in the early 1950s as a cytopathogenic agent from primary cell cultures derived from human adenoids and respiratory secretions of patients with acute respiratory illnesses *(23,24)*. This virus was actually a group of nonenveloped viruses containing linear, double-stranded DNA encapsulated in an icosahedral protein capsid. To date, more than 100 types of adenoviruses that infect a wide range of mammalian and avian hosts have been identified *(25)*. At least 51 human adenovirus serotypes have been isolated; they are classified into six subgroups (A to F) *(25,26)* on the basis of their ability to agglutinate red blood cells *(27)*. Except for the group C and E viruses, other human adenoviruses can induce tumors in rats and hamsters, yet no evidence has been found that links adenoviruses to cancers in humans *(25)*. Adenovirus infections in humans usually result in mild signs and symptoms of respiratory illness, conjunctivitis, or gastroenteritis *(25)*. However, an adenovirus infection can be fatal in immunocompromised individuals *(26)*.

Most of the adenovectors used in gene therapy are based on adenovirus serotypes 2 and 5 (Ad2 and Ad5) [subgroup C], whose total DNA content is about 36-kb in length. The base sequences of these two viruses are more than 95% identical *(28,29)*. At each end of the DNA strand there is an identical inverted terminal repeat that is required for viral DNA to replicate. Reading the DNA from 5′ to 3′, next to this inverted terminal repeat is a DNA sequence of about 160 bp that is required for viral DNA to be packaged into viral particles *(30–32)*. More than 40 proteins are encoded by various genes, which have been termed early (E1 through E4) and late (L1 through L5) regions, depending on whether they are expressed before or after the initiation of viral DNA replication (Fig. 1). Eleven of these proteins, four in the core of the virus and seven in the outer shell, combine with the viral DNA to form an icosahedral viral particle that is approx 150-MDa in molecular weight and approx 90-nm in diameter *(25,33)*. The outer

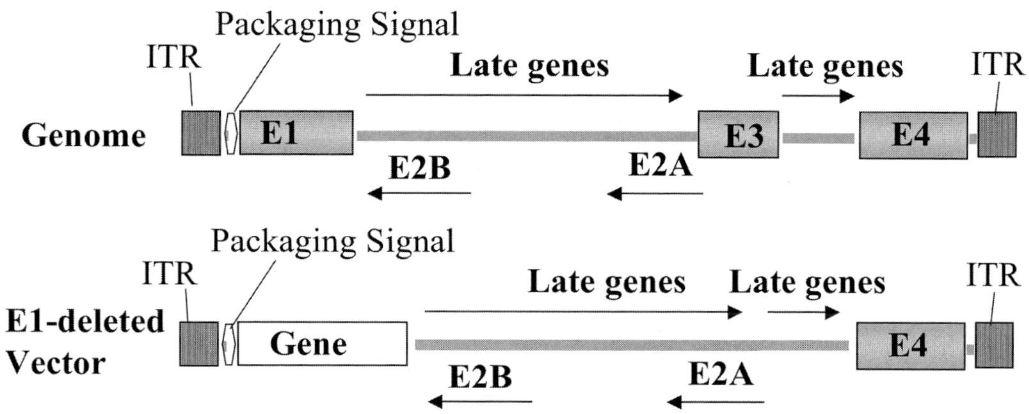

Fig. 1. Simplified diagrams of adenoviral genome and E1-deleted adenovector. Most of adenovectors are constructed by replacing E1 gene with a therapeutic gene.

shell capsid is organized into hexon and penton subunits *(25)*. Projecting from the penton base is the fiber formed from a trimeric fiber protein that interacts with a cellular receptor protein to attach the virus. The cellular receptor for Ad5 and most other adenovirus serotypes is the coxsackievirus and adenovirus receptor (CAR) *(34)*. After attachment, the virion is then internalized by endocytosis through the interaction of its penton base with αvβ3 and αvβ5 integrins on the host cell surface *(35)*. Studies have shown that some major histocompatibility molecules may serve as receptors for Ad5 fiber and that other integrin molecules may interact with the penton base. Once inside a cell, the virion undergoes a stepwise disassembly, releasing the DNA into the cell's nucleus *(36)*. Expression of *E1*, *E2*, and *E4* genes in host cells is required for viral DNA replication and for the expression of late genes, which encode structure proteins used for encapsidation of viral DNA. One lytic cycle of adenovirus replication typically takes between 36 and 48 h. One cell can produce as many as 10^4 viral particles, which are released at the end of each lytic cycle.

3. REPLICATION-DEFECTIVE ADENOVECTORS

Most replication-defective adenovectors are generated by replacing the E1 region with a therapeutic gene (Fig. 1). Up to 3.2 kb of an E1 region can be removed. Adenoviruses can effectively package 105% of the length of the wild-type gene genome *(37,38)*. Removal of the E1 region provides a total of packaging capacity about 5 kb for foreign inserts *(39)*. Removal of the E3 region may provide another 2.7 kb of packaging space without producing dramatic effects on replication and viral stability *(38,39)*. Although the genes in the E3 region are dispensable for the viral life cycle, those in the E1 region function as transactivators for other viral gene expression and are required for viral replication. Removal of the E1 region renders a virus defective in lytic replication. Therefore, whereas a vector can express the genes it carries, it cannot replicate in most cells. Nevertheless, vectors can be generated and propagated in packaging cells, such as 293 and 911 cells, those which provide E1 region functions in trans *(40,41)*. Several methods have been reported for generating such vectors, including homologous recombination in packaging cells *(42)*, homologous recombination in bacteria *(43)*, and in vitro ligation *(44,45)*.

Various in vivo studies have demonstrated that an E1-deleted adenovector can efficiently deliver transgenes to a variety of tissues in various animal models, including mouse, rat, rabbit, swine, dog, and monkey. However, these studies have also revealed that the transgene expression and therapeutic effects that occur in adenovirus-mediated gene transfer in immunocompetent animals are transient, primarily because of the host immune response to the E1-deleted recombinant adenoviral vectors and to the transgene product expressed in transduced cells *(46–48)*. This transient expression suggests that repeated administration would be required for treating most genetic disorders and cancers. Unfortunately, in these studies host humoral immune responses to the vectors abrogated any therapeutic effects of the adenovirus-mediated gene transfer after repeated systemic administration *(47,49)*.

Because of this problem, numerous efforts have been made to modify adenovectors by removing or inactivating other viral genes, including those in the E2 *(50)* and E4 regions *(51–53)* and in most of the entire viral coding regions *(54–56)*. A packaging cell line for adenovectors in which most of an encoding region or the entire region has been removed is not available. Adenovectors with such large deletions are produced using a helper virus that contains all the viral genes required for replication but that has a conditional defect in its packaging *(54,56)*. In immunocompetent animals, these modified vectors have been shown to be less toxic and have less immunogenicity and mediated prolonged transgene expression *(57,58)*.

Additional strategies for improving adenoviral vector-based gene delivery systems have also been explored. For example, chemically or genetically modified capsid proteins to enhance the transduction efficiency in CAR-defective cells or to redirect vector tropisms have been rigorously tested and it has been reported that the formulation of an adenovector in protamine or other pharmaceutical excipients enhance in vivo transduction in the lung after systemic administration, intratracheal instillation, or aerosolized vector delivery *(59,60)*. Furthermore, several small molecules, such as Syn3 and some anticancer agents *(61,62)*, have been reported to dramatically enhance adenovector-mediated gene delivery. Treating animals with low-dose etopside can suppress the formation of neutralizing antibodies and thus enhance intratumoral transgene expression in immunized animals *(63)*. Moreover, the modification of adenovectors with polyethylene glycol *(64–68)* and formulations of adenoviral vectors in a collagen-based matrix *(69)*, in a liposome, and in a synthetic surfactant *(70–72)* have all been reported to improve gene transfer in animals with antiadenovirus immunity. Several clinical trials have also demonstrated favorable outcomes in patients treated with adenovector-mediated cancer gene therapy plus conventional chemotherapy or radiation therapy. Although the mechanisms are yet to be determined, gene delivery by such a combination regimen has been shown to be enhanced in vitro in a cultured cell system.

4. ONCOLYTIC ADENOVIRUSES

The use of conditional replication-competent adenoviruses (CRADs) for cancer gene therapy gained much attention after a report published in 1996 stated that an adenovirus with a mutation in the E1B region (designated dl1520 or ONYX-015) replicates specifically in *p53*-mutated tumors *(73)*. It is therefore conceivable that the destructive effect of a replication-competent adenovirus would be beneficial for cancer therapy as long as this destructive effect was limited to tumors. Because *p53* is the most frequently mutated gene in human cancers *(74)*, an adenovirus that would specifically destroy *p53*-negative or-mutant cells would thus be regarded as a powerful anticancer agent. However, subsequent studies indicated that a lytic infection of cells with an E1B-mutated adenovirus did not depend on the cellular *p53* status and that *p53* might play a necessary part in mediating cellular destruction via a productive adenovirus infection *(75,76)*. Nevertheless, the notion that *in situ* amplification of CRADs and the resulting burst of viral progeny from the lysed cancer cells could enhance the local spread and penetration of these vectors, thereby greatly increasing therapeutic efficacy, spurred the creation and testing of various other CRADs for cancer therapy. This is because pre-clinical and clinical studies have shown that one of the major limitations of a replication-defective adenovector was the incomplete transduction of target cells because of poor vector penetration in tumor tissue. Indeed, the intratumoral injection of E1-deleted vectors often resulted in the transduction of only a small portion of the tumor cells surrounding a needle track. CRADs are believed to overcome this problem by producing cycles of replication, oncolysis, and local dissemination within tumor tissues that will ultimately eradiate all the cancer cells. It is noteworthy that CRAD and E1-deleted vectors are alike in most ways except for replication capability. Thus, resistance to an adenovirus infection resulting from lack of CAR expression, inflammatory response, or immune response which have all been observed in E1-deleted vectors, may also cause resistance to CRADs. However, these problems may be overcome through use of the same strategies used to enhance the transduction efficiency of E1-deleted vectors.

Two techniques have been used to create CRADs. In the first, a tumor-specific promoter is used to control the expression of an essential early gene, most frequently E1A. Several CRADs whose E1A gene is driven by a tissue-specific promoter have been reported to elicit tumor-specific cell lysis *(77)*. The promoters used in these studies included the prostate-specific antigen (PSA) promoter for prostate cancer *(77)*, the α-fetoprotein promoter for liver cancer, and human telomerase reverse transcriptase for various cancers *(78)*. Similarly, expressing the viral E1B and E2 genes from the promoters controlled by the Tcf4 transcription factor targeted CRADs to colon cancers, which resulted in the constitutive activation of the *wnt* signaling pathway *(79)*.

In the second approach, viral mutants with defective functions that are required for viral replication in normal cells but that are dispensable for replication in cancer cells are explored for virotherapy. Because mutations or deletions of the *p53* and retinoblastoma (*Rb*) genes are frequently found in cancers, CRADs that selectively replicate in cells with *p53* or *Rb* defects have been sought for anticancer therapy *(19,73,80)*. For example, E1A protein binds to *Rb* to trigger cell-cycle progression into the S phase. An adenovirus (Ad-δ24) with a deletion of eight animo acids from the *Rb* binding region of the E1A protein was reported to replicate specifically in *Rb*-defective cells *(80)*. It was also reported that a virus associated-I (VAI) RNA mutant adenovirus can be used for Ras-dependent oncolytic virotherapy *(81)*. It is noteworthy, however, that even though the E1-deleted adenovirus is generally regarded as replication defective, certain cancer cells may express E1-like factors that can accommodate replication of the E1-defective vectors *(51,82,83)*. In fact, it has been reported that E1-deleted adenoviruses were able to replicate in HeLa and H1299 cells when the cells were infected with high multiplicities of infections *(51,82)*.

It should be noted, however, that the outburst, or release, of CRADs from the cells in which they replicate may also depend on their ability to induce cell death during a late stage of infection. Indeed, it has been found that many cancer cells that have a defective *p53* pathway do not support CRAD-induced cell death, whereas exogenous expression of *p53* in human cancer cells during adenovirus replication augmented viral progeny release and increased antitumor potency. For example, a clinical trial of the ONYX-015 vector showed that even though the vector was present and replicating in tumors as much as a week after intralesional injection, no obvious tumor necrosis or apoptosis was detected *(84)*, suggesting that replication alone is not sufficient to induce cell death. On the other hand, a *p53*-expressing CRAD, Addl24-p53, was shown to have an advantage over Addl24, which does not express *p53 (85,86)*. Similarly, a CRAD over-expressing the adenovirus death protein (ADP), a 11.6-kDa protein from the E3 region, was found to be more effective in killing tumor cells than the CRAD lacking ADP *(87)*.

5. VECTOR-RELATED TOXICITY AND SAFETY ISSUES

Local administration of adenovectors for cancer therapy is generally well tolerated. However, the death of a young man in 1999 who had been enrolled in a clinical trial of the adenovector-mediated transfer of ornithine transcarbamylase gene raised much concern about adenovector-related toxicity. Because of this death the Office of Biotechnology Activities (OBA) at the National Institute of Health (NIH) established the Working Group on Adenoviral Vector Safety and Toxicity (AdSAT) to investigate the incident. This group has now completed a comprehensive review and analysis of scientific, safety, and ethical issues associated with adenovector-based human gene transfer; and concluded that the man's death was caused by a systemic, adenovirus vector-induced shock syndrome, which resulted from a cytokine cascade that led to disseminated intravascular coagulation, acute respiratory distress, and multiorgan failure *(20,22)*. The toxicity was dose related and had occurred over a very narrow dose range. The AdSAT working group also concluded that human gene transfer experiments using adenovectors should continue, though with caution *(22)*. In particular, they stated that it was advisable to have arithmetic rather than logarithmic dose escalations in trials designed to measure the dose range of toxicity. Another NIH group, The Recominant DNA Advisory Committee, also recommended the development of standards for vector potency (e.g., particle number, titer, dose), vector strength (e.g., transgene expression, transduction efficiency, and specificity), vector quality (e.g., identity, purity, integrity, and homogeneity), and vector-or treatment-related toxicity. They also advocated the development of a centralized database for collecting and organizing of safety and toxicity data *(22)*. Several additional recommendations were made to improve the safety of clinical studies and their participants, including rigorous pharmaceutical analyses, inclusion of vector controls, a rigorous analysis of each participant's immune status, and other procedures *(22)*.

The acute toxic effects of adenovectors administered systemically typically begin within minutes of administration and peak around 6 h later. This toxicity is mediated by the interaction of vectors with reticuloendothelial cells and the release of several pro-inflammatory cytokines, such as interleukin 6 (IL-6), tumor necrosis factor-α (TNF-α), IL-8, and granulocyte macrophage-colony stimulating factors (GM-CSF) *(88)*. Within a few days, the expression of the transgenes, or adenoviral genes, leads to inflammatory and immune responses mediated by the infiltration of lymphocytes and the formation of antibodies. A lethal response, which includes severe endothelial injury, disseminated intravascular coagulopathy, or both, may occur in an individual treated with a high dose *(21)*. Nevertheless, adenoviruses administered locally via different routes (e.g., nasal epithelium, bronchial epithelium, percutaneous to solid tumor, intradermal, epicardial injection of the myocardium, and skeletal muscle) have been reported to be well tolerated, with only 0.7% of the incidences of the major adverse events likely caused by an adenovector *(17,89,90)*. For example, one study found that *Adp53* could be delivered by bronchoalveolar lavage in doses as high as 2×10^{12} vp/cycle and that as many as 14 cycles administered to all lobes of the lung were well tolerated *(17)*.

6. VECTOR TARGETING

In cancer therapy, the cytotoxic/oncolytic agents must be targeted directly to the cancer to minimize toxicity reactions. One way to do this is by local or locoregional delivery of a therapeutic gene. Unfortunately, local administration in clinical settings has limited application. In fact, it is applicable only in situations in which a local, unresectable tumor is the major problem, as is the case in some head and neck, lung, brain, pancreatic, and liver cancers. Thus, many investigators have tried to develop other strategies for the use of targeted cancer gene therapy. Generally, such strategies have fallen into two categories: using vectors that specifically transduce cancer cells (targeted transduction) and controlling transgene expression with tumor-specific promoters (after nonspecific transduction).

6.1. Targeted Transduction

Various studies have found that viral particles can be modified by reshaping preformed vector particles with bispecific conjugates, a process resulting in viral particles with altered tropism *(91,92)*. Bi-specific conjugates are molecules that can bridge vectors and target cells by binding specifically to surface molecules on the vectors and the target cells. Various forms of bispecific conjugates have been used for targeting adenovectors to various cell types. Examples include the antiadenovirus knob antibody and its Fab fragment conjugated with folate *(93)*, with growth factor *(94,95)*, and with antibodies against growth factor receptor *(96,97)*. Recombinant fusion proteins containing a single-chain antibody (scFV) against knob and against epidermal growth factor or antigrowth factor receptor scFV have also been used for retargeting adenovectors *(96,98–100)*.

Vector targeting can also be achieved by modifying the genes encoding the viral capsid proteins, a process that results in viral particles with modified surface proteins or incorporated ligands. Fibers of adenovectors can be modified to redirect vector tropism. For example, in one study, an adenoviral vector that contained a chimeric fiber of Ad3 and Ad5 is reported to enhance the transduction efficiency in certain cell lines *(101)*. In another study, replacing Ad5 fiber with Ad35 fiber led to increased tropism in hematopoietic cells *(102)*. Other researchers found that ligands can be added to adenoviral fiber genetically. For example, adding polylysine to the fiber by erasing the stop codon targeted a viral vector to broadly expressed, heparin-containing cellular receptors *(103)*. Such a vector can effectively transduce a variety of cell types that are CAR defective or unreceptive to commonly used Ad2 or Ad5 vectors *(103,104)*. Alternatively, peptides containing arginine-glycine-aspartatic acid (RGD) sequences can be added to the knob of anadenoviral fiber. Adenovectors with an RGD fiber can effectively bind αv-integrin-positive cells, leading to the enhanced transduction of endothelial cells, dendritic cells, smooth muscle cells, and various cancer cells in vitro and in vivo *(105–108)*.

However, despite these promising advances in the genetic engineering of tumor-specific adenoviruses numerous hurdles and obstacles remain. For example, to genetically engineer such a vector, it is necessary to abrogate the native tropism of the virus, incorporate a tumor-specific ligand into the capsid proteins, and generate a cell line permissive for the production of the vector *(91)*. Moreover, it is sometimes difficult to find candidate receptors present in cancer cells only because of their scarcity. Generally, even classical tumor receptors, like folate receptors, or growth factor receptors overexpressed in certain types of cancer cells are also present in a variety of normal cells and, thus, nonspecific. To identify peptides that can specifically bind to cancer cells or cancer vasculature, several groups have used phage display libraries and other techniques *(109–112)*. For example, the RGD-4C motif for αv integrins *(113)* and NGR motif for aminopeptidase N (CD13) *(114)* can specifically bind to tumor blood vessels *(109)*. Moreover, adenovectors with RGD-4C incorporated into their fiber can effectively target primary tumor cells *(106)*. Nevertheless, incorporating such a targeting ligand may increase transduction in refractory cells but doing so is not necessary to block the natural tropism of a vector. There may be several reasons that account for this. First, the ligand for natural tropism is not abolished by the modification in the targeting vector *(115)*. Second, vector-host cell interaction may not completely depend on ligand-receptor interaction. Rather, nonspecific adsorption of targeted vector particles to cells could be sufficient for transduction *(116)*. Finally, the in vivo distribution and tropism of a vector depend largely on the bioavailability of the vector in a specific site or organ. The difficulty of a vector passing through blood vessels and reaching the target cells imposes a major limitation for in vivo targeting via vector transduction. The large molecular size of gene-based medicines decreases their extravasation from blood into tissue and increases their clearance by macrophages, immunoglobulins, and complements. Thus, even if adenovectors are ablated of the capacity to bind to CAR, their in vivo distribution is quite similar to that of commonly used Ad5 vectors, most of which end up in the liver *(117)*.

6.2. Targeted Transcription

The use of tissue- or tumor-specific promoters for selective transgene expression after nonselective gene delivery has also been zealously pursued in cancer gene therapy *(118,119)*. A number of promoters have been identified as being more active in cancer cells than their normal counterparts. These include the carcinoembryonic antigen promoter for colon and pancreatic cancers *(120,121)*, the α-feto-protein promoter for hepatic cancers *(122,123)*, the probasin promoter and prostate-specific antigen promoter for prostate carcinoma *(124,125)*, the mucin-secreting 1 promoter for mucin-secreting adenocarcinoma *(126)*, and the E2F promoter for cancers with a defective retinoblastoma gene *(127)*. The completion of the human genome project and the development of new technologies will undoubtedly lead to the identification of more genes that are overexpressed in cancer cells and whose promoters can be used for targeted cancer gene therapy.

Nevertheless, despite this promising outlook, there are also limitations for promoter-based targeting. First, most promoters are tissue specific rather than tumor specific. Vectors generated with these tissue-specific promoters are applicable only to certain types of tumors and cannot be used broadly in tumors of different origins. Second, most of these promoters are much weaker than commonly used viral promoters, such as the cytomegalovirus early promoter. Strong promoters are key to highly efficient, noninflammatory, and noncytotoxic adenoviral-mediated transgene delivery in vivo *(128)*. Fortunately, these two limitations can be overcome by using promoters that are active in a variety of cancer types and by using transcriptional factors to augment transgene expression.

Evidence has shown that human telomerase reverse transcriptase (hTERT) promoter *(129)* can be used to target proapoptotic genes to cancer cells *(130,131)*. Telomerase is a specialized type of reverse transcriptase that is responsible for the replication of chromosomal ends, or telomeres *(132,133)*. It is highly active in immortalized cell lines and in 85% of human cancer cells but silent in differentiated normal human somatic cells *(134–136)*. A growing body of evidence suggests that the catalytic subunit, telomerase reverse transcriptase (TERT), plays a key role in the activation of telomerase *(137–139)* and that the gene for TERT is expressed at high levels in primary tumors in the cells of various cancer cell lines, and telomerase-positive cells. Thus, the hTERT promoter may be able to function as a universal tumor-specific promoter. In vitro studies have shown that the hTERT promoter is highly active in human and murine cancer cells derived from carcinomas of the lung, colon, liver, breast, ovary, and brain *(130,140–144)*. It is not active in normal human fibroblasts *(130)*; in normal human epithelial cells from the trachea *(130)*, breast *(144)*, and ovary *(142)*; in normal human primary hepatocytes *(143)*; in normal human $CD34^+$ progenitor cells *(140)*; or in normal mouse fibroblasts *(140)*. In vivo studies have shown that systemic administration of adenovectors expressing proapoptotic genes, such as Bax or TRAIL, from the hTERT promoter results in no detectable transgene product or liver toxicity *(130,143)*, suggesting that the hTERT promoter is indeed dormant in adult somatic tissues *(130,140)* and may be used to target cancer cells. Thus far, the hTERT promoter has been used for the tumor-specific expression of proapoptotic/cytotoxic proteins *(130,140,143,145)*, and cytokine/chemokines, and for E1A expression in CRAD vectors *(146,147)*.

It has been reported that transgene expression from a weak, tumor-specific promoter can be dramatically augmented using a transcriptional factor *(148,149)*. This augmentation happens because a small amount of a potent transcriptional factor, such as a GAL4/VP16 *(150)* or a tetR/VP16 (tTA) *(151)* fusion protein, expressed from a tumor-specific promoter is sufficient to activate their target promoters upstream of a transgene and so increase transgene expression. Findings in our laoratory showed that the GAL4 gene regulatory system could augment transgene expression from the carcino-embryonic antigen (CEA) promoter could be augmented up to 100-fold, both in vitro or in vivo, without the loss of its specificity *(148)*. Similarly, the levels of *lacZ* gene expression from the hTERT promoter via the GAL4 regulatory system were dramatically augmented *(152)*. An adenovector expressing the TRAIL gene from the hTERT promoter via the GAL4 regulatory system (Ad/gTRAIL) has also been shown to induce high levels of transgene expression and apoptosis in various human cancer cells *(142–144)*. In vitro and in vivo studies have also shown that Ad/gTRAIL causes relatively little transgene expression and apoptosis induction in human fibroblasts, human primary hepatocytes, mammary epithelial cells, and ovarian epithelial cells in culture *(142–144)*.

7. CLINICAL TRIALS

As previousely discussed, adenovectors can effectively transduce in both dividing and nondividing cells in vivo and because long-term transgene expression is not a common prerequisite for cancer therapy, adenovectors are the most commonly used vector in cancer gene therapy (Journal of Gene Medicine Website, www.wiley.co.uk/genmed/clinical). The genes used in adenovector-mediated cancer therapy include tumor-suppressor genes (e.g., *p53*, *Rb*, and *p16*), prodrug activator or suicide genes (*TK* and *CD*), and genes encoding cytokine (GM-CSF, IL-2, IL-12, interferon [IFN]- α, IFN-β, IFN-γ, IL-7, MDA-7, and CD40L), tumor antigens or costimulatory molecules (MART-1, pg100, PSA, AFP, B7-1), and the single-chain antibody for erbB2. Among these genes, those encoding p53, herpes-simplex tyrosine-kinase (HSV-*tk*) and GM-CSF are the most frequently used in clinical trials. In addition, the replication-competent adenovector, ONYX-015, has also been used extensively in clinical trials. The results of several of these trials have already been published .

7.1. Adp53 *Gene Therapy*

A phase I trial enrolled 28 non-small-cell lung carcinoma (NSCLC) patients whose cancers were unresponsive to conventional treatments. Gene transfer was demonstrated in 80% of evaluable patients *(153)*. Gene expression was detected in 46%; apoptosis was demonstrated in all but one of the patients expressing the gene; no clinically significant toxicity was observed. More than a 50% reduction in tumor size was observed in two patients, with one patient remaining free of tumor more than 1 yr after concluding therapy and another experiencing nearly complete regression of a chemotherapy and radiotherapy resistant upper lobe endobronchial tumor.

A phase I study of 33 patients with head and neck squamous cell carcinoma (HNSCC) showed that transfer of the *Adp53* construct caused little toxicity. Clinical response was observed in 9 out of 18 clinically evaluable patients *(154)*. A subsequent phase II clinical trial of *Adp53* in over 200 recurrent or refractory HNSCC patients resulted in demonstration of complete or partial responses in approx10% of patients, with minor responses or stabilization observed in 60% of patients *(155,156)*.

Twenty-four NSCLC patients with tumors that did not respond to conventional treatment were enrolled in a phase I trial of Ad*p53* in sequence with cisplatin *(157)*. Seventy-five percent of the patients had previously experienced tumor progression on cisplatin or carboplatin containing regimens. Up to six monthly courses of intravenous cisplatin, each followed 3 d later with intratumoral injection of *Adp53*, resulted in 17 patients remaining stable for at least 2 mo, 2 patients achieving partial responses, 4 patients continuing to exhibit progressive disease, and 1 patient unevaluable as a result of progressive disease. Seventy-nine percent of tumor biopsies showed an increase in number of apoptotic cells, 7% demonstrated a decrease in apoptosis, and 14% indicated no change.

A phase II clinical trial evaluated two comparable metastatic lesions in each NSCLC patient enrolled in the study *(158)*. All patients received chemotherapy, either three cycles of carboplatin plus paclitaxel or three cycles of cisplatin plus vinorelbine, and then *Adp53* was injected directly into one lesion. *Adp53* treatment resulted in minimal vector related toxicity and no overall increase in chemotherapy related adverse events. Detailed statistical analysis of the data indicated that patients receiving carboplatin plus paclitaxel, the combination of drugs providing the greatest benefit on its own, did not realize additional benefit from *Adp53* gene transfer, however, patients treated with the less successful cisplatin and vinorelbine regimen experienced significantly greater mean local tumor regression, as measured by size, in the *Adp53* injected lesion as compared with the control lesion.

A phase I/II clinical study of recurrent ovarian cancer patients by Buller and coworkers demonstrated safety and tolerability of single dose and multiple dose intraperitoneal *Adp53* in combination with platinum-based chemotherapy *(159)*. Long-term follow-up of these patients indicated that those individuals receiving multiple dose *Adp53* with chemotherapy had a median survival of 12 to 13 mo, whereas those treated with a single dose of *Adp53* had a median survival of only 5 mo *(159)*. More than 20 mo after conclusion of multiple-dose treatment for recurrent disease there were 10 long-term survivors, whereas only 2 patients receiving a single dose of *Adp53* were long-term survivors.

Preclinical studies suggesting that *p53* gene replacement might confer radiation sensitivity to some tumors *(160–162)* led to a phase II clinical trial of *p53* gene transfer in conjunction with radiation therapy *(163)*. Data from 19 patients with localized NSCLC revealed a complete response in one patient (5%), partial responses in 11 patients (58%), stable disease in 3 patients (16%), and progressive disease in 2 patients (11%), whereas two patients (11%) were nonevaluable as a result of tumor progression or early death. Three months following completion of therapy, biopsies showed no viable tumor in 12 patients (63%) and viable tumor in 3 (16%). The tumors of 4 patients (21%) were not biopsied because of tumor progression, early death, or poor performance status. The 1-yr progression-free survival rate was 45.5%. Among 13 evaluable patients after 1 yr, 5 patients (39%) had a complete response and 3 (23%) had a partial response or disease stabilization. Most treatment failures were caused by metastatic disease.

Recently, the first randomized clinical trial of *p53* gene therapy was reported. Ninety patients with squamous cell carcinoma of the head and neck were randomly allocated to receive intratumoral injection of *Adp53* (10^{12} VP/dose/wk for a total of 8 wk) in combination with radiation therapy (70 GY/8 wk) or radiation therapy alone. Complete remission was seen in 64.7% of patients receiving *Adp53* combined with radiation therapy compared with 20% of patients receiving radiation therapy alone, which was highly significant statistically *(164)*.

*7.2. HSV-***tk** *Gene Therapy*

In another study, the HSV-*tk* gene was delivered by both retrovirus-packaging cells and adenoviruses as therapy for malignant glioma in combination with ganciclovir *(165)*. Intratumoral injection of the adenovirus resulted in a substantial increase in anti-adenovirus antibodies and the frequency of epileptic seizures in some patients. Mean survival times for the retrovirus, adenovirus, and control groups were 7.4, 15.0, and 8. 3 mo, respectively *(165)*. In addition, a phase I trial was reported of the HSV-*tk* expressing adenovector (AdHSV-*tk*) injected intratumorally in combination with ganciclovir administered intravenously to treat patients with metastatic colorectal adenocarcinoma in the liver *(166)*. Sixteen patients were treated with an adenovector dose ranging from 1.0×10^{10} to 1.0×10^{13} virus particles/patient. The results indicated that AdHSV-*tk* could be safely administered by percutaneous intratumoral injection in patients with hepatic metastases at doses of up to 1.0×10^{13} virus particles/patient. The toxic effects observed in some patients included grade 1 elevation in serum aminotransferase levels, grade 2–3 fevers, grade 3 thrombocytopenia, and grade 2 leucopenia. Most of these effects resolved within 1 wk, suggesting that HSV-*tk* gene therapy is safe and well tolerated. However, no partial or complete response was observed in this trial. Similarly, a phase I/II trial of combined radiotherapy and *in situ* Ad-mediated HSV-*tk* gene/valacyclovir with or without hormonal therapy for the treatment of prostate cancer also showed that this combination therapy was safe and well tolerated *(167)*.

7.3. ONYX-015 Gene Therapy

More than 200 cancer patients have been treated with the replication-competent virus ONYX-015 in more than 10 clinical trials. Intratumorally injecting the virus into head and neck cancers or into intrahepatic and intrapancreatic tumor masses revealed no maximal tolerated dose or dose-limiting toxicity after doses as high as 2×10^{12} viral particles/injection *(18,168,169)*. No clinically significant incidence of hepatitis or pancreatitis was seen. The most frequently reported adverse events were fever, chills, injection site pain, asthenia, and nausea. In addition to intratumoral injection, the intraperitoneal, intra–hepatic arterial, and intravenous administration routes have also been used with this vector *(18,168,169)*. Intraperitoneal administration was feasible at doses as high as 10^{13} viral particles divided over 5 d. The most common toxic effects included fever; abdominal pain; nausea, vomiting, or both; and bowel-motility changes (i.e., diarrhea and constipation). No dose-limiting toxicities were seen for doses as high as 2×10^{12} viral particles/single dose with intra–hepatic arterial administration or 2×10^{13} particles/cycle (single injection/week for 3 wk) with intravenous administration *(18,168)*. Nevertheless, the treatment of patients with head and neck cancer with five intratumoral injections of ONYX-015 a day resulted in an unconfirmed response (≥50% shrinkage at a single time point) rate of only about 13%. No objective responses were demonstrated for intratumoral injections into pancreatic or gastrointestinal carcinomas or with intraperitoneal, intra–hepatic arterial, and intravenous administration in patients with metastatic carcinomas *(18,168)*. In a phase II trial of intratumorally injected ONYX-015 combined with standard intravenously administered cisplatin and fluorouracil in patients with recurrent head and neck cancer, about 60% responded to the combination therapy. Two of the four chemotherapy-refractory tumors responded to subsequent therapy with ONYX-015 combined with the same chemotherapy to which the tumors had previously been resistant *(19)*. In another trial, 15 patients with colorectal carcinoma who failed to respond to ONYX-015 alone or to chemotherapy alone were treated with a combination of intra–hepatic arterial infusion of ONYX-015 and intravenous administration of 5-fluorouracil combined with leukovorin. One patient had a partial response, and 10 experienced stabilization of their disease for 2 to 7 mo *(18)*. However, none of the patients responded who had been given doses of less than 6×10^{11} viral particles in combination with chemotherapy *(170)*.

8. FUTURE PROSPECTUS

In spite of the promising results obtained from preclinical studies of adenovector-mediated cancer gene therapy, the response rates in clinical trials of this vector as a single agent have continued to be very low. One possible reason for this is that most of the reported clinical trials have been phase I or phase I/II trials that examined toxicity and dose escalation. Most of the patients entered in these trials either were at a terminal stage or had failed to respond to chemotherapy, radiotherapy, or both. It is also evident that improvements in this vector system are critically needed for the future success of clinical studies. Two major obstacles remaining in adenovector-mediated cancer gene therapy are the incomplete transduction of target cells resulting from limited penetration and distribution of the adenovirus within tumor tissues and the resistance of the target cells to an adenovirus infection caused by a loss of CAR expression. Possible solutions to these problems include the development of a replication-competent vector or a CRAD carrying an additional therapeutic gene, the modification of the capsid protein for efficient or specific transduction of tumor cells, the enhancement of tumor-specific therapeutic gene expression, and the development of vector formulations to improve vector quality and in vivo transduction. Furthermore, methods for noninvasive in vivo monitoring of vector distribution, vector penetration, and transgene expression will facilitate pharmacokinetic evaluations of gene-based medicine. Monitoring immune responses and host-vector interactions in both immunocompetent and immunocompromised conditions is also important, especially for CRAD vectors. Clinical studies have also shown that the combination of conventional chemotherapy or radiotherapy with gene therapy greatly improves the antitumor potency of the gene therapy delivered using the both replication-defective and replication-competent adenovectors, indicating that combinational therapy should be studied further.

ACKNOWLEDGMENTS

We thank Gayle Nesom for editorial review and Jesse Null and Carrie Langford for assistance in preparation of this manuscript.

This work was supported in part by grants from the National Institute of Health (RO1 CA92487-01A1 and RO1 CA98582-01 A1 to BF and P01 CA78778-01A1 and P50-CA 70907 to JAR).

REFERENCES

1. Massie B, Gluzman Y, Hassell JA. Construction of a helper-free recombinant adenovirus that expresses polyomavirus large T antigen. Mol Cell Biol 1986;6:2872–2883.
2. Davis AR, Kostek B, Mason BB, et al. Expression of hepatitis B surface antigen with a recombinant adenovirus. Proc Natl Acad Sci U S A 1985;82:7560–7564.
3. Yamada M, Lewis JA, Grodzicker T. Overproduction of the protein product of a nonselected foreign gene carried by an adenovirus vector. Proc Natl Acad Sci U S A 1985;82:3567–3571.
4. Stratford-Perricaudet LD, Levrero M, Chasse JF, Perricaudet M, Briand P. Evaluation of the transfer and expression in mice of an enzyme-encoding gene using a human adenovirus vector. Hum Gene Ther 1990;1:241–256.
5. Griffith TS, Anderson RD, Davidson BL, Williams RD, Ratliff TL. Adenoviral-mediated transfer of the TNF-related apoptosis-inducing ligand/Apo-2 ligand gene induces tumor cell apoptosis. J Immunol 2000;165:2886–2894.
6. Andrews KJ, Ribas A, Butterfield LH, et al. Adenovirus-interleukin-12-mediated tumor regression in a murine hepatocellular carcinoma model is not dependent on CD1-restricted natural killer T cells. Cancer Res 2000;60:6457–6464.
7. Bui LA, Butterfield LH, Kim JY, et al. In vivo therapy of hepatocellular carcinoma with a tumor-specific adenoviral vector expressing interleukin-2 [see comments]. Hum Gene Ther 1997;8:2173–2182.
8. Lesoon-Wood LA, Kim WH, Kleinman HK, Weintraub BD, Mixson AJ. Systemic gene therapy with p53 reduces growth and metastases of a malignant human breast cancer in nude mice. Hum Gene Ther 1995;6:395–405.
9. Rosenberg SA, Blaese RM, Brenner MK, et al. Human gene marker/therapy clinical protocols. Hum Gene Ther 2000;11:919–979.
10. Vollmer CM, Ribas A, Butterfield LH, et al. p53 selective and nonselective replication of an E1B-deleted adenovirus in hepatocellular carcinoma. Cancer Res 1999;59:4369–4374.
11. Anonymous. Human gene marker/therapy clinical protocols (complete updated listings). Hum Gene Ther 2001;12:2251–2337.
12. Roth JA, Cristiano RJ. Gene therapy for cancer: what have we done and where are we going? J Natl Cancer Inst 1997;89:21–39.
13. Roth JA, Swisher SG, Merritt JA, et al. Gene therapy for non-small cell lung cancer: a preliminary report of a phase I trial of adenoviral p53 gene replacement. Sem Oncol 1998;25:33–37.
14. Habib NA, Hodgson HJ, Lemoine N, Pignatelli M. A phase I/II study of hepatic artery infusion with wtp53-CMV-Ad in metastatic malignant liver tumours. Hum Gene Ther 1999;10:2019–2034.
15. Herman JR, Adler HL, Aguilar-Cordova E, et al. *In situ* gene therapy for adenocarcinoma of the prostate: a phase I clinical trial. Hum Gene Ther 1999;10:1239–1249.
16. Roth JA, Grammer SF, Swisher SG, et al. Gene therapy approaches for the management of non-small cell lung cancer. Sem Oncol 2001;28:50–56.

17. Swisher SG, Roth JA, Carbone DP. Genetic and immunologic therapies for lung cancer. Sem Oncol 2002;29:95–101.
18. Kirn D. Clinical research results with dl1520 (ONYX-015), a repication-selective adenovirus for the treatment of cancer: what have we learned. Gene Ther 2001;8:89–98.
19. Khuri FR, Nemunaitis J, Ganly I, et al. A controlled trial of intratumoral ONYX-015, a selectively-replicating adenovirus, in combination with cisplatin and 5-fluorouracil in patients with recurrent head and neck cancer. Nat Med 2000;6:879–885.
20. Raper SE, Yudkoff M, Chirmule N, et al. A pilot study of in vivo liver-directed gene transfer with an adenoviral vector in partial ornithine transcarbamylase deficiency. Hum Gene Ther 2002;13:163–175.
21. Morral N, O'Neal WK, Rice K, et al. Lethal toxicity, severe endothelial injury, and a threshold effect with high doses of an adenoviral vector in baboons. Hum Gene Ther 2002;13:143–154.
22. Anonymous. NIH Report±Assessment of adenoviral vector safety and toxicity: Report of the National Institutes of Health Recombinant DNA Advisory Committee. Hum Gene Ther 2002;13: 3–13.
23. Rowe WP, Huebner RJ, Gilmore LK, Parrot RH, Ward TG. Isolation of a cytopathogenic agent from human adenoids undergoing spontaneous degeneration in tissue culture. Proc Soc Exp Biol Med 1953;84:570–573.
24. Hilleman MR, Werner JH. Recovery of new agents from patients with acute respiratory illness. Proc Soc Exp Biol Med 1954;85:183–188.
25. Shenk T. Adenoviridae: the viruses and their replication. In: Fundamental Virology, Third Edition Fields BN, Knipe DM, Howley PM, eds Philadelphia: Lippincott-Raven, 1996; pp. 979–1016.
26. Kojaoghlanian T, Flomenberg P, Horwitz MS. The impact of adenovirus infection on the immuno-compromised host. Rev Med Virol 2003;13:155–171.
27. Hierholzer JC. Further subgrouping of the human adenoviruses by differential hemagglutination. J Infect Dis 1973;128:541–550.
28. Roberts RJ, O'Neill KE, Yen CT. DNA sequences from the adenovirus 2 genome. J Biol Chem 1984;259:13,968–13,975.
29. Chroboczek J, Bieber F, Jacrot B. The sequence of the genome of adenovirus type 5 and its comparison with the genome of adenovirus type 2. Virology 1992;186:280–285.
30. Hammarskjold ML, Winberg G. Encapsidation of adenovirus 16 DNA is directed by a small DNA sequence at the left end of the genome. Cell 1980;20:787–795.
31. Grable M, Hearing P. cis and trans requirements for the selective packaging of adenovirus type 5 DNA. J Virol 1992;66:723–731.
32. Hearing P, Samulski RJ, Wishart WL, Shenk T. Identification of a repeated sequence element required for efficient encapsidation of the adenovirus type 5 chromosome. J Virol 1987;61:2555–2558.
33. San Martin C, Burnett RM. Structural studies on adenoviruses. Curr Topic Microbiol Immunol 2003;272:57–94.
34. Bergelson JM, Cunningham JA, Droguett G, et al. Isolation of a common receptor for Coxsackie B viruses and adenoviruses 2 and 5. Science 1997;275:1320–1323.
35. Wickham TJ, Mathias P, Cheresh DA, Nemerow GR. Integrins alpha v beta 3 and alpha v beta 5 promote adenovirus internalization but not virus attachment. Cell 1993;73:309–319.
36. Greber UF, Willetts M, Webster P, Helenius A. Stepwise dismantling of adenovirus 2 during entry into cells. Cell 1993;75:477–486.
37. Graham FL. Covalently closed circles of human adenovirus DNA are infectious. EMBO J 1984;3:2917–2922.
38. Bett AJ, Prevec L, Graham FL. Packaging capacity and stability of human adenovirus type 5 vectors. J Virol 1993;67:5911–5921.
39. Bett AJ, Haddara W, Prevec L, Graham FL. An efficient and flexible system for construction of adenovirus vectors with insertions or deletions in early regions 1 and 3. Proc Natl Acad Sci U S A 1994;91:8802–8806.
40. Graham FL, Smiley J, Russell WC, Nairn R. Characteristics of a human cell line transformed by DNA from human adenovirus type 5. J Gen Virol 1977;36:59–74.
41. Fallaux FJ, Kranenburg O, Cramer SJ, et al. Characterization of 911: a new helper cell line for the titration and propagation of early region 1-deleted adenoviral vectors. Hum Gene Ther 1996;7:215–222.
42. Graham FL, Prevec L. Methods for construction of adenovirus vectors. Mol Biotech 1995;3:207–220.
43. He TC, Zhou S, da Costa LT, Yu J, Kinzler KW, Vogelstein BA. Simplified system for generating recombinant adenoviruses. Proc Natl Acad Sci U S A 1998;95:2509–2514.

44. Mizuguchi H, Kay MA, Hayakawa T. Approaches for generating recombinant adenovirus vectors. Adv Drug Rev 2001;52:165–176.
45. Mizuguchi H, Kay MA, Hayakawa T. In vitro ligation-based cloning of foreign DNAs into the E3 and E1 deletion regions for generation of recombinant adenovirus vectors. Biotechniques 2001;30:1112–1114.
46. Yang Y, Nunes FA, Berencsi K, Furth EE, Gonczol E, Wilson JM. Cellular immunity to viral antigens limits E1-deleted adenoviruses for gene therapy. Proc Natl Acad Sci U S A 1994;91:4407–4411.
47. Fang B, Eisensmith RC, Li XH, et al. Gene therapy for phenylketonuria: phenotypic correction in a genetically deficient mouse model by adenovirus-mediated hepatic gene transfer. Gene Ther 1994;1:247–254.
48. Kay MA, Landen CN, Rothenberg SR, et al. In vivo hepatic gene therapy: complete albeit transient correction of factor IX deficiency in hemophilia B dogs. Proc Natl Acad Sci U S A 1994;91: 2353–2357.
49. Fang B, Eisensmith RC, Wang H, et al. Gene therapy for hemophilia B: host immunosuppression prolongs the therapeutic effect of adenovirus-mediated factor IX expression. Hum Gene Ther 1995;6:1039–1044.
50. Zhou H, O'Neal W, Morral N, Beaudet AL. Development of a complementing cell line and a system for construction of adenovirus vectors with E1 and E2a deleted. J Virol 1996;70:7030–7038.
51. Fang B, Koch P, Roth JA. Diminishing adenovirus gene expression and viral replication by promoter replacement. J Virol 1997;71:4798–4803.
52. Armentano D, Sookdeo CC, Hehir KM, et al. Characterization of an adenovirus gene transfer vector containing an E4 deletion. Hum Gene Ther 1995;6:1343–1353.
53. Brough DE, Lizonova A, Hsu C, Kulesa VA, Kovesdi I. A gene transfer vector-cell line system for complete functional complementation of adenovirus early regions E1 and E4. J Virol 1996;70: 6497–6501.
54. Mitani K, Graham FL, Caskey CT, Kochanek S. Rescue, propagation, and partial purification of a helper virus-dependent adenovirus vector. Proc Natl Acad Sci U S A 1995;92:3854–3858.
55. Morsy MA, Gu M, Motzel S, et al. An adenoviral vector deleted for all viral coding sequences results in enhanced safety and extended expression of a leptin transgene. Proc Natl Acad Sci USA 1998;95:7866–7871.
56. Parks RJ, Chen L, Anton M, Sankar U, Rudnicki MA, Graham FL. A helper-dependent adenovirus vector system: removal of helper virus by Cre-mediated excision of the viral packaging signal. Proc Natl Acad Sci U S A 1996;93:13,565–13,570.
57. Ji L, Bouvet M, Price RE, Roth JA, Fang B. Reduced toxicity, attenuated immunogenicity and efficient mediation of human p53 gene expression in vivo by an adenovirus vector with deleted E1, E3 and inactivated E4 by GAL4-TATA promoter replacement. Gene Ther 1999;6:393–402.
58. Morral N, O'Neal W, Rice K, et al. Administration of helper-dependent adenoviral vectors and sequential delivery of different vector serotype for long-term liver-directed gene transfer in baboons. Proc Natl Acad Sci U S A 1999;96:12,816–12,821.
59. Lin T, Gu J, Zhang L, et al. Enhancing adenovirus-mediated gene transfer in vitro and in vivo by addition of protamine and hydrocortisone. J Gene Med 2003;5:868–875.
60. Croyle MA, Cheng X, Sandhu A, Wilson JM. Development of novel formulations that enhance adenoviral-mediated gene expression in the lung in vitro and in vivo. Mol Ther 2001;4:22–28.
61. Connor RJ, Engler H, Machemer T, et al. Identification of polyamides that enhance adenovirus-mediated gene expression in the urothelium. Gene Ther 2001;8:41–48.
62. Li Y, Okegawa T, Lombardi DP, Frenkel EP, Hsieh JT. Enhanced transgene expression in androgen independent prostate cancer gene therapy by taxane chemotherapeutic agents. J Urol 2002;167:339–346.
63. Bouvet M, Fang B, Ekmekcioglu S, et al. Suppression of the immune response to an adenovirus vector and enhancement of intratumoral transgene expression by low-dose etoposide. Gene Ther 1998;5:189–195.
64. Croyle MA, Chirmule N, Zhang Y, Wilson JM. "Stealth" adenoviruses blunt cell-mediated and humoral immune responses against the virus and allow for significant gene expression upon readministration in the lung. J Virol 2001;75:4792–4801.
65. Croyle MA, Yu QC, Wilson JM. Development of a rapid method for the PEGylation of adenoviruses with enhanced transduction and improved stability under harsh storage conditions. Hum Gene Ther 2000;11:1713–1722.
66. Ohsawa T, Nakamura T, Mihara M, Sato K. Enhancement of adenovirus-mediated gene transfer into dermal fibroblasts in vitro and in vivo by polyethylene glycol 6000. J Dermatol 2000;27:244–251.

67. O'Riordan CR, Lachapelle A, Delgado C, et al. PEGylation of adenovirus with retention of infectivity and protection from neutralizing antibody in vitro and in vivo. [see comments]. Hum Gene Ther 1999;10:1349–1358.
68. Chillon M, Lee JH, Fasbender A, Welsh MJ. Adenovirus complexed with polyethylene glycol and cationic lipid is shielded from neutralizing antibodies in vitro. Gene Ther 1998;5:995–1002.
69. Siemens DR, Elzey BD, Lubaroff DM, et al. Cutting edge: restoration of the ability to generate CTL in mice immune to adenovirus by delivery of virus in a collagen-based matrix. J Immunol 2001;166: 731–735.
70. Kukowska-Latallo JF, Chen C, Eichman J, Bielinska AU, Baker JR, Jr. Enhancement of dendrimer-mediated transfection using synthetic lung surfactant exosurf neonatal in vitro. Biochem Biophys Res Comm 1999;264:253–261.
71. Raczka E, Kukowska-Latallo JF, Rymaszewski M, Chen C, Baker JR, Jr. The effect of synthetic surfactant Exosurf on gene transfer in mouse lung in vivo. Gene Ther 1998;5:1333–1339.
72. Matthews C, Jenkins G, Hilfinger J, Davidson B. Poly-L-lysine improves gene transfer with adenovirus formulated in PLGA microspheres. Gene Ther 1999;6:1558–1564.
73. Bischoff JR, Kirn DH, Williams A, et al. An adenovirus mutant that replicates selectively in p53-deficient human tumor cells. Science 1996;274:373–376.
74. Hollstein M, Sidransky D, Vogelstein B, Harris CC. p53 mutations in human cancers. Science 1991;253:49–53.
75. Hall AR, Dix BR, O'Carrol SJ, Braithwaite AW. p53-dependent cell death/apoptosis is required for a productive adenovirus infection [see comments]. Nat Med 1998;4:1068–1072.
76. Goodrum FD, Ornelles DA. p53 status does not determine outcome of E1B 55-kilodalton mutant adenovirus lytic infection. J Virol 1998;72:9479–9490.
77. Rodriguez R, Schuur ER, Lim HY, Henderson GA, Simons JW, Henderson DR. Prostate attenuated replication competent adenovirus (ARCA) CN706: a selective cytotoxic for prostate-specific antigen-positive prostate cancer cells. Cancer Res 1997;57:2559–2563.
78. Hallenbeck PL, Chang YN, Hay C, et al. A novel tumor-specific replication-restricted adenoviral vector for gene therapy of hepatocellular carcinoma. Hum Gene Ther 1999;10:1721–1733.
79. Brunori M, Malerba M, Kashiwazaki H, Iggo R. Replicating adenoviruses that target tumors with constitutive activation of the wnt signaling pathway. J Virol 2001;75:2857–2865.
80. Fueyo J, Alemany R, Gomez-Manzano C, et al. Preclinical characterization of the antiglioma activity of a tropism-enhanced adenovirus targeted to the retinoblastoma pathway. J Natl Cancer Inst 2003;95:652–660.
81. Cascallo M, Capella G, Mazo A, Alemany R. Ras-dependent oncolysis with an adenovirus VAI mutant. Cancer Res 2003;63:5544–5550.
82. Shenk T, Jones N, Colby W, Fowlkes D. Functional analysis of adenovirus-5 host-range deletion mutants defective for transformation of rat embryo cells. Cold Spring Harbor Symposia on Quantitative Biology, 1980;44 Pt 1, 367–375.
83. Zhao T, Rao XM, Xie X, et al. Adenovirus with insertion-mutated E1A selectively propagates in liver cancer cells and destroys tumors in vivo. Cancer Res 2003;63:3073–3078.
84. Wadler S, Yu B, Tan JY, et al. Persistent replication of the modified chimeric adenovirus ONYX-015 in both tumor and stromal cells from a patient with gall bladder carcinoma implants. Clin Cancer Res 2003;9:33–43.
85. Van Beusechem VW, van den Doel PB, Grill J, Pinedo HM, Gerritsen WR. Conditionally replicative adenovirus expressing p53 exhibits enhanced oncolytic potency. Cancer Res 2002;62:6165–6171.
86. Sauthoff H, Pipiya T, Heitner S, et al. Late expression of p53 from a replicating adenovirus improves tumor cell killing and is more tumor cell specific than expression of the adenoviral death protein. Hum Gene Ther 2002;13:1859–1871.
87. Doronin K, Toth K, Kuppuswamy M, Ward P, Tollefson AE, Wold WS. Tumor-specific, replication-competent adenovirus vectors overexpressing the adenovirus death protein. J Virol 2000;74:6147–6155.
88. Higginbotham JN, Seth P, Blaese RM, Ramsey WJ. The release of inflammatory cytokines from human peripheral blood mononuclear cells in vitro following exposure to adenovirus variants and capsid. Hum Gene Ther 2002;13:129–141.
89. Crystal RG, Harvey BG, Wisnivesky JP, et al. Analysis of risk factors for local delivery of low- and intermediate-dose adenovirus gene transfer vectors to individuals with a spectrum of comorbid conditions. Hum Gene Ther 2002;13:65–100.
90. Harvey BG, Maroni J, O'Donoghue KA, et al. Safety of local delivery of low- and intermediate-dose adenovirus gene transfer vectors to individuals with a spectrum of morbid conditions. Hum Gene Ther 2002;13:15–63.

91. Wickham TJ. Targeting adenovirus. Gene Ther 2000;7:110–114.
92. Barnett BG, Crews CJ, Douglas JT. Targeted adenoviral vectors. [Review] [162 refs]. Biochimica Biophysica Acta 2002;1575:1–14.
93. Douglas JT, Rogers BE, Rosenfeld ME, Michael SI, Feng M, Curiel DT. Targeted gene delivery by tropism-modified adenoviral vectors. Nat Biotechnol 1996;14:1574–1578.
94. Gu DL, Gonzalez AM, Printz MA, et al. Fibroblast growth factor 2 retargeted adenovirus has redirected cellular tropism: evidence for reduced toxicity and enhanced antitumor activity in mice. Cancer Res 1999;59:2608–2614.
95. Goldman CK, Rogers BE, Douglas JT, et al. Targeted gene delivery to Kaposi's sarcoma cells via the fibroblast growth factor receptor. Cancer Res 1997;57:1447–1451.
96. Van Beusechem VW, Grill J, Mastenbroek DC, et al. Efficient and selective gene transfer into primary human brain tumors by using single-chain antibody-targeted adenoviral vectors with native tropism abolished. J Virol 2002;76:2753–2762.
97. Miller CR, Buchsbaum DJ, Reynolds PN, et al. Differential susceptibility of primary and established human glioma cells to adenovirus infection: targeting via the epidermal growth factor receptor achieves fiber receptor-independent gene transfer. Cancer Res 1998;58:5738–5748.
98. Nettelbeck DM, Miller DW, Jerome V, et al. Targeting of adenovirus to endothelial cells by a bispecific single-chain diabody directed against the adenovirus fiber knob domain and human endoglin (CD105). Molecular Therapy: J Am Soc Gene Ther 2001;3:882–891.
99. Wesseling JG, Bosma PJ, Krasnykh V, et al. Improved gene transfer efficiency to primary and established human pancreatic carcinoma target cells via epidermal growth factor receptor and integrin-targeted adenoviral vectors. Gene Ther 2001;8:969–976.
100. Dmitriev I, Kashentseva E, Rogers BE, Krasnykh V, Curiel DT. Ectodomain of coxsackievirus and adenovirus receptor genetically fused to epidermal growth factor mediates adenovirus targeting to epidermal growth factor receptor-positive cells. J Virol 2000;74:6875–6884.
101. Stevenson SC, Rollence M, Marshall-Neff J, McClelland A. Selective targeting of human cells by a chimeric adenovirus vector containing a modified fiber protein. J Virol 1997;71:4782–4790.
102. Yotnda P, Onishi H, Heslop HE, et al. Efficient infection of primitive hematopoietic stem cells by modified adenovirus. Gene Ther 2001;8:930–937.
103. Wickham TJ, Roelvink PW, Brough DE, Kovesdi I. Adenovirus targeted to heparan-containing receptors increases its gene delivery efficiency to multiple cell types. Nat Biotechnol 1996;14: 1570–1573.
104. Pearson AS, Koch PE, Atkinson N, et al. Factors limiting adenovirus-mediated gene transfer into human lung and pancreatic cancer cell lines. Clin Cancer Res 1999;5:4208–4213.
105. Wickham TJ, Tzeng E, Shears LL 2nd, Roelvink PW, et al. Increased in vitro and in vivo gene transfer by adenovirus vectors containing chimeric fiber proteins. J Virol 1997;71:8221–8229.
106. Dmitriev I, Krasnykh V, Miller CR, et al. An adenovirus vector with genetically modified fibers demonstrates expanded tropism via utilization of a coxsackievirus and adenovirus receptor-independent cell entry mechanism. J Virol 1998;72:9706–9713.
107. Lamfers ML, Grill J, Dirven CM, et al. Potential of the conditionally replicative adenovirus Ad5-Delta24RGD in the treatment of malignant gliomas and its enhanced effect with radiotherapy. Cancer Res 2002;62:5736–5742.
108. Asada-Mikami R, Heike Y, Kanai S, et al. Efficient gene transduction by RGD-fiber modified recombinant adenovirus into dendritic cells. Jap J Cancer Res 2001;92:321–327.
109. Arap W, Pasqualini R, Ruoslahti E. Cancer treatment by targeted drug delivery to tumor vasculature in a mouse model. Science 1998;279:377–380.
110. Koivunen E, Arap W, Valtanen H, et al. Tumor targeting with a selective gelatinase inhibitor. Nat Biotechnol 1999;17:768–774.
111. Nicklin SA, White SJ, Watkins SJ, Hawkins RE, Baker AH. Selective targeting of gene transfer to vascular endothelial cells by use of peptides isolated by phage display. Circulation 2000;102:231–237.
112. Kolonin M, Pasqualini R, Arap W. Molecular addresses in blood vessels as targets for therapy. Curr Opin Chem Biol 2001;5:308–313.
113. Pasqualini R, Koivunen E, Ruoslahti EA. Peptide isolated from phage display libraries is a structural and functional mimic of an RGD-binding site on integrins. J Cell Biol 1995;130:1189–1196.
114. Pasqualini R, Koivunen E, Kain R, et al. Aminopeptidase N is a receptor for tumor-homing peptides and a target for inhibiting angiogenesis. Cancer Res 2000;60:722–727.
115. Roelvink PW, Mi LG, Einfeld DA, Kovesdi I, Wickham TJ. Identification of a conserved receptor-binding site on the fiber proteins of CAR-recognizing adenoviridae. Science 1999;286:1568–1571.

116. Pizzato M, Blair ED, Fling M, et al. Evidence for nonspecific adsorption of targeted retrovirus vector particles to cells. Gene Ther 2001;8:1088–1096.
117. Leissner P, Legrand V, Schlesinger Y, et al. Influence of adenoviral fiber mutations on viral encapsidation, infectivity and in vivo tropism. Gene Ther 2001;8:49–57.
118. Nettelbeck DM, Jerome V, Muller R. Gene therapy: designer promoters for tumour targeting. Trends Genet 12000;6:174–181.
119. Clary BM, Lyerly HK. Transcriptional targeting for cancer gene therapy. [Review] [21 refs]. Surg Oncol Clin North Am 1998;7:565–574.
120. Osaki T, Tanio Y, Tachibana I, et al. Gene therapy for carcinoembryonic antigen-producing human lung cancer cells by cell type-specific expression of herpes simplex virus thymidine kinase gene. Cancer Res 1994;54:5258–5261.
121. Richards CA, Austin EA, Huber BE. Transcriptional regulatory sequences of carcinoembryonic antigen: identification and use with cytosine deaminase for tumor-specific gene therapy. Hum Gene Ther 1995;6:881–893.
122. Ido A, Nakata K, Kato Y, et al. Gene therapy for hepatoma cells using a retrovirus vector carrying herpes simplex virus thymidine kinase gene under the control of human alpha-fetoprotein gene promoter. Cancer Res 1995;55:3105–3109.
123. Kaneko S, Hallenbeck P, Kotani T, et al. Adenovirus-mediated gene therapy of hepatocellular carcinoma using cancer-specific gene expression. Cancer Res 1995;55:5283–5287.
124. Andriani F, Nan B, Yu J, et al. Use of the probasin promoter ARR2PB to express Bax in androgen receptor-positive prostate cancer cells. J Natl Cancer Inst 2001;93:1314–1324.
125. Gotoh A, Ko SC, Shirakawa T, et al. Development of prostate-specific antigen promoter-based gene therapy for androgen-independent human prostate cancer. J Urol 1998;160:220–229.
126. Chen L, Chen D, Manome Y, Dong Y, Fine HA, Kufe DW. Breast cancer selective gene expression and therapy mediated by recombinant adenoviruses containing the DF3/MUC1 promoter. J Clin Invest 1995;96:2775–2782.
127. Parr MJ, Manome Y, Tanaka T, et al. Tumor-selective transgene expression in vivo mediated by an E2F-responsive adenoviral vector. Nat Med 1997;3:1145–1149.
128. Gerdes CA, Castro MG, Lowenstein PR. Strong promoters are the key to highly efficient, noninflammatory and noncytotoxic adenoviral-mediated transgene delivery into the brain in vivo. Mol Ther J Am Soc Gene Ther 2000;2:330–338.
129. Takakura M, Kyo S, Kanaya T, et al. Cloning of human telomerase catalytic subunit (hTERT) gene promoter and identification of proximal core promoter sequence essential for transcriptional activation in immortalized and cancer cells. Cancer Res 1999;59:551–557.
130. Gu J, Kagawa S, Takakura M, et al. Tumor-specific transgene expression from the human telomerase reverse transcriptase promoter enables targeting of the therapeutic effects of the Bax gene to cancers. Cancer Res 2000;60:5359–5364.
131. Komata T, Kondo Y, Kanzawa T, et al. Treatment of malignant glioma cells with the transfer of constitutively active caspase-6 using the human telomerase catalytic subunit (human telomerase reverse transcriptase) gene promoter. Cancer Res 2001;61:5796–5802.
132. Morin GB. The human telomere terminal transferase enzyme is a ribonucleoprotein that synthesizes TTAGGG repeats. Cell 1989;59:521–529.
133. Blackburn EH. Telomerases. [Review] [31 refs]. Ann Rev Biochem 1992;61:113–129.
134. Kim NW, Piatyszek MA, Prowse KR, et al. Specific association of human telomerase activity with immortal cells and cancer. Science 1994;266:2011–2015.
135. Counter CM, Avilion AA, LeFeuvre CE, et al. Telomere shortening associated with chromosome instability is arrested in immortal cells which express telomerase activity. EMBO J 1992;11:1921–1929.
136. Shay JW, Bacchetti S. A survey of telomerase activity in human cancer. [Review] [51 refs]. Eur J Cancer 1997;33:787–791.
137. Nakamura TM, Morin GB, Chapman KB, et al. Telomerase catalytic subunit homologs from fission yeast and human. Science 1997;277:955–959.
138. Nakayama J, Tahara H, Tahara E, et al. Telomerase activation by hTRT in human normal fibroblasts and hepatocellular carcinomas. Nat Genet 1998;18:65–68.
139. Meyerson M, Counter CM, Eaton EN, et al. hEST2, the putative human telomerase catalytic subunit gene, is up-regulated in tumor cells and during immortalization. Cell 1997;90:785–795.
140. Gu J, Andreeff M, Roth JA, Fang B. hTERT Promoter Induces Tumor-Specific Bax Gene Expression and Cell Killing in Syngenic Mouse Tumor Model and Prevents Systemic Toxicity . Gene Ther 2002; 9:30–37.

141. Gu J, Zhang L, Huang X, et al. A novel single tetracycline-regulative adenoviral vector for tumor-specific Bax gene expression and cell killing in vitro and in vivo. Oncogene 2002;21:4757–4764.
142. Huang X, Lin T, Gu J, et al. Combined TRAIL and Bax gene therapy prolonged survival in mice with ovarian cancer xenograft. Gene Ther 2002;9:1379–1386.
143. Lin T, Gu J, Zhang L, et al. Targeted expression of green fluorescent protein/Tumor necrosis factor-related apoptosis-inducing ligand fusion protein from human telomerase reverse transcriptase promoter elicits antitumor activity without toxic effect on primary human hepatocytes. Cancer Res 2002;62:3620–3625.
144. Lin T, Huang X, Gu J, et al. Long-term tumor-free survival from treatment with the GFP-TRAIL fusion gene expressed from the hTERT promoter in breast cancer cells. Oncogene 2002;21:8020–8028.
145. Koga S, Hirohata S, Kondo Y, et al. A novel telomerase-specific gene therapy: gene transfer of caspase-8 utilizing the human telomerase catalytic subunit gene promoter. Hum Gene Ther 2000;11:1397–1406.
146. Huang TG, Savontaus MJ, Shinozaki K, Sauter BV, Woo SL. Telomerase-dependent oncolytic adenovirus for cancer treatment. Gene Ther 2003;10:1241–1247.
147. Wirth T, Zender L, Schulte B, et al. A telomerase-dependent conditionally replicating adenovirus for selective treatment of cancer. Cancer Res 2003;63:3181–3188.
148. Koch P, Guo ZS, Kagawa S, Gu J, Roth JA, Fang B. Augmenting transgene expression from carcinoembryonic antigen (CEA) promoter via a GAL4 gene regulatory system. Mol Ther J Am Soc Gene Ther 2001;3:278–283.
149. Qiao J, Doubrovin M, Sauter BV, et al. Tumor-specific transcriptional targeting of suicide gene therapy. Gene Ther 2002;9:168–175.
150. Sadowski I, Ma J, Triezenberg S, Ptashne M. GAL4-VP16 is an unusually potent transcriptional activator. Nature 1988;335:563–564.
151. Gossen M, Bujard H. Tight control of gene expression in mammalian cells by tetracycline-responsive promoters. Proc Natl Acad Sci U S A 1992;89:5547–5551.
152. Gu J, Fang B. Telomerase promoter-driven cancer gene therapy. Cancer Biol Ther 2003;2:S64–S70.
153. Swisher SG, Roth JA, Nemunaitis J, et al. Adenovirus-mediated p53 gene transfer in advanced non-small-cell lung cancer. J Natil Cancer Inst 1999;91:763–771.
154. Clayman GL, el Naggar AK, Lippman SM, et al. Adenovirus-mediated p53 gene transfer in patients with advanced recurrent head and neck squamous cell carcinoma. J Clin Oncol 1998;16:2221–2232.
155. Bier-Laning CM, VanEcho D, Yver A, Dreiling LK. A phase II multicenter study of AD5CMV-P53 administered intratumorally to patients with recurrent head and neck cancer. Proc Am Sco Clin Oncol 1999;18:444a.
156. Goodwin WJ, Esser D, Clayman GL, Nemunaitis J, Yver A, Dreiling LK. Randomized phase II study of intratumoral injection of two dosing schedules using a replication-deficient adenovirus carrying the p53 gene (AD5CMV-P53) in patients with recurrent/refractory head and nech cancer. Proc Am Sco Clin Oncol 1999;19:445a.
157. Nemunaitis J, Swisher SG, Timmons T, et al. Adenovirus-mediated p53 gene transfer in sequence with cisplatin to tumors of patients with non-small-cell lung cancer. J Clin Oncol 2000;18:609–622.
158. Schuler M, Herrmann R, De Greve JL, et al. Adenovirus-mediated wild-type p53 gene transfer in patients receiving chemotherapy for advanced non-small-cell lung cancer: results of a multicenter phase II study. J Clin Oncol 2001;19:1750–1758
159. Buller RE, Shahin MS, Horowitz JA, et al. Long term follow-up of patients with recurrent ovarian cancer after Adp53 gene replacement with SCH58500. Cancer Gene Ther 2002;9:567–572.
160. Broaddus WC, Liu Y, Steele LL, et al. Enhanced radiosensitivity of malignant glioma cells after adenoviral p53 transduction. J Neurosurg 1999;91:997–1004.
161. Jasty R, Lu J, Irwin T, Suchard S, Clarke MF, Castle VP. Role of p53 in the regulation of irradiation-induced apoptosis in neuroblastoma cells. Mol Genet Metab 1998;65:155–164.
162. Spitz FR, Nguyen D, Skibber JM, Meyn RE, Cristiano RJ, Roth JA. Adenoviral-mediated wild-type p53 gene expression sensitizes colorectal cancer cells to ionizing radiation. Clin Cancer Res 1996;2:1665–1671.
163. Swisher SG, Roth JA, Komaki R, et al. Induction of p53-regulated genes and tumor regression in lung cancer patients after intratumoral delivery of adenoviral p53 (INGN 201) and radiation therapy. Clin Cancer Res 2003;9:93–101.
164. Peng Z, Han D, Zhang S, et al. Clinical evaluation of safety and efficacy of intratumoral administration of a recombinant adenoviral-p53 anticancer agent (Genkaxin). Mol Ther 2003;7:S422.
165. Sandmair AM, Loimas S, Puranen P, et al. Thymidine kinase gene therapy for human malignant glioma, using replication-deficient retroviruses or adenoviruses. Hum Gene Ther 2000;11:2197–2205.

166. Sung MW, Yeh HC, Thung SN, et al. Intratumoral adenovirus-mediated suicide gene transfer for hepatic metastases from colorectal adenocarcinoma: results of a phase I clinical trial. Mol Ther J Am Soc Gen Ther 2001;4:182–191.
167. Shalev M, Kadmon D, Teh BS, et al. Suicide gene therapy toxicity after multiple and repeat injections in patients with localized prostate cancer. J Urol 2000;163:1747–1750.
168. Nemunaitis J, Cunningham C, Buchanan A, et al. Intravenous infusion of a replication-selective adenovirus (ONYX-015) in cancer patients: safety, feasibility and biological activity. Gene Ther 2001;8:746–759.
169. Habib NA, Sarraf CE, Mitry RR, et al. E1B-deleted adenovirus (dl1520) gene therapy for patients with primary and secondary liver tumors. Hum Gene Ther 2001;12:219–226.
170. Reid T, Galanis E, Abbruzzese J, et al. Intra-arterial administration of a replication-selective adenovirus (dl1520) in patients with colorectal carcinoma metastatic to the liver: a phase I trial. Gene Ther 2001;8:1618–1626.

2 Efficacy, Toxicity, and Immunogenicity of Adenoviral Vectors

Dmitry M. Shayakhmetov, PhD

CONTENTS

Summary

To date, over 60% of all gene therapy clinical trials in the United States have focused on the development and validation of new therapies for cancer. Many of these trials utilize Ad vectors as novel anticancer therapeutics. In recent years, however, initial enthusiasm and high expectations for successful clinical application of Ad-based vectors as efficient anticancer therapeutics has been dampened based on the data obtained during a series of clinical trials. Along with the major concerns over the safety of systemic Ad application, which was found to be associated with immediate innate and inflammatory host responses and can also lead to fatalities, such issues as rapid clearance of the bulk of administered vector by cells of the reticulo-endothelial system, neutralization of virus particles by highly prevalent pre-existing antibodies, and poor transduction of primary tumors resulting from low-level Ad receptor expression and/or anatomical barriers, including extracellular matrix surrounding tumors, have established a great need for research to further improve existing Ad vectors and unravel their true therapeutic potential as anticancer agents. This chapter reviews and discusses the current status, limitations and future challenges for the Ad vector development field with respect to their efficacy, toxicity and immunogenicity.

Key Words: Adenovirus vectors; oncolytic viruses; innate antiviral response; disseminated tumors; pathways of adenovirus infection; intravascular virus administration.

1. INTRODUCTION

Adenoviruses (Ad) are promising vectors for therapeutic interventions in humans. To date, over 60% of all gene therapy clinical trials in the United States have focused on the development and validation of new therapies for cancer, and many of these trials utilize Ad vectors as novel anticancer therapeutics *(1)*. Over recent years, however,

From: *Cancer Drug Discovery and Development: Gene Therapy for Cancer*
Edited by: K. K. Hunt, S. A. Vorburger, and S. G. Swisher © Humana Press Inc., Totowa, NJ

initial enthusiasm and high expectations for successful clinical application of Ad-based vectors as efficient anticancer therapeutics has been dampened based on the data obtained during a series of clinical trials. Along with the major concerns over the safety of systemic Ad application, which was found to be associated with immediate innate and inflammatory host responses and can also lead to fatalities *(2,3)*, such issues as rapid clearance of the bulk of administered vector by cells of the reticulo-endothelial system, neutralization of virus particles by highly prevalent pre-existing antibodies, and poor transduction of primary tumors resulting from low-level Ad receptor expression and/or anatomical barriers, including extracellular matrix surrounding tumors, have established a great need for further research to improve existing Ad vectors and unravel their true therapeutic potential as anticancer agents. This chapter reviews and discusses the current status, limitations, and future challenges for the Ad vector development field with respect to Ad efficacy, toxicity and immunogenicity.

2. FACTORS AFFECTING EFFICACY OF AD AS AN ANTICANCER AGENT

Initial attempts to utilize Ads as anticancer therapeutics were undertaken shortly after their discovery in early 1950s *(4)*. Administration of wild-type Ads into patients with cervical carcinomas did not demonstrate significant efficacy. As a result, further development of Ad-based anticancer therapeutics was essentially abandoned for four decades. By the mid-1990s, accumulated data on the virus genome organization and protein expression coupled with significant insights into mechanisms governing Ad-host cell interactions revived the idea of using Ad for the therapy of cancer in humans resulting primarily from the following three remarkable features of the virus: (1) its great efficiency in killing infected cells during virus replication, (2) it's ability to infect a variety of primary human cells in vitro, and (3) it's relative safety and ease of propagation and large-scale production in the laboratory.

A number of academic research teams and companies worldwide have focused their efforts on developing Ad-based cancer therapeutics. Three major strategies are primarily being pursued: (1) delivery of genes cytotoxic for tumor cells or restriction of virus replication exclusively to tumor cells; (2) enhancement of virus potential to spread through the tumor mass, and (3) restriction of viral infection in the body only to the tumor cell via modification of virus–host cell interactions.

2.1. Restriction of Virus Replication to Cancer Cells

Initially, mutants with deletions in one or more critical viral genes (located within the E1 and E3 regions) were constructed as replication-incompetent vectors to deliver genes exerting antitumor activity (e.g., *p53*, prodrug-activating enzymes) *(5–8)*. As a next step, Ads were engineered to replicate selectively within tumor cells in vivo, so-called conditionally replicating Ads (CRADs) (*see* Chapter 1) *(5)*.

One of the most studied CRAD is ONYX-015 (*dl*1520), which lacks the expression of the functional E1B-55kD gene *(9)*. In wild-type Ad this gene interacts with the host cell to suppress its p53 mediated cell-cycle arrest or apoptosis, which would then abrogate viral amplification. Hence, efficient replication of this E1B-devoid vector is thought to be restricted to cells with p53-deficient phenotype *(9–12)*. Because more than 50% of tumors possess no functional p53 protein, there has been considerable enthusiasm for the use of ONYX-015 as a selective anticancer agent. In phase I and II clinical trials, both intratumoral and intravascular administrations of ONYX-015 were demonstrated to be safe at doses up to 2×10^{13} viral-particles (vp) *(13)*. However, using the intravascular route of administration only 14% of patients in one study *(14)* and none in the other *(15)* demonstrated tumor regression, whereas progressive disease was eventually found in all participants of the trials. In a phase II clinical trial in patients with gastrointestinal carcinoma metastatic to the liver *(14)*, intravascular administration of 2×10^{12} vp of ONYX-015 by hepatic artery injection (two injections with a 7-d interval), resulted in partial tumor regression in 3 out 27 patients. Using an intratumoral route of administration in patients with advanced head and neck squamous cell carcinoma *(16)* (multiple injections of 2×10^{11} vp), 14% of patients demonstrated partial to complete tumor regression. Importantly, virus replication was clearly detected in tumor biopsies between 5 and 14 d post-treatment, and its efficiency was, indeed, dependent on the p53 status of the tumor.

Another approach to limit the replication of oncolytic viruses to tumor cells is by transcriptional regulation of the expression of genes essential for virus replication (e.g., E1A, E4, or both). Most CRADs developed using this strategy possess E1A or a combination of E1A and E4 genes under the control of tumor- or tissue-specific promoters, like the human telomerase reverse transcriptase (hTERT) *(17)*, the prostate-specific antigen (PSA) *(18)*, and the α-feto-protein (AFP) *(19)*. Thus, by using the α-fetoprotein promoter to control E1A gene expression, selective replication of CRADs in human hepatocellular carcinoma cells was demonstrated *(19,20)*. Similarly, using rat probasin *(21)* or human PSA promoters *(22)*, Ad vectors were generated that replicated specifically in prostate cancer cells. Despite the fact that the feasibility of these approaches has been convincingly demonstrated in multiple preclinical animal models of human cancers *(8,23–26)*, a series of clinical trials with multiple tumor types and routes of administration demonstrated limited efficacy in humans to date *(27–29)*. In a dose-ranging phase I study of a prostate-specific, replication-restricted Ad for the treatment of prostate cancer, the safety and activity of intraprostatic delivery of CV706 virus has been shown *(30)*. Twenty patients in five groups were treated with 1×10^{11} to 1×10^{13} vp. No severe virus associated toxicity was reported, and in the patients receiving the highest virus doses, reduction of serum PSA has been demonstrated, suggesting, thus, some efficacy of the direct intratumoral application of CRADs.

2.2. Enhancing Virus Spread in the Tumor Tissue

Whereas virus replication in cancer cells can be efficiently regulated by controlling the expression of a relatively small number of genes (e.g., E1A, E1B, E4), boosting virus spread through the tumor mass is, apparently, a more complex task. To date, there are only preclinical data on using Ad mutants, which are capable of efficiently spreading through the tumor resulting from specific genetic modifications. So far, the best evidence for improved oncolytic potential of Ad via boosting intratumoral virus spread was provided by Doronin et al. *(31,32)*. In Ad vectors KD1 and KD3, the E3 region of the Ad genome was modified to overexpress Ad death protein (ADP), which facilitates cell lysis during later stages of virus life cycle. In comparison with parental vectors, KD1-SPB variants demonstrated superior antitumor efficacy in a human H441 cell xenograft model *(33)*. An alternative approach to boost virus spread through the tumor, which was also investigated in preclinical model systems, is to induce apoptosis of virus infected cancer cells during late stages of virus replication *(34)*. Although potentially advantageous, none of the vectors with improved efficacy of intratumoral spread to date has been tested in clinical trials. This is, among other factors, partly the reuslt of concerns that the enhanced spreading of Ad is not limited to the tumor mass, but that it could also lead to increased toxicity as a result of leakage from the oncolytic virus to the surrounding (healthy) tissue.

2.3. Restriction of Viral Infection by Modification of Virus-Host Cell Interactions

Analysis of Ad entry into cells, and, specifically, approaches to target Ad infection selectively to tumor cells has been an area of major investigation recently. Whereas understanding of the Ad infection process in vitro has been greatly increased since the mid 1990s, there are still a very limited number of examples where these fundamental findings have been successfully applied to improve antitumor efficiency of existing Ads. Because the spectrum of initial virus-host interactions is dictated by Ad capsid proteins (*see* Chapter 12), genetic modification of these proteins, which alters the natural tropism of Ad represents the main approach to achieve virus targeting to tumor cells. Currently, two targeting ligands have been successfully incorporated into the fiber protein of tumor targeted Ads—polylysine and short RGD motif-containing peptides. Addition of twenty lysine residues to the C-terminus of the Ad fiber knob domain (F/K20 fiber) resulted in improved infectivity of the Ad toward human malignant glioma cell lines, which express heparan sulfate proteoglycans, a putative receptor for F/K20 fibers *(35,36)*. Combination of F/K20 fiber modification with E1B gene mutation in one vector enhanced both the oncolytic properties in vitro and the antitumor activity in preclinical models, using U373-MG human glioma cells *(36)*. Incorporation of the RGD motif-containing peptides into the Ad fiber HI-loop allowed efficient infection of a variety of αv-integrin-expressing cancer cells *(37–39)*. Importantly, combination of this capsid modification with genetic modification of E1A (Ad5-Δ24RGD *[40,41]* and Δ-24RGD *[26]*) (*see* Chapter 19) was found to increase oncolytic potential of Ad vectors toward human lung carcinoma and glioma cells in preclinical models in vivo.

Summarizing the existing clinical data, it is evident that despite encouraging results obtained from preclinical studies, the clinical trials involving Ads as sole anticancer agents demonstrated their poor efficacy. Whereas direct intratumoral administration was found to be safe, intravascular administration of existing vectors is limited by the severe and potentially lethal side effects, caused by the host antiviral innate and inflammatory responses. These side effects limit the vector load that can be delivered safely to patients via the intravascular route (about 6×10^{11} vp/kg), suggesting that improvement of the Ad antitumor efficacy cannot be achieved by merely escalating the administered amount of vectors *(42)*. Mathematical modeling of oncolytic Ad interactions with the tumor and analysis of the critical parameters affecting vector efficacy demonstrated that tumor eradication requires widespread distribution of the virus within the tumor at the time of initial infection, a goal that is rarely achieved with existing Ad vectors *(43)*. It was also speculated that inefficient replication and cell lysis, slow speed of virus spread through the tumor, and the presence of an innate immune response could severely affect the ability of virus to "control" and/or eradicate the tumor. The validity of these initial assumptions and the importance of identified factors find their conformation in experimental data obtained from model systems in animals and clinical trials in humans. The efficacy of oncolytic 01/PEME virus, possessing multiple genetic modifications to restrict replication to tumor cells and boost virus spread through the tumor, was analyzed in a mouse model with subcutaneous PC3 prostate cancer tumors using both intratumoral and intravascular routes of vector administration *(44)*. This study clearly demonstrated that Ad applied intratumorally was more than 1000 times more efficient at tumor eradication than the same vector applied via the vasculature. Moreover, it was found that the levels of vector replication in the tumor might not be a reliable parameter to predict the Ad antitumor efficacy. Instead, the authors concluded that efficient initial distribution of Ad to the tumor site is one of the most immportant parameter affecting the efficacy of oncolytic Ads.

In summary, whereas great progress has undoubtedly been made with regard to both developing Ad vectors capable of selective replication within a variety of tumor cells in vitro and of efficient spread through the three-dimensional tumor architecture, disappointingly little has been achieved in targeting efficient virus infection to tumor cells in vivo, especially via the intravascular route of administration. Therefore, future studies are needed to improve our understanding of the mechanisms governing the infectivity and toxicity of Ad in vivo in order to improve the performance of the currently existing oncolytic vectors.

3. PATHWAYS OF AD INFECTION IN VITRO AND IN VIVO

According to the currently accepted model, which is based primarily on in vitro data, Ad infects cells in a two-step process *(45–47)*. The first step is the fiber coat protein-mediated binding of Ad to the primary cell surface receptor. Ads belonging to subgroups A through F, except subgroup B, can utilize coxsackie and Ad receptor, CAR, as a primary attachment receptor for infection *(48–51)*. We and others have recently found that the ubiquitously expressed complement regulatory protein, CD46, represents a major subgroup B Ad receptor on human cells *(52,53)*. As CAR lacking its intracellular domain is sufficient to mediate virus infection *(54)*, the role of signaling downstream of CAR upon its binding to Ad is currently considered to be negligible for efficient virus infection. However, the role of signaling downstream of CAR in the initiation of innate in vivo responses to Ad requires further investigation.

Following initial attachment, RGD motifs within the Ad penton base interact with cellular integrins, allowing for the internalization of attached virus particles into the cell *(55)*. It has been shown that a number of RGD motif-interacting integrins ($\alpha v\beta 1$, $\alpha v\beta 3$, $\alpha v\beta 5$, $\alpha v\beta 6$, $\alpha 5\beta 1$, $\alpha_M\beta 2$,$\alpha_L\beta 2$) can serve as secondary receptors, promoting Ad internalization into different cell types in vitro *(47,55–59)*. Viral interaction with cellular integrins initiates downstream signaling through the activation of two independent but synergistic pathways *(60)*. The first pathway includes the lipid kinase phospho-inositol-3-kinase (PI3K), the small G proteins cdc42 and rac1, and p38 kinase mitogen activated protein kinase (MAPK) *(61–64)*. The second pathway involves signal transduction through focal adhesion kinase, Raf-1 and ERK1/2 protein kinases *(65–68)*. The signal transduction through either of these pathways can induce actin polymerization near the site of the virus attachment triggering endocytosis *(60)*. Importantly, the activation of p38 MAPK and ERK1/2 was linked to the translocation of NF-κB into the nucleus and the initiation of proinflammatory cytokine and chemokine gene expression *(60,69–71)*.

Upon acidification of the intraendosomal environment, Ad escapes to the cytosol by disrupting endocytic vesicles, and the particles then engage in bidirectional movement along microtubules *(72,73)*, ultimately leading to the docking of partially disassembled capsids to the nuclear pore complexes and the translocation of virus genomic DNA into the nucleus. Recent studies have shown that Ad internalization into cells expressing β5-integrins with mutated cytoplasmic domains occurred normally; however, the virus was unable to efficiently escape from the endosomes *(74)*. The authors suggested that signaling downstream of the β5-integrin subunit is important for the endosome escape step of virus infection. These data also imply that integrin-mediated signaling may involve different target/adaptor molecules upon virus internalization and upon its escape from the endosome into the cytoplasm. Clearly, binding of Ad to integrins, which varies dramatically in different tissues, may contribute to the diverse cellular responses to virus infection. It was previously found that integrins can have several activation states and their adaptor/signal transduction molecules may be involved in activation of the early cellular response genes (e.g., β1-integrin signaling through integrin linked kinase [ILK] was associated with NF-κB-dependent activation of the proinflammatory genes, including interleukin-1 (IL-1) and tumor necrosis factor α (TNF-α)*(75–79)*.

Although cellular CAR expression levels correlate well with susceptibility to Ad infection in vitro, most recent data demonstrate that disrupting CAR binding does not appreciably impact the level and pattern of Ad distribution in vivo *(80–84)*. These data indicate that the presence of CAR on cells is not a critical factor in determining their susceptibility to group C Ad infection in vivo. Recently, a number of novel moieties, including heparin sulfate glycosaminoglycans and dipalmitoyl phosphatidylcholines, were characterized as potential Ad5 primary attachment receptors; however, their roles in governing Ad infectivity in vivo remains unknown *(85,86)*. It has also been reported that Ad binding to integrins is not necessary for efficient hepatocyte transduction in mice and rats *(87)*.

Numerous studies of Ad pharmacokinetics in animals after systemic administration have shown that within the first minutes more than 99% of an injected dose is cleared from the circulation *(27,88)*. The cells of the hepatic reticulo-endothelial system, in particular the Kupffer cells, are believed to be responsible for the rapid clearance of Ad from the blood *(82,88–90)*. Because of the natural kinetics of Ad clearance, the liver is the predominant organ in the body transduced with Ad after systemic application. Following Ad administration, transduction of liver cells is directly associated with a strong innate immune response and systemic toxicity that can be fatal for the host *(91,92–95)*. In this regard, it has been demonstrated that inactivation of Kupffer cells prior to Ad injection can partially reduce the manifestations of this acute toxicity and increase the levels and prolong the duration of the vector-encoded transgene expression *(96,97)*. Thus, in clinical settings, where specific delivery of therapeutic genes or anti-tumor Ad vectors to multiple organs or metastases is necessary, rapid liver-mediated removal of the virus from the circulation and related manifestations of viral toxicity represent the major hindrances to safety and efficacy.

Different approaches to avoid liver mediated clearance of Ad from the blood have been tested, including intraperitoneal vector application or modification of the Ad fiber shaft domain *(81a,98,99)*. Although data obtained from these studies are encouraging, the molecular mechanisms responsible for these phenomena require further investigation. Our recent analyses of factors responsible for the liver-mediated clearance of Ad from the blood revealed that the rapid deposition of Ad5-based vectors in the liver does not correlate with liver cell transduction and occurs independently of Ad fiber knob-mediated interactions with liver cells receptors *(100)*. On the contrary, the levels of the innate and inflammatory responses to systemically administered Ads correlated well with the efficiency of Ad hepatocyte transduction. These data demonstrated that different molecular mechanisms are likely to be responsible for liver-mediated clearance of Ad from the blood and for liver cell transduction. Systematic analyses of proteins interacting with Ad fiber knob domain in mouse and human plasma revealed that several blood factors (including coagulation factor IX) can bind Ad5 fiber protein and target the virus infection to hepatocytes and Kupffer cells in vivo via interaction with heparin sulfate proteoglycans and low-density lipoproteins (LDL) receptor-related protein, LRP *(101)*. Although these findings are helpful in understanding the biodistribution of systemically applied Ad vectors, the relationship between these new mechanisms of virus infection and vector-associated innate toxicity remain unknown.

4. UNDERSTANDING THE HOST RESPONSES TO NATURAL AD INFECTION

Ad infections occur worldwide as epidemic, endemic, and sporadic infections. Of the 51 human Ad serotypes currently known, the most common in clinical materials are the respiratory types of subgenus C (Ad1, Ad2, Ad5) and subgenus B (Ad3 and Ad7) *(102,103)*. Along with being an important cause of respiratory tract infections, Ad can also cause conjunctivitis and gastrointestinal disease. Ads have been implicated in aseptic meningitis, encephalitis, hepatitis, and hemorrhagic cystitis and may cause severe disseminated infections in immunocompromised patients of all ages *(104)*. In humans, the majority of Ad infections in immunocompetent hosts are subclinical, meaning that no apparent symptoms are present. This feature has made Ad an attractive platform for numerous gene therapy applications, including cancer. However, like most human virus pathogens, Ads possess a substantial genetic armamentarium to interfere with the immune system of the host to ensure their evolutionary survival *(105–108)*. Infection with Ad results in inhibition of cellular macromolecular synthesis leading to cell damage and death. To avoid clearance from the host, Ads express a number of viral genes that interfere with responses of both the innate and adaptive immune systems. It has been shown that the early Ad genes E1B-55K and E1B-19K inhibit intrinsic p53- and BAX-mediated apoptosis of infected cells *(109,110)*. Expression of virus associated VAI-RNA and E1A genes results in inhibition of cellular responses to interferons *(111,112)*. The Ad E3-19K protein binds major histocompatability complex (MHC) class I molecules in the endoplasmic reticulum, reducing their transport to the cell surface *(113,114)* and thus preventing the detection and killing of infected cells by cytotoxic T-lymphocytes (CTLs). Lastly, E3-RID, E3-14.7K and E1B-19K proteins interfere with TNF signaling and inhibit cellular apoptosis induced through the death domains *(108,115,116)*.

The data on the immune response to natural Ad infection in humans are scarce. In children with fatal Ad infection, TNFα, IL-6, and IL-8 were detected in the serum *(117)*. However, in patients with only mild disease, none of these cytokines were found at elevated levels in the blood. In a cotton rat model of Ad infection, which closely resemble the pathology of virus infection observed in humans *(118,119)*, two phases in the pathogenesis of Ad2- and Ad5-caused pneumonia have been described. The early histopathologic changes, which are induced by TNF-α and reach the maximum 3 to 5 d after infection, are characterized by mild to moderate injury to bronchial epithelial cells and infiltration of monocytes/macrophages, neutrophils and lymphocytes into peribroncheal and alveolar regions. During the late phases, 5 to 10 d after infection, a peribroncheal and perivascular infiltration is mostly composed of CD8+ lymphocytes, reflecting a virus-specific cytotoxic T-cell response to infected cells. Ad infection induces the formation of neutralizing antibodies that granted protection against reinfection with the same serotype. In the human population, the prevalence of anti-Ad5 neutralizing antibodies is approx 50 to 80% *(120)*. The high prevalence of pre-existing antibodies is one of the factors that may limit significantly the efficacy of proposed Ad-based gene therapy. A number of approaches are currently under development to avoid neutralization of therapeutic Ad vectors by pre-existing immunity. One of them is conjugation of virus particles to polyethylene glycol (PEG), that was found to protect Ad from antibody binding *(121,122)*. Another approach is the construction of therapeutic vectors using alternative Ad serotypes. Analyses of the prevalence of neutralizing antibodies to different Ad serotypes revealed that neutralizing antibodies to group B Ad11 and Ad35 are least prevalent in human populations (less that 10%) *(123)*. Therefore, significant efforts have been made to construct Ad vectors based on these human serotypes *(124,125)*. Alternatively, vectors based on different animal Ad serotypes (canine Ad, CAV1-3, bovine Ad, BAV-3, chimpanzee Ads) are currently being developed to avoid pre-existing neutralizing immunity *(126–130)*.

5. INNATE IMMUNE RESPONSE TO SYSTEMICALLY APPLIED AD

Even though natural infections with Ads are largely harmless in humans, intravenous Ad administration for gene delivery purposes, especially at high doses, stimulates strong innate and adaptive immune responses and can be fatal for the host *(91a,92,94)*. It is currently recognized that the initiation of this acute systemic inflammation depends on interactions of the Ad capsid with host cells. Upon systemic application of Ads in rodents, rhesus monkeys, and humans, a rapid liver-mediated vector removal from the circulation was observed *(5a,88a,89a,93)*. Despite significant knowledge regarding Ad interactions with cells in vitro, the molecular mechanisms governing Ad biodistribution, hepatic tropism and toxicity in vivo remain poorly understood.

Systemically applied Ads induce two phases of inflammatory gene expression in the liver. The first phase of acute inflammation depends entirely on virus capsid interactions with host cells and occurs within 24 h after virus administration *(2,60a)*. The second phase begins 3 to 4 d after Ad administration and requires viral gene expression *(96)*. In animal models, intravenous Ad administration has been shown to induce transcription and release of a number of cytokines and chemokines, including IL-6, TNF-α, RANTES, IP-10, IL-8, MIP-1α, MIP-1β, and MIP-2 into the serum *(64a,69a,70a,95,96,131,132)*. Macrophages, including tissue residential macrophages (e.g., Kupffer cells in the liver), and dendritic cells throughout the body are considered to be the primary source of these cytokines and chemokines following their transduction with Ads *(60a)*. Additionally, rapid clearance of Ad from the circulation by Kupffer cells may have a protective role against the dissemination of Ads to the lymphoid organs, therefore reducing systemic inflammation. In several gene therapy clinical trials it has been found that after systemic Ad administration at high doses ($2 \times 10^{12} - 4 \times 10^{13}$ vp), serum levels of IL-6, IL-10 and IL-1 were elevated *(133–136)*. However the role of these cytokines in the initiation of an immediate innate immune response remains, so far, unclear. Histological evaluation of tissues, including lung, liver, and spleen, revealed areas of leukocyte and neutrophil infiltration as well as microinfarctation, indicating that most tissues in the body are involved in the inflammatory response to systemically applied Ad (our unpublished observation) *(132,137)*. However, it is apparent that Ad-mediated liver damage plays a central role in the pathogenesis of acute systemic inflammation caused by intravenous Ad administration. To this end, it has been found that activation of the MIP-2 chemokine is critical for neutrophil attraction to the liver tissue, and inactivation of MIP-2 with an anti-MIP-2 antibody reduces observed liver pathology and markedly decreased systemic Ad toxicity *(132)*. To date, it is not known which cell type(s) in the liver tissue or other organs (such as spleen, lung and lymph nodes) are primarily responsible for the initiation of the systemic anti-Ad innate immune response. Interestingly, significant Ad-induced systemic inflammation was also observed in splenectomized or Kupffer cell-depleted mice (own observation) *(131,138)*. Recently, a role for liver sinusoid endothelial cells in the initiation of an anti-Ad innate immune response has been suggested *(138)*. However, because the primary mediators of the antivirus inflammatory response in vivo remain unidentified, this hypothesis still awaits substantiation.

It is conceivable that the cell types transduced by Ad upon intravascular administration directly participate in initiation of antiviral innate response. Therefore, if the administration of a therapeutic tumor-targeted Ad results in transduction of splenocytes, cells of bone marrow, or lung and liver residential macrophages, the toxicity profile of such a vector would be suboptimal because of this "nontarget" cell transduction. Because multiple pathways and cell surface receptors are utilized by different virus serotypes for the Ad entry into cells, identification of pathways, and ablation of virus interaction with nontargeted cell types is a promising approach to improve the toxicity profiles of existing oncolytic and tumor-targeted vectors. An alternative approach to reduce innate immune and inflammatory responses to systemically applied Ads is to pharmacologically interfere with molecular and/orsignaling pathways involved in the initiation or maintenance of these responses. Toietta et al. demonstrated that administration of anti-TNF-α antibody into mice prior to Ad delivery allows reduction of inflammatory responses toward Ads *(139)*. Our recent data also suggested that IL-1 participates in initiation of an anti-Ad inflammatory response and that pharmacological interference with IL-1 signaling pathways using anti-IL-1 antibody allows for significant improvement of the Ad toxicity profile following systemic application *(145)*.

6. ANIMAL MODELS FOR THE ANALYSIS OF INNATE IMMUNE AND INFLAMMATORY RESPONSES TO SYSTEMICALLY APPLIED AD

Animal models have proven to be an invaluable tool for the analysis of both Ad-mediated immune responses and the antitumor efficacy of Ad vectors. Because of ethical, regulatory, and practical issues (such as a large amount of clinical grade vector stocks), the conduction of routine studies in humans to analyze mechanisms of host response and optimize existing vectors is not an acceptable option. However, although being useful, animal models eventually provide only limited knowledge regarding vector performance in humans. As a result of natural and as yet uncharacterized species-specific factors, human Ads do not replicate efficiently in mice. This fact significantly complicates strategies for the analysis of oncolytic vector efficacy in preclinical mouse models. The use of large animal models (i.e., dogs and primates) is limited as a result of the relatively few immunochemical reagents on the market (i.e., antibodies for specific assays), the large amounts of vectors required for each administration, and the costs of large animal maintenance. The most abundant data on Ad performance in vivo was obtained in mice. Numerous studies of Ad pharmacokinetics after systemic administration have shown that within the first minutes of intravenous virus delivery in mice, more than 99% of the infectious particles are removed from the circulation *(27a,88a)*. Although the kinetics of virus clearance from the blood in primates (and humans) is somewhat slower than in mice, the liver remains the predominant organ in the body transduced with Ad after systemic application *(2,27a,88a,140)*. Upon intravenous Ad administration, serum levels of IL-6 and TNF-α are increased with similar kinetics in both mice and humans *(60a,141)*. Moreover, hepatic injury plays a key role in the pathogenesis of systemic Ad toxicity observed in mice *(60a,131)*. It is important to note that immune responses to Ad vary significantly among different mouse strains and between different species *(142)*. Whereas Ad-induced hepatitis following systemic vector application has been observed in all species, the dose of virus that resulted in severe toxicity (calculated as particles/kg) differed dramatically. In addition, it has to be considered that mice and non-human primates are much more resistant to activation of innate immunity than humans *(42a)*. Considering the limitations of the each particular animal model, it is apparent that intravenous Ad administration in mice will continue to be a valuable model for the analysis of cell types, virus capsid-host interactions, and molecular mechanisms involved in the initiation and maintenance of anti-Ad immune responses. At the same time, the development of novel small animal models that reflect more adequately human responses to Ad is highly desirable for the analysis of antitumor efficacy of Ads. Initials steps toward adapting mouse models for analysis of the oncolytic potential of Ads have already been taken, and more studies are currently underway *(143)*.

7. SUMMARY

Currently, data from clinical trials demonstrate relatively low-antitumor efficacy of existing Ad vectors as a sole therapeutic agent. For vectors applied intravenously, rapid clearance from the blood by the liver and subsequent systemic toxicity resulting from inflammatory responses are the major hindrances for its safe and effective use in humans. Whereas intratumoral vector administration was shown to be efficient for some types of cancers (e.g., gliomas, head and neck cancer), eradication of disseminated cancer cells in metastatic disease will, ultimately, require the systemic application of the therapeutic vector *(26a,27a,30a,144)*. Hence, the prevention of liver-mediated Ad sequestration would represent a major step toward development of safe and effective systemically applicable tumor-targeted Ad vectors for the treatment of local and disseminated metastatic disease.

In recent years, a significant body of data on the mechanisms of Ad-host cell interactions in vitro has been accumulated. However, it is currently unknown how these new findings relate to the pathogenesis of systemic toxicity in animals and humans after intravenous Ad administration. Although it is largely accepted that the immediate innate immune response toward Ad is initiated upon virus capsid interactions with host cells and, hence, does not require viral gene expression, the precise step(s) of virus–host interactions, the cell types involved and the primary mediators of this response remain unknown. The development of improved Ad-based therapeutics will ultimately require additional efforts to further our understanding of the fundamental mechanisms involved in host response toward systemically applied viral vectors. To this end, the identification of cell types or molecular pathways initiating innate anti-Ad immune response and the development of vectors unable to infect these cell types should represent a rational approach to improve the safety profile of existing antitumor Ads. Moreover, these studies should significantly improve our understanding of fundamental mechanisms of the host defense against viral pathogens, creating a basis for the development of safe and efficient Ad vectors for the therapy of a wide range of inborn and acquired human diseases, including cancer.

REFERENCES

1. Journal of Gene Medicine website, www.wiley.co.uk/genmed/clinical/.
2. Brunetti-Pierri N, Palmer DJ, Beaudet AL, Carey KD, Finegold M, Ng P. Acute toxicity after high-dose systemic injection of helper-dependent adenoviral vectors into nonhuman primates. Hum Gene Ther 2004;15:35–46.
3. Nunes FA, Furth EE, Wilson JM, Raper SE. Gene transfer into the liver of nonhuman primates with E1-deleted recombinant adenoviral vectors: safety of readministration. Hum Gene Ther 1999; 10:2515–2526.
4. Huebner RJ, Rowe WP, Schatten WE, Smith RR, Thomas LB. Studies on the use of viruses in the treatment of carcinoma of the cervix. Cancer 1956;9:1211–1218.
5. Kirn D, Martuza RL, Zwiebel J. Replication-selective virotherapy for cancer: Biological principles, risk management and future directions. Nat Med 2001;7:781–787.
6. McCormick F. Cancer gene therapy: fringe or cutting edge? Nat Rev Cancer 2001;1:130–141.
7. Roth JA, Cristiano RJ. Gene therapy for cancer: what have we done and where are we going? J Natl Cancer Inst 1997;89:21–39.
8. Qiao J, Doubrovin M, Sauter BV, et al. Tumor-specific transcriptional targeting of suicide gene therapy. Gene Ther 2002;9:168–175.
9. Bischoff JR, Kirn DH, Williams A, et al. An adenovirus mutant that replicates selectively in p53-deficient human tumor cells. Science 1996;274:373–376.
10. Heise C, Sampson-Johannes A, Williams A, McCormick F, Von Hoff DD, Kirn DH. ONYX-015, an E1B gene-attenuated adenovirus, causes tumor-specific cytolysis and antitumoral efficacy that can be augmented by standard chemotherapeutic agents. Nat Med 1997;3:639–645.
11. Heise CC, Williams AM, Xue S, Propst M, Kirn DH. Intravenous administration of ONYX-015, a selectively replicating adenovirus, induces antitumoral efficacy. Cancer Res 1999;59:2623–2628.
12. Heise CC, Williams A, Olesch J, Kirn DH. Efficacy of a replication-competent adenovirus (ONYX-015) following intratumoral injection: intratumoral spread and distribution effects. Cancer Gene Ther 1999;6:499–504.
13. Kirn D. Clinical research results with dl1520 (Onyx-015), a replication-selective adenovirus for the treatment of cancer: what have we learned? Gene Ther 2001;8:89–98.
14. Reid T, Galanis E, Abbruzzese J, et al. Hepatic arterial infusion of a replication-selective oncolytic adenovirus (dl1520): phase II viral, immunologic, and clinical endpoints. Cancer Res 2002; 62:6070–6079.
15. Nemunaitis J, Cunningham C, Buchanan A, et al. Intravenous infusion of a replication-selective adenovirus (ONYX-015) in cancer patients: safety, feasibility and biological activity. Gene Ther 2001; 8:746-59.
16. Nemunaitis J, Khuri F, Ganly I, et al. Phase II trial of intratumoral administration of ONYX-015, a replication-selective adenovirus, in patients with refractory head and neck cancer. J Clin Oncol 2001; 19:289–298.
17. Huang J, Bai YX, Han SW, et al. A human TERT C-terminal polypeptide sensitizes HeLa cells to H2O2-induced senescence without affecting telomerase enzymatic activity. Biochem Biophys Res Commun 2003;301:627–632.
18. Yu DC, Sakamoto GT, Henderson DR. Identification of the transcriptional regulatory sequences of human kallikrein 2 and their use in the construction of calydon virus 764, an attenuated replication competent adenovirus for prostate cancer therapy. Cancer Res 1999;59:1498–1504.
19. Hallenbeck PL, Chang YN, Hay C, et al. A novel tumor-specific replication-restricted adenoviral vector for gene therapy of hepatocellular carcinoma. Hum Gene Ther 1999;10:1721–1733.
20. Li Y, Yu DC, Chen Y, et al. A hepatocellular carcinoma-specific adenovirus variant, CV890, eliminates distant human liver tumors in combination with doxorubicin. Cancer Res 2001;61:6428–6436.
21. Yu DC, Chen Y, Seng M, Dilley J, Henderson DR. The addition of adenovirus type 5 region E3 enables calydon virus 787 to eliminate distant prostate tumor xenografts. Cancer Res 1999; 59:4200–4203.

22. Rodriguez R, Schuur ER, Lim HY, Henderson GA, Simons JW, Henderson DR. Prostate attenuated replication competent adenovirus (ARCA) CN706: a selective cytotoxic for prostate-specific antigen-positive prostate cancer cells. Cancer Res 1997;57:2559–2563.
23. Post DE, Khuri FR, Simons JW, Van Meir EG. Replicative oncolytic adenoviruses in multimodal cancer regimens. Hum Gene Ther 2003;14:933–946.
24. Rasmussen H, Rasmussen C, Lempicki M, et al. TNFerade Biologic: preclinical toxicology of a novel adenovector with a radiation-inducible promoter, carrying the human tumor necrosis factor alpha gene. Cancer Gene Ther 2002;9:951–957.
25. Steinwaerder DS, Carlson CA, Otto DL, Li ZY, Ni S, Lieber A. Tumor-specific gene expression in hepatic metastases by a replication-activated adenovirus vector. Nat Med 2001;7:240–243.
26. Fueyo J, Alemany R, Gomez-Manzano C, et al. Preclinical characterization of the antiglioma activity of a tropism-enhanced adenovirus targeted to the retinoblastoma pathway. J Natl Cancer Inst 2003;95:652–660.
27. Reid T, Warren R, Kirn D. Intravascular adenoviral agents in cancer patients: lessons from clinical trials. Cancer Gene Ther 2002;9:979–986.
28. Hermiston TW, Kuhn I. Armed therapeutic viruses: strategies and challenges to arming oncolytic viruses with therapeutic genes. Cancer Gene Ther 2002;9:1022–1035.
29. Bauzon M, Castro D, Karr M, Hawkins LK, Hermiston TW. Multigene expression from a replicating adenovirus using native viral promoters. Mol Ther 2003;7:526–534.
30. DeWeese TL, van der Poel H, Li S, et al. A phase I trial of CV706, a replication-competent, PSA selective oncolytic adenovirus, for the treatment of locally recurrent prostate cancer following radiation therapy. Cancer Res 2001;61:7464–7472.
31. Doronin K, Toth K, Kuppuswamy M, Ward P, Tollefson AE, Wold WS. Tumor-specific, replication-competent adenovirus vectors overexpressing the adenovirus death protein. J Virol 2000; 74:6147–6155.
32. Doronin K, Toth K, Kuppuswamy M, Krajcsi P, Tollefson AE, Wold WS. Overexpression of the ADP (E3-11.6K) protein increases cell lysis and spread of adenovirus. Virology 2003;305:378–387.
33. Doronin K, Kuppuswamy M, Toth K, et al. Tissue-specific, tumor-selective, replication-competent adenovirus vector for cancer gene therapy. J Virol 2001;75:3314–3324.
34. Mi J, Li ZY, Ni S, Steinwaerder D, Lieber A. Induced apoptosis supports spread of adenovirus vectors in tumors. Hum Gene Ther 2001;12:1343–1352.
35. Yoshida Y, Sadata A, Zhang W, Saito K, Shinoura N, Hamada H. Generation of fiber-mutant recombinant adenoviruses for gene therapy of malignant glioma. Hum Gene Ther 1998;9:2503–2515.
36. Shinoura N, Yoshida Y, Tsunoda R, et al. Highly augmented cytopathic effect of a fiber-mutant E1B-defective adenovirus for gene therapy of gliomas. Cancer Res 1999;59:3411–346.
37. Volk AL, Rivera AA, Kanerva A, et al. Enhanced adenovirus infection of melanoma cells by fiber-modification: incorporation of RGD peptide or Ad5/3 chimerism. Cancer Biol Ther 2003;2:511–515.
38. Dehari H, Ito Y, Nakamura T, et al. Enhanced antitumor effect of RGD fiber-modified adenovirus for gene therapy of oral cancer. Cancer Gene Ther 2003;10:75–85.
39. Nagel H, Maag S, Tassis A, Nestle FO, Greber UF, Hemmi S. The alphavbeta5 integrin of hematopoietic and nonhematopoietic cells is a transduction receptor of RGD-4C fiber-modified adenoviruses. Gene Ther 2003;10:1643–1653.
40. Suzuki K, Fueyo J, Krasnykh V, Reynolds PN, Curiel DT, Alemany R. A conditionally replicative adenovirus with enhanced infectivity shows improved oncolytic potency. Clin Cancer Res 2001; 7:120–126.
41. Bauerschmitz GJ, Lam JT, Kanerva A, et al. Treatment of ovarian cancer with a tropism modified oncolytic adenovirus. Cancer Res 2002;62:1266–1270.
42. Raper SE, Chirmule N, Lee FS, et al. Fatal systemic inflammatory response syndrome in a ornithine transcarbamylase deficient patient following adenoviral gene transfer. Mol Genet Metab 2003; 80:148–158.
43. Wein LM, Wu JT, Kirn DH. Validation and analysis of a mathematical model of a replication-competent oncolytic virus for cancer treatment: implications for virus design and delivery. Cancer Res 2003;63:1317–1324.
44. Demers GW, Johnson DE, Tsai V, et al. Pharmacologic indicators of antitumor efficacy for oncolytic virotherapy. Cancer Res 2003;63:4003–4008.
45. Nemerow GR. Cell receptors involved in adenovirus entry. Virology 2000;274:1–4.
46. Bergelson JM. Receptors mediating adenovirus attachment and internalization. Biochem Pharmacol 1999;57:975–979.

47. Meier O, Greber UF. Adenovirus endocytosis. J Gene Med 2003;5:451–462.
48. Roelvink PW, Lizonova A, Lee JG, et al. The coxsackievirus-adenovirus receptor protein can function as a cellular attachment protein for adenovirus serotypes from subgroups A, C, D, E, and F. J Virol 1998;72:7909–7915.
49. Roelvink PW, Mi Lee G, Einfeld DA, Kovesdi I, Wickham TJ. Identification of a conserved receptor-binding site on the fiber proteins of CAR-recognizing adenoviridae. Science 1999;286:1568–1571.
50. Bergelson JM, Cunningham JA, Droguett G, et al. Isolation of a common receptor for Coxsackie B viruses and adenoviruses 2 and 5. Science 1997;275:1320–1323.
51. Tomko RP, Xu R, Philipson L. HCAR and MCAR: the human and mouse cellular receptors for subgroup C adenoviruses and group B coxsackieviruses. Proc Natl Acad Sci U S A 1997;94:3352–3356.
52. Gaggar A, Shayaklumetov DM, Lieber A. CD46 is a cellular receptor for group B adenoviruses. Nature Medicine 2003;9:1408–1412.
53. Segerman A, Atkinson JP, Marttila M, Dennerquist V, Wadell G, Arnberg N. Adenovirus type 11 uses CD46 as a cellular receptor. J Virol 2003;77:9183–9191.
54. Wang X, Bergelson JM. Coxsackievirus and adenovirus receptor cytoplasmic and transmembrane domains are not essential for coxsackievirus and adenovirus infection. J Virol 1999;73:2559–2562.
55. Wickham TJ, Mathias P, Cheresh DA, Nemerow GR. Integrins alpha v beta 3 and alpha v beta 5 promote adenovirus internalization but not virus attachment. Cell 1993;73:309–319.
56. Li E, Brown SL, Stupack DG, Puente XS, Cheresh DA, Nemerow GR. Integrin alpha(v)beta1 is an adenovirus coreceptor. J Virol 2001;75:5405–5409.
57. Davison E, Diaz RM, Hart IR, Santis G, Marshall JF. Integrin alpha5beta1-mediated adenovirus infection is enhanced by the integrin-activating antibody TS2/16. J Virol 1997;71:6204–6207.
58. Davison E, Kirby I, Whitehouse J, Hart I, Marshall JF, Santis G. Adenovirus type 5 uptake by lung adenocarcinoma cells in culture correlates with Ad5 fibre binding is mediated by alpha(v)beta1 integrin and can be modulated by changes in beta1 integrin function. J Gene Med 2001;3:550–559.
59. Huang S, Kamata T, Takada Y, Ruggeri ZM, Nemerow GR. Adenovirus interaction with distinct integrins mediates separate events in cell entry and gene delivery to hematopoietic cells. J Virol 1996;70:4502–4508.
60. Liu Q, Muruve DA. Molecular basis of the inflammatory response to adenovirus vectors. Gene Ther 2003;10:935–940.
61. Li E, Stupack D, Klemke R, Cheresh DA, Nemerow GR. Adenovirus endocytosis via alpha(v) integrins requires phosphoinositide-3-OH kinase. J Virol 1998;72:2055–2061.
62. Li E, Stupack D, Bokoch GM, Nemerow GR. Adenovirus endocytosis requires actin cytoskeleton reorganization mediated by Rho family GTPases. J Virol 1998;72:8806–8812.
63. Suomalainen M, Nakano MY, Boucke K, Keller S, Greber UF. Adenovirus-activated PKA and p38/MAPK pathways boost microtubule-mediated nuclear targeting of virus. Embo J 2001;20:1310–1319.
64. Bhat NR, Fan F. Adenovirus infection induces microglial activation: involvement of mitogen-activated protein kinase pathways. Brain Res 2002;948:93–101.
65. Nemerow GR, Stewart PL. Role of alpha(v) integrins in adenovirus cell entry and gene delivery. Microbiol Mol Biol Rev 1999;63:725–734.
66. Li E, Stupack DG, Brown SL, Klemke R, Schlaepfer DD, Nemerow GR. Association of p130CAS with phosphatidylinositol-3-OH kinase mediates adenovirus cell entry. J Biol Chem 2000; 275:14,729–14,735.
67. Tibbles LA, Spurrell JC, Bowen GP, et al. Activation of p38 and ERK signaling during adenovirus vector cell entry lead to expression of the C-X-C chemokine IP-10. J Virol 2002;76:1559–1568.
68. Bruder JT, Kovesdi I. Adenovirus infection stimulates the Raf/MAPK signaling pathway and induces interleukin-8 expression. J Virol 1997;71:398–404.
69. Bowen GP, Borgland SL, Lam M, Libermann TA, Wong NC, Muruve DA. Adenovirus vector-induced inflammation: capsid-dependent induction of the C-C chemokine RANTES requires NF-kappa B. Hum Gene Ther 2002;13:367–379.
70. Borgland SL, Bowen GP, Wong NC, Libermann TA, Muruve DA. Adenovirus vector-induced expression of the C-X-C chemokine IP-10 is mediated through capsid-dependent activation of NF-kappaB. J Virol 2000;74:3941–3947.
71. Tamanini A, Rolfini R, Nicolis E, Melotti P, Cabrini G. MAP kinases and NF-kappaB collaborate to induce ICAM-1 gene expression in the early phase of adenovirus infection. Virology 2003;307: 228–242.
72. Suomalainen M, Nakano MY, Keller S, Boucke K, Stidwill RP, Greber UF. Microtubule-dependent plus- and minus end-directed motilities are competing processes for nuclear targeting of adenovirus. J Cell Biol 1999;144:657–672.

73. Mabit H, Nakano MY, Prank U, et al. Intact microtubules support adenovirus and herpes simplex virus infections. J Virol 2002;76:9962–9971.
74. Wang K, Guan T, Cheresh DA, Nemerow GR. Regulation of adenovirus membrane penetration by the cytoplasmic tail of integrin beta5. J Virol 2000;74:2731–2739.
75. Brakebusch C, Fassler R. The integrin-actin connection, an eternal love affair. Embo J 2003; 22:2324–2333.
76. Yurochko AD, Liu DY, Eierman D, Haskill S. Integrins as a primary signal transduction molecule regulating monocyte immediate-early gene induction. Proc Natl Acad Sci U S A 1992;89:9034–9038.
77. Ritzenthaler JD, Roman J. Interleukin-1beta gene transcription in U937 cells is modulated by type I collagen and cytoskeletal integrity via distinct signaling pathways. J Interferon Cytokine Res 2001; 21:105–116.
78. Roman J, Ritzenthaler JD, Perez RL, Roser SL. Differential modes of regulation of interleukin-1beta expression by extracellular matrices. Immunology 1999;98:228–237.
79. Roman J, Ritzenthaler JD, Fenton MJ, Roser S, Schuyler W. Transcriptional regulation of the human interleukin 1beta gene by fibronectin: role of protein kinase C and activator protein 1 (AP-1). Cytokine 2000;12:1581–1596.
80. Mizuguchi H, Koizumi N, Hosono T, et al. CAR- or alphav integrin-binding ablated adenovirus vectors, but not fiber-modified vectors containing RGD peptide, do not change the systemic gene transfer properties in mice. Gene Ther 2002;9:769–776.
81. Akiyama M, Roelvink P, Einfeld D, Kovesdi I, King CR. Effect of Ablating CAR and integrin binding on the biodistribution and cellular localization of adenovirus vectors following intravenous or intraperitoneal delivery. Mol Ther 2003;7(5):S173.
82. Alemany R, Curiel DT. CAR-binding ablation does not change biodistribution and toxicity of adenoviral vectors. Gene Ther 2001;8:1347–1353.
83. Fechner H, Haack A, Wang H, et al. Expression of coxsackie adenovirus receptor and alphav-integrin does not correlate with adenovector targeting in vivo indicating anatomical vector barriers. Gene Ther 1999;6:1520–1535.
84. Smith T, Idamakanti N, Kylefjord H, et al. In vivo hepatic adenoviral gene delivery occurs independently of the coxsackievirus-adenovirus receptor. Mol Ther 2002;5:770–779.
85. Dechecchi MC, Melotti P, Bonizzato A, Santacatterina M, Chilosi M, Cabrini G. Heparan sulfate glycosaminoglycans are receptors sufficient to mediate the initial binding of adenovirus types 2 and 5. J Virol 2001;75:8772–8780.
86. Balakireva L, Schoehn G, Thouvenin E, Chroboczek J. Binding of adenovirus capsid to dipalmitoyl phosphatidylcholine provides a novel pathway for virus entry. J Virol 2003;77:4858–4866.
87. Hautala T, Grunst T, Fabrega A, Freimuth P, Welsh MJ. An interaction between penton base and alpha v integrins plays a minimal role in adenovirus-mediated gene transfer to hepatocytes in vitro and in vivo. Gene Ther 1998;5:1259–1264.
88. Alemany R, Suzuki K, Curiel DT. Blood clearance rates of adenovirus type 5 in mice. J Gen Virol 2000;81:2605–269.
89. Tao N, Gao GP, Parr M, et al. Sequestration of adenoviral vector by Kupffer cells leads to a nonlinear dose response of transduction in liver. Mol Ther 2001;3:28–35.
90. Worgall S, Wolff G, Falck-Pedersen E, Crystal RG. Innate immune mechanisms dominate elimination of adenoviral vectors following in vivo administration. Hum Gene Ther 1997;8:37–44.
91. Raper SE, Yudkoff M, Chirmule N, et al. A pilot study of in vivo liver-directed gene transfer with an adenoviral vector in partial ornithine transcarbamylase deficiency. Hum Gene Ther 2002;13:163–175.
92. Assessment of adenoviral vector safety and toxicity: Report of the National Institutes of Health Recombinant DNA Advisory Committee. Hum Gene Ther 2002;13:3–13.
93. Lozier JN, Csako G, Mondoro TH, et al. Toxicity of a first-generation adenoviral vector in rhesus macaques. Hum Gene Ther 2002;13:113–124.
94. Morral N, O'Neal WK, Rice K, et al. Lethal toxicity, severe endothelial injury, and a threshold effect with high doses of an adenoviral vector in baboons. Hum Gene Ther 2002;13:143–154.
95. Schnell MA, Zhang Y, Tazelaar J, et al. Activation of innate immunity in nonhuman primates following intraportal administration of adenoviral vectors. Mol Ther 2001;3:708–722.
96. Lieber A, He CY, Meuse L, et al. The role of Kupffer cell activation and viral gene expression in early liver toxicity after infusion of recombinant adenovirus vectors. J Virol 1997;71:8798–8807.
97. Schiedner G, Hertel S, Johnston M, Dries V, van Rooijen N, Kochanek S. Selective depletion or blockade of Kupffer cells leads to enhanced and prolonged hepatic transgene expression using high-capacity adenoviral vectors. Mol Ther 2003;7:35–43.

98. Vigne E, Dedieu JF, Brie A, et al. Genetic manipulations of adenovirus type 5 fiber resulting in liver tropism attenuation. Gene Ther 2003;10:153–162.
99. Smith TA, Idamakanti N, Rollence ML, et al. Adenovirus serotype 5 fiber shaft influences in vivo gene transfer in mice. Hum Gene Ther 2003;14:777–787.
100. Shayakhmetov D. M. Z-YL, S. Ni, A Lieber. Analysis of adenovirus sequestration in the liver, transduction of hepatic cells, and innate toxicity after injection of fiber-modified vectors. J Virol 2004; 78:5368–5381.
101. Shayakhmetov DM, Gaggar A, Ni S, Li ZY, Lieber A. Adenovirus binding to blood factors results in liver cell infection and hepatotoxicity. J Virol 2005;79:7478–7491.
102. Ruuskanen O MO, Akusjarvi G. Adenoviruses. 2002:515–534.
103. Shenk T. Adenoviridae. in *Field's Virology* (D.M. Nipe and P.M. Howley, Eds.) 2001:2265–2328.
104. Kojaoghlanian T, Flomenberg P, Horwitz MS. The impact of adenovirus infection on the immunocompromised host. Rev Med Virol 2003;13:155–171.
105. Mahanty S, Hutchinson K, Agarwal S, McRae M, Rollin PE, Pulendran B. Cutting edge: impairment of dendritic cells and adaptive immunity by Ebola and Lassa viruses. J Immunol 2003;170: 2797–2801.
106. Benedict CA, Norris PS, Ware CF. To kill or be killed: viral evasion of apoptosis. Nat Immunol 2002;3:1013–1018.
107. Benedict CA, Banks TA, Ware CF. Death and survival: viral regulation of TNF signaling pathways. Curr Opin Immunol 2003;15:59–65.
108. Wold WS, Doronin K, Toth K, Kuppuswamy M, Lichtenstein DL, Tollefson AE. Immune responses to adenoviruses: viral evasion mechanisms and their implications for the clinic. Curr Opin Immunol 1999;11:380–386.
109. Yasuda M, Theodorakis P, Subramanian T, Chinnadurai G. Adenovirus E1B-19K/BCL-2 interacting protein BNIP3 contains a BH3 domain and a mitochondrial targeting sequence. J Biol Chem 1998; 273:12,415–12,421.
110. Martin ME, Berk AJ. Adenovirus E1B 55K represses p53 activation in vitro. J Virol 1998; 72:3146–3154.
111. Leonard GT, Sen GC. Effects of adenovirus E1A protein on interferon-signaling. Virology 1996; 224:25–33.
112. Mathews MB, Shenk T. Adenovirus virus-associated RNA and translation control. J Virol 1991; 65:5657–5662.
113. Feuerbach D, Etteldorf S, Ebenau-Jehle C, Abastado JP, Madden D, Burgert HG. Identification of amino acids within the MHC molecule important for the interaction with the adenovirus protein E3/19K. J Immunol 1994;153:1626–1636.
114. Beier DC, Cox JH, Vining DR, Cresswell P, Engelhard VH. Association of human class I MHC alleles with the adenovirus E3/19K protein. J Immunol 1994;152:3862–3872.
115. Benedict CA, Norris PS, Prigozy TI, et al. Three adenovirus E3 proteins cooperate to evade apoptosis by tumor necrosis factor-related apoptosis-inducing ligand receptor-1 and -2. J Biol Chem 2001; 276:3270–3278.
116. Tollefson AE, Hermiston TW, Lichtenstein DL, et al. Forced degradation of Fas inhibits apoptosis in adenovirus-infected cells. Nature 1998;392:726–730.
117. Mistchenko AS, Diez RA, Mariani AL, et al. Cytokines in adenoviral disease in children: association of interleukin-6, interleukin-8, and tumor necrosis factor alpha levels with clinical outcome. J Pediatr 1994;124:714–20.
118. Ginsberg HS, Prince GA. The molecular basis of adenovirus pathogenesis. Infect Agents Dis 1994; 3:1–8.
119. Prince GA, Porter DD, Jenson AB, Horswood RL, Chanock RM, Ginsberg HS. Pathogenesis of adenovirus type 5 pneumonia in cotton rats (Sigmodon hispidus). J Virol 1993;67:101–111.
120. Garnett CT, Erdman D, Xu W, Gooding LR. Prevalence and quantitation of species C adenovirus DNA in human mucosal lymphocytes. J Virol 2002;76:10,608–10,616.
121. Croyle MA, Chirmule N, Zhang Y, Wilson JM. PEGylation of E1-deleted adenovirus vectors allows significant gene expression on readministration to liver. Hum Gene Ther 2002;13:1887–1900.
122. O'Riordan CR, Lachapelle A, Delgado C, et al. PEGylation of adenovirus with retention of infectivity and protection from neutralizing antibody in vitro and in vivo. Hum Gene Ther 1999;10: 1349–1358.
123. Nwanegbo E, Vardas E, Gao W, et al. Prevalence of neutralizing antibodies to adenoviral serotypes 5 and 35 in the adult populations of The Gambia, South Africa, and the United States. Clin Diagn Lab Immunol 2004;11:351–357.

124. Sakurai F, Mizuguchi H, Yamaguchi T, Hayakawa T. Characterization of in vitro and in vivo gene transfer properties of adenovirus serotype 35 vector. Mol Ther 2003;8:813–821.
125. Vogels R, Zuijdgeest D, van Rijnsoever R, et al. Replication-deficient human adenovirus type 35 vectors for gene transfer and vaccination: efficient human cell infection and bypass of preexisting adenovirus immunity. J Virol 2003;77:8263–8271.
126. Hemminki A, Kanerva A, Kremer EJ, et al. A canine conditionally replicating adenovirus for evaluating oncolytic virotherapy in a syngeneic animal model. Mol Ther 2003;7:163–173.
127. Soudais C, Skander N, Kremer EJ. Long-term in vivo transduction of neurons throughout the rat CNS using novel helper-dependent CAV-2 vectors. Faseb J 2004;18:391–393.
128. Renaut L, Colin M, Leite JP, Benko M, D'Halluin JC. Abolition of hCAR-dependent cell tropism using fiber knobs of Atadenovirus serotypes. Virology 2004;321:189–204.
129. Wu Q, Tikoo SK. Altered tropism of recombinant bovine adenovirus type-3 expressing chimeric fiber. Virus Res 2004;99:9–15.
130. Cohen CJ, Xiang ZQ, Gao GP, Ertl HC, Wilson JM, Bergelson JM. Chimpanzee adenovirus CV-68 adapted as a gene delivery vector interacts with the coxsackievirus and adenovirus receptor. J Gen Virol 2002;83:151–155.
131. Zhang Y, Chirmule N, Gao GP, et al. Acute cytokine response to systemic adenoviral vectors in mice is mediated by dendritic cells and macrophages. Mol Ther 2001;3:697–707.
132. Muruve DA, Barnes MJ, Stillman IE, Libermann TA. Adenoviral gene therapy leads to rapid induction of multiple chemokines and acute neutrophil-dependent hepatic injury in vivo. Hum Gene Ther 1999;10:965–976.
133. Reid T, Galanis E, Abbruzzese J, et al. Intra-arterial administration of a replication-selective adenovirus (dl1520) in patients with colorectal carcinoma metastatic to the liver: a phase I trial. Gene Ther 2001;8:1618–1626.
134. Crystal RG, Harvey BG, Wisnivesky JP, et al. Analysis of risk factors for local delivery of low- and intermediate-dose adenovirus gene transfer vectors to individuals with a spectrum of comorbid conditions. Hum Gene Ther 2002;13:65–100.
135. Ben-Gary H, McKinney RL, Rosengart T, Lesser ML, Crystal RG. Systemic interleukin-6 responses following administration of adenovirus gene transfer vectors to humans by different routes. Mol Ther 2002; 6:287–297.
136. Mickelson CA. Department of Health and Human Services National Institutes of Health Recombinant DNA Advisory Committee. Minutes of meeting March 8–10, 2000. Hum Gene Ther 2000; 11:2159–2192.
137. McCoy RD, Davidson BL, Roessler BJ, et al. Pulmonary inflammation induced by incomplete or inactivated adenoviral particles. Hum Gene Ther 1995;6:1553–1560.
138. Liu Q, Zaiss AK, Colarusso P, et al. The role of capsid-endothelial interactions in the innate immune response to adenovirus vectors. Hum Gene Ther 2003;14:627–643.
139. Toietta G MV, Pastore L, Finegold MJ, Ng P, Beaudet AL, Lee B. Determinants of and pharmacologic modulation of acute toxicity associated with systemic administration of first feneration and helper-dependent adenovirus vectors. Mol. Therapy 2003;7:S162.
140. Smith TA, Idamakanti N, Marshall-Neff J, et al. Receptor interactions involved in adenoviral-mediated gene delivery after systemic administration in non-human primates. Hum Gene Ther 2003; 14:1595–1604.
141. George JS. Gene therapy progress and prospects: adenoviral vectors. Gene Ther 2003;10:1135–1141.
142. Ginsberg HS, Moldawer LL, Sehgal PB, et al. A mouse model for investigating the molecular pathogenesis of adenovirus pneumonia. Proc Natl Acad Sci U S A 1991;88:1651–1655.
143. Wang Y, Hallden G, Hill R, et al. E3 gene manipulations affect oncolytic adenovirus activity in immunocompetent tumor models. Nat Biotechnol 2003;21:1328–1335.
144. Nemunaitis J, Ganly I, Khuri F, et al. Selective replication and oncolysis in p53 mutant tumors with ONYX-015, an E1B-55kD gene-deleted adenovirus, in patients with advanced head and neck cancer: a phase II trial. Cancer Res 2000;60:6359–6366.
145. Shayakhmetov DM, Li ZY, Ni S, Lieber A. Interference with the IL-1 signaling pathway improves the toxicity profile of systemically applied adenovirus vectors. J Immunol 2005;174:7310–7319.

3 Lentiviral and Retroviral Vector Systems

Renata Stripecke, PhD *and*
Noriyuki Kasahara, MD, PhD

CONTENTS

Summary

Retroviruses have been widely used as gene transfer vectors, and in fact represent the vector system used in the majority of clinical gene therapy trials for cancer to date. In an ex vivo setting, conventional replication-defective oncoretrovirus vectors can reliably and efficiently achieve permanent gene transfer which is selective for dividing cells; however, successful application of these vectors in vivo has been difficult because of their relatively low-transduction efficiency. Recently, however, the field has been revitalized by the advent of significant improvements in basic retrovirus vector technology, including the development of lentivirus-based vectors which are capable of efficient gene transfer even to quiescent nondividing cells, and tumor-selective replication-competent retrovirus vectors which progressively transduce cancer cells as the virus spreads through the tumor. This chapter reviews these important recent developments and their potential utility for gene therapy of cancer.

Key Words: Retrovirus; lentivirus; vector; cancer; gene therapy.

1. INTRODUCTION

The development of effective gene transfer methods in the early 1980s, which exploited the natural mechanisms of viruses for cellular entry and expression of genetic material, represented an enabling technology that catalyzed the rapid progress of gene therapy from a distant vision to a clinically feasible therapeutic modality. Among the first viruses to be converted from pathogenic to therapeutic agent in this manner was Moloney murine leukemia virus (MMLV), a simple retrovirus with a diploid RNA genome, which was one of the first viral genomes to be cloned and sequenced in its entirety. Numerous studies over almost two decades have demonstrated the utility of these vectors for stable gene transfer to mammalian cells in culture and in small animal models. However, efforts to translate the results from animal studies to clinical trials have thus far generally proved disappointing, and the successes in human gene therapy

From: *Cancer Drug Discovery and Development: Gene Therapy for Cancer*
Edited by: K. K. Hunt, S. A. Vorburger, and S. G. Swisher © Humana Press Inc., Totowa, NJ

using retrovirus vectors have often been sporadic, equivocal, and/or subtherapeutic. Issues with regard to their low production titers, intrinsic inability to infect quiescent cells, and overall low transduction efficiency in vivo represent significant technical obstacles to the success of retrovirus-mediated gene therapy, and many investigators have sought other, more efficient viruses as vectors for use in clinical trials.

Nevertheless, retrovirus vectors remain the most frequently utilized clinical gene delivery modality that is clearly capable of permanent integration into host cells, and thus far have been used in the majority of human gene therapy trials; in fact, MMLV-based retrovirus vectors represent the only gene transfer modality to have progressed to large-scale phase III clinical trials for cancer, even though the results proved disappointing. Recently, however, methodological advances in the clinical application of retrovirus vectors have now yielded highly promising results, particularly in the ex vivo setting, including the amelioration of X-linked severe combined immunodeficiency (SCID) syndrome, arguably one of the leading success stories of human gene therapy to date but which has also been associated with a sobering reminder of the potential for risk as well as benefit. Many such successes have resulted from a progressive understanding of the characteristic limitations of MMLV-based vectors, which in turn has spurred the development of numerous incremental but cumulative improvements in vector production and transduction methods, as well as judicious and rational application to the most relevant clinical scenarios. Significant improvements in basic retrovirus vector technology are also being actively pursued; among the most promising of these in recent years has been the development of lentivirus-based vector systems. Additionally, significant improvements have been made in the areas of vector design, pseudotyping and envelope modification, transcriptional regulation, and conditionally replicating vectors; these developments promise to further enhance the usefulness of this classic vector system, particularly for gene therapy of cancer. This chapter reviews the basic technology of retrovirus- and lentivirus-based gene delivery systems, and provides an overview of ex vivo and in vivo applications to genetic and immunomodulatory treatments for cancer in preclinical and clinical studies (Table 1).

2. BASIC PRINCIPLES OF RETROVIRAL VECTOR TECHNOLOGY

2.1. Oncoretroviral Vectors: The Basic Technology

Retroviruses are enveloped viruses that contain a diploid positive-strand RNA genome, whose life cycle is characterized by their use of reverse transcriptase to convert the RNA genome to double-stranded DNA, which is then permanently integrated into the chromosomes of the host cell. As noted above, most retroviral vectors in current use are traditionally based on Moloney murine leukemia virus (MMLV), a simple oncoretrovirus that contains 5′- and 3′-long terminal repeat (LTR) sequences flanking only three gene loci: *gag*, *pol*, and *env*, which encode capsid/matrix, reverse transcriptase/integrase, and envelope proteins, respectively (*see* Fig. 1). Assembly of these viral proteins to form a virion is initiated by a *cis*-acting sequence located next to the 5′-LTR; identification of this sequence (Ψ) as the dominant signal for viral packaging (*see* Fig. 2) enabled the development of trans-complementing systems for packaging of replication-defective viral genomes in which the natural coding sequences have been replaced by therapeutic genes of interest (*see* Fig. 3). Once the replication-defective vector RNA has been packaged into the nucleocapsid, the nascent virion buds from the cell surface, thereby encoating itself with the lipid bilayer membrane of the host cell, in

Table 1
Strategies for Gene Therapy of Cancer Using Retrovirus and Lentivirus Vectors

A. Ex vivo gene therapy *Target cell population*	*Strategy*	*Transgenes*
Hematopoietic stem cells Hematopoietic progenitor cells	Myeloprotection during high-dose chemotherapy	Chemotoxin pump proteins (e.g., MDR-1) Chemotoxin metabolizing enzymes (e.g., DHFR, MGMT)
Hematopoietic stem cells	Elimination of oncoproteins (e.g., BCR-ABL)	Antisense RNA, ribozymes, siRNA directed against target mRNA
Cytotoxic T-lymphocytes	Abrogation of GVHD after transplantation to achieve GVL effect	Suicide genes (e.g., HSV-*tk*)
Cytotoxic T-lymphocytes	Tumor antigen-specific immunocytotoxicity	Tumor antigen-specific, engineered T-cell receptors
DCs, DC progenitor cells (e.g., monocytes), other APCs (e.g., macrophages, Kupffer cells, microglia)	Tumor antigen presentation, potentiation of antitumoral immune response	Tumor-specific antigens Immunostimulatory cytokines (e.g., GM-CSF, IL-4, CD40L)
Leukemia/lymphoma cells, Other explantable tumor cells	Tumor cell vaccine	Immunostimulatory cytokines (e.g., GM-CSF, IL-2, IL-12, IFNs) Costimulatory molecules (e.g., CD80, CD86, 4-1-BB)

B. In vivo gene therapy *Target cell population*	*Strategy*	*Transgenes*
Tumor cells	Direct cell killing by introduction of vector or vector producer cells	Suicide genes (e.g., HSV-*tk*, yCD, *E. coli* PNP) Proapoptotic genes (e.g., BAX) Toxin genes (e.g., Diphtheria toxin, HIV-vpr, hyperfusogenic GALV envelope)
Tumor cells	Over-expression of genes with tumor suppressor activity	Tumor suppressor genes (e.g., p53, BRCA-1, p16, PTEN, MDA-7/IL-24) Cell-cycle inhibitors (dominant-negative cyclin G1)
Tumor cells	Inhibition of oncogenes	Antisense RNA, ribozymes, siRNA directed against target mRNA
Tumor cells Tumor infiltrating immunocytes and APCs	Potentiation of antitumoral immune response	Immunostimulatory cytokines (e.g., GM-CSF, IL-2, IL-12, IFNs) Costimulatory molecules (e.g., CD80, CD86, 4-1-BB) Inhibitors of immunosuppressive factors (e.g., dominant-negative TGF-β receptor)
DCs, DC progenitor cells (e.g., monocytes), other antigen	Tumor antigen presentation, viral antitumor	Tumor-specific antigens (e.g., MART-1. NY-ESO-1)

(*Continued*)

Table 1 (*Continued*)

Target cell population	*Strategy*	*Transgenes*
presenting cells (e.g., macrophages, Kupffer cells, microglia)	vaccine delivered by direct in vivo injection	
Tumor cells Tumor endothelial cells	Inhibition of tumor neovasculature	Antiangiogenic factors (e.g., endostatin, angiostatin, thrombospondin-1, soluble VEGF receptor)

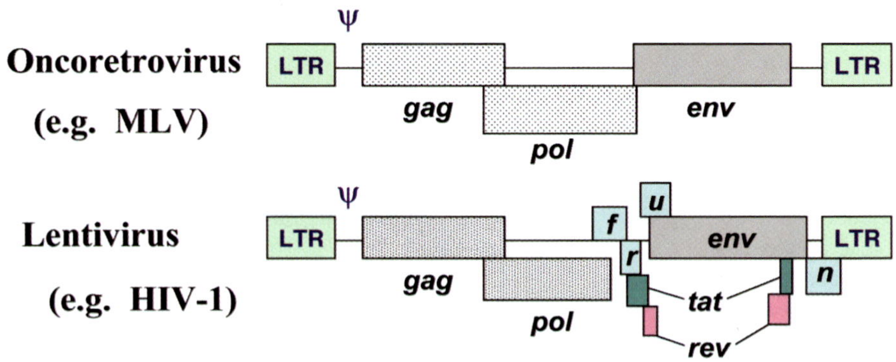

Fig. 1. Comparison of oncoretrovirus vs lentivirus genomes. Both types of retrovirus are characterized by LTR sequences flanking the viral structural genes. Oncoretroviruses such as MMLV have relatively simple genome configurations, with only three structural gene loci: *gag* (which encodes viral capsid and matrix proteins), *pol* (which encodes viral protease, reverse transcriptase, and integrase proteins), and *env* (encoding the viral envelope protein). Lentiviruses such as HIV-1 are more complex and contain additional open reading frames encoding "accessory genes" such as *tat* (viral transcription factor), *rev* (facilitates nuclear export of viral mRNA), and various virulence factors (f: *vif*, r: *vpr*, u: *vpu*, n: *nef*). Both oncoretrovirus and lentivirus genomes contain specific packaging signal sequences (ψ), located just downstream of the LTR and generally extending into the 5′ sequence of *gag*, that allow encapsidation of the viral genomic RNA.

which the viral envelope proteins are embedded (*see* Fig. 4). The envelope proteins mediate cellular entry by binding to receptors on the target cell surface. This binding event triggers a conformational change that activates virus-cell membrane fusion, allowing the nucleocapsid complex to be released into the cytoplasm. Reverse transcription of the viral RNA yields the double-stranded DNA proviral form, which is then permanently integrated at relatively random locations in the host cell genome, and is therefore present in all progeny cells derived from the initially infected host. With wild-type MMLV, the proviral genome then transcribes additional copies of viral genomic RNA as well as a spliced message that specifically encodes the *env* gene (*see* Fig. 2). However, with replication-defective vectors, these sequences have been replaced by therapeutic genes, which are expressed in the host cell and all progeny instead (*see* Fig. 4).

The generation of high titer retroviral stocks for the efficient transduction of target cells is an important technical goal for a range of gene transfer applications. This was first made feasible through the development of packaging cell lines that *trans*-complement vector genomes with the MMLV *gag*, *pol*, and *env* proteins required for virus assembly *(1)*. Replication-defective retroviral vector genomes containing the Ψ encapsidation

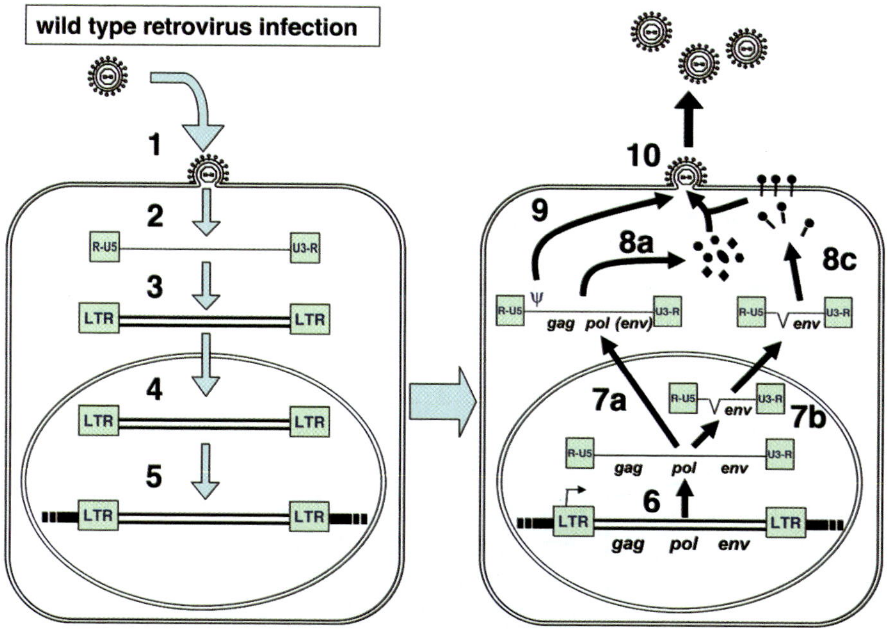

Fig. 2. Molecular events associated with infection by a replication-competent (wild-type) retrovirus. The schematic of the infected cell on the left depicts events occurring during infection, the schematic on the right depicts events after infection has been established. **1:** Virion adsorption via interaction between viral envelope protein and cell surface receptor, followed by virus–cell lipid membrane fusion. **2:** Entry of viral nucleocapsid complex into cytoplasm. **3:** Reverse transcription of viral genomic RNA (single line) to double-stranded DNA (double lines), U3 and U5 sequences duplicated at 5′- and 3′-ends, respectively, to convert R-U5 and U3-R into matching LTR sequences flanking viral genome. **4:** Entry into cell nucleus, either by passive diffusion upon nuclear membrane breakdown during mitosis (oncoretrovirus) or uptake by active transport (lentivirus). **5:** Integration of proviral DNA into host cell chromosome. **6:** Transcription of viral mRNA, encoding *gag*, *pol*, and *env* structural gene loci. **7:** Nuclear export of viral genomic mRNA (7a), and splicing and nuclear export of viral *env* mRNA (7b). **8:** Viral genomic sequence serves as mRNA for translation of *gag* and *pol* proteins (8a), viral *env* mRNA directs expression of viral envelope proteins on cell membrane. **9:** Virion assembly: viral proteins encapsidate viral genomic RNA by recognition of its packaging signal (ψ). **10:** Budding of virion from cell surface membrane, encoated by viral envelope proteins.

signal can be introduced into these packaging cells by by transient transfection with an appropriate plasmid, or in some cases by viral transduction (*see* Fig. 3). To obtain retroviral stocks of the highest titers, it is necessary to establish additional virus producer cell lines that not only contain the *gag-pol* and *env* cassettes, but also have the proviral vector genome stably integrated. To identify the highest producing lines, many subclones may then need to be screened, as greatly varying titers are observed between different subclones. This screening process can take several weeks and the cell lines so established may lose their packaging ability as they are passaged. As a simpler alternative system for the production of retroviral stocks without the use of packaging lines, many groups now utilize a packaging systems for production of high titer helper-free virus stocks by transient transfection *(2)*. Generally, human embryonic kidney-derived 293T cells are used as they are highly transfectable, and a three-plasmid transient cotransfection method is used to express: (1) a packaging plasmid expressing *gag-pol*;

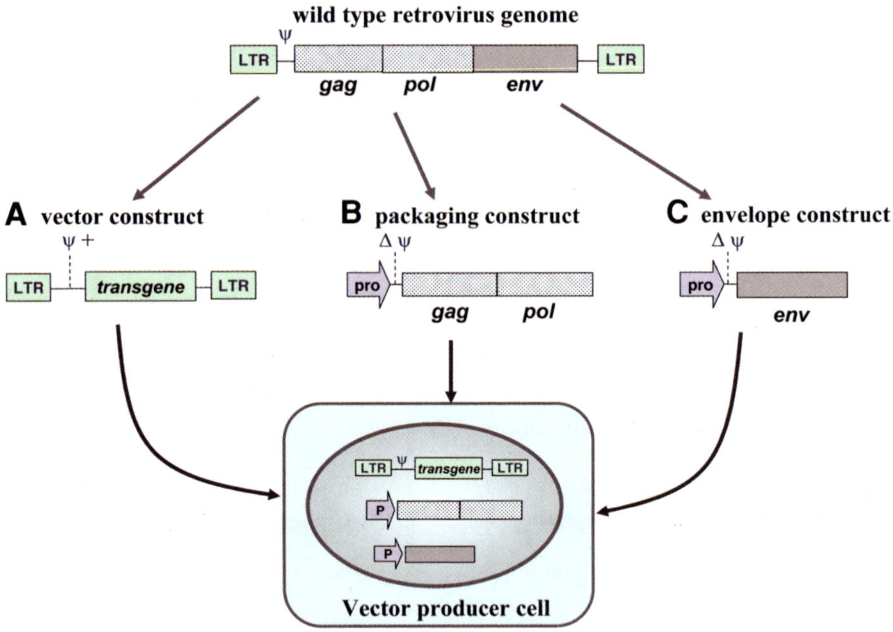

Fig. 3. ABCs of constructing conventional replication-defective retrovirus vectors. (**A**) The structural genes of the virus are removed and replaced with a transgene expression cassette, which remains flanked by the viral LTR sequences. This "vector construct" retains the viral packaging signal (ψ+), which allows encapsidation of the vector RNA. (**B**) The *gag-pol* structural genes are generally expressed together as a "packaging construct" that can be placed under the control of a heterologous promoter (pro). (**C**) The viral envelope protein can be expressed by itself as a separate "envelope construct." Separating the *env* gene from the *gag-pol* genes facilitates the use of heterologous envelopes from other species to virus to encoat the vector ("pseudotyping"), and reduces the likelihood of recombination events that might lead to the reconstitution of replication-competent wild-type virus. Note that the packaging signal is deleted or mutated (Δψ) in the packaging and envelope constructs so that these mRNAs cannot be encapsidated. All three constructs are expressed together within a permissive cell ("vector producer cell" or VPC) to generate the virus vector.

(2) an envelope plasmid expressing the envelope glycoprotein *env* (generally the MMLV amphotropic envelope, which binds to a highly conserved inorganic phosphate transporter, PiT-2, and hence exhibits broad host species binding tropism, including human); and (3) the transfer vector plasmid expressing the replication-defective retroviral vector construct containing the gene of interest. Transient cotransfection methods can be optimized to achieve titers of up to 10^6 helper-free viral/mL stocks within 48 h without the need to establish and maintain packaging cell lines or stable producer lines, thereby allowing rapid production of high titer retroviral vectors for subsequent cellular transduction by a convenient, rapid and reproducible method, and enables rapid characterization of multiple vectors containing different genes of interest.

As vehicles for the delivery of genes into eukaryotic cells, retroviruses have several advantages *(3,4)*: (1) gene transfer is relatively efficient, particularly in a cell culture or ex vivo setting, as most retroviral vectors are produced from packaging cells at titers on the order of 10^{6-7} plaque-forming units (pfu)/mL; (2) stable integration into the host cell DNA is a natural part of the retroviral life cycle, and therefore the integrated provirus is passed on to all daughter cells and continues to direct the nonlytic production of its encoded products; and (3) replication-defective vectors can

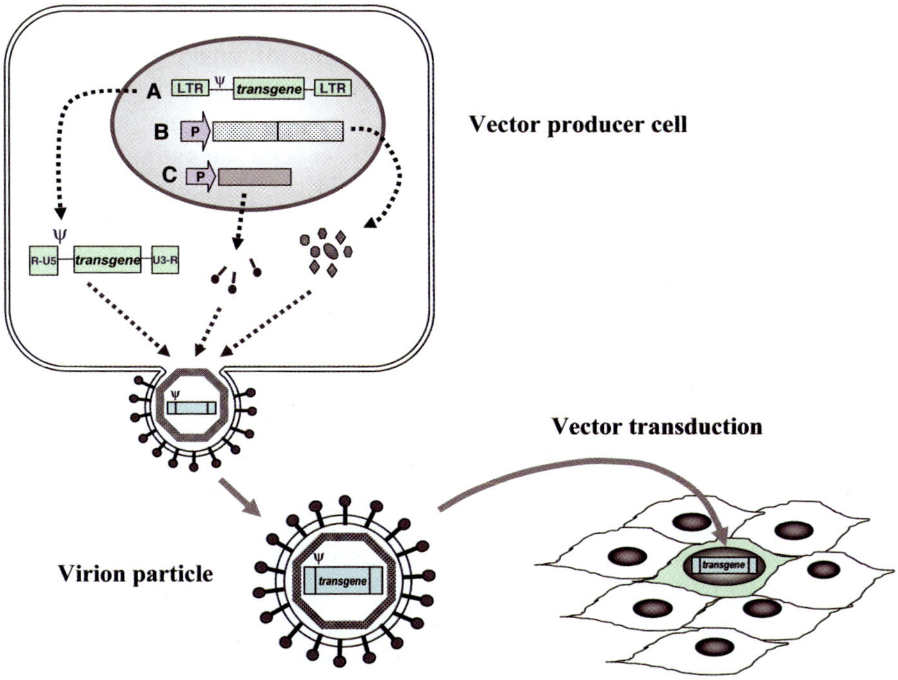

Fig. 4. ABCs of constructing conventional replication-defective retrovirus vectors, part 2. Viral vector (**A**), packaging (**B**), and envelope (**C**) constructs are introduced into the producer cell, generally by simultaneous co-transfection for transient production of virus. Alternatively, cell lines that have been stably transfected with the packaging and/or envelope construct ("packaging cell lines"), as well as with specific vector constructs ("producer cell lines"), can be prepared for constitutive virus production. Only the RNA transcribed from the vector construct (**A**) contains a packaging signal (ψ), allowing encapsidation by the viral proteins expressed from the packaging construct (**B**) and envelope construct (**C**). The virion particle thus assembled buds from the cell surface, and because there are no viral structural genes present in the vector, only the transgene of interest is transmitted to the target cell upon infection ("vector transduction").

easily be created by deletion of all essential viral genes, which renders the vectors incapable of secondary infection. An additional characteristic specific to MMLV is that it requires cell division during infection so that the nucleocapsid complex can gain access to the host cell genome, and hence cannot infect nondividing cells. As many cell types are considered to be largely quiescent in vivo, the traditional application, which has been adopted for MMLV-based retroviral vectors has been to transduce cell lines in culture; when animal studies have been performed using retroviral gene delivery, this has usually been accomplished by viral infection of primary cells in culture by the ex vivo method, followed by reimplantation of the transduced cells. This approach requires surgical acquisition, isolation, and culture of autologous cells. This is labor intensive and invasive and limits the scope of ex vivo retroviral gene transfer to those cell types that can be readily accessed, manipulated in culture, and reimplanted (e.g., hematopoietic cells, skin fibroblasts, and hepatocytes). On the other hand, this absolute selectivity for actively dividing cells results in preferential infection of malignant cells, which can be advantageous for cancer-related research and therapeutics.

2.2. Lentiviral Vectors: The Next Generation

The lentiviridae are complex retroviruses that contain additional regulatory and pathogenicity-enhancing "accessory" genes in addition to the *gag*, *pol* and *env* structural proteins expressed by oncoretroviruses. For human immunodeficiency virus (HIV), for example, the additional regulatory genes are *tat* and *rev*, and the pathogenicity-enhancing accessory genes are *vif, vpr, vpu* and *nef* (*see* Fig. 1). Furthermore, although the overall life cycle of lentiviruses is similar to that of oncoretroviruses, there are several major differences. As noted above, vectors based on oncoretroviruses such as MMLV can only transduce cells that divide shortly after infection, because the MMLV preintegration complex cannot achieve chromosomal integration in the absence of nuclear envelope breakdown during mitosis.

In contrast, lentiviruses can infect nonproliferating cells, owing to the karyophilic properties of the lentiviral preintegration complex, which allows recognition by the cell nuclear import machinery. Correspondingly, lentiviral vectors can transduce cell lines that are growth arrested in culture, as well as terminally differentiated primary cells including hematopoietic stem cells, neurons, hepatocytes, cardiomyocytes, endothelium, alveolar pneumocytes, keratinocytes and dendritic cells *(5–13)*. Hence, there has been a keen interest in the development of vector systems based on a wide variety of lentiviruses, including HIV), simian immunodeficiency virus (SIV), feline immunodeficiency virus (FIV), and equine infectious anemia virus (EIAV) recently. This chapter focuses primarily on HIV-based lentiviral vectors as this technology has progressed most rapidly and is already in clinical trials.

Furthermore, the possible toxicity of HIV accessory genes retained in lentiviral vector constructs, as well as the possibility of recombination leading to generation of wild-type virus, has also been raised as a safety concern. Considerable effort has been invested in the generation of more efficient and safer vectors *(14,15)*. The lentiviral packaging system was originally developed by Naldini et al. following a tripartite transient transfection procedure *(5)* and later evolved into the "second generation" lentiviral vectors, where the four accessory genes of HIV (*vif, vpr, vpu*, and *nef*) were deleted from the viral packaging system without affecting viral titers or transduction efficiency *(15)*. The only remaining auxiliary gene in this system was, therefore, *rev*, which, along with the Rev response element (RRE) as its cognate binding sequence, is required for efficient export of the vector and packaging construct RNAs from the nucleus during virus production. Thus both toxicity as well as the likelihood of recombination are reduced in these second- and third-generation lentiviral vector systems (*see* Fig. 5). More recently, further optimization of packaging systems for HIV and other lentiviruses has aimed at minimizing the risk of homologous recombination with HIV by splitting the *gag-pol* genes *(16)* and by cross-packaging configurations (i.e. using the packaging system of HIV to encapsidate transfer vectors from other lentiviral origins [SIV, HIV-2, FIV]) *(17,18)*.

In most cases, the vectors are pseudotyped (i.e., encoated with a heterologous envelope protein) with vesicular stomatitis virus glycoprotein (VSV-G), which is a rhabdovirus envelope protein that is reported to bind to cell-surface phospholipids thereby achieving a wide host range. However, the VSV-G protein is highly fusogenic, and even with the use of inducible promoters, it has proven difficult to generate high titer stable packaging cell lines expressing VSV-G as a result of its cytotoxicity. Hence, transient transfection is the most commonly employed method for lentiviral vector production, and the use of transiently produced vectors has been approved in the first clinical trial of lentiviral gene

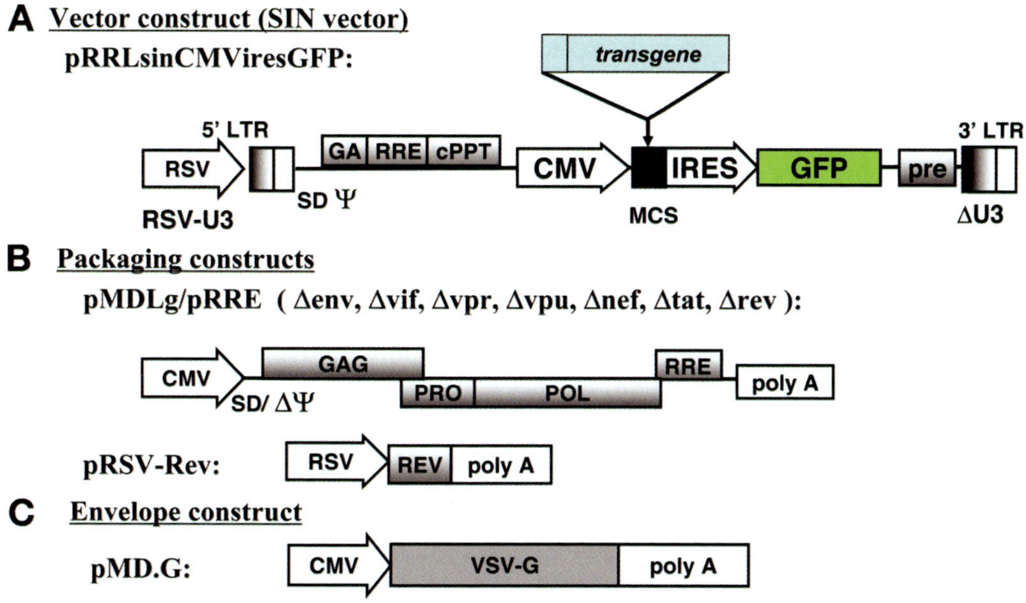

Fig. 5. Components required for production of 3rd generation lentiviral vectors, based on constructs developed by Zufferey et al. (**A**) The vector construct pRRLsinCMViresGFP contains a modified 5′-LTR sequence in which the *tat*-dependent viral promoter in the U3 region has been replaced with the constitutively active Rous sarcoma virus (RSV) promoter, and a modified 3′-LTR in which most of the U3 region has been deleted (ΔU3). This U3 deletion is copied to the 5′-LTR upon reverse transcription, making this a "self-inactivating" vector in which transgene expression relies entirely upon an internal promoter (CMV: cytomegalovirus promoter). The packaging signal (Ψ) spans the region from viral splice donor (SD) sequence and the 5′-end of the *gag* gene (ga). The Rev response element (RRE) is attached immediately downstream from the truncated *gag* 5′ sequence and facilitates nuclear export of the unspliced full-length genomic RNA during virus production and assembly, as does the woodchuck hepatitis virus PRE element (pre) inserted just upstream of the 3′-LTR. Addition of the central polypurine tract (cPPT) sequence further enhances titer by facilitating nuclear import and reverse transcription during viral transduction of the target cell. The transgene expression cassette includes a multiple cloning site (MCS) for insertion of the therapeutic transgene of interest, and a linked marker gene cassette consisting of the encephalomyocarditis virus (EMCV) internal ribosome entry site (IRES) and the Aequorea jellyfish GFP gene. (**B**) Packaging constructs for the third generation system are split into the pMDLg/pRRE construct, which expresses the HIV *gag-pol* loci driven by the CMV promoter, and the pRSV-*Rev* construct, which expresses the accessory gene *Rev* driven by the RSV promoter. The pMDLg/pRRE construct is deleted of all accessory genes (Δ*env*, Δ*vif*, Δ*vpr*, Δ*vpu*, Δ*nef*, Δ*tat*, Δ*rev*) and the packaging signal (Ψ). SD: splice donor, RRE: Rev response element, polyA: polyadenylation signal. (**C**) The envelope construct pMD.G contains a CMV promoter driving expression of the vesicular stomatitis virus glycoprotein (VSV-G) envelope, which pseudotypes the vector virion and provides broad host cell tropism.

therapy for acquired immunodeficiency syndrome (AIDS). As with MMLV-based vectors, the lentiviral vector construct is transiently cotransfected along with the lentiviral *gag-pol* packaging construct and VSV-G *env* construct into 293T cells to produce virus (*see* Fig. 5), thereby enabling high-level expression of viral proteins and efficient packaging of vector genomes without the need for long-term maintenance of stable packaging cell lines and without the attendant risk of recombination leading to generation of helper virus over time.

In parallel with improvements in the packaging system has been the development of self-inactivating (SIN) lentivirus vector designs, which generally contain a 400 nucleotide deletion in the 3′-long terminal repeat (LTR) *(15)* (*see* Fig. 5). Through the process of reverse transcription, this deletion is copied to the 5′-LTR, thereby abolishing the 5′-LTR promoter activity and hampering recombination with wild-type HIV in an infected host *(15)*. Therefore, the risk of vector mobilization with the wild-type virus and subsequent production of replication competent lentiviral vectors is drastically reduced for the SIN vectors. The self-inactivating vectors with a *tat*-independent promoter have been termed "third generation" lentiviral vectors, which could be considered as appropriate candidates for clinical trials in humans. Subsequently, it was observed that a sequence within *pol*, which is thought to be required *in cis* to promote more efficient reverse transcription, nuclear entry and integration of lentiviral vectors, had been removed from the lentiviral vector backbone. It was found that restoring this central polypurine tract and termination sequence (cPPT/CTS, a 118-bp element) in some of the newer lentiviral vector designs did, indeed, result in transduction of several types of human primary cells at a much higher efficiency *(19–21)* (*see* Fig. 5).

3. APPLICATIONS OF RETROVIRAL GENE TRANSFER FOR CANCER THERAPY

3.1. Ex Vivo Gene Therapy Using Retroviral and Lentiviral Vectors

3.1.1. Retroviral Gene Transfer to Hematopoietic Cells: General Considerations

The use of hematopoietic stem cells (HSC) in bone marrow transplantation approaches have convincingly demonstrated the potential of this approach to repopulate the different hematologic lineages in mice and in humans, and has found application not only in the treatment of hereditary diseases but also in myelo-reconstitution after high-dose chemotherapy and in controlling graft vs host disease. Because it was shown that HSC can be persistently transduced ex vivo with retroviral vectors *(22)*, these vectors have been extensively used in gene replacement or augmentation and anticancer strategies involving the hematopoietic system.

Numerous technical refinements developed over more than a decade have greatly increased the efficiency of murine retroviral vectors for transduction of HSC, as reflected by the recent clinical utility of this approach *(23,24)*. In a study performed by Alain Fischer and colleagues in Paris, an optimized protocol for ex vivo gene transfer into hematopoietic progenitor cells was employed to achieve successful retroviral vector-mediated expression of the interleukin receptor common γ (γc) chain, a component of several cytokine receptors that is defective in severe combined immunodeficiency-X1 (SCID-X1) disease *(25)*. Building on a decade of experience, that has led to incremental yet cumulative improvements in the efficiency of retrovirus-mediated gene transfer to hematopoietic progenitors, Fischer and colleagues applied the appropriate cytokine-mediated stimulation including, stem cell factor (SCF), Flt-3 ligand, megakaryocyte growth and differentiation factor (M-GDF), and interleukin-3 (IL-3), to induce $CD34^+$ proliferation without loss of lymphoid or myeloid potential, resulting in increased transduction efficiency *(26)*. Transduction of γc-deficient bone marrow cells was performed using a retrovirus containing the γc gene based on the simple MFG vector backbone produced from ΨCRIP packaging cells and optimized procedures including immobilization of the vector and target cells on fibronectin-coated tissue culture plates. Subsequent transplantation into a SCIDX1 mouse model resulted in normal levels of immunoglobulins, normal T- and B-cell interaction, and the presence of lymphocytes 47 wk post-treatment *(25)*.

This success has further been extended to include the full correction of SCIDX1 in humans. The $CD34^+$ cells taken from bone marrow of two patients, aged 8 and 11 mo, were transduced with an efficiency of between 20 and 40% *(23)*. Two weeks after replacement of the transduced cells, the γc transgene was detected in the blood and T-cell levels had increased *(23)*. At 10 mo post-treatment, both patients exhibited T and NK cells expressing the γc transgene and functioning at levels similar to normal controls of identical age *(23)*. Since then, an additional nine patients have been treated in this manner, with successful reconstitution with corrected cells in all but one case. This was also the first demonstration of a selective growth advantage for genetically corrected cells reintroduced into humans, a hitherto hypothetical idea, that previously had not been possible to definitively demonstrate in the adenosine deaminase (ADA) gene therapy trials because of the continued administration of polyetylene glycol (PEG)-ADA. Long-term follow-up will be necessary to determine how much transduction was achieved in the earliest multipotent, self-renewing hematopoietic stem cell population. Nevertheless, this success illustrated the usefulness of MMLV vectors applied using optimized ex vivo transduction procedures in the setting of a well-thought-out clinical application in which even relatively low levels of corrected cells can achieve therapeutic efficacy through conferral of a selective advantage. Unfortunately, this trial also demonstrated for the first time in humans the potential for retroviral insertional events to contribute to the development of oncogenesis; an aspect, which will be discussed below and in other chapters separately.

More recently, however, it has become evident that lentiviral vectors are more efficient at transducing quiescent HSC than murine retroviral vectors. Thus, some of the specific applications of hematopoietic gene transfer with implications for cancer gene therapy using retroviral vectors are presented below, with emphasis on lentiviral vectors.

3.1.2. Efficiency of Retroviral/Lentiviral Vector Gene Delivery Into Long-Term Repopulating Hematopoietic Progenitors

As noted above, HSC are predominantly quiescent cells in the G0/G1 phase of the cell cycle. It has been demonstrated convincingly by several groups that lentiviral vectors, which encode proteins that permit active import of the viral genome into the nucleus of nondividing cells, are a more efficient system for gene transfer to HSCs than other retroviral vectors. Early observations based on the initially available generations of lentiviral vectors used to transduce purified human HSC, showed higher rates of ex vivo gene delivery by lentiviral vectors compared with retroviral vectors whether in the presence or absence of growth factors *(27–29)*. Subsequently, animal models of hematopoietic reconstitution showed that $CD34^+$ cells transduced with lentiviral vectors were capable of stable, long-term reconstitution of nonobese diabetic/severe combined immunodeficient (NOD/SCID) mice. These studies have shown long-term expression of marker genes from 15 to 22 wk in lymphoid, myeloid, and erythroid progeny and also engrafted human cells that retained the $CD34^+$ phenotype *(30,31)*. Importantly, analysis of human progenitor cells isolated from bone marrow of NOD/SCID recipient animals showed that the overall percentage of gene marking in colony-forming cells by microscopy was equivalent to the percentage of provirus sequences by polymerase chain reaction (PCR) analysis, indicating minimal transgene silencing in vivo *(32)*. Later, repopulating assays in NOD/SCID mice with lentivirus-transduced human HSC cells included dose-response analyses to determine the minimal MOI (and hence lower numbers of virus integrants/cell) required to produce consistent gene marking in serial transplantation assays, demonstrating that even at low MOI *(3)* and in the absence of cytokines, lentiviral vectors were able to consistently produce marking in self-renewing, multi-potent and long-term repopulating hematopoietic cells *(33–35)*. It is interesting to note that lentiviral vectors and MMLV vectors seem to transduce mouse HSC (lineage-negative cells obtained from bone marrow) with similar efficiency when performed in the presence of growth factors (IL-3, IL-6, and stem cell factor), demonstrating that, although not totally essential for transduction, entry into the cell cycle favors optimal lentiviral transduction *(36,37)*. The comparison of lentiviral and oncoretroviral vectors has further been extended to nonhuman primate models. In baboons, efficient lentiviral gene transfer of HSC was dependent on the presence of cytokines during transduction *(38)*. Surprisingly, as the result of a postentry restriction to HIV infection in rhesus macaques, although low levels of marking in rhesus cells could be detected, it was generally poor *(39–41)*. Further studies assessing lentiviral vector-mediated gene transfer into HSC and transplantation into primates are currently being performed by several groups to allow long-term evaluation of safety, maintenance of gene expression, and potential immune responses against transgene products in large animal models. Notably, in one recent study, it was noted that mobilized $CD34^+$ cells transduced with lentiviral vectors expressing enhanced green fluorescent protein (EGFP) transplanted into myeloablated rhesus macaques resulted in the induction of specific immunological tolerance toward the foreign transgene *(42)*.

3.1.3. Approaches Exploring Hematopoietic Reconstitution for Cancer Gene Therapy

Retrovirus-mediated gene transfer and overexpression of cytostatic drug-resistance genes has been envisaged as a myeloprotective strategy that would permit chemotherapeutic dose escalation beyond normally tolerated levels following bone marrow transplantation (BMT) and reconstitution with transduced hematopoietic progenitors. When used to express the human multiple drug resistance (MDR-1) gene, retroviral vectors significantly improved protection to cytostatic drugs *in vitro* in transduced hematopoietic cell lines and in HSC transplanted into mice *(43,44)*.

When MDR-1 transduced HSC were injected into nonirradiated mice, high levels of long-term engraftment and conferral of chemoprotection were observed *(45,46)*. Interestingly, it appears that MDR-1 overexpression may somehow alter the ability of HSC to respond to cytokines in culture, as significant expansion of the repopulating cell fraction of HSC after MDR-1 transduction at high-copy-number by retroviral gene transfer has been reported during ex vivo culture in the presence of IL-3, IL-6, and SCF, but without any drug selection; in contrast, such expansion was not observed after retroviral gene transfer of the dihyfrofolate reductase (DHFR) gene, also a drug selection marker *(47)*. However, mice transplanted with these expanded stem cells developed a myeloproliferative disorder characterized by high peripheral white blood cell counts and splenomegaly *(47)*. These preclinical results demonstrate that enforced stem cell self-renewal divisions can have adverse consequences. Nonetheless, using transduced HSC with significantly lower copies of MDR integrations per cell (about 1–2 vs >10), studies by other groups did not show any signs of myeloproliferative disorder in transplanted mice *(46)*. Therefore, the rationale for conducting clinical trials with optimized retroviral vectors containing drug resistance genes such as MDR-1 to prevent chemotherapy-induced myelosuppression is still under consideration *(46)*, although this elegant approach faces intense scrutiny prior to clinical implementation.

In this context, it should also be noted that this general strategy for in vivo drug selection and amplification of transduced hematopoietic progenitors is now being further explored with other drug resistance genes, such as the P140K variant methylguanine methyl transferase gene (MGMT). This drug resistance gene confers resistance to O^6-benzylguanine (BG) and temozolomide (TMZ), as well as 1,3-bis (2-chloroethyl)-1-nitrosourea (BCNU), allowing efficient in vivo selection of transduced hematopoietic cells even without extensive prior myeloablation *(48,49)*. In some studies, it has been reported that this strategy can achieve such efficient amplification and 80 to 90% of circulating cells are found to be transduced *(50,51)*, to confer protection against chemotherapy-induced myelosuppression and therapeutically relevant levels of donor chimerism even in an allogeneic transplant setting *(51)*. Dose-limiting hematopoietic toxicity of conventional chemotherapy remains a major problem, as observed in a recent phase II trial of BG/BCNU in patients with nitrosourea-resistant glioma *(52)*, hence the pursuit of innovative gene transfer strategies to confer myeloprotection are certainly warranted.

Another interesting concept to improve the efficacy of anticancer treatments with gene therapy is to manipulate the immune response after hematologic transplants. Following allogeneic BMT or HSC transplantation in leukemia/lymphoma treatment, donor lymphocytes are known to mediate a graft-vs-leukemia effect (GVL). However, a major problem with this approach is the potential development of graft-vs-host diseases (GVHD). One promising solution to prevent GVHD is to genetically modify donor T-cells with a suicide mechanism that can be activated by administration of a prodrug if this life-threatening complication should occur. This strategy has been confirmed preclinically by several groups using retroviral vector-mediated gene transfer of the herpes simplex virus thymidine kinase (HSV-*tk*) suicide gene, which encodes an enzyme that phosphorylates and thereby activates the antiviral prodrug ganciclovir (GCV) *(53–55)*. The clinical utility of this system was recently confirmed in a phase 1 study with eight leukemia/lymphoma patients who relapsed and were subsequently treated with donor lymphocytes transduced with the HSV-*tk* suicide gene. The transduced lymphocytes survived for up to 12 mo, resulting in antitumor activity in five patients. Three patients developed GVHD, which could be effectively controlled by GCV-induced elimination of the transduced cells *(56)*.

Another potential scenario for the utilization of retroviral gene transfer is to "repair" genetic damage caused by translocations, widely seen in hematologic malignancies. Chronic myelogenous leukemia (CML) and Philadelphia-positive acute lymphoblastic leukemia (Ph^+ ALL) are malignant diseases caused by gene rearrangement resulting in the formation of the abnormal fusion protein BCR/ABL. Despite the high remission rate initially obtained by the advent of new drugs such as Gleevec, a small molecule inhibitor of BCR/ABL kinase activity, it has become increasingly clear that the emergence of drug resistant clones eventually results in relapse; hence, more definitive treatment strategies are still being sought. The presence of the BCR/ABL oncoprotein is a necessary event for malignant transformation seen in CML and Ph^+ ALL. Thus, genetic modification of HSC in order to eliminate expression of BCR/ABL might render transduced CML and Ph^+ ALL stem and progenitor cells functionally normal. This approach has been successfully shown to work by the use of retroviral vectors expressing antisense RNA *(57)*, ribozymes *(58)*, and RNAi *(59,60)*. More recently, third-generation lentiviral vectors expressing ribozymes directed specifically against the fusion joint in the BCR/ABL transcript were used to transduce primary Ph^+ ALL and $CD34^+$ cells, resulting in growth inhibition and apoptosis specifically in the leukemic blasts *(61)*. Thus, allied with the high efficiency of the lentiviral vector system to transduce HSC, this technology has the potential to develop into a realistic treatment modality for patients with CML or Ph^+ ALL.

3.1.4. Transduction of Dendritic Cells for Anticancer Vaccines

Dendritic cells (DCs) provide the most potent pathway for initiating T- and B-cell immune responses *(62)*. Myeloid DC precursors derived from peripheral blood, bone marrow or cord blood can be differentiated in vitro and used for immunization with peptides, protein, cDNA, RNA, or cell extracts *(63,64)*. $CD14^+$ monocytes are a naturally abundant cell population in the peripheral blood, which is an easily accessible source for production of DCs. Plastic-adherent peripheral blood monocytes can differentiate into "immature DCs" if a mixture of cytokines is added to the culture *(65,66)*. After differentiation, DCs do not proliferate, and therefore attempts to transduce them with MMLV vectors were not successful.

Thus, adenoviral vectors, which are capable of transducing nonreplicating cells, have been traditionally used to transduce DCs. To reach efficient transduction, however, adenoviral vectors have to be used at high multiplicity of infection (MOI = 100–1000) *(67–69)* which can produce cytopathic and cytotoxic effects. Furthermore, the commonly used adenoviral vectors are themselves highly immunogenic in humans, which may hamper immune responses to weaker "self" tumor antigens *(70)*, or trigger the rejection of transduced cells coexpressing adenoviral antigenic determinants *(71)*. In addition, it was shown that transduction of mouse DCs with *null* adenoviral vectors at high MOI (>100) induces some degree of activation by itself *(72)*, with unpredictable effects on the instruction of immune responses by these DC in vivo.

In contrast to these potential unwanted side effects of using the adenoviral vector system, lentiviral vectors offer an approach by which simple, efficient, persistent, nontoxic, and nonimmunogenic gene delivery into monocytes and DCs may be obtained. HIV-1 is naturally effective in infecting dendritic cells and monocytes, and a number of groups, including our own, have demonstrated that lentiviral vector transduction is a suitable methodology for efficient and persistent gene delivery into ex vivo differentiated DCs *(13,73–75)*, and into monocytes obtained from peripheral blood mononuclear cells (PBMC) *(76)*. Transduction of DCs with lentiviral vectors expressing the green fluorescent protein (GFP) did not alter their viability, immunophenotype or the ability to differentiate into mature DCs capable of stimulating autologous T-cell responses *(75)*. In a demonstration of their immunostimulatory functionality, lentivirus-transduced DCs expressing an antigenic HLA-A2.1 restricted Flu peptide were able to effectively activate autologous Flu-specific CTL responses *(74)*. We have shown that improved and safer third-generation self-inactivating lentiviral vectors very efficiently delivered GFP and CD40L genes into DCs with an average transduction efficiency of 70% *(13)*. After transduction, DC maturation and activation was stimulated only by the vector containing the CD40L immunocytokine transgene, but not by a control vector expressing only the GFP marker transgene, indicating that

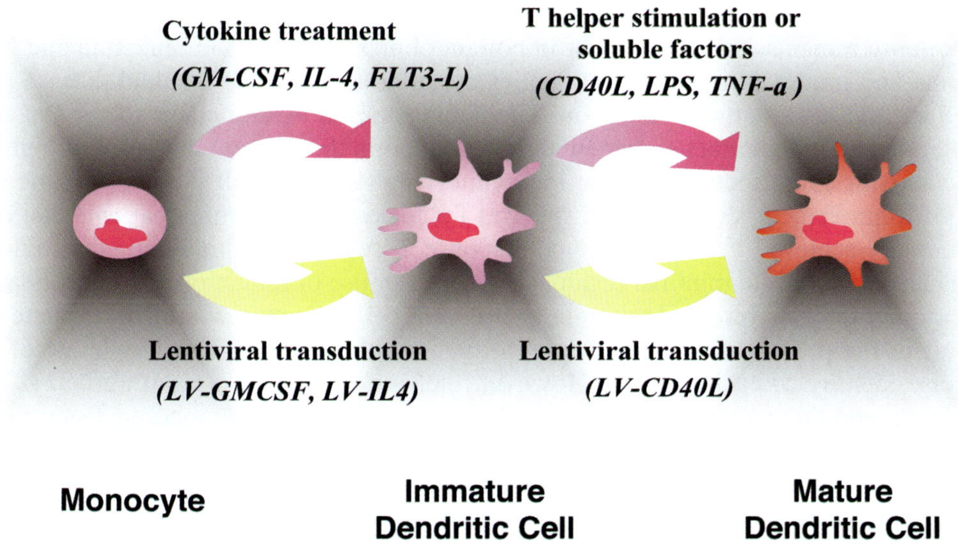

Fig. 6. Lentiviral vector-mediated genetic modification of dendritic cell precursors or immature dendritic cells. Conventional methods for dendritic cell differentiation and maturation require treatment with recombinant cytokines and stimulation with T-helper cells or other soluble factors (upper arrows). Instead, lentivirus-mediated gene transfer (lower arrows) can be used to achieve endogenous production of immunomodulators, thereby triggering autonomous differentiation.

lentiviral transduction *per se* is unlikely to cause DCs to differentiate, mature, activate, or otherwise engage in unpredictable immune stimulation. Transduction of DCs with the RRL-CD40L vector correlated with a mature DC phenotype as shown by morphology, upregulation of CD83 and other immunological relevant markers and production of IL-12 *(13)* (*see* Fig. 6). Autologous responses against an HLA-A2-restricted tumor associated antigenic peptide (gp100) and against an influenza peptide (Flu-M1) were significantly enhanced at non-saturating effector/target ratios when CD40L transduced DCs were used as antigen-presenting cells for in vitro stimulation of $CD8^+$ cytotoxic T-lymphocytes *(13)*.

Recently, we have evaluated a one-hit lentiviral transduction approach for genetic modification of monocytes in order to promote autocrine and paracrine production of factors required for their differentiation into immature DCs *(76)*. High-titer third-generation self-inactivating lentiviral vectors expressing granulocyte-macrophage colony stimulating factor (GM-CSF) and interleukin-4 (IL-4) efficiently achieved simultaneous and persistent codelivery of the transgenes into purified human $CD14^+$ monocytes (*see* Fig. 6). Coexpression of GM-CSF and IL-4 in monocytes was sufficient to induce their differentiation into lentivirus-modified DCs ("DC/LVs"), as evidenced by their morphology, immunophenotype, and immune-function. Mixed lymphocyte reactions showed that the T-cell stimulating activity of DC/LVs was superior to that of DCs grown by conventional methods. DC/LVs displayed efficient antigen-specific, major histocompatability complex (MHC) Class-I restricted stimulation of autologous $CD8^+$ T-cells, as shown by interferon (IFN)-γ production and CTL assays. Importantly, DC/LVs exhibited a longer lifespan in culture and could be maintained metabolically active and viable in culture for 2 to 3 wk in the absence of exogenously added growth factors, compared with DCs cultured by conventional methods *(76)*.

3.1.5. Autologous Leukemia/Lymphoma Cell Vaccines

Relapse remains one of the most important clinical problems in leukemia and lymphoma and immune therapeutic strategies designed to eradicate residual disease hold promise and are an attractive option. The demonstration of immune responses against leukemia and lymphoma associated antigens supports the concept that normal immune mechanisms can effectively target leukemia/lymphoma cells. It is thus possible that major improvements in long-term survival for leukemia/lymphoma patients could be potentially achieved if a host immune response to several leukemia antigens could be enhanced to eradicate minimal residual disease after use of induction and consolidation chemotherapy. Therefore, leukemia/lymphoma cell vaccines would be expected to result in the presentation of multiple antigens without requiring knowledge of the precise identity of each antigen. However, inefficient antigen presenting cell (APC) function, and the poor reactivity of autologous anti-leukemia/lymphoma T-cell mediated immunity, are associated with the inability of leukemia/lymphoma cells to provide sufficient co-stimulation to autologous T-cells. Indeed, we and others have found that requisite immune costimulators such as CD80 (B7.1) are frequently lacking leukemic cells. This provides the rationale to modify leukemia/lymphoma cells into efficient APCs by genetic manipulation, which has been tested and confirmed preclinically in a variety of models (for review see *[77]*).

As human leukemia/lymphoma cell vaccines have moved towards clinical trials, different types of vectors to genetically engineer human leukemia cells have been tested, including those based on MMLV *(78)*, herpesviruses *(79)*, adenoviruses *(80)*, and plasmids *(78)*, but none of those proved to be efficient or consistent enough for clinical application to the development of autologous cell vaccines. However, primary leukemia/lymphoma cells are good candidates for lentiviral vector transduction, as they show poor proliferation in vitro *(81)*. Thus, we and others have been able to show that HIV-derived lentiviral vectors pseudotyped with the VSV-G envelope were capable of efficiently transducing human leukemia cells and hematopoietic progenitor cells *(78,82–84)*.

In our first endeavor to deliver CD80 and GM-CSF genes into human ALL cells, we used a second-generation lentiviral vector packaging system (*see* Fig. 7). Functional experiments were performed to evaluate the response of the patients' autologous T-cells against their lentivirus transduced leukemia cells *(82)*. The stimulatory activity of non-transduced and transduced ALL cells was compared in primary and secondary autologous T-cell stimulation assays. These showed that ALL/CD80 cells, but not ALL/Mock or ALL/GFP, stimulated significant T-cell proliferation, which could be abrogated in the presence of an anti-CD80 blocking antibody or the fusion protein CTLA4-Ig, which blocks the engagement of CD28 by CD80 *(82)*. These results demonstrated that the transduction of CD80 into ALL cells was capable of converting the leukemia cells into competent APC. Subsequently, we evaluated a third generation SIN lentiviral vector coexpressing GM-CSF and CD80 for transduction of primary acute myeloid leukemia (AML) cells *(83)*. Allogeneic and autologous T-cell stimulation experiments demonstrated that transduction with RRL-CD80, RRL-GM-CSF and RRL-GM-CSF/CD80 significantly increased allogeneic T-cell proliferation, in contrast to a smaller increase in the autologous T-cell proliferation *(83)*. We have more recently evaluated the insertion of the central polypurine tract and the central termination sequence (cPPT/CTS) into a SIN lentiviral vector encoding for GM-CSF and CD80 *(77)*. Expression levels of GM-CSF and CD80 were consistently and significantly

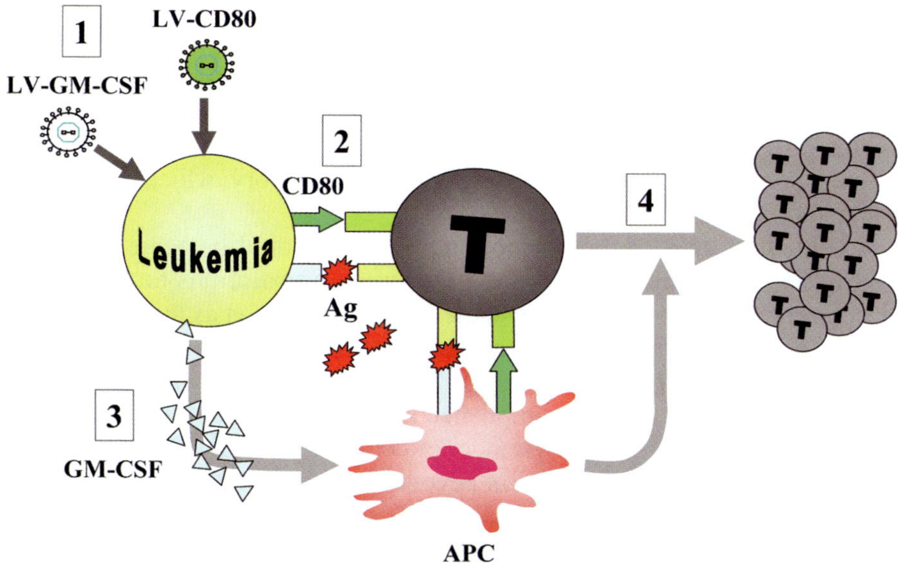

Fig. 7. Lentiviral vector-mediated genetic modification of primary leukemia cells. **1:** Lentiviral vectors expressing CD80 and GM-CSF are used to transduce leukemic cells, which frequently evade the immune response as a result of down-regulation of the CD80 costimulator molecule. **2:** CD80 re-expression mediates direct co-stimulation of T-cells recognizing tumor antigens (Ag). **3:** Expression of GM-CSF from transduced leukemia cells induces recruitment and activation of professional antigen presenting cells (APCs), such as dendritic cells. **4:** Activation and proliferation of tumor antigen-specific cytotoxic T-cells.

superior for the RRL-cPPT-GM/CD vector. Therefore, "re-insertion" of the cPPT/CTS element into self-inactivating vectors provided higher transduction rates in primary AML cells, which we now consider the "state-of-the-art" lentiviral vector design for future studies of leukemia cell vaccine development.

It should be noted that recently, other malignant hematopoietic cell types that have been notoriously difficult to genetically modify have also been successfully transduced through the use of lentiviral vectors (e.g., T-cell lymphoma *[85]* and myeloma cells *[86]*), further attesting to the promise of this approach for immunogenetic therapy.

3.2. In Vivo Vancer Gene Therapy

3.2.1. Lessons From Clinical Trials of Retroviral Gene Therapy for Cancer

Clinical trials involving retroviral gene therapy have thus far yielded mixed results, often disappointing, but in some recent cases highly promising. Application of retrovirus vectors in vivo initially focused on delivery of suicide genes into solid tumors. Introduction of vector producer cells (VPCs) for transduction of the HSV-*tk* gene into murine gliomas, followed by administration of the nucleoside analog GCV, resulted in regression or elimination of the cancerous cells *(87,88)*. However, application to human glioblastoma multiforme has yielded less successful results. A recent report evaluated the results of a phase III clinical trial of retrovirus-mediated HSV-*tk*/GCV treatment in malignant gliomas, the largest randomized and controlled study of gene therapy for cancer conducted to date *(89)*. Patients receiving simultaneous surgical resection and tumor-site injections of HSV-*tk* retrovirus VPCs, followed by GCV and radiation treatments, were identical to control patients undergoing conventional surgical resection and radiation therapy with respect to median time to tumor progression, clinical deterioration and death, as well as 12-mo overall survival rates. These disappointing results are most likely the result of the inability of the viral vectors to diffuse more than a few cell diameters from the injection site, and the highly infiltrative nature of human glioblastomas, resulting in inadequate levels of gene delivery, which were reported to be less than 0.002% *(89)*.

It is possible that increased transduction efficiency could be achieved through the simple expedient of further concentrating retrovirus preparations to achieve a higher titer, particularly with the use of more stable pseudotypes such as the VSV-G envelope. In fact, it has been reported that by rather labor-intensive measures it is possible to concentrate retrovirus vectors to titers of 10^{10}–10^{11} pfu/mL, allowing gene transfer of HSV-*tk* to mouse gliomas to be accomplished at an efficiency of less than 10%, resulting in complete eradication by the bystander effect in 80% of the tumors *(90)*. However, given the low level of vector penetration beyond the injection site by simple diffusion, it is not clear whether this strategy can be successfully applied to human tumors. Alternatively, it is possible that improved results could be achieved even with current titers by repeat administration of retrovirus vectors or VPCs. However, in a recent phase I/II clinical trial assessing repeat instillation of VPCs via Ommaya reservoir into the resected tumor cavity, it was concluded that although feasible, this procedure was associated with significant potential for complications; more than half of the patients enrolled in the study experienced adverse events, including a total of 8 out of 30 patients who developed Ommaya reservoir complications such as infection or blockage, or acute ventricular/meningeal reactions immediately upon VPC reinfusion *(91)*. In this study, 6 out of 30 patients survived longer than one year (median survival 492 d, range 390–703 d) but subsequently died from disease progression, and an additional patient remained alive and progression-free more than 5 yr after enrollment, but specific conclusions regarding the antitumoral efficacy of this approach could not be drawn because of the small sample size *(91)*.

Other phase I trials evaluating tumor suppressive strategies by direct in vivo administration of retroviral vectors, including retroviral gene transfer of p53 by intratumoral injection in patients with lung cancer *(92)* and multiple intraperitoneal infusions of retrovirus vectors expressing a tumor-inhibitory splice variant of BRCA1 via indwelling catheter in patients with ovarian cancer *(93)*, have also been reported to show initial promise. However, these approaches have largely been abandoned in favor of the greater gene transfer efficiency afforded by adenoviral vectors *(94)*, or as a result of their failure to fulfill therapeutic expectations in subsequent phase II trials *(95)*. More recently, daily intravenous administration of a von Willebrand factor-targeted retrovirus vector carrying dominant-negative cyclin G1 at doses of up to 3×10^{11} pfu was reported to show promise in a phase I clinical trial of pancreatic cancer conducted in the Philippines *(96)*.

However, given the generally poor levels of in vivo transduction that have been achieved thus far using conventional retrovirus vectors, a more promising approach may be to deliver therapeutic genes encoding secreted proteins. If sufficient levels of secretion could be achieved, transduction of even a small number of target cells in vivo could result in therapeutic efficacy. This approach has been adapted to the delivery of genes encoding a wide variety of secreted proteins, and may prove to be most useful in the case of cytokines, which can exert a potent immunostimulatory effect if sufficiently high local concentrations can be achieved. An early gene therapy trial reported promising results with retrovirus-mediated gene transfer of IL-2 to tumor infiltrating lymphocytes, which were reinfused into the chest cavity of patients with advanced lung cancer *(97)*. Subsequently, Nemunaitis et al. *(98)* have tested intratumoral administration of retroviral vectors for delivery of the interferon-γ gene in patients with metastatic melanoma. All 8 patients who received multiple injections exhibited stable or improved disease status, as opposed to 1 of 9 who received a single injection. Additionally, patients who received multiple injections showed immune reactivity and a survival time twice that of the single injection group *(98)*. In other studies, peritumoral injection of autologous primary dermal fibroblasts transduced with a retrovirus vector expressing human interleukin 12 (IL-12) was evaluated by Lotze and colleagues in parallel phase I dose-escalation trials conducted at the University of Pittsburgh and at the Samsung Medical Center in Seoul *(97,99)*. They reported transient but clear reductions of tumor sizes, with some instances of hemorrhagic necrosis, at injected as well as non-injected sites in melanoma patients. None of the above clinical studies showed any evidence of retroviral recombination or generation of replication competent revertants, attesting to the safety of retroviral gene therapy in vivo.

3.2.2. Improving In Vivo Cancer Gene Therapy: Application of Lentiviral Vectors

The low efficiency of in vivo gene delivery by conventional replication-defective onco-retroviral vectors is largely a consequence of the fact that a large number of the cells in the tissues of the adult body are quiescent. With the development of lentiviral vectors, a new optimism emerged in the field, leading to preclinical testing of lentiviral vector administration in vivo by several groups. These studies explored high titer lentiviral vectors pseudotyped with the VSV-G protein driving the expression of marking genes (GFP or LacZ) by constitutive promoters (CMV or PGK), which have shown repetitively that intravenous injections of lentivirus vectors lead to conspicuous gene transfer into liver and spleen *(101–105)* and in some cases bone marrow as well *(104,105)*. Early studies with lentiviral vectors lacking the cPPT-CTS element were problematic, as gene delivery into spleen or liver could only be assessed with confidence through the use of very sensitive methods such as quantitative real-time PCR *(104)* or if additional procedures for liver regeneration were employed *(101)*. Studies using the SIN configuration vector with the cPPT-CTS element, however, have consistently demonstrated that intravenous injection of 10^8–10^9 infective particles in mice can elicit significant marking of cells in the spleen (15–25%) and liver (5–15%) *(102)*. For liver, marking was observed predominantly in hepatocytes whereas for spleen, APCs (DCs and B cells) were mostly transduced *(102)*, although lentiviral gene marking has also been observed in stromal and parenchymal cells of several organs *(104)*. In addition to these positive biodistribution results, no significant toxicity was observed and transgene expression could be followed for several months. Hence lentiviral gene transfer may now deliver the potential of direct gene corrections or insertions directly in vivo.

As a logical progression towards the safety and specificity of lentiviral vectors, the use of tissue specific promoters for expression targeting has been actively explored: for example, vectors containing the promoter and enhancer sequences from the Tie-2 gene demonstrated specific expression in endothelial cells in vitro and in vivo *(103)*, whereas the albumin gene promoter restricted lentiviral expression to hepatocytes *(104)*. Successful targeted expression in hepatocytes has been shown to contribute to long-term expression of Factor IX in mice by intravenous injection of lentiviral vectors was achieved, which intriguingly limited the immune responses to the transgene *(105)*.

Of interest to immunotherapy for cancer, direct in vivo administration of lentiviral vectors by systemic injection has also been successfully explored as a vaccination approach. Intravenous administration of lentiviral vectors expressing melanoma antigens induced potent melanoma-specific CTL responses in mice *(106,107)*, which is probably correlated with the high capability of lentiviral vectors to transduce APCs in the spleen *(102)*. Additionally, lentiviral vector injection into the foot-pad of mice directly transduced DCs in vivo, which migrated to the draining lymph node and spleen, leading to antigen-specific CTL responses *(108)*.

Naturally, another potential application is to extend the previous work on retroviral gene delivery *in situ* into the tumor, as lentiviral vectors would potentially achieve more efficient gene transfer into both the nonproliferating as well as the actively proliferating cell fractions within the tumor. Thus, in an ovarian carcinoma mouse model, lentiviral vectors pseudotyped with VSV-G delivered GFP 10-fold more efficiently to ovarian cancer cells growing ip in SCID mice than conventional replication-defective MMLV-based retroviral vectors with the same envelope and comparable doses *(109)*. In addition, injection of ex vivo transduced tumor cells, sorted for GFP expression, indicated that the lentiviral vector was more resistant to in vivo silencing in comparison with the retroviral vector *(109)*. High levels of marking using the GFP transgene were also documented after in vivo injection of high doses of lentiviral vectors into subcutaneous or orthotopic masses of PC3 and DU145 prostate cancer cells grown in NOD/SCID mice *(110)*. In another prostate cancer model, lentiviral vectors driving GFP expression from a probasin promoter (ARR(2)PB) injected into tumors expressed GFP in prostate LNCaP tumors, but not in A-549 lung or CaKi-2 kidney tumors *(111)*. Antitumor effects of lentiviral vectors expressing HSV-*tk* or HSV-*tk*/GFP fusions combined with GCV treatment showed that this suicide gene therapy approach could inhibit tumor growth and increase survival in animal models for ovarian tumor *(112)* and hepatocellular carcinoma *(113)*. Insertion of toxic genes as diphtheria toxin A *(114)*, HIV-1 *vpr* *(115)* and the gibbon ape leukemia virus envelope fusogenic membrane glycoprotein *(116)* into lentiviral vectors to reduce tumor masses in vivo have also shown success.

Nonetheless, lentiviral gene transfer into tumors is still restricted by limited diffusion of the vectors away from the injection site, and in our own studies we have observed transduction levels only on the order of a few percent in many solid tumors after a single injection (Shichinohe, Sazawa et al. 2004, submitted). Thus, for any replication-defective retroviral or lentiviral vector system, is would seem advisable to employ a transgene which can induce a potent bystander effect, or encoding a secreted protein product (e.g., such as a cytokine as discussed above, or an antiangiogenic peptide *(9)*, in order to achieve the most optimal therapeutic effect relative to the achievable transduction efficiency.

3.2.3. Improving In Vivo Cancer Gene Therapy: Application of RCR Vectors

As the inability of standard replication-defective retroviral vectors to achieve effective transduction of tumors in vivo has been a major obstacle to cancer gene therapy, more efficient transduction could be achieved if a replication-competent retrovirus (RCR) were used. With an RCR vector, the virus would then replicate and multiply after the initial infection event and each infected tumor cell would, in effect, become a virus producer cell.

In fact, the idea of using replication competent viruses as oncolytic agents dates back almost a century, and a number of different viruses were employed in patients with advanced cancer during the period from 1950 to the early 1970s. These early attempts, using wild type viruses that could only be manipulated by classical virological culture techniques available at the time, generally met with discouraging results, characterized by initial tumor reduction, only to be followed by recurrence in conjunction with an antiviral immune response. With the advent of modern chemotherapeutic drugs, the concept of oncolytic virotherapy was largely abandoned.

Now, with advances over the past 25 yr in our understanding of the molecular mechanisms involved in viral pathogenesis and in our ability to more precisely manipulate viral genomic sequences through recombinant DNA technology, and with the realization that conventional gene therapy approaches employing replication-defective vectors have largely failed to achieve significant therapeutic benefit, there has recently been a renewed interest in the use of conditionally replication-competent viruses for the treatment of cancer. Replicating forms of a number of different virus species, including adenovirus, paramyxoviruses, herpes virus, reovirus, poliovirus, and vesicular stomatitis virus are now being developed as oncolytic agents, particularly for locally advanced or recurrent cancer. However, these all represent cytotoxic viruses that do not permanently integrate into the host cells, and hence, as previously, long-term therapeutic benefit had been elusive because of rapid virus clearance by the host and tumor recurrence.

In contrast, MMLV-based RCR vectors can achieve highly efficient and persistent gene transfer preferentially to replicating cancer cells, and we have found that this system has significant advantages over other replicating viruses as an oncolytic agent. First of all, MMLV is a simple and well-characterized retrovirus for which the mechanisms mediating viral replication are well understood. The MMLV capsid contains no nuclear localization signals for active uptake across an intact nuclear membrane, and so the initial rationale for use of retroviral vectors in cancer gene therapy still holds true for RCR vectors (i.e., MMLV-based vectors can only transduce cells that are actively dividing). Because the majority of normal cells in many adult tissues are quiescent, preferential transduction of tumor cells can be achieved.

We have already demonstrated that MMLV-based RCR vectors containing transgene cassettes inserted precisely at the env-3′ UTR border (*see* Fig. 8) can efficiently transduce and stably propagate over multiple infection cycles, thereby achieving a tremendous *in situ* amplification effect after initial administration of a small inoculum. As predicted from their robust replicative capabilities, we have found that intratumoral injection of as little as 10^4 total infectious units of RCR vector was found to be capable of spreading and transmitting an inserted transgene throughout entire solid tumor masses in vivo, achieving greater than 99% transduction in xenograft models using a variety of different human cancer cell lines *(117,118)*.

Notably, after direct intratumoral injection, systemic spread of vectors was undetectable in immunocompetent animals by sensitive real-time PCR assays in all normal tissues examined, including bone marrow, spleen, intestine, and skin. We have also successfully tested strategies to further enhance safety and efficiency by targeting RCR vectors specifically to cancer cells, via modifications of viral envelope tropism *(119)* or incorporation into a targetable hybrid vector system *(120)*, and insertion of tissue-specific or inducible transcriptional regulatory elements *(121)*.

As an intrinsically noncytolytic virus, MMLV is less likely to cause acute toxicity as a direct consequence of viral infection; however, MMLV-based RCR vectors can readily be engineered with suicide genes for synchronous killing of tumor cells triggered by prodrug administration. Using this approach, we have achieved highly efficient killing of cancer cells in culture and in tumor models in vivo. Interestingly, stable integration by MMLV appears to result in long-term persistence of viral infection that follows

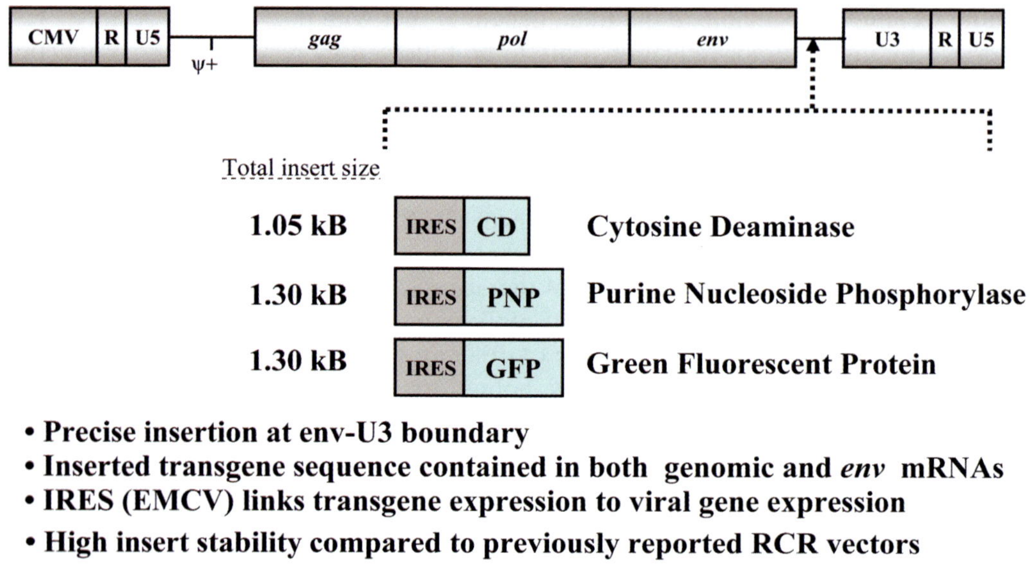

Fig. 8. An improved design strategy for replication-competent retrovirus (RCR) vectors. The U3 region of the 5′-LTR has replaced with the CMV promoter for higher levels of initial virus production. Expression cassettes consisting of the encephalomyocarditis virus (EMCV) internal ribosome entry site (IRES) sequence and therapeutic transgenes such as the yeast cytosine deaminase (CD) or *Escherichia coli* purine nucleoside phosphorylase (PNP) suicide genes, or marker genes such as the jellyfish GFP, are inserted precisely at the 3′ end of the viral *env* gene, just upstream from the 3′ untranslated region of the virus genome. All other abbreviations are as described in **Fig. 1**.

cancer cells even as they metastasize to new sites, thus enabling multiple rounds of prodrug administration to achieve further prolongation of survival. A multicycle prodrug regimen after a single dose of RCR vector expressing a suicide gene in an intracranial U-87 human glioma xenograft model continuously prolonged survival for more than 120 d, compared with 0% survival of control groups in less than 40 d ($p < 0.0001$ *(118)* (*see* Fig. 9).

Thus, RCR-vectors can achieve highly efficient, tumor-restricted, and therapeutically efficacious gene transfer, and we propose that the use of such vectors would be well justified in clinical scenarios involving highly aggressive and rapidly progressive solid tumors which arise from a normally quiescent tissue such as localized brain tumors. Stable genomic integration by RCR vectors enables greater long-term therapeutic efficacy, as continuous virus production allows persistent spread of the virus even as tumor cells migrate to ectopic foci, and continuous suicide gene expression allows multiple cycles of prodrug administration to be performed even after a single injection of the vector (*see* Fig. 9).

4. SAFETY OF RETROVIRAL/LENTIVIRAL VECTORS

The safety of conventional replication-defective retrovirus vectors has been well established over the past decade of clinical trials. However, as retrovirus technology improves and transduction levels in vivo increase, so will the potential for adverse effects. It is already recognized, for example, that the use of human packaging cells

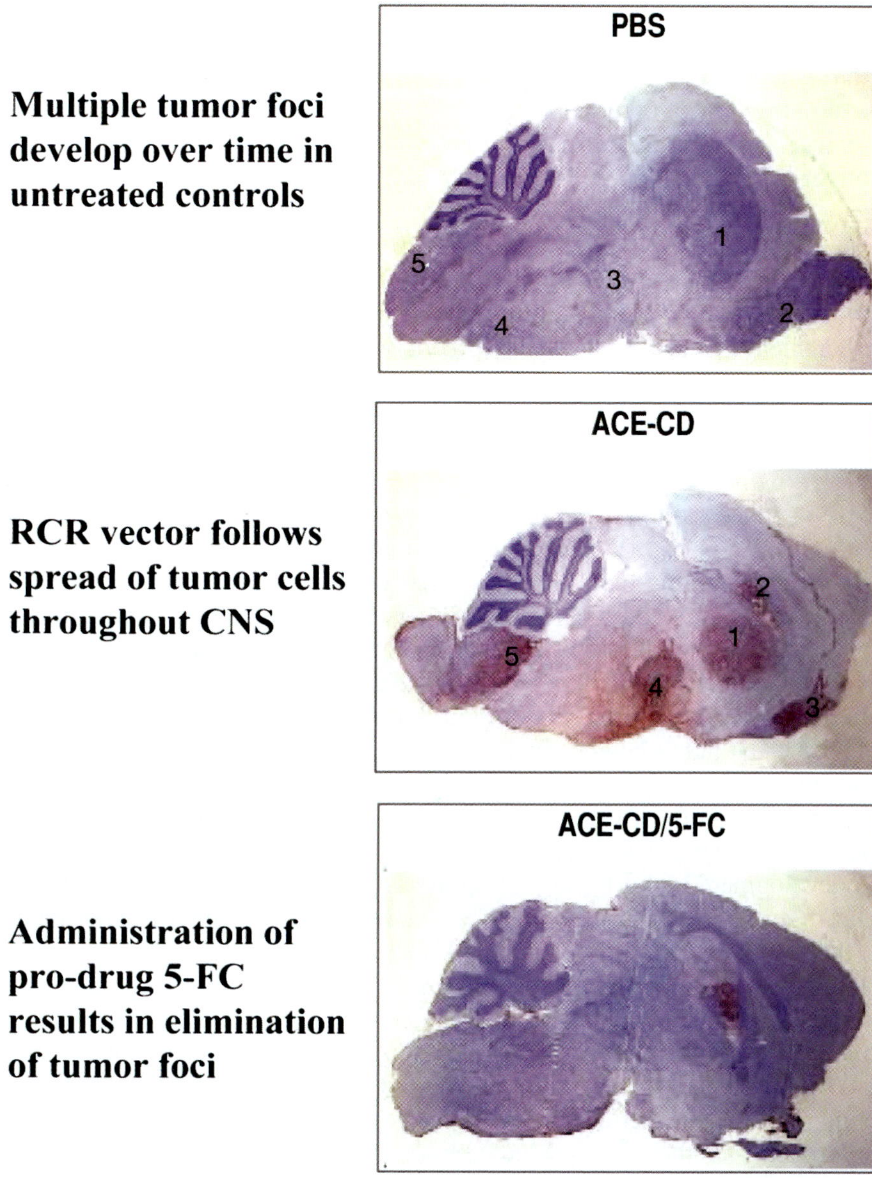

Fig. 9. Suicide gene RCR vectors achieve significant inhibition of intracranial gliomas and persistent expression in migrating tumor foci. *Upper panel:* Brain section from athymic mouse 5 wk after intracerebral inoculation of U-87 human glioma cells, showing development of multiple tumor foci (numbered) after control treatment with saline (PBS). Primary tumor inoculation site is designated as 1. *Middle panel:* Brain section from athymic mouse with U-87 glioma after single injection of RCR vector carrying the yeast cytosine deaminase suicide gene (ACE-CD). Immunohistochemical staining with a retrovirus-specific antibody shows vector has spread throughout all visible tumor foci, but does not infect normal brain tissue because of the inability of the retrovirus to infect quiescent cells. *Lower panel:* Brain section from athymic mouse with U-87 glioma after single injection of ACE-CD vector followed by administration of the specific pro-drug, 5-fluorocytosine (5-FC). This pro-drug is enzymatically converted by yeast cytosine deaminase to the active chemotoxin 5-fluorouracil (5-FU) only in the RCR-transduced glioma cells, resulting in selective killing of the tumor foci.

will significantly reduce serum inactivation of retrovirus particles, as the presence of β-galactose epitopes on proteins produced by nonhuman cells is now known to be the primary target of such inactivation by preformed anti-β-galactose antibodies present in human serum, the same antibodies that are responsible for hyperacute rejection in xenotransplantation *(122)*. Hence retroviral vectors produced in human packaging cells will persist longer in vivo, and so will their attendant risks *(123)*.

4.1. Genotoxicity and Potential for Carcinogenesis

One major concern for retroviral vectors including lentivirus is, that inappropriate retroviral integration might lead to insertional mutagenesis and malignancies. This concern was heightened following the development of fatal lymphomas in 3 out of 10 rhesus macaque recipients of bone marrow cells contaminated with RCR *(124)*. It should be noted that the macaques that developed malignancies were severely immunocompromised, and similar experiments using less severe immunosuppression showed no evidence of any pathology resulting from systemic inoculation of wild type MMLV *(125,126)*. Nonetheless, the potential for such adverse events now has clinical precedent *(127)*, with recent reports of clonal T-cell proliferation in 2 out of 11 immunodeficient pediatric patients emerging more than 2 yr after correction of interleukin receptor common γ-chain deficiency SCID. This serious adverse event has caused major effect on clinical gene therapy trials worldwide. As described above, in this trial, the patients received hematopoietic stem cells that had been transduced with an oncoretroviral vector expressing a functional γc gene product. Common denominators for these two patients were thought to represent potential contributory factors to these serious adverse events *(128)*. First, viral integration in the clonally proliferating cells occurred in the *LMO2* gene in both cases. Second, both of these patients received relatively high dose of transduced hematopoietic stem cells. Third, the patients were treated about 3 mo after birth and the leukemia development had a latency of approx 30 mo. Additionally, at least one of the patients had a family history of malignancies and showed cytogenetic abnormalities that predated the clonal proliferation event. With these considerations, a worldwide hold on clinical trials of retroviral gene therapy was gradually lifted, and the original trial as well as various similar trials in the United States and the United Kingdom were resumed with some protocol modifications (number of administered cells, inclusion criteria, age of the patients to be enrolled, etc.) aimed at reducing the risk of insertional oncogenesis.

Since the restart of their clinical trial, one new patient has been treated by the Fischer group in Paris, and another trial conducted by Adrian Thrasher and colleagues *(129)* has shown functional immunological recovery in another four children with no evidence of any serious adverse event. Moreover, recent studies in large animal models indicated that retroviral integration at the copy numbers achieved using standard protocols were unlikely to result in leukemogenesis, and suggested that patient- or transgene-specific factors most likely contributed to the occurrence of leukemia in the SCID-X1 gene therapy trial *(130)*. However, in January 2005, the Agence Française de Securite Sanitaire des Produits de Sante (AFSSAPS) reported that a third child in the Fischer trial has been diagnosed with T-cell proliferation (*http://afssaps.sante.fr/ang/indang.htm*). This child was 9 mo old when receiving retroviral gene therapy for SCID-X1 in April 2002. At present, it is not clear whether an *LMO2* insertion event was involved, and the molecular characteristics of this third adverse event are currently under investigation.

The risk factors involved in retroviral gene transfer include the number of integration hits, the specific integration sites, the nature of the insertional mutagenesis event (e.g., disruption of a tumor suppressor or activation of an adjacent proto-oncogene), ubiquitous vs controlled gene expression, nature of the target cell, cell dose, host immune competence, host genetic background, and transgene function. Therefore, preclinical scrutiny of the potential effects of insertional mutagenesis will be a prerequisite for further clinical development of onco-retroviral and lentiviral vectors *(131,132)*. Of course, however, the multistep nature of carcinogenesis makes it unlikely that retroviral insertion leading to activation of a proto-oncogene was the sole causative event, and presumably other factors such as the potent in vivo selective growth advantage caused by correction of this growth factor receptor deficiency, and a familial predisposition to cancer documented in at least one of the patients might also represent potential contributory factors. Thus, it will be mandatory to seek a deeper understanding of the risk factors predisposing retroviral vector-mediated gene therapy to malignancies.

In addition to understanding (and thereby, presumably, avoiding) relevant risk factors, additional strategies to avoid the occurrence of insertional activation events are now being explored. Many of these strategies were initially proposed many years ago but have rarely been applied to vectors used in clinical trials, including the use of self-inactivating vectors *(133,134)*, incorporation of chromatin "insulator" domains *(135,136)*, and the routine addition of suicide genes to future generations of vectors. However, it is becoming increasingly evident that each of these approaches is not without potential flaws *(137,138)*. Thus, additional strategies for more stringent control of vector expression, and ultimately, devising methods to achieve site-specific targeting of viral integration *(139)* may be necessary to ensure the safety of retroviral and lentiviral gene transfer, particularly to hematopoietic cells.

4.2. Specific Safety Considerations for Lentiviral Vectors

Specifically with regard to lentiviral vectors, it should be noted that genome-wide analyses of viral integration sites have recently demonstrated that lentivirus tends to integrate more within active genes but less frequently upstream of transcriptionally active promoter regions compared with MMLV-based retrovirus *(140,141)* [(further information on retroviral insertion sites in murine hematopoietic tumors is now available online at the Retroviral Tagged Cancer Gene Database (*http://RTCGD.ncifcrf.gov*)], and therefore lentiviral vectors may be less prone to causing insertional activation of adjacent proto-oncogenes. Furthermore, it has now been reported that multicopy integration after HIV-derived lentivirus vector transduction of murine hematopoietic stem cells with a single round of infection at a multiplicity of 1, 3, 10, or 30 does not appear to promote clonal proliferation in primary or secondary mouse recipients *(141a)*. Thus, overall, it appears that lentiviral vectors may be both more efficient and safer than conventional MMLV-based vectors.

Of course, a major concern with the use of HIV-derived lentiviral vector system clinically has also been its association with AIDS, with the idea that inadvertent contamination by replication competent lentivirus (RCL) in clinical vector preparations used to treat patients could potentially cause some variant AIDS-related disease. Actually, the altered tropism imparted by the VSV-G envelope used to pseudotype most HIV-based lentiviral vectors (and the absence of the natural CD4-tropic gp160 HIV envelope in third-generation packaging systems) would seem to make such a scenario relatively unlikely even if some type of RCL were to emerge. Nonetheless, there has been discussion as to whether it might be better to develop vectors from alternative lentiviral species that primarily infect nonhuman hosts (e.g., FIV, EIAV, BIV) and that are not known to cause human disease; conversely, it can also be argued that engineering of previously benign viruses into high titer vectors might result in novel zoonoses should RCL contaminants be generated.

Ultimately, the biosafety implications of lentivirus-mediated gene transfer for human gene therapy are still not well known, as these vectors have not yet been sufficiently explored in clinical trials. A phase-1 clinical trial with HIV-derived lentiviral vectors has been initiated for HIV-infected patients (*www.aegis.com/news/PR/2003/PR030761.html*) and other applications for lentiviral vectors will soon be explored clinically for neuronal diseases (*www.biomedica.co.uk/news/2003-ob-14.htm*). These clinical trials will be pivotal in establishing whether currently available generations of lentiviral vectors are sufficiently safe for clinical application.

4.3. Specific Safety Considerations for RCR Vectors

If even replication-defective vectors can initiate the process of clonal proliferation, one would assume that uncontrolled spread of replication-competent virus certainly has the potential to result in insertional mutagenesis and carcinogenesis, particularly in the context of immunosuppression, predisposing genetic risk factors, and positive selection for transduced cells with a proliferative advantage. However, in contrast to gene replacement therapy, a number of considerations mitigate this concern when contemplating the use of retroviral vector-mediated suicide gene transfer for cancer therapy. Certainly, the possibility of generating replication-competent revertants during production of retroviral vectors has been a foremost concern of investigators in the field. Again, however, the initial rationale for use of retroviral vectors in cancer gene therapy would still hold true even for RCR vectors (i.e., MMLV-based vectors can only transduce cells that are actively dividing, and transduction is preferential for replicating tumor cells). Thus, compared with direct transduction and re-infusion of hematopoietic stem cells as performed in the γc-SCID trial, intratumoral injection is less likely to result in significant transduction of hematopoietic progenitors leading to leukemia. Furthermore, particularly in the case of terminal malignancies such as glioblastoma, the lack of effective therapeutic options and the dismal prognosis may render relatively moot the concerns over potential late-onset risks.

In fact, as noted above, we have already demonstrated that intratumoral injection of RCR vectors can, indeed, mediate highly efficient transduction throughout solid tumors in various xenograft models without detectable spread to normal tissues by PCR analysis *(117,118)*. A recent study by Klatzmann and coworkers did report transduction of bone marrow and spleen at levels quantitated as 0.0037–0.21 copies/cell by real-time PCR, but only after direct intravenous injection of replicating MMLV vectors and only in immunodeficient nude mice; importantly, no such transduction was observed in any tissue after intravenous injection in immunocompetent Balb/c mice *(142)*. Furthermore, antiretroviral drugs such as 3′-azido-3′-deoxythymidine (AZT) can readily terminate replication of wild-type MMLV *(143)* as well as MMLV-based RCR vectors *(118,142)*, and in fact, the low-level contamination of bone marrow and spleen by wild type MMLV after direct intravenous injection in nude mice mentioned above was shown to be completely suppressed by AZT *(142)*. Finally, the incorporation of a suicide gene into the RCR vector would itself constitute a self-destruct mechanism and hence provides a built-in safeguard, as even noncancerous cells infected by the vector would generally be eliminated by treatment, although escape mechanisms against suicide genes in retroviral vectors have also been observed *(144)*. In summary, RCR vector spread to extratumoral sites should be inherently limited in immunocompetent hosts and readily abrograted by antiretroviral agents and suicide gene function, but certainly the risk vs benefit ratio of this novel and still experimental therapeutic approach remains to be fully elucidated.

5. CONCLUSION

Retrovirus vectors have long been a reliable workhorse for cancer gene therapy strategies, and this vector system still retains considerable advantages including a well-documented safety record in phase III clinical trials, established methods for large-scale manufacturing with the use of constitutive producer cell lines, and the ability to permanently integrate into the host cell genome. Whereas initial clinical trials of retrovirus-mediated cancer gene therapy proved disappointing, new strategies for application of traditional MMLV-based oncoretrovirus and newer HIV-based lentivirus vectors, based on a clear understanding of their characteristic limitations and advantages with optimization of ex vivo and in vivo transduction procedures, are actively being pursued in preclinical and clinical studies. More radical innovations also show promise, including the development of replication-competent retrovirus vectors for application to cancer gene therapy. Even as true therapeutic success was achieved in clinical trials employing ex vivo retroviral gene transfer, the real risk of insertional mutagenesis leading to malignancy became manifest, providing a sobering lesson pointing to the need for on-going efforts to improve not only the efficiency but also the safety of retroviral/lentiviral gene therapy.

REFERENCES

1. Mann R, Mulligan RC, Baltimore D. Construction of a retrovirus packaging mutant and its use to produce helper-free defective retrovirus. Cell 1983;33:153–159.
2. Soneoka Y, Cannon PM, Ramsdale EE, et al. A transient three-plasmid expression system for the production of high titer retroviral vectors. Nucleic Acids Res 1995;23(4):628–633.
3. Gunzburg WH, Salmons B. Virus vector design in gene therapy. Mol Med Today 1995;1(9):410–417.
4. Weber E, Anderson WF, Kasahara N. Recent advances in retrovirus vector-mediated gene therapy: teaching an old vector new tricks. Curr Opin Mol Ther 2001;3(5):439–453.
5. Naldini L, Blomer U, Gallay P, et al. In vivo gene delivery and stable transduction of nondividing cells by a lentiviral vector. Science 1996;272(5259):263–267.
6. Blomer U, Naldini L, Kafri T, Trono D, Verma IM, Gage FH. Highly efficient and sustained gene transfer in adult neurons with a lentivirus vector. J Virol 1997;71(9):6641–6649.
7. Kafri T, Blomer U, Peterson DA, Gage FH, Verma IM. Sustained expression of genes delivered directly into liver and muscle by lentiviral vectors. Nat Genet 1997;17(3):314–317.
8. Sakoda T, Kasahara N, Hamamori Y, Kedes L. A high-titer lentiviral production system mediates efficient transduction of differentiated cells including beating cardiac myocytes. J Mol Cell Cardiol 1999;31(11):2037–2047.
9. Shichinohe T, Bochner BH, Mizutani K, et al. Development of lentiviral vectors for antiangiogenic gene delivery. Cancer Gene Ther 2001;8(11):879–889.
10. Borok Z, Harboe-Schmidt JE, Brody SL, et al. Vesicular stomatitis virus G-pseudotyped lentivirus vectors mediate efficient apical transduction of polarized quiescent primary alveolar epithelial cells. J Virol 2001;75(23):11,747–11,754.
11. Li W, Nadelman C, Gratch NS, Chen M, Kasahara N, Woodley DT. An important role for protein kinase C-delta in human keratinocyte migration on dermal collagen. Exp Cell Res 2002;273(2): 219–228.
12. Chen M, Kasahara N, Keene DR, et al. Restoration of type VII collagen expression and function in dystrophic epidermolysis bullosa. Nat Genet 2002;32(4):670–675.
13. Koya RC, Kasahara N, Favaro PM, et al. Potent maturation of monocyte-derived dendritic cells after CD40L lentiviral gene delivery. J Immunother 2003;26(5):451–460.

14. Zufferey R, Nagy D, Mandel RJ, Naldini L, Trono D. Multiply attenuated lentiviral vector achieves efficient gene delivery in vivo. Nat Biotechnol 1997;15(9):871–875.
15. Dull T, Zufferey R, Kelly M, et al. A third-generation lentivirus vector with a conditional packaging system. J Virol 1998;72(11):8463–8471.
16. Kawakami Y, Dang N, Wang X, et al. Recognition of shared melanoma antigens in association with major HLA-A alleles by tumor infiltrating T lymphocytes from 123 patients with melanoma. J Immunother 2000;23(1):17–27.
17. Goujon C, Jarrosson-Wuilleme L, Bernaud J, Rigal D, Darlix JL, Cimarelli A. Heterologous human immunodeficiency virus type 1 lentiviral vectors packaging a simian immunodeficiency virus-derived genome display a specific postentry transduction defect in dendritic cells. J Virol 2003;77 (17):9295–9304.
18. Browning MT, Schmidt RD, Lew KA, Rizvi TA. Primate and feline lentivirus vector RNA packaging and propagation by heterologous lentivirus virions. J Virol 2001;75(11):5129–5140.
19. Follenzi A, Ailles LE, Bakovic S, Geuna M, Naldini L. Gene transfer by lentiviral vectors is limited by nuclear translocation and rescued by HIV-1 pol sequences. Nat Genet 2000;25(2):217–222.
20. Sirven A, Pflumio F, Zennou V, et al. The human immunodeficiency virus type-1 central DNA flap is a crucial determinant for lentiviral vector nuclear import and gene transduction of human hematopoietic stem cells. Blood 2000;96(13):4103–4110.
21. Dardalhon V, Herpers B, Noraz N, et al. Lentivirus-mediated gene transfer in primary T cells is enhanced by a central DNA flap. Gene Ther 2001;8(3):190–198.
22. Anderson WF, Blaese RM, Culver K. The ADA human gene therapy clinical protocol: Points to Consider response with clinical protocol, July 6, 1990. Hum Gene Ther 1990;1(3):331–362.
23. Cavazzana-Calvo M, Hacein-Bey S, de Saint Basile G, et al. Gene therapy of human severe combined immunodeficiency (SCID)-X1 disease. Science 2000;288(5466):669–672.
24. Aiuti A, Slavin S, Aker M, et al. Correction of ADA-SCID by stem cell gene therapy combined with nonmyeloablative conditioning. Science 2002;296(5577):2410–2413.
25. Soudais C, Shiho T, Sharara LI, et al. Stable and functional lymphoid reconstitution of common cytokine receptor gamma chain deficient mice by retroviral-mediated gene transfer. Blood 2000;95 (10):3071–3077.
26. Hacein-Bey S, Gross F, Nusbaum P, et al. Optimization of retroviral gene transfer protocol to maintain the lymphoid potential of progenitor cells. Hum Gene Ther 2001;12(3):291–301.
27. Sutton RE, Wu HT, Rigg R, Bohnlein E, Brown PO. Human immunodeficiency virus type 1 vectors efficiently transduce human hematopoietic stem cells. J Virol 1998;72(7):5781–5788.
28. Uchida N, Sutton RE, Friera AM, et al. HIV, but not murine leukemia virus, vectors mediate high efficiency gene transfer into freshly isolated G0/G1 human hematopoietic stem cells. Proc Natl Acad Sci U S A 1998;95(20):11,939–11,944.
29. Case SS, Price MA, Jordan CT, et al. Stable transduction of quiescent CD34(+)CD38(-) human hematopoietic cells by HIV-1-based lentiviral vectors. Proc Natl Acad Sci U S A 1999;96(6): 2988–2993.
30. Miyoshi H, Smith KA, Mosier DE, Verma IM, Torbett BE. Transduction of human CD34+ cells that mediate long-term engraftment of NOD/SCID mice by HIV vectors. Science 1999;283(5402): 682–686.
31. Gao Z, Golob J, Tanavde VM, Civin CI, Hawley RG, Cheng L. High levels of transgene expression following transduction of long-term NOD/SCID-repopulating human cells with a modified lentiviral vector. Stem Cells 2001;19(3):247–259.
32. Gatlin J, Padgett A, Melkus MW, Kelly PF, Garcia JV. Long-term engraftment of nonobese diabetic/severe combined immunodeficient mice with human CD34+ cells transduced by a self-inactivating human immunodeficiency virus type 1 vector. Hum Gene Ther 2001;12(9):1079–1089.
33. Woods NB, Fahlman C, Mikkola H, et al. Lentiviral gene transfer into primary and secondary NOD/SCID repopulating cells. Blood 2000;96(12):3725–3733.
34. Ailles L, Schmidt M, Santoni de Sio FR, et al. Molecular evidence of lentiviral vector-mediated gene transfer into human self-renewing, multi-potent, long-term NOD/SCID repopulating hematopoietic cells. Mol Ther 2002;6(5):615–626.
35. Scherr M, Battmer K, Blomer U, et al. Lentiviral gene transfer into peripheral blood-derived CD34+ NOD/SCID-repopulating cells. Blood 2002;99(2):709–712.
36. Barrette S, Douglas JL, Seidel NE, Bodine DM. Lentivirus-based vectors transduce mouse hematopoietic stem cells with similar efficiency to moloney murine leukemia virus-based vectors. Blood 2000;96(10):3385–3391.

37. Mikkola H, Woods NB, Sjogren M, et al. Lentivirus gene transfer in murine hematopoietic progenitor cells is compromised by a delay in proviral integration and results in transduction mosaicism and heterogeneous gene expression in progeny cells. J Virol 2000;74(24):11,911–11,918.
38. Horn PA, Morris JC, Bukovsky AA, et al. Lentivirus-mediated gene transfer into hematopoietic repopulating cells in baboons. Gene Ther 2002;9(21):1464–1471.
39. An DS, Wersto RP, Agricola BA, et al. Marking and gene expression by a lentivirus vector in transplanted human and nonhuman primate CD34(+) cells. J Virol 2000;74(3):1286–1295.
40. Hanawa H, Hematti P, Keyvanfar K, et al. Efficient gene transfer into rhesus repopulating hematopoietic stem cells using a simian immunodeficiency virus-based lentiviral vector system. Blood 2004;103(11):4062–4069.
41. Kootstra NA, Munk C, Tonnu N, Landau NR, Verma IM. Abrogation of postentry restriction of HIV-1-based lentiviral vector transduction in simian cells. Proc Natl Acad Sci U S A 2003;100(3): 1298–1303.
42. Kung SK, An DS, Bonifacino A, et al. Induction of transgene-specific immunological tolerance in myeloablated nonhuman primates using lentivirally transduced CD34+ progenitor cells. Mol Ther 2003;8(6):981–991.
43. O'Shaughnessy JA, Cowan KH, Nienhuis AW, et al. Retroviral mediated transfer of the human multidrug resistance gene (MDR-1) into hematopoietic stem cells during autologous transplantation after intensive chemotherapy for metastatic breast cancer. Hum Gene Ther 1994;5(7):891–911.
44. Carpinteiro A, Peinert S, Ostertag W, et al. Genetic protection of repopulating hematopoietic cells with an improved MDR1-retrovirus allows administration of intensified chemotherapy following stem cell transplantation in mice. Int J Cancer 2002;98(5):785–792.
45. Schiedlmeier B, Wermann K, Kuhlcke K, et al. Human multidrug resistance-1 gene transfer to long-term repopulating human mobilized peripheral blood progenitor cells. Bone Marrow Transplant 2000;25 Suppl 2:S118–124.
46. Laufs S, Baum C, Fruehauf S. Transplantation of human hematopoietic progenitor cells transduced with a retroviral vector containing the human multidrug-resistance-1 gene for myeloprotective gene therapy. Transplant Proc 2002;34(6):2325–2329.
47. Bunting KD, Galipeau J, Topham D, Benaim E, Sorrentino BP. Transduction of murine bone marrow cells with an MDR1 vector enables ex vivo stem cell expansion, but these expanded grafts cause a myeloproliferative syndrome in transplanted mice. Blood 1998;92(7):2269–2279.
48. Zielske SP, Reese JS, Lingas KT, Donze JR, Gerson SL. In vivo selection of MGMT(P140K) lentivirus-transduced human NOD/SCID repopulating cells without pretransplant irradiation conditioning. J Clin Invest 2003;112(10):1561–1570.
49. Pollok KE, Hartwell JR, Braber A, et al. In vivo selection of human hematopoietic cells in a xenograft model using combined pharmacologic and genetic manipulations. Hum Gene Ther 2003;14(18): 1703–1714.
50. Persons DA, Allay ER, Sawai N, et al. Successful treatment of murine beta-thalassemia using in vivo selection of genetically modified, drug-resistant hematopoietic stem cells. Blood 2003;102(2):506–513.
51. Neff T, Horn PA, Peterson LJ, et al. Methylguanine methyltransferase-mediated in vivo selection and chemoprotection of allogeneic stem cells in a large-animal model. J Clin Invest 2003;112(10): 1581–1588.
52. Quinn JA, Pluda J, Dolan ME, et al. Phase II trial of carmustine plus O(6)-benzylguanine for patients with nitrosourea-resistant recurrent or progressive malignant glioma. J Clin Oncol 2002;20(9): 2277–2283.
53. Junker K, Koehl U, Zimmerman S, et al. Kinetics of cell death in T lymphocytes genetically modified with two novel suicide fusion genes. Gene Ther 2003;10(14):1189–1197.
54. Bordignon C, Bonini C, Verzeletti S, et al. Transfer of the HSV-tk gene into donor peripheral blood lymphocytes for in vivo modulation of donor anti-tumor immunity after allogeneic bone marrow transplantation. Hum Gene Ther 1995;6(6):813–819.
55. Litvinova E, Maury S, Boyer O, et al. Graft-versus-leukemia effect after suicide-gene-mediated control of graft-versus-host disease. Blood 2002;100(6):2020–2025.
56. Marktel S, Magnani Z, Ciceri F, et al. Immunologic potential of donor lymphocytes expressing a suicide gene for early immune reconstitution after hematopoietic T-cell-depleted stem cell transplantation. Blood 2003;101(4):1290–1298.
57. Zhao RC, McIvor RS, Griffin JD, Verfaillie CM. Gene therapy for chronic myelogenous leukemia (CML): a retroviral vector that renders hematopoietic progenitors methotrexate-resistant and CML progenitors functionally normal and nontumorigenic in vivo. Blood 1997;90(12):4687–4698.

58. Tanabe T, Kuwabara T, Warashina M, Tani K, Taira K, Asano S. Oncogene inactivation in a mouse model. Nature 2000;406(6795):473–474.
59. Wilda M, Fuchs U, Wossmann W, Borkhardt A. Killing of leukemic cells with a BCR/ABL fusion gene by RNA interference (RNAi). Oncogene 2002;21(37):5716–5724.
60. Scherr M, Battmer K, Winkler T, Heidenreich O, Ganser A, Eder M. Specific inhibition of bcr-abl gene expression by small interfering RNA. Blood 2003;101(4):1566–1569.
61. Soda Y, Tani K, Bai Y, et al. A novel maxizyme vector targeting a bcr-abl fusion gene induced specific cell death in Philadelphia chromosome-positive acute lymphoblastic leukemia. Blood 2004;104 (2):356–363.
62. Banchereau J, Steinman RM. Dendritic cells and the control of immunity. Nature 1998;392(6673): 245–252.
63. Schuler G, Steinman RM. Dendritic cells as adjuvants for immune-mediated resistance to tumors. J Exp Med 1997;186(8):1183–1187.
64. Ribas A, Butterfield LH, Hu B, et al. Generation of T-cell immunity to a murine melanoma using MART-1-engineered dendritic cells. J Immunother 2000;23(1):59–66.
65. Romani N, Gruner S, Brang D, et al. Proliferating dendritic cell progenitors in human blood. J Exp Med 1994;180(1):83–93.
66. Sallusto F, Lanzavecchia A. Efficient presentation of soluble antigen by cultured human dendritic cells is maintained by granulocyte/macrophage colony-stimulating factor plus interleukin 4 and downregulated by tumor necrosis factor alpha. J Exp Med 1994;179(4):1109–1118.
67. Kirk CJ, Mule JJ. Gene-modified dendritic cells for use in tumor vaccines. Hum Gene Ther 2000;11(6):797–806.
68. Ranieri E, Herr W, Gambotto A, et al. Dendritic cells transduced with an adenovirus vector encoding Epstein- Barr virus latent membrane protein 2B: a new modality for vaccination. J Virol 1999;73(12):10,416–10,425.
69. Ribas A, Butterfield LH, Amarnani SN, et al. CD40 cross-linking bypasses the absolute requirement for CD4 T cells during immunization with melanoma antigen gene-modified dendritic cells. Cancer Res 2001;61(24):8787–8793.
70. Molnar-Kimber KL, Sterman DH, Chang M, et al. Impact of preexisting and induced humoral and cellular immune responses in an adenovirus-based gene therapy phase I clinical trial for localized mesothelioma. Hum Gene Ther 1998;9(14):2121–2133.
71. Jooss K, Yang Y, Fisher KJ, Wilson JM. Transduction of dendritic cells by DNA viral vectors directs the immune response to transgene products in muscle fibers. J Virol 1998;72(5):4212–4223.
72. Korst RJ, Mahtabifard A, Yamada R, Crystal RG. Effect of adenovirus gene transfer vectors on the immunologic functions of mouse dendritic cells. Mol Ther 2002;5(3):307–315.
73. Schroers R, Sinha I, Segall H, et al. Transduction of human PBMC-derived dendritic cells and macrophages by an HIV-1-based lentiviral vector system. Mol Ther 2000;1(2):171–179.
74. Dyall J, Latouche JB, Schnell S, Sadelain M. Lentivirus-transduced human monocyte-derived dendritic cells efficiently stimulate antigen-specific cytotoxic T lymphocytes. Blood 2001;97(1): 114–121.
75. Gruber A, Kan-Mitchell J, Kuhen KL, Mukai T, Wong-Staal F. Dendritic cells transduced by multiply deleted HIV-1 vectors exhibit normal phenotypes and functions and elicit an HIV-specific cytotoxic T- lymphocyte response in vitro. Blood 2000;96(4):1327–1333.
76. Koya RC, Weber JS, Kasahara N, et al. Making dendritic cells from the inside out: lentiviral vector-mediated gene delivery of granulocyte-macrophage colony-stimulating factor and interleukin 4 into CD14+ monocytes generates dendritic cells in vitro. Hum Gene Ther 2004;15(8):733–748.
77. Stripecke R, Koya RC, Ta HQ, Kasahara N, Levine AM. The use of lentiviral vectors in gene therapy of leukemia: combinatorial gene delivery of immunomodulators into leukemia cells by state-of-the-art vectors. Blood Cells Mol Dis 2003;31(1):28–37.
78. Mascarenhas L, Stripecke R, Case SS, Xu D, Weinberg KI, Kohn DB. Gene delivery to human B-precursor acute lymphoblastic leukemia cells. Blood 1998;92(10):3537–3545.
79. Dilloo D, Rill D, Entwistle C, et al. A novel herpes vector for the high-efficiency transduction of normal and malignant human hematopoietic cells. Blood 1997;89(1):119–127.
80. Anderson R, Macdonald I, Corbett T, Hacking G, Lowdell MW, Prentice HG. Construction and biological characterization of an interleukin-12 fusion protein (Flexi-12): delivery to acute myeloid leukemic blasts using adeno-associated virus. Hum Gene Ther 1997;8(9):1125–1135.
81. Planken EV, Willemze R, Kluin-Nelemans JC. The role of the CD40 antigen on malignant B cells. Leuk Lymphoma 1996;22(3-4):229–235.

82. Stripecke R, Cardoso AA, Pepper KA, et al. Lentiviral vectors for efficient delivery of CD80 and granulocyte- macrophage- colony-stimulating factor in human acute lymphoblastic leukemia and acute myeloid leukemia cells to induce antileukemic immune responses. Blood 2000;96(4):1317–1326.
83. Koya RC, Kasahara N, Pullarkat V, Levine AM, Stripecke R. Transduction of acute myeloid leukemia cells with third generation self- inactivating lentiviral vectors expressing CD80 and GM-CSF: effects on proliferation, differentiation, and stimulation of allogeneic and autologous anti-leukemia immune responses. Leukemia 2002;16(9):1645–1654.
84. Bonamino M, Serafini M, D'Amico G, et al. Functional transfer of CD40L gene in human B-cell precursor ALL blasts by second-generation SIN lentivectors. Gene Ther 2004;11(1):85–93.
85. Thaler S, Burger AM, Schulz T, Schnierle BS. MLV/HIV-pseudotyped vectors: a new treatment option for cutaneous T cell lymphomas. Mol Ther 2003;8(5):756–761.
86. De Vos J, Bagnis C, Bonnafoux L, et al. Comparison of murine leukemia virus, human immunodeficiency virus, and adeno-associated virus vectors for gene transfer in multiple myeloma: lentiviral vectors demonstrate a striking capacity to transduce low-proliferating primary tumor cells. Hum Gene Ther 2003;14(18):1727–1739.
87. Ezzeddine ZD, Martuza RL, Platika D, et al. Selective killing of glioma cells in culture and in vivo by retrovirus transfer of the herpes simplex virus thymidine kinase gene. New Biologist 1991;3(6):608–614.
88. Culver KW, Ram Z, Wallbridge S, Ishii H, Oldfield EH, Blaese RM. In vivo gene transfer with retroviral vector-producer cells for treatment of experimental brain tumors. Science 1992;256 (5063):1550–1552.
89. Rainov NG. A phase III clinical evaluation of herpes simplex virus type 1 thymidine kinase and ganciclovir gene therapy as an adjuvant to surgical resection and radiation in adults with previously untreated glioblastoma multiforme. Hum Gene Ther 2000;11(17):2389–2401.
90. Tamura K, Tamura M, Ikenaka K, et al. Eradication of murine brain tumors by direct inoculation of concentrated high titer-recombinant retrovirus harboring the herpes simplex virus thymidine kinase gene. Gene Ther 2001;8(3):215–222.
91. Prados MD, McDermott M, Chang SM, et al. Treatment of progressive or recurrent glioblastoma multiforme in adults with herpes simplex virus thymidine kinase gene vector-producer cells followed by intravenous ganciclovir administration: a phase I/II multi-institutional trial. J Neurooncol 2003;65(3):269–278.
92. Roth JA, Nguyen D, Lawrence DD, et al. Retrovirus-mediated wild-type p53 gene transfer to tumors of patients with lung cancer. Nat Med 1996;2(9):985–991.
93. Tait DL, Obermiller PS, Redlin-Frazier S, et al. A phase I trial of retroviral BRCA1sv gene therapy in ovarian cancer. Clin Cancer Res 1997;3(11):1959–1968.
94. Moon C, Oh Y, Roth JA. Current status of gene therapy for lung cancer and head and neck cancer. Clin Cancer Res 2003;9(14):5055–5067.
95. Tait DL, Obermiller PS, Hatmaker AR, Redlin-Frazier S, Holt JT. Ovarian cancer BRCA1 gene therapy: Phase I and II trial differences in immune response and vector stability. Clin Cancer Res 1999;5(7):1708–1714.
96. Gordon EM, Cornelio GH, Lorenzo CC, 3rd, et al. First clinical experience using a 'pathotropic' injectable retroviral vector (Rexin-G) as intervention for stage IV pancreatic cancer. Int J Oncol 2004;24(1):177–185.
97. Tan Y, Xu M, Wang W, et al. IL-2 gene therapy of advanced lung cancer patients. Anticancer Res 1996;16(4A):1993–1998.
98. Nemunaitis J, Buchanan A, Jolly DJ. Long-term follow-up of retroviral vector-administered interferon-gamma (IFN-gamma) gene in metastatic melanoma. Cancer Gene Ther 2000;7(10): 1297–1298.
99. Kang WK, Park C, Yoon HL, et al. Interleukin 12 gene therapy of cancer by peritumoral injection of transduced autologous fibroblasts: outcome of a phase I study. Hum Gene Ther 2001;12(6): 671–684.
100. Pan D, Gunther R, Duan W, et al. Biodistribution and toxicity studies of VSVG-pseudotyped lentiviral vector after intravenous administration in mice with the observation of in vivo transduction of bone marrow. Mol Ther 2002;6(1):19–29.
101. Ohashi K, Park F, Schwall R, Kay M. Efficient gene transduction to cultured hepatocytes by HIV-1 derived lentiviral vector. Transplant Proc 2002;34(5):1431–1433.
102. VandenDriessche T, Thorrez L, Naldini L, et al. Lentiviral vectors containing the human immunodeficiency virus type-1 central polypurine tract can efficiently transduce nondividing hepatocytes and antigen-presenting cells in vivo. Blood 2002;100(3):813–822.

103. De Palma M, Venneri MA, Naldini L. In vivo targeting of tumor endothelial cells by systemic delivery of lentiviral vectors. Hum Gene Ther 2003;14(12):1193–1206.
104. Follenzi A, Sabatino G, Lombardo A, Boccaccio C, Naldini L. Efficient gene delivery and targeted expression to hepatocytes in vivo by improved lentiviral vectors. Hum Gene Ther 2002;13(2):243–260.
105. Follenzi A, Battaglia M, Lombardo A, Annoni A, Roncarolo MG, Naldini L. Targeting lentiviral vector expression to hepatocytes limits transgene-specific immune response and establishes long-term expression of human antihemophilic factor IX in mice. Blood 2004;103(10):3700–3709.
106. Firat H, Zennou V, Garcia-Pons F, et al. Use of a lentiviral flap vector for induction of CTL immunity against melanoma. Perspectives for immunotherapy. J Gene Med 2002;4(1):38–45.
107. Palmowski MJ, Lopes L, Ikeda Y, Salio M, Cerundolo V, Collins MK. Intravenous injection of a lentiviral vector encoding NY-ESO-1 induces an effective CTL response. J Immunol 2004;172(3):1582–1587.
108. Esslinger C, Chapatte L, Finke D, et al. In vivo administration of a lentiviral vaccine targets DCs and induces efficient CD8(+) T cell responses. J Clin Invest 2003;111(11):1673–1681.
109. Indraccolo S, Habeler W, Tisato V, et al. Gene transfer in ovarian cancer cells: a comparison between retroviral and lentiviral vectors. Cancer Res 2002;62(21):6099–6107.
110. Bastide C, Maroc N, Bladou F, et al. Expression of a model gene in prostate cancer cells lentivirally transduced in vitro and in vivo. Prostate Cancer Prostatic Dis 2003;6(3):228–234.
111. Yu D, Jia WW, Gleave ME, Nelson CC, Rennie PS. Prostate-tumor targeting of gene expression by lentiviral vectors containing elements of the probasin promoter. Prostate 2004;59(4):370–382.
112. Kong B, Wang W, Liu C, et al. Efficacy of lentivirus-mediated and MUC1 antibody-targeted VP22-TK/GCV suicide gene therapy for ovarian cancer. In Vivo 2003;17(2):153–156.
113. Gerolami R, Uch R, Faivre J, et al. Herpes simplex virus thymidine kinase-mediated suicide gene therapy for hepatocellular carcinoma using HIV-1-derived lentiviral vectors. J Hepatol 2004;40(2):291–297.
114. Zheng JY, Chen D, Chan J, Yu D, Ko E, Pang S. Regression of prostate cancer xenografts by a lentiviral vector specifically expressing diphtheria toxin A. Cancer Gene Ther 2003;10(10):764–770.
115. Pang S, Kang MK, Kung S, et al. Anticancer effect of a lentiviral vector capable of expressing HIV-1 Vpr. Clin Cancer Res 2001;7(11):3567–3573.
116. Diaz RM, Bateman A, Emiliusen L, et al. A lentiviral vector expressing a fusogenic glycoprotein for cancer gene therapy. Gene Ther 2000;7(19):1656–1663.
117. Logg CR, Tai CK, Logg A, Anderson WF, Kasahara N. A uniquely stable replication-competent retrovirus vector achieves efficient gene delivery in vitro and in solid tumors. Hum Gene Ther 2001;12(8):921–932.
118. Wang WJ, Tai CK, Kasahara N, Chen TC. Highly efficient and tumor-restricted gene transfer to malignant gliomas by replication-competent retroviral vectors. Hum Gene Ther 2003;14(2):117–127.
119. Tai CK, Logg CR, Park JM, Anderson WF, Press MF, Kasahara N. Antibody-mediated targeting of replication-competent retroviral vectors. Hum Gene Ther 2003;14(8):789–802.
120. Soifer H, Higo C, Logg CR, et al. A novel, helper-dependent, adenovirus-retrovirus hybrid vector: stable transduction by a two-stage mechanism. Mol Ther 2002;5(5 Pt 1):599–608.
121. Logg CR, Logg A, Matusik RJ, Bochner BH, Kasahara N. Tissue-specific transcriptional targeting of a replication-competent retroviral vector. J Virol 2002;76(24):12,783–12,791.
122. Takeuchi Y, Porter CD, Strahan KM, et al. Sensitization of cells and retroviruses to human serum by (alpha 1-3) galactosyltransferase. Nature 1996;379(6560):85–88.
123. DePolo NJ, Harkleroad CE, Bodner M, et al. The resistance of retroviral vectors produced from human cells to serum inactivation in vivo and in vitro is primate species dependent. J Virol 1999;73(8):6708–6714.
124. Donahue RE, Kessler SW, Bodine D, et al. Helper virus induced T cell lymphoma in nonhuman primates after retroviral mediated gene transfer. J Exp Med 1992;176(4):1125–1135.
125. Cornetta K, Moen RC, Culver K, et al. Amphotropic murine leukemia retrovirus is not an acute pathogen for primates. Hum Gene Ther 1990;1(1):15–30.
126. Cornetta K, Morgan RA, Gillio A, et al. No retroviremia or pathology in long-term follow-up of monkeys exposed to a murine amphotropic retrovirus. Hum Gene Ther 1991;2(3):215–219.
127. Marshall E. Clinical research. Gene therapy a suspect in leukemia-like disease. Science 2002;298(5591):34–35.
128. Hacein-Bey-Abina S, Von Kalle C, Schmidt M, et al. LMO2-associated clonal T cell proliferation in two patients after gene therapy for SCID-X1. Science 2003;302(5644):415–419.

129. Gaspar HB, Parsley KL, Howe S, et al. Gene therapy of X-linked severe combined immunodeficiency by use of a pseudotyped gammaretroviral vector. Lancet 2004;364(9452):2181–2187.
130. Kiem HP, Sellers S, Thomasson B, et al. Long-term clinical and molecular follow-up of large animals receiving retrovirally transduced stem and progenitor cells: no progression to clonal hematopoiesis or leukemia. Mol Ther 2004;9(3):389–395.
131. Sadelain M. Insertional oncogenesis in gene therapy: how much of a risk? Gene Ther 2004;11(7): 569–573.
132. Baum C, von Kalle C, Staal FJ, et al. Chance or necessity? Insertional mutagenesis in gene therapy and its consequences. Mol Ther 2004;9(1):5–13.
133. Yu SF, von Ruden T, Kantoff PW, et al. Self-inactivating retroviral vectors designed for transfer of whole genes into mammalian cells. Proc Natl Acad Sci USA 1986;83(10):3194–3198.
134. Zufferey R, Dull T, Mandel RJ, et al. Self-inactivating lentivirus vector for safe and efficient in vivo gene delivery. J Virol 1998;72(12):9873–9880.
135. Chung JH, Bell AC, Felsenfeld G. Characterization of the chicken beta-globin insulator. Proc Natl Acad Sci U S A 1997;94(2):575–580.
136. Ramezani A, Hawley TS, Hawley RG. Performance- and safety-enhanced lentiviral vectors containing the human interferon-beta scaffold attachment region and the chicken beta-globin insulator. Blood 2003;101(12):4717–4724.
137. Logan AC, Haas DL, Kafri T, Kohn DB. Integrated self-inactivating lentiviral vectors produce full-length genomic transcripts competent for encapsidation and integration. J Virol 2004;78(16): 8421–8436.
138. Jakobsson J, Rosenqvist N, Thompson L, Barraud P, Lundberg C. Dynamics of transgene expression in a neural stem cell line transduced with lentiviral vectors incorporating the cHS4 insulator. Exp Cell Res 2004;298(2):611–623.
139. Bushman FD. Integration site selection by lentiviruses: biology and possible control. Curr Top Microbiol Immunol 2002;261:165–177.
140. Schroder AR, Shinn P, Chen H, Berry C, Ecker JR, Bushman F. HIV-1 integration in the human genome favors active genes and local hotspots. Cell 2002;110(4):521–529.
141. Mitchell RS, Beitzel BF, Schroder AR, et al. Retroviral DNA integration: ASLV, HIV, and MLV show distinct target site preferences. PLoS Biol 2004;2(8):E234.
141a. American Society of Hematology Meeting. Blood 2004;104(11):579a.
142. Solly SK, Trajcevski S, Frisen C, et al. Replicative retroviral vectors for cancer gene therapy. Cancer Gene Ther 2003;10(1):30–39.
143. Ruprecht RM, Chou TC, Chipty F, et al. Interferon-alpha and 3′-azido-3′-deoxythymidine are highly synergistic in mice and prevent viremia after acute retrovirus exposure. J Acquir Immune Defic Syndr 1990;3(6):591–600.
144. Frank O, Rudolph C, Heberlein C, et al. Tumor cells escape suicide gene therapy by genetic and epigenetic instability. Blood 2004;104(12):3543–3549.

4 Vaccinia and Pox-Virus

Sricharan Chalikonda, MD
and David L. Bartlett, MD

CONTENTS

Summary

Vaccinia virus has been studied extensively since its discovery as a smallpox vaccine in 1798. Its use as a smallpox vaccine documented its safety profile. It was later found that its large size and ability to accept large fragments of DNA combined with its natural tumor affinity make it an attractive agent for cancer therapy.

This chapter discusses the history of the vaccinia, the various strains available, the biology of the virus as well as the steps in creating recombinants. The various clinical and safety considerations will be addressed. We will also discuss the various methods used to treat cancer using the vaccinia virus and will review the recent clinical trials using vaccinia in the treatment of cancer.

Key Words: Vaccinia; pox viruses; oncolytic viruse; extracellular enveloped virus; intracellular mature virus.

1. INTRODUCTION

The concept of tumor directed viral therapy has been extensively studied over the past few decades. Creating a tumor-specific cytotoxic virus that has minimal toxicity to the host has long been considered the "holy grail" amongst researchers and clinicians alike. There are several viruses that are currently being studied as possible vectors for tumor directed therapy including adenovirus, herpes simplex, reovirus, Newcastle disease virus, and the vaccinia virus. The use of vaccinia as a cancer treatment modality is a focus of many ongoing laboratory and clinical research projects. Several avenues are

From: *Cancer Drug Discovery and Development: Gene Therapy for Cancer*
Edited by: K. K. Hunt, S. A. Vorburger, and S. G. Swisher © Humana Press Inc., Totowa, NJ

currently being explored including: (1) vaccinia as vector for gene delivery; (2) vaccinia as a tumor vaccine; and (3) vaccinia as an oncolytic agent.

2. CHARACTERISTICS

Vaccinia virus is a member of the pox family of viruses. It comprises a family of complex DNA viruses that replicate in the cytoplasm of both vertebrate and invertebrate cells. They can be classified into two subfamilies based on host species: chordopoxvirinae (vertebrate poxviruses) and entomopoxvirinae (insect poxviruses) *(1–3)*. Its clinical use dates back more than 150 yr to 1798, when Edward Jenner demonstrated that vaccination with the cowpox virus offered protection from smallpox. Vaccinia was used for widespread vaccination against smallpox until 1978 when smallpox was declared eradicated.

Vaccinia virus has many attributes which make it an attractive vector for tumor directed therapy including: (1) a quick lifecycle with the ability to form mature virions within 6 h of infection; (2) the ability to spread from cell to cell efficiently; (3) a large genome which allows it to accept large fragments of DNA without deletion; (4) the ability to achieve high levels of transgene expression; and (5) most importantly, it can infect a large range of human tissues without causing any known human disease *(4)*. Another very interesting quality of vaccinia virus is its affinity to replicate selectively in tumor tissue making it potentially valuable for tumor targeting strategies. This tumor affinity combined with the properties mentioned above make the vaccinia virus the focus of ongoing anticancer research worldwide.

3. BIOLOGY OF VACCINIA VIRUS

The vaccinia virus exists in two infectious forms. The intracellular mature virus (IMV) is released upon cellular disruption during the viral purification process, which is the form found in vitro. It has a single outer membrane derived from the *trans*-golgi network membrane. The extracellular enveloped virus (EEV) is responsible for cell–cell spread in vivo. It incorporates an outer membrane derived from the cell membrane. The EEV is not able to be purifed in vitro as a result of the fragility of its outer envelope which does not withstand the purification process *(5)*.

The mechanism of attachment and uptake of the vaccinia virus remains unclear because of its various infectious forms and variety of cellular receptors and viral proteins *(1,9,10)*. No definite cellular receptor for vaccina virus has been identified. Confocal microscopy has shown that IMV and EEV enter cells by different mechanisms *(11)*. Both attach to cells via different proteins allowing the virus to enter by membrane fusion. The IMV envelope proteins A17L, A27L, and D8L may be instrumental in viral attachment. The D8L protein was one of the earliest IMV membrane proteins identified and is thought to mediate IMV binding to cell surface chondroitin sulfate *(12,13)*. The A27L protein may mediate vaccinia attachment through cell surface heparin sulfate; this was shown by demonstrating a 60% viral inhibition in the presence of soluble heparin sulfate *(7)*. The EEV is the infectious form responsible for cell–cell transmission in vivo. To date, 6 EEV specific membrane proteins (A33R, A34R, A36R, A56R, B5R, and F13L) have been identified *(1)*. It has been found that the A56R protein can be mutated without affecting infectivity *(14)*.

Vaccinia have been engineered to circumvent the normal cell receptor requirements by binding to alternate cell-surface molecules. Expression of an ScFv to erbB2 on the

these cytokines naturally suppress the host response to vaccinia. IL-10 knockout mice thereby exhibited greater inhibition of viral replication than IL-4 deficient mice. When the effects of each cytokine was examined in the infection with recombinant vaccinia virus constructs, local expression of IL-4 showed a much greater inhibition of host responses. In fact, whereas the absence of IL-10 resulted in improved clearance of IL-6 and IL-1, the local expression of IL-10 had little to no effect on viral clearance. Similarly, Deonarain et al. have shown that IFN-α/β knockout mice demonstrate markedly enhanced susceptibility to vaccinia viral infection *(53)*. Other studies have shown that IL-12 and IL-18 act synergistically to clear vaccinia infection and that virus clearance involves NK and T-cells *(54)*.

6. STRATEGIES IN VACCINIA GENE THERAPY TO EVADE IMMUNE CLEARANCE

The clearance of the virus in vivo needs to be overcome in order to deliver an adequate amount of virus to the tumor and allow time for viral replication. Several strategies have been tested to overcome this barrier. The first strategy is to create a virus that is less recognizable by the immune system. The problem with this method is that the vaccinia virus presents a broad spectrum of antigens to the host. Hence, one or two mutations in the viral envelope would probably not be sufficient to avoid detection by the immune system. The other issue with altering the viral envelope is that the alteration may result in decrease infectivity of the virus.

The second strategy involves developing other pox viruses that are able to selectively infect and lyse human tumor cells without crossreacting with vaccinia. Examples include Yatapox virus, Yaba like disease virus, and Avian poxvirus. The problem with these alternative viruses is that they do not replicate in human cells and are less efficient vectors *(55–57)*.

The third strategy involves using immunosuppressive agents to increase the viral load and the time of expression in tumor cells. Unpublished studies from our group have found that immunosuppressive therapy increased viral recovery and tumor response in animal models without increasing the pathogenicity. Because of the knowledge gained from transplantation, specific agents are now availablet that allow for targeting of the immune system selectively on various effector pathways. The use of immune modulation to overcome preformed antibodies may be useful in the future for treating patients with prior smallpox vaccination.

7. CLINICAL SAFETY

There is extensive data regarding the overall safety of the vaccinia virus, which was generated during its use in the eradication of smallpox. The complications associated with vaccinia virus include encephalitis, vaccinia necrosum, and eczema vaccinatum. These complications are more prevalent in immunocomprimised individuals and infants (*see* Fig. 2) *(34–36)*.

Vaccinia associated encephalitis results from infection of the central nervous system (CNS). Studies have shown viral recovery from the CNS of patients suffering from vaccinia associated encephalitis *(35)*. This dreaded complication can be avoided by use of a tumor selective vaccinia virus.

Vaccinia necrosum is a progressive necrotic ulcer caused by the vaccinia virus. It is more common in immunosuppressed patients and can destroy significant amounts of

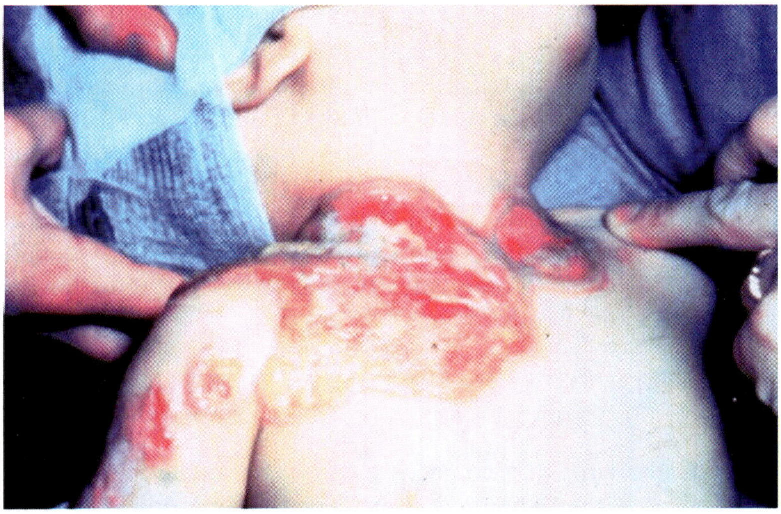

Fig. 2. Vaccinia necrosum. This picture illustrates the complication related to the administration of vaccinia virus. This followed smallpox vaccination in a young child.

tissue producing significant morbidity. The extensive tissue loss may require reconstruction with tissue grafts and can sometimes require amputation. Surprisingly, this dramatic local infection does not cause a systemic viral spread.

Eczema vaccinatum originates from the infection of eczematous skin throughout the body by vaccinia. It causes a large viral load that induces viremia with fever and malaise and can sometimes progress to death. Although rare, the side effects of vaccinia virus have been the focus of multiple laboratory experiments and animal models suggest a role of inflammatory cytokines in the pathogenicity of viral infection.

8. VACCINIA AS A CANCER VACCINE

The experience with vaccinia in the eradication of smallpox led to research into its use as an antitumor vaccine. Vaccinia was engineered to express tumor antigens and serve as a cancer vaccine. The size of the potential transgene that can be put into the vaccinia vector allows for flexibility in engineering, such that immune enhancing genes and antigenetic genes can be recombined into the genome. The immunostimulatory effects and efficient transcriptional machinery of the virus were utilized to create various cancer vaccine vectors (Table 2).

Recently, a phase I clinical trial of vaccinia expressing prostate specific antigen (PSA) in prostate cancer patients was published. In this trial the Wyeth strain virus was delivered intradermally every 4 wk for three doses without producing significant systemic toxicities. A cutaneous reaction, consistent with viral replication was seen in all patients treated with the virus at a dose of 2.65×10^7 pfu. Several patients developed T-cell immune responses to PSA associated with prolonged periods before disease progression *(55)*. Another phase II clinical trial by the NCI examines the potential of three strains of recombinant vaccinia virus expressing either PSA, B7.1, or of the fowlpox virus expressing PSA. Vaccinia expressing the tumor antigen carcino embryonic antigen (CEA) has been studied clinically as a priming vaccine followed by a boost with avipox expressing CEA. This regimen consisted of 1×10^7 pfu Wyeth strain vaccinia

Table 2
Recent Clinical Trials

First author	*Vector*	*Results*
Mastrangelo *(58)*	Vaccinia-GM-CSF	Regression of injected lesions.
Marshall *(56)*	Vaccinia-CEA	No clinical response.
Mukherjee *(68)*	Vaccinia-IL-2	No clinical response.
Eder *(55)*	Vaccinia-PSA	Stabilization of PSA levels.
Sanda *(69)*	Vaccinia-PSA	Stabilization of PSA levels.
Conry *(70)*	Vaccinia-CEA	No clinical response.
Tsang *(71)*	Vaccinia-CEA	No clinical response.
Adams *(67)*	Vaccinia-HPV	Response in cervical cancer.
Rochlitz *(60)*	MVA-Muc1	Response in metastatic disease.
Greiner *(57)*	rV-CEA TRICOM	Safe.

injected intradermally. Although specific T-cell immune responses were generated and the regimen was well tolerated, there were no positive clinical responses noted *(56)*. Rochlitz et al. published their phase I trial of a modifed vaccinia (MVA strain) expressing human MUC1 for antigen specific immunotherapy in patients with advanced MUC 1 positive cancers *(60)*. They found that patients tolerated repeated doses of the virus with minimal side effects and 1 of the 13 patients with advanced cancer showed a marked decrease in the size of his metastasis that lasted 14 mo. Greiner et al. developed a vaccinia expressing a triad of costimulatory molecules including B7.1, intercellular adhesion molecule-1 (ICAM-1), and leukocyte function-associated antigen-3 combined with CEA to produce a vaccine against CEA expressing cancers. This virus, known as rV-CEA TRICOM or a recombinant vaccinia vector that carries a triad of costimulatory molecules, has been encouraging in preclinical studies and is now the focus of clinical trials *(57)*.

9. VACCINIA AS A VECTOR FOR TUMOR DIRECTED GENE DELIVERY

The properties that make vaccinia attractive as vector for gene delivery were described earlier and the use of vaccinia as a vector for gene delivery is now being investigated in clinical trials. Mastrangelo et al. have reported their phase I clinical trial using vaccinia expressing granulocyte-macrophage colony-stimulating factor (GM-CSF). Patients underwent intratumoral injections of up to 2×10^7 pfu per lesion and 8×10^7 pfu per session twice weekly over 6 wk. Systemic toxicities were limited to mild flu-like symptoms and local inflammation at the injection site with doses greater than 10^7 pfu/lesion. All patients were vaccinated against the vaccinia within weeks prior to receiving the vaccinia-GM-CSF. Interesting positive responses were reported in five of the seven patients treated. Three patients had mixed responses with complete regression of treated and untreated dermal metastases, one patient had partial response with regression of injected and uninjected regional dermal metastasis and onr patient had complete remission of multiple dermal metastasis *(58,59)*.

Vaccinia has also been engineered to express suicide and tumor suppressor genes. The suicide gene therapy involves the combination of a nonmammalian enzyme such as cytosine deaminase and the nontoxic prodrug 5-fluorocytosine, which is catalyzed to 5-FU by the cytosine deaminase. Vaccinia expressing the suicide genes cytosine deaminase and 5-fluorocytosine has shown promising results in both in vitro and mouse models *(64)*. Another approach in which vaccina vectors were used to transfer the tumor suppressor gene *p53* into gliomas and bladder tumors that expressed mutated p53 induced apoptotic cell death and showed some antitumor efficacy *(65,66)*.

10. VACCINIA AS AN ONCOLYTIC VIRUS FOR CANCER THERAPY

The concept of a tumor selective oncolytic virus that can be safely administered is very appealing and is the focus of current research by multiple laboratories. The advantages of the vaccinia virus as an oncolytic virus have been described earlier in the chapter. The most important advantage is the efficiency of viral replication, cell to cell spread and ability to destroy tissue.

Development of an oncolytic virus has focused on genetic alterations of the WR strain of virus to achieve a tumor selective replicating virus *(4)*. It has been previously demonstrated that an intradermal injection of 10^6 pfu of the wild-type WR strain of vaccinia into nonhuman primates leads to a necrotic ulcer of 108 cm^2 in only 8 d without systemic spread of the virus (unpublished data). This ability to quickly spread and its ability to produce high levels of trangene expression is extremely promising, as one of the limiting factors in antitumor gene therapy is the limitation of vector distribution throughout fibrinous tumors. Animal models studying the distribution of a systemically delivered tumor-selective mutant vaccinia virus have shown the highest levels of virus in the tumor whereas little to no virus has been detected in other organs. The most promising mutant has been a virus deleted of the TK and vaccinia growth factor (VGF) genes (*see* Fig. 3).

LTK is important for vaccinia nucleotide and DNA synthesis and it is almost essential in normal cells where the host nucleotide pool is low. VGF is a protein that is expressed early by vaccinia virus and is secreted by infected cells. It binds growth factor receptors on surrounding resting cells and stimulates them to proliferate. This increases the available nucleotides and primes them for vaccinia infection. By deleting both the VGF and TK genes the replication of vaccinia in normal cells can be completely abrogated without decreasing the ability of the vaccinia to replicate in tumor cells. This double deleted virus has been tested and found to preferentially replicate in tumor cells and ovarian tissue with little or replication in nontumor tissue *(4)*. Experiments using nude mice injected systemically with 1×10^9 pfu of the double deleted vaccinia showed a marked response in established tumors with no pathogenecity *(61)*. Primate studies showed no pathogenecity of 10^9 pfu of vaccinia delivered intravenously (unpublished data).

Puhlman et al. demonstrated that systemic administration of a TK-deleted vaccinia virus expressing the suicide gene purine nucleoside phosphorylase in combination with 6-methylpurine deoxyribose treatment led to a complete response in 50% of mice with hepatic metastases *(62,63)*. We are currently exploiting another strategy by deleting the antiapoptotic genes *spi*-1 and *spi*-2 to improve tumor selectivity and oncolysis. Ultimately, the combination of genetic deletions and expression of antitumor genes may prove to be more successful to inhibit tumor growth than the strains available at present.

11. SUMMARY

Vaccinia virus is a member of the pox family of viruses. Viral recombinants are made with relative ease and their natural tumor affinity make them attractive vectors for tumor directed therapy. It has a proven safety profile from its use as a smallpox vaccine and its

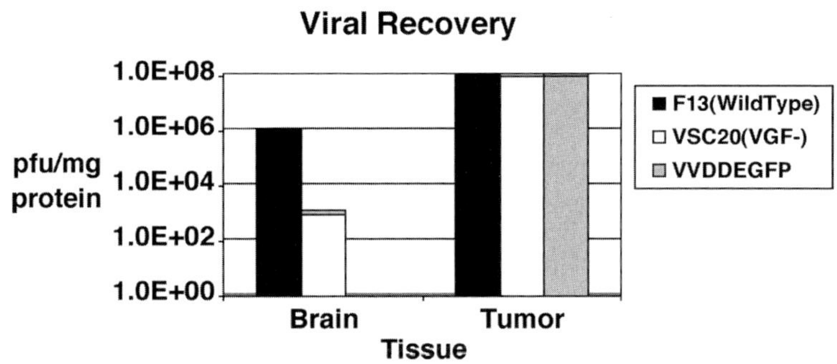

Fig. 3. Differential viral recovery. Vaccinia titers recovered from brain and tumor 4 d after injection of virus intraperitoneally in MC38 subcutaneous tumor bearing mice. Data represents median of 5 values. No recoverable titers are seen in brain tissue form the double deleted virus (VVDDEGFP) whereas the tumor has equivalent titers to wild type.

immunogenic and oncolytic properties combined with its effectiveness to spread through tissues make it an attractive vector for future development of tumor directed therapies. Ongoing clinical trials focusing on these properties are beginning to show its potential in the treatment of cancer.

REFERENCES

1. Moss B. Poxviridae: The viruses and Their Replication. In: Fields Virology. Fields BN, Knipe DM, Howley PM, Lippincott Raven, Philadelphia, USA (1996): 2637–2671.
2. Guo ZS, Bartlett DL. Vaccinia as a vector for gene delivery. Expert Opin Biol Ther 2004;4(6):1–17.
3. Fenner F, Wittek R, Dumbell KR. Vaccinia virus: The tool for smallpox eradication. In: The Orthopoxviruses. Fenner F, Wittek R, Dumbell, eds. New York: Academic Press, Inc., 1989:143–170.
4. Zeh HJ, Bartlett DL. Development of a replication-selective, oncolytic poxvirus for the treatment of human cancers. Cancer Gene Therapy 2002;9:1001–1012.
5. Smith GL, Vanderplasschen A. Extracellular enveloped vaccinia virus: entry, egress, and evasion. In: Coronaviruses and Arteriviruses. Enjuanes A, ed. New York:Plenum Press, 1998:395–414.
6. Hsaio JC, Chung CS, Chang W. Vaccinia virus envelope D8L protein binds to cell surface chondroitin sulfate and mediates the adsorption of intracellular mature virions to cells. J Virol 1999;73:8750–8761.
7. Chung CS, Hsiao JC, Chang YS, Chang W. A27L protein mediates vaccinia virus interaction with cell surface heparin sulfate. J Virol 1998;72:1577–1585
8. Salzman NP. The rate of formation of vaccinia deoxyribonucleic acid and vaccinia virus. Virology 1960;10:150–152.
9. Payne LG. Adsorption and penetration of enveloped and naked vaccinia virus particles. J Virol 1978;27:19–27.
10. Vanderplasschen A, Hollinshead M, Smith GL. Intracellular and extracellular vaccinia virions enter cells by different mechanisms. J Gen Virol 1998;79:877–887.
11. Vanderplasschen A, Smith GL. A novel binding assay using confocal microscopy: demonstration that the intracellular and extracellular vaccinia virions bind to different cellular receptors. J Virol 1997;71:4032–4041.
12. Hsaio JC, Chung CS, Chang W. Vaccinia virus envelope D8L protein binds to cell surface chondroitin sulfate and mediates the adsorption of intracellular mature virions to cells. J Virol 1999;73:8750–8761.
13. Sodeik B, Cudmore S, Ericsson M, Esteban M, Niles EG, Griffiths G. Assembly of vaccinia virus: incorporation of p14 and p32 into the membrane of the intracellular mature virus. J Virol 1999;73:8750–8761.
14. Galmiche MC, Rindisbacher L, Wels W, Wittek R, Buchegger F. Expression of a functional single chain antibody on the surface of extracellular enveloped vaccinia virus as a step towards selective tumor cell targeting. J Gen Virol 1997;78:3019–3027.
15. Katz E, Wolffe EJ, Moss B. The ctuoplasmic and transmemvrane domains of the vaccinia virus b5R protein target a chimeric human immunodeficiency virus type 1 glycoprotein to the outer envelope of nascent vaccinia virions. J Virol 1997;71(4):3178–3187.

16. Beaud G. Vaccinia virus DNA replication: a short review. Biochimie 1995;77(10):774–779.
17. Tolonen N, Doglio L, Scheich S, Locker JK. Vaccinia virus DNA replication occurs in endoplasmic reticulum enclosed mini nuclei. Mol Biol Cell 2001;12:2031–2046.
18. Sodeik B, Krijnse-Locker J. Assembly of vaccinia virus revisited: de novo membrane synthesis or acquisition from the host? Trends Microbiol 2002;10:15–24.
19. Sutter G, Moss B. Novel vaccinia vector derived from the host range restricted and highly attenuated MVA strain of vaccinia virus. Dev Biol Stand 1995;84:195–200.
20. Moss B. Vaccinia virus: a tool for research and vaccine development. Science 1991;252:1662–1667.
21. Carroll, Moss B. Poxviruses as expression vectors. Curr Opin Biotech 1997;8:573–577.
22. Domi A, Moss B. Cloning the vaccinia virus genome as a bacterial artificial chromosome in Escherichia coli and recovery of infectious virus in mammalian cells. Proc Natl Acad Sci U S A 2002; 99:12,415–12,420.
23. Yao XD, Evans DH. High frequency genetic recombination and reactivation of orthopoxviruses from DNA fragments transfected into lepoporipoxvirus-infected cells. J Virol 2003;77:7281–7290.
24. Yuen L, Moss B. Oligonucleotide sequence signaling transcriptional termination of vaccinia virus early genes. Proc Natl Acad Sci U S A 1987;84:6417–6421.
25. Buller RML, Chakrabarti S, Cooper JA, Twardzik DR, Moss B. Deletion of the vaccinia virus growth factor gene reduces virus virulence. J Virol 1988;62:866–874.
26. Faithi Z, Dyster LM, Seto J, Condit RC, Niles EG. Intragenic and intergenic recombination between temperature-sensitive mutants of vaccinia virus. J Gen.Virol 1991;72:2733–2737.
27. Davison AJ, Moss B. Structure of vaccinia virus early promoters. J Mol Biol 1989;210:749–769.
28. Davison AJ, Moss B. Structure of vaccinia virus late promoters. J Mol Biol 1989;210(4):771–784.
29. Chakrabarti S, Sisler JR, Moss B. Compact, synthetic, vaccinia virus early/late promoter for protein expression. BioTechniques 1997;23:1094–1097.
30. Earl PL, Moss B. Expression of Proteins in Mammalian Cells Using Vaccinia Viral Vectors. In: Current Protocols in Molecular Biology. Ausubel FM, Kinston RE, Moore DD, Seidman JG, Smith JA et al., eds. New York: Green/Wiley Interscience, 1998:16.
31. Boyle DB, Coupar BE. A dominant selectable marker for the construction of recombinant poxviruses. Gene 1988;65(1):123–128.
32. Perkus ME, Limbach K, Paoletti E. Cloning and expression of foreign genes in vaccinia virus, using a host range selection system. J Virol 1989;63(9):3829–3836.
33. Moss B. Vaccinia Virus. A Tool for Research and Vaccine Development. Science 1991;252:1662–1667.
34. Fulginiti VA, Papier A, Lane JM, Neff JM, Henderson DA. Smallpox vaccination: a review, part II. Adverse events. Clin Infect Dis 2003;37:251–271.
35. Gurvich EB, Vilesova IS. Vaccinia virus in postvaccinal encephalitis. Acta Virol 1983;27(2):154–159.
36. Enserink M. Public Health. Treating vaccine reactions: two lifelines, but no guarantees. Science 2002;298:2313.
37. Enserink M. Bioterrorism. In search of a kindler, gentler vaccine. Science 2002:296:1594.
38. Smith GL, Symons JA, Khanna A, Vanderplasschen A, Alcami A. Vaccinia virus immune evasion. Immunol Rev 1997;159:137–154.
39. Smith GL, Vanderplasschen A, Law M. The formation and function of extra cellular enveloped vaccinia virus. J Gen Virol 2002;83:2915–2931.
40. McCart JA, Puhlmann M, Lee J, et al. Complex interactions between the replicating oncolytic effect and the enzyme/prod rug effect of vaccinia mediated tumor regression. Gene Ther 2000;7:1217–1223.
41. Puhlman M, Brown CK, Gnant M, et al. Vaccinia as a vector for tumor directed gene therapy: biodistribution of a thymidine kinas deleted mutant. Cancer Gene Ther 2000;7:66–73.
42. Alcami A, Smith GL. The vaccinia virus soluble alpha/beta interferon(IFN) receptor binds to the cell surface and protects cells from the antiviral effects of IFN. J Virol 2000;74(23):11,230–11,239.
43. Colamonici OR, Domanski P, Sweitzer SM, Larner A, Buller RM. Vaccinia virus B18R gene encodes a type I interferon-binding protein that blocks and interferon alpha transmembrane signaling. J Biol Chem 1995;270(27):15,974–15,978.
44. Alcami A, Smith GL. The vaccinia virus soluble interferon-gamma receptor is homodimer. J Gen Virol 2002;83:545–549.
45. Seet BT, McFadden G. Viral chemokine-binding proteins. J Leukoc Biol 2002;72(1):24–34.
46. Alcami A, Symons JA, Collins PD, Williams TJ, Smith GL. Blockade of chemokine activity by a soluble chemokine binding protein from vaccinia virus. J Immunol 1998;160(2):624–633.
47. Mahalingam S, Karupiah G. Modulation of chemokines by poxvirus infections. Curr Opin Immunol 2000;12(4):409–412.

48. Smith VP, Byant NA, Alcami A. Ectromelia, vaccinia and coxpox viruses encode secreted interleukin-18 binding proteins. J Gen Virol 2000;81:1223–1230.
49. Calderara S, Xiang Y, Moss B. Orthopoxvirus IL-18 binding proteins: affinities and antagonistic activities. Virology 2001;279:22–26.
50. Angelini G, Gardella S, Ardy M, et al. Antigen-presenting dendritic cells provide the reducing extracellular microenvironment required for T lymphocyte activation. Proc Natl Acad Sci U S A 2002;99:1491–1496.
51. Novick D, Kim SH, Fantuzzi G, Reznikov LL, Dinarello CA, Rubinstein M. Interleukin-18 binding protein: a novel modulator of the Th1 cytokine response. Immunity 1999;10:127–136.
52. Van Den Broek M, Bachmann MF, Kohler G, et al. IL-4 and IL-10 antagonize IL-12 mediated protection against acute vaccinia virus infection with a limited role of IFN gamma and nitric oxide synthetase 2. J Immunol 2000;164:371–378.
53. Deonarain R, Alcami A, Alexiou M, Dallman MJ, Gewert DR, Porter AC. Impaired antiviral response and alpha/beta interferon induction in mice lacking beta interferon. J Virol 2003;84:1962–1972.
54. Gherardi MM, Ramirez JC, Esteban M. IL-12 and IL-18 act in synergy to clear vaccinia virus infection: involvement of innate and adaptive components of the immune system. J GenVirol 2003;84:1961–1972.
55. Eder JP, Kantoff PW, Roper K. A phase I trial of recombinant vaccinia virus expressing prostate-specific antigen in advanced prostate cancer. Clin Cancer Res 2000;6:1632–1638.
56. Marshall JL, Hoyer RJ, Toomey MA, et al. Phase I study in advanced cancer patients of a diversified prime and boost vaccination protocol using recombinant vaccinia virus and recombinant non replicating avipox virus to elicit anti-carcinoembroyinic antigen immune responses. J Clin Oncol 2000;18:3964–3973.
57. Greiner JW, Zeytin H, Anver MR, Schlom J. Vaccine based therapy directed against carcinoembryonic antigen demonstrates antitumor activity on spontaneous intestinal tumors in the absence of autoimmunity. Cancer Res 2000;62:6944–6951.
58. Mastrangelo MJ, Maguire HC, Jr, Eisenlohr LC, et al. Intratumoral recombinant GM-CSF-encoding virus as gene therapy in patients with cutaneous melanoma. Cancer Gene Ther 1998;6:409–422.
59. Mastrangelo MJ, Maguire HC, Jr, Lattime EC. Intralesional vaccinia/GM-CSF recombinant virus in the treatment of metastatic melanoma. Adv Exp Med Biol 2000;465:391–400.
60. Rochlitz C, Figlin R, Squiban P, et al. Phase I immunotherapy with a modified vaccinia virus (MVA) expressing human MUC1 as antigen specific immunotherapy in patients with MUC 1 advanced cancer. J Gene Med 2003;5:690–699.
61. McCart JA, Ward JM, Lee J, et al. Systemic cancer therapy with a tumor selective vaccinia virus mutant lacking thymidine kinase and vaccinia growth factor genes. Cancer Res 2001;61:8751–8757.
62. Puhlman M, Gnant M, Brown CK, Alexander HR, Bartlett DL. Thymidine kinase-deleted vaccinia virus expressing purine nucleoside phosphorylase as a vector for tumor-directed gene therapy. Human Gene Ther 1999;10:649–657.
63. Mullen JT, Tanabe KT. Viral Oncolysis for Malignant Liver Tumors. Annal Surg Oncol 2003;10:596–605.
64. Gnant M, Puhlman MD, Bartlett DL, Alexander HR. Regional versus Systemic Delivery of Recombinant Vaccinia Virus as Suicide Gene Therapy for Murine Liver Metastases. Annal Surg 1999;230: 352–361.
65. Fodor I, Timiryasova T, Denes B, Yoshida J, Ruckle H, Lilly M. Vaccinia virus-mediated p53 gene therapy of bladder cancer in an orthotopic murine model. J Urol 2005;173:604–609.
66. Haghighat P, Timiryasova T, Chen B, Kajioka E, Gridley DS, Fodor I. Antitumor effect of Il-2, p53, and bax gene transfer in C6 glioma cells. Anticancer Res 2000;20:1337–1342.
67. Adams M, Borysiewicz L, Fiander A, et al. Clinical studies of human papilloma vaccines in pre-invasive and invasive cancer. Vaccine 2001 21;19(17–19):2549–2456.
68. Mukherjee S, Haenel T, Himbeck R, et al. Replication-restricted vaccinia as a cytokine gene therapy vector in cancer: Persistent transgene expression despite antibody generation. Cancer Gene Ther 2000;7:663–670.
69. Sanda MG, Smith DC, Charles LG, et al. Recombinant vaccinia-PSA can induce prostatic specific immune response in androgen-modulated human prostate cancer. Urology 1999;53:260–266.
70. Conry RM, Allen KO, Lee S, Moore SE, Shaw DR, LoBuglio AF. Human autoantibodies to CEA induced by a vaccinia-CEA vaccine. Clin Cancer Res 2000;6(1):34–41.
71. Tsang KY, Zaremba S, Nieroda CA, Zhu MZ, Hamilton JM, Schlom J. Generation of human cytotoxic T cells specific for human CEA epitopes form patients immunized with recombinant vaccinia-CEA vaccine. J Natl Caner Inst 1995;87:982–990.

5 Herpes Simplex Virus as a Therapy for Cancer

Ian J. Mohr, PhD

CONTENTS

Summary

Inspired by reports that viral infection might be capable of promoting tumor regression published in the early 20th century, investigators have struggled to identify a suitable virus, which though unable to cause disease, retained the capability to replicate in cancer cells. In principal, the productive growth of the virus would kill or lyse malignant cells and the newly minted viral progeny would spread the infection, resulting ultimately in the destruction of the tumor by a process termed viral oncolysis. Fueled by revolutionary advances in molecular biology that enabled a new understanding of viral virulence at the genetic level, nonpathogenic strains of human viruses have been engineered in the laboratory and their oncolytic ability evaluated in animal models of human cancer. This chapter chronicles the milestones in engineering oncolytic strains of herpes simplex virus type 1,

From: *Cancer Drug Discovery and Development: Gene Therapy for Cancer*
Edited by: K. K. Hunt, S. A. Vorburger, and S. G. Swisher © Humana Press Inc., Totowa, NJ

highlighting different stages of development beginning with the pioneering use of recombinant viruses produced in the laboratory, accompanied by a discussion of key design innovations which upon incorporation into HSV-1 oncolytic strains, substantially improved both their safety and efficacy, and summarizes recent experiences in phase I clinical trials.

Key Words: Oncolytic virus; replication-competent attenuated herpes simplex virus; eIF2α phosphorylation and viral pathogenesis; herpes simplex virus virulence; antitumor therapy.

1. INTRODUCTION

One hundred years ago, the first anecdotal observations correlating viral infection with tumor regression were reported and lead to several investigations over the course of the last century, evaluating the potential of various natural human and animal viruses to treat cancer *(1)*. However, it was the achievements of the last two decades, most notably technical innovation in the area of molecular biology coupled with a heightened understanding of viral replication and pathogenesis at the genetic level, that ushered in the possibility of creating viruses in the laboratory which were selectively pathogenic for neoplastic cells. Through genetic engineering, it was now possible to selectively harness many key attributes of viruses, such as their ability to enter, reproduce, and ultimately destroy their host cells, while dialing out the undesirable properties associated with viral infection, namely their ability to destroy normal cells and cause disease. As a virus engineered in this fashion retains the ability to replicate in and ultimately kill tumor cells, it could potentially propagate a self-limiting infection throughout a tumor mass, resulting in oncolysis or lysis of the cancer cells in the tumor and subsequent tumor regression. Whereas a variety of mutant viruses with such capabilities have been reported, this chapter will focus on the development of herpes simplex virus type 1 (HSV-1) as an oncolytic virus.

2. HERPES SIMPLEX VIRUS FUNDAMENTALS: LIFELONG LATENCY PUNCTUATED BY EPISODES OF PRODUCTIVE GROWTH

"O'er ladies lips, who straight on kisses dream, which oft the angry Mab with blisters plagues, because their breaths with sweetmeats tainted are."

– William Shakespeare, Romeo and Juliet, circa 1595.

Following infection of oral epithelial cells in its human host, HSV-1 invades axons and travels to the nuclei of sensory neurons that innervate this epithelia. Here, the virus establishes a latent infection, characterized by a restricted pattern of viral gene expression, the assembly of the viral genome into a regular chromatin structure, and its maintenance as a circular extrachromosomal element *(2)*. Latency, therefore, results in the permanent colonization of the host by the virus, and the severely limited expression of viral genes functions to shield the virus from host defenses.

In response to a variety of stimuli, these latent infections "reactivate," resulting in episodes of productive viral growth characterized by expression of over 80 viral open reading frames (ORFs) distributed among two unique, single copy segments or within multiple repetitive loci of the large HSV-1 DNA genome. Activation of the productive or lytic gene expression program results in the production of viral particles and the eventual death of the infected cell. Distinct mRNA populations accumulate at discrete times in the productive replication cycle, resulting in the differential expression of viral genes in what has been termed a cascade pattern (*see* Fig. 1) *(2)*. The process is

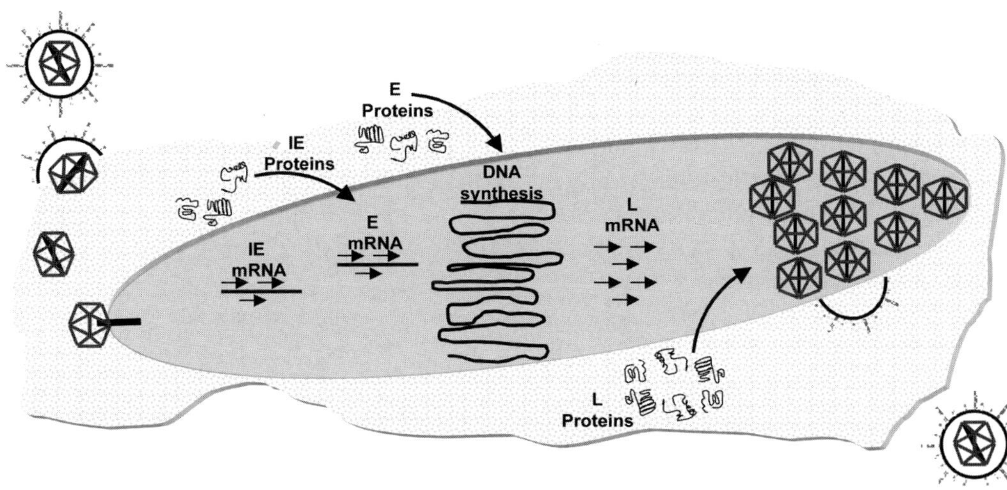

Fig. 1. The HSV-1 productive or lytic replication cycle. Following fusion of the virion envelope with the host plasma membrane, the viral nucleocapsid is deposited into the cytosol along with numerous proteins contained within the virus particle, one of which is the virus encoded transcription factor VP16. After the nucleocapsid docks at the nuclear membrane, viral DNA translocates through the nuclear pore into the nucleus. Transcription from 5 immediate early (IE or α) viral genes commences once the cellular transcription machinery is recruited to the promoters by VP16. Several IE gene products (ICP 4,0,22, and 27) are important for the subsequent expression of the second class of viral genes, the early genes, and return to the nucleus after being synthesized in the cytosol. Early (E or β) mRNAs predominately encode proteins involved in nucleotide metabolism and DNA synthesis. Replicating viral DNA accumulates as a large concatamer in the nucleus, where multiple genome segments are joined end to end, and is subsequently processed into unit length genomes concomitant with packaging into newly assembled nucleocapsids. In addition, DNA synthesis marks the transition from the early phase of the lifecycle to the late or γ_2 phase, and is associated with an increase in late γ_2 mRNAs. Late genes (L or γ) encode virion structural proteins along with virion components required for subsequent rounds of infection (i.e., VP16). Once assembled in the nucleus, capsids acquire an envelope by budding from the nuclear membrane. One proposed pathway for HSV-1 egress suggests enveloped capsids between the inner and outer leaflets of the nuclear membrane fuse with the outer nuclear membrane, releasing unenveloped capsids into the perinuclear region. These capsids transit through the cytosol and are thought to acquire other virion protein components and their final lipid envelope by budding into a post-golgi compartment prior to exiting the cell.

initiated by VP16, a transcription factor carried within the viral particle that recruits cellular transcription factors along with the RNA polymerase II holoenzyme to the promoters of five viral immediate-early (IE or α) genes. Whereas one of these IE gene products dampens the host immune response by inhibiting the presentation of peptide antigens in conjunction with major histocompatability complex (MHC) class I molecules, the remaining four IE proteins are important for the subsequent expression of the next class of viral genes, the early or β genes. Viral early polypeptides primarily encode functions required for nucleotide metabolism and viral DNA synthesis, the initiation of which signals entry into the final late or γ phase of the viral life cycle. Two classes of late genes have been identified based upon their transcription in the presence of viral DNA synthesis inhibitors. Whereas transcription of a subset of γ genes, the γ_2 class, requires viral DNA synthesis, expression of γ_1 genes is not completely dependent upon viral DNA replication and is only modestly reduced in the presence of inhibitors. Included among the late gene products are polypeptides critical for assembling infectious virus, virion components that function following entry but before IE gene expression, and proteins that regulate the host response to infection. Reactivation of a latent infection in a sensory neuron results in antereograde transport of viral progeny back to the portal of entry followed by the ensuing infection of epithelial cells, mobilization of the cellular immune response, and the formation of a fever blister or cold sore. Rarely, HSV-1 can enter and replicate within the central nervous system (CNS), causing encephalitis.

Although many HSV-1 genes are required for the virus to productively infect an established cultured monkey kidney cell line used extensively in many virology laboratories, it is striking that viral replication can in fact proceed quite efficiently in the absence of numerous HSV-1 gene products. This class of genes, though dispensable for viral replication in cell culture, is thought to be important for replication in specialized cell types, encode functions that are redundant or overlapping with other viral gene products, or affect pathogenesis in animals. In support of this proposal, HSV-1 genes important for modulating the host immune response, the spread of the virus from peripheral sites of inoculation to the CNS (neuroinvasiveness), and replication within CNS tissues (neurovirulence) have been identified *(2)*; moreover, these genetic determinants of pathogenesis figure prominently in the development of safe, oncolytic HSV-1 strains.

3. TAKING THE FIRST STEP: ENGINEERING ONCOLYTIC HSV-1 STRAINS

Ground breaking studies by Martuza and colleagues were the first to demonstrate the therapeutic promise of an engineered oncolytic HSV-1 strain, the thymidine kinase (tk) negative HSV-1 mutant, *dl*sptk *(3)*. This mutant derivative was chosen because tk mutants replicate effectively in actively dividing cells such as those found in tumors, but are relatively impaired for replication in nondividing cells, such as neurons and therefore display reduced neurovirulence compared with wild-type strains upon introduction into the CNS of adult mice *(4–8)*. The tumor selected for oncolytic therapy was malignant glioma, as the outcome for patients with this devastating brain tumor is grim, remaining essentially unchanged over the past 50 yr despite advances in surgery, radiation, and chemotherapy. Direct injection of *dl*sptk into established tumors inhibited the growth of human glioma implants (subcutanteous or subrenal) in athymic mice and prolonged survival of mice with intracranial gliomas as well. However, fatal encephalitis was still observed in 70 to 100% of the treated mice despite the fact that the tk mutant was significantly less neurovirulent than wild-type HSV-1 *(3)*. In subsequent years, the oncolytic potential of HSV-1 derivatives with mutations in the viral ribonucleotide reductase large subunit (hr3) or DNA polymerase genes (AraA) was evaluated. Unlike the tk mutant *dl*sptk, these strains were sensitive to acyclovir, an extremely effective, safe antiviral drug adding a component of safety to control the infection if necessary. However, despite their ability to inhibit tumor growth and responsiveness to antiviral chemotherapy, these viral strains were still not adequately attenuated to merit further investigation. Thus, whereas it proved possible to use HSV-1 as an oncolytic virus to destroy cancer cells, the understanding of virulence was not sufficiently advanced to render the virus safe.

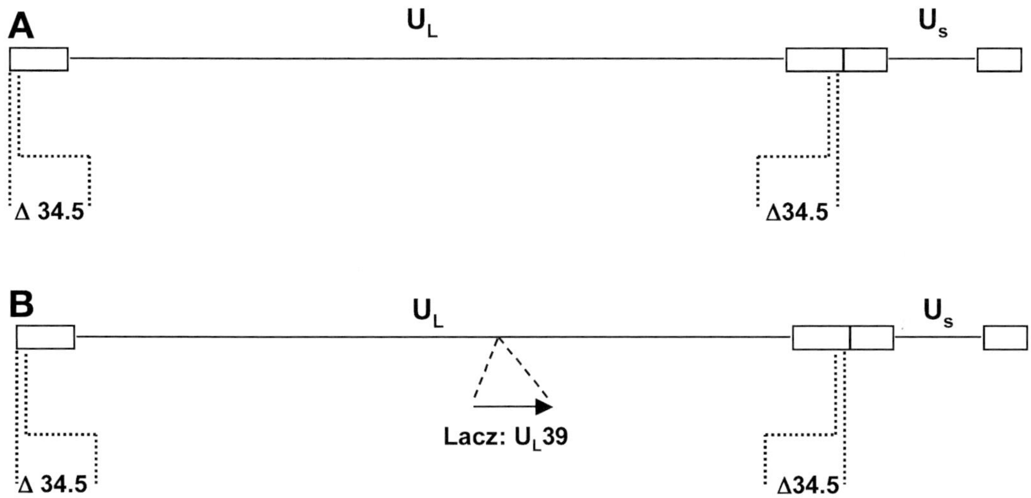

Fig. 2. Genetic structure of oncolytic HSV-1 γ34.5 mutant derivatives. The HSV-1 genome is 152-Kb in length and is composed of a unique long segment (UL), a unique short segment (Us), and several reiterated components (rectangles). The γ34.5 gene is contained within these repetitive components that flank the UL segment and is therefore diploid. (**A**) Δ34.5 null mutant where both copies of the γ34.5 gene have been deleted. The recombinants R3616 (strain F) and 1716 (strain 17) represent this class of simple deletion mutations. (**B**) A multimutated strain that contains a bacterial β-galactosidase (lacZ) expression cassette disrupting the viral UL39 gene in addition to a deletion affecting both copies of the γ34.5 gene. This Δ34.5 null mutant is also unable to produce the large subunit of the viral ribonucleotide reductase, the UL39 gene product. The recombinants G207 and MGH1 (both strain F) are of this genotype.

4. FINDING THE ACHILLE'S HEEL: THE $\gamma_1$34.5 GENE CONTROLS HSV-1 NEUROVIRULENCE

The breakthrough in creating attenuated HSV-1 strains resulted from characterizing viruses containing engineered mutations in the $\gamma_1$34.5 genes. Embedded within a repetitive genome component (*see* Fig. 2A), the $\gamma_1$34.5 gene is expressed with γ_1 late kinetics and is not required for growth in cultured monkey kidney cells. Strikingly, its impact on viral neurovirulence is greater than any single HSV-1 gene identified to date *(11–13)*. Although the LD_{50} of many wt HSV-1 strains is less than 300 pfu following intracranial delivery, it is not possible to accurately measure the LD_{50} for γ34.5 mutant viruses. Indeed, upwards of 10^6–10^7 pfu of γ34.5 mutant viruses have been safely injected intracranially into mouse, non-human primate, and human brains *(11–18)*. In studies designed to examine the efficacy with which γ34.5 mutants were able to destroy human or murine gliomas implanted into mice, not only had the attenuation problem been solved, but the treated mice survived longer than their untreated counterparts and no longer developed viral encephalitis. Long-term surviving animals (usually in the vicinity of 60–80 d) were produced with efficiencies ranging from 10 to 50% of the treated animals depending on the tumor model and treatment regimen *(9,19–23)*. γ34.5 mutants were also tk+ and therefore retained their sensitivity to acyclovir, which could be used, if necessary, to control viral encephalitis. Despite reports of $\gamma_1$34.5 mutants replicating to varying degrees in CNS tissue depending on the viral strain and the immune status of the mice, encephalitis has not been observed in numerous studies performed with $\gamma_1 34.5$ mutants in different viral genetic backgrounds *(24–26)*. To further restrict viral replication to actively dividing cells, additional mutations in the UL39 ribonucleotide reductase gene (*see* Fig. 2B) or the UL2 uracil DNA glycosidase gene were introduced into the $\gamma 34.5$ mutant background *(14,27,28)*. Although each of these non-neurovirulent, multimutated viruses could still reduce subcutaneous tumor growth and extend the survival of mice with intracranial tumors, more than 80% of the treated subjects still succumbed, emphasizing a different problem limiting the efficacy and outcome of treatment. Whereas encephalitis was no longer observed in animals treated with any of these $\gamma_1 34.5$ mutant derivatives, the $\gamma_1 34.5$ deletion, either alone or in conjunction with additional mutations, impaired the replicative ability of these viruses in many human tumor cells, allowing the growth of residual glioma cells which ultimately killed the animals. Thus, the successful attenuation of HSV-1 left in its wake another problem for investigators to grapple with: engineered mutants that were sufficiently safe had lost a substantial amount of their replicative efficacy, impairing their oncolytic ability.

5. REDUCED ONCOLYTIC ABILITY OF $\gamma_1 34.5$ MUTANT DERIVATIVES RESULTS FROM A TRANSLATIONAL BLOCK

After the initial reports established that the $\gamma_1 34.5$ gene was a major determinant of HSV-1 neurovirulence nonessential for growth in cultured monkey kidney cells, further investigation revealed that $\gamma_1 34.5$ mutants actually behaved like classical viral host range mutants, exhibiting restricted growth in some lines of cultured cells but not others. Thus, whereas a standard line of monkey kidney cells were permissive or supported the replication $\gamma_1 34.5$ mutants, many human tumor cells were in fact nonpermissive, or did not support the growth of $\gamma_1 34.5$ mutant derivatives. Upon infection of a nonpermissive human tumor cell with a $\gamma_1 34.5$ mutant strain, all of the events in the viral life cycle proceeded normally up to and including viral DNA replication and the accumulation of γ_2 late mRNA transcripts. These viral late mRNAs encoding key structural proteins required to complete the viral life cycle and assemble the next generation of viral progeny, however, were never translated resulting from a block at the level of protein synthesis, effectively interrupting the viral life cycle prior to the assembly and release of viral particles *(29)*. Subsequent biochemical analysis demonstrated that the $\gamma_1 34.5$ gene product was required to prevent accrual of phosphorylated eIF2, a critical translation initiation factor inactivated by phosphorylation of its alpha subunit *(30)*.

6. eIF2α, HOST DEFENSES AND INNATE IMMUNITY

As obligate intracellular parasites, viruses are completely dependent upon the translational machinery resident in their host cells. It is not surprising, therefore, that a major host defense component centers on impeding viral mRNA translation. Indeed, one of at least four stress responsive eIF2α kinases present in mammalian cells, the double stranded RNA dependent protein kinase PKR is induced by the antiviral cytokines interferon α/β. It has been proposed that abundant dsRNA, a replicative intermediate formed in the replication of RNA viruses and a by-product of overlapping transcription units on opposite DNA strands of DNA viruses, is a signature of viral infection. PKR binds dsRNA and in the presence of this activating ligand forms a dimer whereupon each subunit phosphorylates the other. It is this activated, phosphorylated form of PKR that then goes on to phosphorylate other substrates, including eIF2α, the regulatory subunit of eIF2 *(31)*.

eIF2 is a heterotrimeric G protein, forming a ternary complex composed of its α,β, and γ subunits bound to GTP along with the initiator tRNA, that is responsible for chaperoning the initiator tRNA to the 40S ribosomal subunit, forming what is known as the 48S complex (*see* Fig. 3A) *(32)*. Like many G proteins, a GTPase activating protein (eIF5) and a guanine nucleotide exchange factor (eIF2B) regulate its activity. Normally, eIF5 promotes GTP hydrolysis following the joining of the 60S ribosomal subunit to form an 80S ribosome, releasing eIF2 bound to GDP. To participate in subsequent rounds of polypeptide chain initiation, the GDP form of eIF2 requires the activity of eIF2B in order to exchange GDP for GTP. However, phosphorylation of eIF2α leads to a strong association between eIF2B and eIF2, effectively preventing eIF2B from catalyzing the nucleotide exchange reaction (*see* Fig. 3B). As the quantity of eIF2B present in cells is limiting, phosphorylation of small amounts of eIF2α by PKR can have relatively large effects on translation by sequestering eIF2B, hindering nucleotide exchange, and inhibiting translation. Unchecked, PKR activated by dsRNA in virus infected cells would therefore effectively deplete active eIF2, inhibit ternary complex formation, and prevent viral and cellular protein synthesis. Should cells initially infected succeed in inhibiting translation, the viral invader would effectively be stopped in its tracks, denied access to the cellular translational apparatus it needs to complete its life cycle. This arm of the innate host response then is designed to sacrifice the initially infected cells for the benefit of the larger population. However, numerous viruses, including HSV-1, have captured a variety of functions to counter this cellular response *(32)*. This struggle for control of the translational machinery is often an integral component of viral pathogenesis *(33–35)*.

Normally, the $\gamma_1$34.5 gene product prevents the accumulation of phosphorylated eIF2α by recruiting a cellular phosphatase, protein phosphatase 1α (PP1α), to remove phosphate from eIF2α *(36)*. Interestingly, the domain of the $\gamma_1$34.5 protein that contains this activity is homologous to a domain in the GADD34 protein, a cellular PP1α binding protein that promotes eIF2α dephosphorylation in response to other forms of cell stress *(37)*. Besides their defect in protein synthesis, $\gamma_1$34.5 mutant derivatives are hypersensitive to interferon α, and therefore more sensitive to this arm of innate host defenses that serve to limit viral replication in the host *(38,39)*. This hypothesis is supported by reports demonstrating that $\gamma_1$34.5 mutant viruses, whereas neuroattenuated in normal mice and mice with deficiencies in their acquired immune response, exhibit restored neurovirulence in mice with deficiencies in innate immunity *(33,34)*.

Ensuing genetic studies revealed that HSV-1 actually encodes multiple functions to control eIF2α phosphorylation, as the dsRNA binding protein specified by the true late Us11 gene prevents PKR activation *(40–43)*. Analysis of a panel of $\gamma_1$34.5 and Us11 mutants established that both Us11 and $\gamma_1$34.5 gene products act at different times in the productive growth cycle to regulate eIF2α phosphorylation in infected cells *(44)* (*see* Fig. 3C). Importantly, Us11 expressed in its natural context as a late γ_2 protein is required to properly regulate PKR activation, eIF2α phosphorylation, and viral translation. Thus, because late proteins are not produced in nonpermissive tumor cells infected with a $\gamma_1$34.5 mutant virus, the $\gamma_1$34.5 mutant is actually doubly deficient in that it also fails to translate the γ_2 Us11 mRNA. Moreover, the interferon sensitivity of $\gamma_1$34.5 mutants, previously attributed solely to the absence of $\gamma_1$34.5 function, likewise results from the absence of the $\gamma_1$34.5 protein and the failure to synthesize the Us11 polypeptide *(45)*.

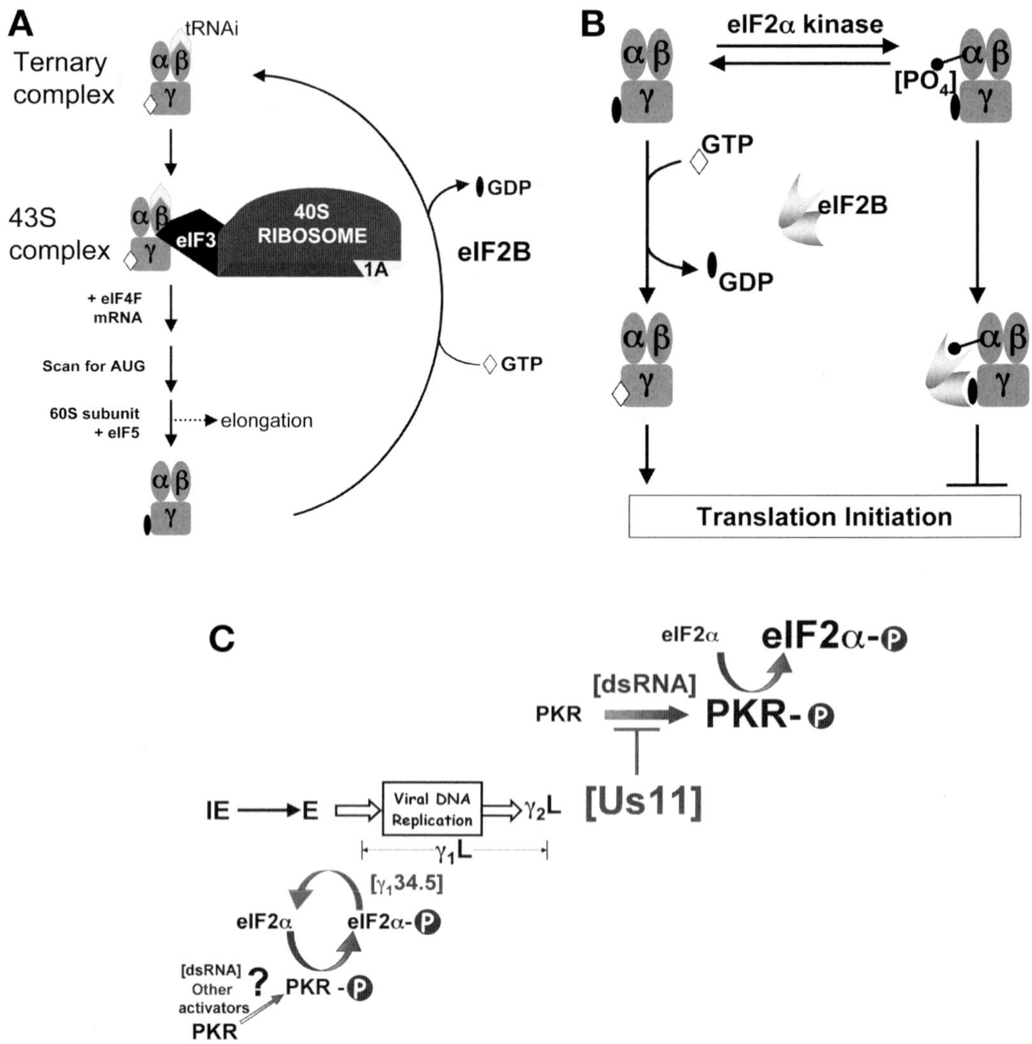

Fig. 3. Regulation of translation by phosphorylation of eIF2, a critical translation initiation factor. (**A**) Composed of α,β, and γ subunits, eukaryotic translation initiation factor 2 (eIF2) forms a ternary complex with GTP and the initiator tRNA (tRNAi). This complex associates with the 40S ribosomal subunit bound to eIF3, and recognizes the 5′-end of the mRNA through an association with eIF4F. Once the AUG codon in the mRNA has been identified by a unidirectional translocation process termed scanning, GTP hydroylsis stimulated by eIF5 and the subsequent release of the eIF2·GDP complex facilitate the joining of the 60S ribosome subunit and translation elongation commences. The guanine nucleotide exchange factor eIF2B is required to exchange the GDP bound to eIF2 and replace it with GTP, thus recycling the active form of eIF2. (**B**) After phosphorylation of eIF2 on its α subunit by PKR, an eIF2α kinase, eIF2B remains tightly bound and cannot exchange the GDP bound to eIF2 for GTP. This failure to recycle eIF2 to its active, GTP bound form inhibits the initiation of translation. (**C**) Regulation of eIF2α phosphorylation by different functions that act during discrete phases in the HSV-1 lifecycle. Early in the HSV-1 lifecycle, small quantities of dsRNA, or perhaps other effectors that remain to be identified activate the normally dormant cellular PKR kinase. After assembling a dimer of PKR on dsRNA, each subunit of the multimer phosphorylates the other (PKR–P). Because PKR is activated in cells infected with a $\gamma_1$34.5 mutant virus, preventing the translation of γ_2 mRNAs, we propose that the $\gamma_1$34.5 gene product, through its interaction with PP1α, is able to adequately dephosphorylate the quantities of phosphorylated eIF2α (eIF2α–P)

7. WORKING WITH WHAT YOU HAVE: TACTICS TO AUGMENT THE ONCOLYTIC ABILITY OF $\gamma_1$34.5 MUTANT DERIVATIVES

Although $\gamma_1$34.5 mutant derivatives appeared safe in preclinical animal studies, their restricted replication resulting from their inability to counter components of the innate host response needed to be addressed if they were to emerge as efficacious oncolytic agents. One approach to deal with this concern combines conventional chemotherapy and radiotherapy with oncolytic virus treatment of mice with human tumor implants, taking advantage of specific properties associated with each treatment modality *(46–50)*. On the one hand, traditional systemic treatments, although highly toxic, are able to effectively debulk a tumor. Oncolytic $\gamma_1$34.5 mutant derivatives, on the other hand, appear safe but have limited replicative ability in many human tumor cells. The question at hand then, was if the two therapeutic components together were more effective than each individual component. In support of this idea, head and neck derived squamous cell carcinomas implanted into mice subcutaneously and treated with a combination of cisplatin and G207 responded better than tumors treated with either single agent *(49)*. In addition, combining G207 treatment with radiation improved its antitumor activity against human colorectal carcinoma xenografts in mice, whereas no additional effects on its ability to reduce the growth of human prostate cancer xenografts in mice and mouse prostate cancer were detected *(48,51)*. Prior exposure to ionizing radiation appears to enhance the replication of the γ34.5 mutant R3616 in human malignant gliomas implanted into athymic mice, but not in subcutaneous tumors composed of human colorectal carcinoma cells *(46,48)*. The differential effects of radiation treatment might be emblematic of the γ34.5 derivatives used in each study (R3616 vs G207), or reflect tissue specific variation in the tumor cell populations. Irrespective of any potential synergistic effects, as viral oncolysis proceeds through a completely different mechanism than chemotherapy or radiotherapy, and should cells resistant to the latter treatments arise, it was thought that they would certainly remain sensitive to the former. Although these initial studies were consistent with this view in that tumor cells resistant to traditional chemotherapy and/or ionizing radiation remained sensitive to HSV-1 oncolysis and did not develop resistance to infection with an HSV-1 oncolytic mutant *(46)*, recent experiments offer a different perspective. Upon selection of a radio-resistant human squamous cell carcinoma by irradiation of athymic mice harboring implanted tumors, upregulation of components of interferon (IFN) related signal pathways was observed. Indeed, these radio-resistant cells no longer supported robust replication of a

produced from the period preceding the initiation of viral DNA synthesis and extending into the initial segment of the late phase (designated as γ_1L). However, late in the viral lifecycle, synthesis of mRNA from γ_2 genes (γ_2L), many of which are transcribed from ORFs located on opposing DNA strands, results in the production of large quantities of viral dsRNA. In the absence of Us11, the increase in dsRNA concentration generates more activated PKR, which in turn phosphorylates eIF2α. The concentration of phosphorylated eIF2α quickly rises beyond the capacity of the $\gamma_1$34.5–PP1α complex to effectively reverse the reaction, accounting for the observed reduction in viral translation rates in cells infected with a Us11 mutant virus. We suggest that although the $\gamma_1$34.5 protein acts downstream of phosphorylated eIF2α and therefore has the potential to counter a variety of eIF2α kinases, Us11 acts late in infection to specifically antagonize PKR activation in response to the copious levels of dsRNA produced in virus infected cells. In this drawing, relative concentrations of PKR -P, dsRNA, and eIF2α–P at earlier, compared with later times in the viral lifecycle, are represented by character size. Panel **C** is reprinted from ref. *44* with permission.

$\gamma_1$34.5 mutant virus *(52)*. This is not surprising, as PKR is an interferon induced gene, and its activation clearly restricts replication of $\gamma_1$34.5 mutant derivatives and potentially limiting their effectiveness when administered as adjuvant agents along with radiation.

An alternative to the joint administration of an oncolytic virus with standard chemo- or radiotherapy involves combining viral oncolysis with the delivery of transgenes designed to potentiate the activation of prodrug chemotherapeutic agents. Oncolytic $\gamma_1$34.5 mutant viruses have been constructed that contain genes encoding either cytochrome P450 2B1 or cytosine deaminase *(53,54)*. Its expression restricted to the liver, cytochrome P450 2B1 is required to generate the active toxic metabolite phosphoramide mustard which is in turn systemically distributed throughout the circulation. Engineered oncolytic HSV-1 derivatives that express cytochrome P450 2B1 have been used to achieve potentially greater concentrations of active metabolites within the local tumor environment, enhancing destruction of cancer cells *(53)*. Likewise, deamination of cytosine to uracil by cytosine deaminase, which is not expressed in mammalian cells, can convert 5-fluorocytosine to 5-fluorouracil, a potent agent used in cancer chemotherapy. The cytosine deaminase gene has been inserted into the HSV-1 ribonucleotide reductase gene, allowing exclusive conversion of systemically administered, nontoxic 5-FC to the toxic 5′-FU in infected tumor cells *(54)*. Importantly, both of these metabolites, while ultimately toxic to cells, appear not to significantly dampen HSV-1 replication. However, all of these adjuvant therapies, designed to enhance overall tumor regression, do nothing to address the underlying replicative deficiencies of oncolytic $\gamma_1$34.5 mutant derivatives.

8. BUILDING A BETTER VIRUS: GENETIC STRATEGIES TO INCREASE VIRULENCE IN TUMOR CELLS

An alternative method for augmenting the oncolytic ability of an HSV-1 $\gamma_1$34.5 mutant serendipitously emerged from further genetic analysis. To learn if other viral components were important in regulating PKR activation and eIF2α phosphorylation, a $\gamma_1$34.5 deletion mutant was sequentially passed in nonpermissive cells to select for isolates with restored capacity to replicate *(40)*. These isolates had all sustained genetic rearrangements where the Us11 γ_2 late promoter and most of the Us12 ORF, including the AUG initiation codon, were deleted (*see* Fig. 4). This extragenic or second-site suppressor mutation resulted in the IE expression of Us11, a dsRNA binding protein that inhibits PKR activation, and allows $\gamma_1$34.5 mutants to replicate efficiently in what were previously nonpermissive cells *(40–43)*. The significant surprise was that although the suppressor mutant was capable of restored growth in cells that failed to support the replication of the $\gamma_1$34.5 parent virus, it essential remained as neuroattenuated as the parental $\gamma_1$34.5 mutant at the doses examined (up to 2×10^7 pfu). This established that it was possible to introduce additional mutations into the genome of an HSV-1 $\gamma_1$34.5 mutant that dramatically improve its replicative ability in cancer cells without increasing neurovirulence in mice *(55)*.

The attenuated neurovirulence profile of the suppressor mutant coupled with its dramatically improved replication properties made it an ideal oncolytic virus candidate. The antitumor activity of the suppressor virus was directly compared with the γ34.5 mutant in three independent studies that utilized an animal model of different human cancers as well as a variety of viral genetic backgrounds *(56–58)*. All of these studies demonstrated that incorporating the suppressor mutation into a γ34.5 mutant virus resulted in

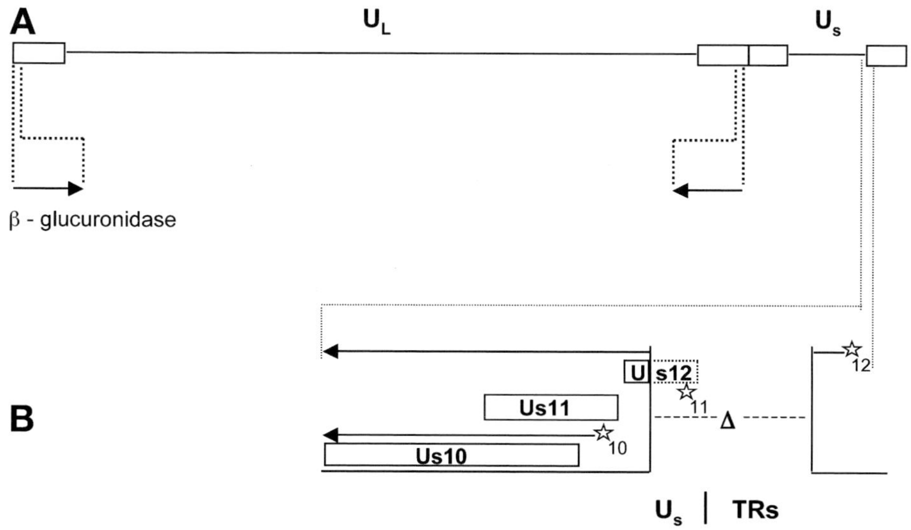

Fig. 4. Genetic structure of an attenuated, oncolytic HSV-1 γ34.5 null virus with an additional growth enhancing mutation. The location of the γ34.5 deletion (**A**) and the additional extragenic suppressor mutation (**B**) is shown on the viral genome. The unique long (UL) region and unique short (Us) region are shown as solid lines. Repetitive regions appear as open rectangles. This neuroattenuated suppressor variant contains two mutations: (1) both copies of the γ34.5 gene have been replaced with sequences encoding β-glucuronidase (**A**); and (2) a 583 bp deletion (Δ) that spans the junction region where the viral Us segment joins the TRs component (**B**). The Us10, Us11, and Us12 open reading frames are shown. The segment of the Us12 open reading frame that is removed by the deletion is represented as a broken rectangle. The two RNA's that are synthesized appear as arrows above the open reading frames. Promoter elements that direct the synthesis of these RNAs appear as stars and each promoter is normally associated with either the Us10, Us11, or Us12 ORF (denoted by the number 10,11, or 12 at the lower right of each star). Note that the suppressor deletion removes the endogenous late Us11 promoter and a large segment of the Us12 ORF, including the ATG codon. This allows the transcript initiating from the immediate-early Us12 promoter in the TRs to direct the synthesis of the Us11 protein. Accumulation of Us11 at immediate-early times allows the suppressor mutant to sustain protein synthesis and thus replicate in nonpermissive cells that do not support the growth of γ34.5 mutants. Furthermore, IE expression of Us11 also renders the virus resistant to interferon α, whereas simple Δ34.5 mutants remain exquisitely sensitive.

a dramatic improvement in the ability of the virus to inhibit tumor growth. A single injection of subcutaneous human prostate cancer tumors with 10^6 pfu of the suppressor virus reduced tumor volume by 50% or more in 60% of the treated animals, whereas animals treated with the γ34.5 mutant were indistinguishable from mock treated animals (*see* Fig. 5) *(56)*. Although inhibition of tumor growth was observed in animals treated with the γ34.5 mutant at 10-fold higher doses of virus, equivalent doses of the suppressor virus still proved more effective. In addition, long-term responders were only seen in animals treated with the suppressor virus *(56)*. A second study arrived at similar conclusions using an independently constructed virus (G47D) that contained a suppressor mutation in a G207 genetic background using a different tumor model. Following two treatments with 10^6 pfu of G47D, 66% of subcutaneous human gliomas implanted into athymic mice completely regressed and exhibited no signs of regrowth during a 3-mo follow-up period whereas only 25% of G207 treated gliomas responded accordingly. Moreover, G47D significantly prolonged the survival of tumor bearing animals *(57)*. Likewise, a third study found that a $\gamma_1$34.5 mutant expressing Us11 as an

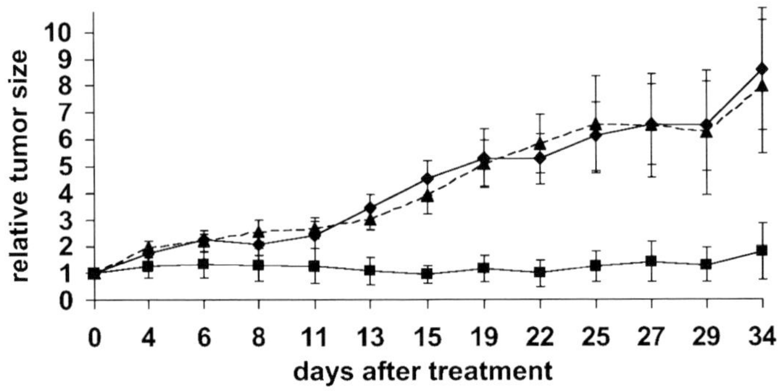

Fig. 5. Evaluation of γ34.5 mutant derivatives that express Us11 at IE times as an antitumor agent in an animal model of human prostate cancer. Balb/c nu/nu mice ($n = 5$ for each treatment group) harboring established, subcutaneous PC3 tumors measuring approximately 50 mm^3 received a single injection containing 2×10^6 pfu of either the γ34.5 deletion mutant Δ34.5 (▲, dotted line) the suppressor mutant SUP (■), or a virus free lysate prepared from mock infected cells (◆). Tumors were measured every 2 d for 34 d and the average normalized values reflecting relative tumor size on each day were plotted. The initial tumor volume immediately prior to treatment was normalized to a relative size of 1.0. Error bars reflect the standard error of the mean. Reprinted with permission from ref. *56*.

IE protein was more effective than a simple $\gamma_1$34.5 deletion mutant in inducing prolonged regression of several different human tumors implanted into athymic mice. Instead of using a laboratory HSV-1 strain, the latter study introduced a $\gamma_1$34.5 deletion, either alone or in conjunction with a suppressor mutation allowing for IE Us11 expression, into a freshly isolated clinical HSV-1 strain *(58)*. Finally, in addition to overcoming the block to protein synthesis seen in cells infected with a $\gamma_1$34.5 mutant derivative, the suppressor mutation, by allowing the production of Us11 as an IE protein, confers interferon resistance and allows a $\gamma_1$34.5 mutant virus to counteract this important arm of innate host defenses *(45)*.

Other avenues to genetically modify $\gamma_1$34.5 mutant derivatives have met with limited success. In one approach, the $\gamma_1$34.5 gene was reintroduced into the viral genome such that it is expressed from a conditional promoter active only in dividing cancer cells. Although this virus demonstrated greater oncolytic activity and remains dramatically more attenuated than wild-type HSV-1, it also was more neurovirulent (LD_{50} 2.7×10^7 pfu) than the parental $\gamma_1$34.5 mutant and serves to illustrate the potential drawbacks of viruses that carry wild-type alleles of the $\gamma_1$34.5 gene *(59,60)*. The oncolytic potential of an engineered virus with a single copy of the $\gamma_1$34.5 gene and a mutation in a repetitive genome component thought to render it non-neuroinvasive has also been explored (*see* Fig. 6). This strain, R7020 and its clonal derivative NV1020, was originally developed as a vaccine candidate that expressed HSV-2 glycoproteins and while non-neuroinvasive, is substantially more neurovirulent than $\gamma_1$34.5 deficient viruses *(61,62)*. Although R7020 and NV1020 replicate more effectively in tumors than a $\gamma_1$34.5 null mutant, they are not suitable for use in CNS tumors *(63)*. A different strategy involved replacing the $\gamma_1$34.5 gene with a hybrid gene encoding a fusion protein where the amino terminus of the $\gamma_1$34.5 protein was joined to the C-terminal segment of the rodent GADD34 gene, myD116. Whereas this recombinant was sufficiently neuroattenuated, it was unable to enhance the survival of mice with syngeneic gliomas beyond that achieved with a $\gamma_1$34.5 mutant virus *(21)*.

Finally $\gamma_1$34.5 mutant derivatives have been constructed that express ectopic transgenes, such as a soluble version of the immunostimulatory molecule B7-1 or the

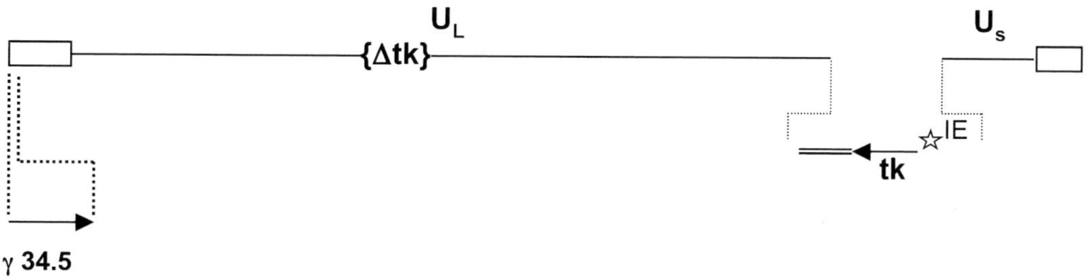

Fig. 6. Genetic structure of a neurovirulent, non-neuroinvasive oncolytic virus suitable for use in non-CNS tumors. R7020, the parent virus of this line, was initially designed as a potential vaccine candidate. These viruses (R7020, NV1020 and transgene containing derivatives in strain F) contain one copy of the γ34.5 gene and a deletion affecting the endogenous thymidine kinase (tk) gene. A cassette that ectopically expresses the viral thymidine kinase gene from an immediate-early (IE) promoter (star) and HSV-2 glycoproteins (double line) replaces the repetitive component containing the second copy of the γ34.5 gene. These viruses therefore produce both the thymidine kinase and γ34.5 gene products.

cytokines interleukin 4 (IL-4), IL-12, granulocyte, macrophage colony stimulating factor (GM-CSF), which are secreted from infected cells and possibly enhance tumor regression without augmenting the replicative ability of the oncolytic virus *(58,64,65)*. In a syngeneic mouse glioma model, animals treated with vehicle or the parent $\gamma_1 34.5$ mutant virus exhibited a mean survival of approximately 19.5 d, whereas animals treated with an IL-12 producing $\gamma_1 34.5$ mutant had a median survival of 50.5 d. IL-12 additionally caused increased infiltration of immune effector cells into the tissue *(65)*. This could potentially augment the antitumor immune response, or alternatively, it might prove problematic, inflicting damage to surrounding normal tissue or hindering oncolysis by promoting enhanced virus clearance. At least in a subcutaneous flank model of murine squamous cell carcinoma treated with an IL-12 expressing NV1020 derivative, which although non-neuroinvasive remains neurovirulent because of the presence of a wild-type $\gamma_1 34.5$ gene, the first of these possibilities appears to prevail. Direct injection of the IL-12 producing NV1020 virus, NV1042, into the tumor not only resulted in greater regression when compared with tumors treated with the parental, noncytokine expressing virus, but also, upon subsequent rechallenge of treated animals with additional cancer cells, was more effective at preventing tumor growth on the contralateral flank. This latter effect required $CD4^+$ and $CD8^+$ T-cells, suggesting that the IL12 expressing virus was able to stimulate a superior antitumor immune response *(66)*.

9. SPREADING THE WORD: CAN ONCOLYTIC VIRUSES DELIVER SYSTEMIC RESULTS?

Whereas direct treatment of the primary tumor is a viable option, it is not always practical; moreover, in many cancers, it is recurrent disease often emerging at distant sites from micrometastases that ultimately prove fatal. With this in mind, other studies have explored alternate modes of administering oncolytic viruses and their effectiveness against disseminated disease. Systemic intravenous delivery of oncolytic HSV-1 strains can regress subcutaneous primary tumors implanted into mice *(50,67)*. Although the mechanism remains unclear, tumor cells seem to exhibit an inherent predilection for infection following the systemic administration of an oncolytic virus *(68)*. In addition, treatment of established intracerebral tumors with IV injection of an oncolytic HSV-1 mutant was markedly enhanced by cobra venom phosphatase mediated complement depletion and cyclophosphamide, an immunosuppressive agent that blocks both the neutralizing antibody as well as innate responses *(50,69)*. Finally, following injection into the primary tumor, HSV-1 can spread through the lymph system to sites of distant, lymphatic metastases *(70)*.

In a different vein, the acquired immune response of the host holds promise to augment the antitumor activity of an oncolytic virus. Although a large fraction of the population is seropositive for HSV-1 by adulthood, this does not appear to significantly hinder the antitumor potential of the virus in HSV-1 seropositive mice with syngeneic tumor implants *(58,71–73)*. In other experiments where syngeneic tumors were bilaterally implanted into HSV-1 naïve mice and only one tumor was injected with G207, both tumors regressed whereas only the injected tumor was positive for lacZ, a marker for G207 infection *(74)*. Intradermal inoculation with G207 did not produce tumor regression, suggesting that this effect was dependent on delivery of the virus to the tumor. Furthermore, a $CD8^+$ cytotoxic T-cell response directed against a dominant tumor specific MHC class I restricted epitope presented by the cancer cells was associated with regression of uninfected tumors *(74)*. This elevated CTL activity directed against the tumor cells persisted for at least 13 mo *(75)*. Thus, oncolytic HSV-1 mutants appear to be capable of fostering a systemic antitumor response in mice, one component of which involves the generation of tumor specific cytotoxic T-lymphocytes (CTLs). Moreover, this ability of oncolytic viruses to induce regression of tumors at distant sites appears to be enhanced by the inclusion of cytokine encoding genes in the viral genome. The efficacy of NV1042, a NV1020 derivative expressing IL-12, a cytokine secreted by antigen producing cells that exhibits antitumor effects in mice, was examined in a mouse model of squamous cell carcinoma with pulmonary metastases *(76)*. Tumor bearing mice treated intravenously with NV1042 displayed a dramatic reduction in pulmonary nodules and enhanced survival compared with mice treated with PBS or NV1023, a virus isogenic to NV1042 that does not express IL-12. Strikingly, 100% survival of animals injected with a low tumor burden (1×10^5 SCC cells) and treated with NV1042 was achieved, whereas only 70% of animals treated with NV1023 survived. The enhanced efficacy of NV1042 relative to NV 1023 was abrogated by depletion of CD4+/8+ T-cells, suggesting that the impact of IL-12 expression required these components of the acquired immune system *(76)*. Likewise, the ability of a $\gamma_1$34.5 suppressor mutant which produces Us11 as an IE protein to induce regression of contralaterally implanted, noninjected tumors was enhanced if the virus also encoded GM-CSF *(58)*. Notably, it was not possible to reestablish tumors in animals where the tumors were successfully eradicated by prior oncolytic virus treatment, suggesting that an antitumor immune response had indeed developed *(58)*.

10. FROM THE LABORATORY TO THE CLINIC: ONCOLYTIC HERPES SIMPLEX VIRUSES APPEAR SAFE IN TRIALS, BUT JUST HOW EFFECTIVE WILL THEY BE?

Within the past few years, two independent dose escalation phase I clinical trials using two different $\gamma_1$34.5 mutant derivatives, G207 (21 patients) and 1716 (9 patients), were completed in patients with recurrent glioblastoma who have failed to respond to conventional therapies *(16,17)*. The oncolytic viruses were generally well tolerated. No adverse events, such as acute toxicity, viral shedding, clinically evident reactivation or encephalitis attributable to virus inoculation or replication were observed in either study at any of the doses, which escalated from 10^3–10^5 pfu with 1716 and 1×10^6–3×10^9 with G207 *(16,17)*. Patient deaths were primarily the reuslt of progressive cancer, with one report of radiation necrosis. Two of the G207 treated patients were alive as of December, 2003 *(77)*. In addition, both studies were unable to establish a maximum tolerated dose *(16,17)*. More recently, evidence has been obtained that is reportedly consistent with replication of 1716 within tumor samples over time, supporting the concept of tumor destruction by viral oncolysis *(78)*. Finally, multiple injections of 1716 directly into skin lesions of a limited number of melanoma patients have proceeded without any harmful effects *(79)*. A phase Ib/II study involving G207 is currently underway open to patients with recurrent glioblastoma that has been refractory to prior chemotherapy (NLM identifier NCT00028158; *www.clinicaltrials.gov*). In the phase Ib segment, doses will escalate from 10^9–10^{10}, and provided no safety issues arise, the phase II component aimed at evaluating efficacy will begin using the highest dose tolerated in the phase Ib study. Studies to determine the efficacy of 1716 treatment are set to proceed as well.

Clinical trials have also commenced using NV1020 to treat colon cancer that has spread to the liver and has not responded to prior chemotherapy (NLM identifier NCT00012155; *www.clinicaltrials.gov*). This study, which is no longer recruiting patients, is a dose escalating protocol designed to evaluate the safety, tolerability, and antitumor activity of a single intrahepatic arterial injection of NV1020. Although this virus replicates more robustly than $\gamma_1 34.5$ null strains, it is substantially more virulent, presumably because it produces the $\gamma_1 34.5$ gene product, and is unsuitable for use in the CNS. As this strain is non-neuroinvasive and cannot gain entry into the CNS, it may be useful in treating non-CNS tumors that are refractory to traditional therapies. Extensive prior study of R7020, the parent of NV1020, as a putative vaccine strain demonstrated its safety for non-CNS administration to rabbits, rodents, and nonhuman primates *(61,62)*. However, one must not lose sight of the fact that this strain is neurovirulent and, unlike strains with $\gamma_1 34.5$ null alleles, could prove harmful if it was somehow introduced into the CNS.

11. MINING THE FINDINGS OF BASIC SCIENCE: SOME THOUGHTS ON FUTURE PROSPECTS

Without a doubt, the development of engineered oncolytic HSV-1 derivatives from the bench to the clinic has been remarkable, feeding off of basic science discoveries, some of them inadvertent, which produced further innovation in the area of designer oncolytic viruses. The fact that $\gamma_1 34.5$ derivatives can safely be introduced into the brains of human patients, many of whom have had immunosuppressive treatments, is truly remarkable, and is of course a prerequisite for their clinical use *(16,17)*. However, the fact that most $\gamma_1 34.5$ mutant derivatives, including both of the mutants in clinical trials, are impaired in their ability to replicate in many types of human cancer cells has been documented in numerous laboratories and clearly compromises their oncolytic activity. This deficiency has only been intensified by the subsequent introduction of additional mutations to create multimutated strains, such as G207. Whereas these additional mutations certainly serve as additional checks on safety, their overriding effect is to reduce the global ability of the virus to replicate and thereby severely diminish its oncolytic potential. Only continued phase II studies in humans will be able to definitively establish their efficacy. Should they successfully stimulate a host immune response against the tumor, they might conceivably display substantial efficacy in the absence of any adjuvant therapy. On the other hand, although a pre-existing, experimentally induced immune response appears not to hinder the oncolytic efficacy of $\gamma_1$34.5 mutant viruses in mice, it does not preclude the possibility that the existing immune response in humans, confronted with numerous episodes of viral reactivation over their lifetime, may adversely impact the oncolytic ability of these viruses. Should this latter scenario prove true, poor replication of these strains may foster the immune mediated clearance of the virus given that most adults are seropositive for HSV-1, thus severely limiting their effectiveness as has been reported for oncolytic adenoviruses lacking the viral E3 immunomodulatory function *(80)*.

Phase I safety trials are also underway using non-neuroinvasive viruses to treat cancers other than CNS malignancies. Whereas viruses such as NV1020 replicate substantially better than $\gamma_1$34.5 mutant derivatives in cancer cells, they remain highly neurovirulent reflecting the fact that they contain a functional $\gamma_1$34.5 gene. True, these strains are susceptible to multiple antiviral agents, and R7020, the NV1020 parent strain, in particular has been subjected to extensive testing in older studies as a vaccine candidate *(61,62)*. However, the presence of a wild-type neurovirulence gene is difficult to overlook and it is somewhat surprising that more efforts have not been made to assess the safety of a neuroattenuated virus with improved growth properties, such as $\gamma_1$34.5 mutant derivatives that express Us11 as an IE protein, in nonhuman primates and if the results warrant into phase I human trials.

$\gamma_1$34.5 mutant derivatives that express Us11 as an IE protein seem to represent an attractive alternative, remaining attenuated because of the complete absence of any $\gamma_1$34.5 genetic material while replicating effectively in human cancer cells. In the absence of the $\gamma_1$34.5 gene product, the Us11 polypeptide is able to prevent PKR activation and the subsequent accumulation of phosphorylated eIF2α, thus overcoming the major obstacle limiting the replicative potential of $\gamma_1$34.5 mutant derivatives in human cancer cells. In addition, IE Us11 expression confers interferon resistance upon a virus that was formerly exquisitely interferon sensitive, allowing the oncolytic virus to resist the onslaught of innate host defenses. Without the ability to counter this arm of host innate immunity, the replicative ability and capacity of a $\gamma_1$34.5 mutant derivative to spread throughout the tumor mass is likely to be severely curtailed. Indeed, $\gamma_1$34.5 mutant derivatives that express Us11 as an IE protein are substantially more effective oncolytic agents in either the genetic background of the multi-mutated G207 strain or simply in the context of a $\gamma_1$34.5 deletion mutant *(56–58)*. Although $\gamma_1$34.5 mutant derivatives that express Us11 as an IE protein and remain neuroattenuated were initially discovered through the isolation of $\gamma_1$34.5 extragenic or second-site suppressor mutations, a lone report describes an altogether different class of $\gamma_1$34.5 variants which exhibit partially restored neurovirulence ($LD_{50} = 4.8 \times 10^5$ pfu) in the absence of alterations to Us11 expression or the Us—TRs region of the genome *(81)*. However, although this could possibly raise concerns that any $\gamma_1$34.5 mutant derivative, including multimutated strains like G207, might sustain additional mutations that enhance virulence to some degree, its significance remains unclear, as the nature of the mutation or mutations responsible for this phenotype has never been identified. Misgivings regarding virulence, although important, seem to have been applied selectively, given that viruses like NV1020 which have advanced into clinical trials for non-CNS tumors are themselves neurovirulent, containing a wt $\gamma_1$34.5 gene, whereas the $\gamma_1$34.5 suppressor mutant that expresses Us11 as an IE polypeptide remains as attenuated as their $\gamma_1 34.5$ counterparts at the doses examined, which escalated up to 2×10^7 pfu, and has never been observed to produce a neurovirulent variant. In due course, provided that they prove safe in aotus monkeys, which are exquisitely sensitive to HSV-1, the utility of $\gamma_1 34.5$ derivatives that express Us11 as an IE protein, may supplant current interest in using HSV-1 strains that carry wt $\gamma_1 34.5$ genetic material as oncolytic agents.

Owing to the location of the Us11 late promoter and the nature of the deletion that removes it, permitting transcripts initiating from the Us12 IE promoter to encode the Us11 polypeptide, $\gamma_1 34.5$ derivatives which express Us11 as an IE protein are also deficient for the Us12 gene product. As an immunomodulatory protein that inhibits the cellular TAP polypeptide, preventing MHC class I molecules from complexing with peptide antigens in the ER lumen, the absence of Us12 function may in fact contribute an unforeseen layer of safety and attenuation upon these oncolytic strains in vivo *(82–84)*. Of course, the absence of Us12 might play itself out in one of two ways. In the first, increased presentation of viral antigens on the surface of infected cells might result in increased clearance of the oncolytic virus, effectively eliminating the infection and its chances of spreading through the tumor. In the second scenario, one may posit desirable consequences resulting from the enhanced presentation of viral antigens, such as the production of a more robust immune response against tumor antigens capable of destroying not only cells within the primary, treated tumor, but micrometastases that have disseminated to distant sites. The reduced efficiency with which Us12 functions in a mouse, regrettably, makes it difficult to assess which of these two possibilities is destined to occur in humans by experimenting with animal models *(85)*.

Whereas all of the oncolytic HSV-1 strains in use to date rely somehow on restricting replication to cancer cells based upon interactions between viral and host proteins inside the cell, a promising alternative approach is to restrict the entry of oncolytic HSV-1 derivatives to malignant cells. This strategy could potentially be applied to create new oncolytic strains, either as a stand-alone modification or engineered into existing attenuated oncolytic strains as an additional level of tumor specificity and safety. Normally, entry of HSV-1 into cells involves an association between heparan sulfate on the cell surface and viral glycoproteins gB along with gC. Interaction of gD with its receptors, HveA and nectin, mediates subsequent membrane fusion *(86)*. Targeted entry of HSV-1 has been achieved by removing the heparan sulfate binding glycoproteins gB/gC, and engineering a gD variant that: (1) can no longer interact with HveA; (2) retains the ability to bind the nectin coreceptor; and (3) contains a new domain conferring alternate receptor binding specificity. Such a strategy was first illustrated by inserting IL13 encoding sequences into the gD gene at codon 24 *(87)*. Importantly, this recombinant virus only replicates in cells expressing the IL13 receptor, a molecule typically abundant on the surface of glioma cells. However, the frequency with which tumor cells resistant to this synthetic mode of HSV-1 entry arise has not been investigated and could severely curtail its utility.

12. CONCLUSION

"We shall not cease from exploration
And the end of all our exploring
Will be to arrive where we started
And know the place for the first time."

– T.S. Eliot, Four Quartets, 1942.

The revolutionary technical developments in molecular biology, coupled with tremendous advances in our understanding of the genetics behind HSV-1 neurovirulence have made the development of engineered, attenuated strains for use as oncolytic viruses possible. Whereas experiments in animal models have revealed both the various strengths and weaknesses that surround each of the strains that have been created in the laboratory, other information can only be learned through advancing these candidates into the clinic. It is extremely encouraging that the first of these agents have been safely administered to an infirm patient population suffering from a truly devastating condition. Completion of phase II trials with G207 and 1716 will be required to learn just how effective they are. Then, of course, their use as adjuvant treatments along with existing therapies can be investigated. Hopefully, successive $\gamma_1$34.5 mutant derivatives with heightened efficacy in animal models will be examined for their safety in nonhuman primates and make their way into phase I trials. One thing, however, is almost certain—that as our understanding of how HSV-1 interfaces with its human host increases we will learn ever more about how the 84 viral genes presently known execute a bewildering array of tasks that completely dominates host cell metabolism. We are likely to uncover, or perhaps more appropriately, stumble upon the unexpected. Perhaps it is the unexpected that will one day put the finishing touches on the genetic alchemy begun in the last decade of the last century, and allow human kind to tame a pathogenic virus. Redirecting its pathogenic gene expression program to a therapeutic end.

ACKNOWLEDGMENTS

I thank Matthew Mulvey for his thoughtful, critical comments on the manuscript and Lynn Koch for assistance with its preparation. Work in my laboratory is supported by grants from the National Institutes of Health and the Department of Defense. Finally, I apologize to those colleagues whose works could not be discussed because of space constraints.

REFERENCES

1. Sinkovics J, Horvath J. New developments in the virus therapy of cancer: a historical review. Intervirology 1993; 36:193–214.
2. Roizman B, Knipe D. Herpes simplex viruses and their replication. In: Knipe DM and Howley PM, eds. Fields Virology, 4th ed., vol. 2., Philadelphia: Lippincott, Williams & Wilkins, 2001: 2399–2460.
3. Martuza RL, Malick A, Markert JM, Ruffner KL, Coen DM. Experimental therapy of human glioma by means of a genetically engineered virus mutant. Science 1991;252:854–856.
4. Field HJ, Wildy P. The pathogenicity of thymidine kinase-deficient mutants of herpes simplex virus in mice. J Hyg (Lond). 1978;81:267–277.
5. Jamieson AT, Gentry GA, Subak-Sharpe JH. Induction of both thymidine and deoxycytidine kinase activity by herpes viruses. J Gen Virol 1974;24:465–480.
6. Field HJ, Darby G. Pathogenicity in mice of strains of herpes simplex virus which are resistant to acyclovir in vitro and in vivo. Antimicrob Agents Chemother 1980;17:209–216.
7. Tenser RB, Miller RL, Rapp F. Trigeminal ganglion infection by thymidine kinase-negative mutants of herpes simplex virus. Science 1979;205:915–917.
8. Coen DM, Kosz-Vnenchak M, Jacobson JG, et al. Thymidine kinase-negative herpes simplex virus mutants establish latency in mouse trigeminal ganglia but do not reactivate. Proc Natl Acad Sci U S A 1989;86:4736–4740.
9. Markert JM, Malick A, Coen DM, Martuza RL. Reduction and elimination of encephalitis in an experimental glioma therapy model with attenuated herpes simplex mutants that retain susceptibility to acyclovir. Neurosurgery 1993;32:597–603.
10. Mineta T, Rabkin SD, Martuza RL. Treatment of malignant gliomas using ganciclovir-hypersensitive, ribonucleotide reductase-deficient herpes simplex viral mutant. Cancer Res 1994;54:3963–3966.

11. Chou J, Kern ER, Whitley RJ, Roizman B. Mapping of herpes simplex virus-1 neurovirulence to gamma (1) 34.5, a gene nonessential for growth in culture. Science 1990;250:1262–1266.
12. Maclean AR, Ul-Fareed M, Robertson L, Harland J, Brown SM. Herpes simplex virus type 1 deletion variants 1714 and 1716 pinpoint neurovirulence-related sequences in Glasgow strain 17+ between immediate early gene 1 and the 'a' sequence. J Gen Virol 1991;72:631–639.
13. Bolovan CA, Sawtell NM, Thompson RL. ICP34.5 mutants of herpes simplex virus type 1 strain 17syn+ are attenuated for neurovirulence in mice and for replication in confluent primary mouse embryo cell cultures. J Virol 1994;68:48–55.
14. Mineta T, Rabkin SD, Yazaki T, Hunter WD, Martuza RL. Attenuated multi-mutated herpes simplex virus-1 for the treatment of malignant gliomas. Nat Med 1995;1:938–943.
15. Hunter WD, Martuza RL, Feigenbaum F, et al. Attenuated, replication-competent herpes simplex virus type 1 mutant G207: safety evaluation of intracerebral injection in nonhuman primates. J Virol 1999;73:6319–6326.
16. Markert JM, Medlock MD, Rabkin SD, et al. Conditionally replicating herpes simplex virus mutant, G207 for the treatment of malignant glioma: results of a phase I trial. Gene Ther 2000;7:867–874.
17. Rampling R, Cruickshank G, Papanastassiou V, et al. Toxicity evaluation of replication-competent herpes simplex virus (ICP 34.5 null mutant 1716) in patients with recurrent malignant glioma. Gene Ther 2000;7:859–866.
18. Sundaresan P, Hunter WD, Martuza RL, Rabkin SD. Attenuated, replication-competent herpes simplex virus type 1 mutant G207: safety evaluation in mice. J Virol 2000;74:3832–3841.
19. Chambers R, Gillespie GY, Soroceanu L, et al. Comparison of genetically engineered herpes simplex viruses for the treatment of brain tumors in a scid mouse model of human malignant glioma. Proc Natl Acad Sci U S A 1995;92:1411–1415.
20. Kesari S, Randazzo BP, Valyi-Nagy T, et al. Therapy of experimental human brain tumors using a neuroattenuated herpes simplex virus mutant. Lab Invest 1995;73:636–648.
21. Andreansky SS, He B, Gillespie GY, et al. The application of genetically engineered herpes simplex viruses to the treatment of experimental brain tumors. Proc Natl Acad Sci U S A 1996;93:11,313–11,318.
22. Andreansky S, Soroceanu L, Flotte ER, et al. Evaluation of genetically engineered herpes simplex viruses as oncolytic agents for human malignant brain tumors. Cancer Res 1997;57:1502–1509.
23. Randazzo BP, Kesari S, Gesser RM, et al. Treatment of experimental intracranial murine melanoma with a neuroattenuated herpes simplex virus 1 mutant. Virology 1995;211:94–101.
24. Kesari S, Lasner TM, Balsara KR, et al. A neuroattenuated ICP34.5-deficient herpes simplex virus type 1 replicates in ependymal cells of the murine central nervous system. J Gen Virol 1998;79:525–536.
25. Lasner TM, Tal-Singer R, Kesari S, Lee VM, Trojanowski JQ, Fraser NW. Toxicity and neuronal infection of a HSV-1 ICP34.5 mutant in nude mice. J Neurovirol 1998;4:100–105.
26. Markovitz NS, Baunoch D, Roizman B. The range and distribution of murine central nervous system cells infected with the gamma(1)34.5-mutant of herpes simplex virus 1. J Virol 1997;71:5560–5569.
27. Kramm CM, Chase M, Herrlinger U, et al. Therapeutic efficiency and safety of a second-generation replication-conditional HSV1 vector for brain tumor gene therapy. Hum Gene Ther 1997;8:2057–2068.
28. Pyles, RB, Warnick RE, Chalk CL, Szanti BE, Parysek LM. A novel multiply-mutated HSV-1 strain for the treatment of human brain tumors. Hum Gene Ther 1997;8:533–544.
29. Chou J, Roizman B. The gamma (1) 34.5 gene of herpes simplex virus 1 precludes neuroblastoma cells from triggering total shutoff of protein synthesis characteristic of programed cell death in neuronal cells. Proc Natl Acad Sci U S A 1992;89:3266–3270.
30. Chou J, Chen JJ, Gross M, Roizman B. Association of a M(r) 90,000 phosphoprotein with protein kinase PKR in cells exhibiting enhanced phosphorylation of translation initiation factor eIF-2 alpha and premature shutoff of protein synthesis after infection with gamma (1) 34.5-mutants of herpes simplex virus 1. Proc Natl Acad Sci U S A 1995;92:10,516–10,520.
31. Kaufman RJ. Double-stranded RNA-activated protein kinase PKR. In: Translational Control. Sonenberg N, Hershey, JWB, Mathews, MB, eds. Cold Spring Harbor, NY: Cold Spring Harbor Laboratory Press 2000:503–528.
32. Schneider RJ, Mohr I. Translation initiation and viral tricks. Trends Biochem Sci 2003;3: 130–136.
33. Leib DA, Harrison TE, Laslo KM, Machalek MA, Moorman NJ, Virgin HW. Interferons regulate the phenotypes of wild - type and mutant herpes simplex viruses in vivo. J Exp Med 1999;189: 663—672.
34. Leib DA, Machalek MA, Williams BR, Silverman RH, Virgin HW. Specific phenotypic restoration of an attenuated virus by knockout of a host resistance gene. Proc Natl Acad Sci U S A 2000;97:6097–6101.
35. Mohr I. Neutralizing innate host defenses to control translation in HSV-1 infected cells. Int. Review of Immunol 2004;23:199–220.

36. He B, Gross M, Roizman B. The gamma(1)34.5 protein of herpes simplex virus 1 complexes with protein phosphatase 1alpha to dephosphorylate the alpha subunit of the eukaryotic translation initiation factor 2 and preclude the shutoff of protein synthesis by double-stranded RNA-activated protein kinase. Proc Natl Acad Sci U S A 1997;94:843–848.
37. Novoa I, Zeng H, Harding HP, Ron D. Feedback inhibition of the unfolded protein response by GADD34-mediated dephosphorylation of eIF2 alpha. J Cell Biol 2001;153:1011–1022.
38. Cheng G, Brett ME, He B. Val^{193} and Phe^{195} of the $\gamma_1$34.5 protein of herpes simplex virus 1 are required for viral resistance to interferon α/β. Virology 2001;290:115–120.
39. Cerveny M, Hessefort S, Yang K, Cheng G, Gross M, He B. Amino acid substitutions in the effector domain of the $\gamma_1$34.5 protein of herpes simplex virus 1 have differential effects on viral response to interferon-α. Virology 2003;307:290–300.
40. Mohr I, Gluzman Y. A herpesvirus genetic element which affects translation in the absence of the viral GADD34 function. EMBO J 1996;15:4759–4766.
41. Mulvey M, Poppers J, Ladd A, Mohr I. A herpesvirus ribosome-associated, RNA-binding protein confers a growth advantage upon mutants deficient in a GADD34-related function. J Virol 1999;73:3375–3385.
42. Poppers J, Mulvey M, Khoo D, Mohr I. Inhibition of PKR activation by the proline-rich RNA binding domain of the herpes simplex virus type 1 Us11 protein. J Virol 2000;74:11,215–11,221.
43. Khoo D, Perez C, Mohr I. Characterization of RNA determinants recognized by the arginine- and proline-rich region of Us11, a herpes simplex virus type 1 encoded double-stranded RNA binding protein that prevents PKR activation. J Virol 2002;76:11,971–11,981.
44. Mulvey M, Poppers J, Sternberg D, Mohr I. Regulation of eIF2α phosphorylation by different functions that act during discrete phases in the HSV-1 lifecycle. J Virol 2003;77:10,917–10,928.
45. Mulvey M, Camarena V, Mohr I. Full resistance of HSV-1 infected primary human cells to interferon α require both the Us11 and $\gamma_1$34.5 gene products. J Virol 2004;78:10,193–10,196.
46. Advani SJ, Sibley GS, Song PY, et al. Enhancement of replication of genetically engineered herpes simplex viruses by ionizing radiation: a new paradigm for destruction of therapeutically intractable tumors. Gene Ther. 1998;5:160–165.
47. Bradley JD, Kataoka Y, Advani S, et al. Ionizing radiation improves survival in mice bearing intracranial high-grade gliomas injected with genetically modified herpes simplex virus. Clin Cancer Res 1999;5:1517–1522.
48. Stanziale SF, Petrowsky H, Joe JK, et al. Ionizing radiation potentiates the antitumor efficacy of oncolytic herpes simplex virus G207 by upregulating ribonucleotide reductase. Surgery 2002;132:353–359.
49. Chahlavi A, Todo T, Martuza RL, Rabkin SD. Replication-competent herpes simplex virus vector G207 and cisplatin combination therapy for head and neck squamous cell carcinoma. Neoplasia 1999;1:162–169.
50. Ikeda K, Ichikawa T, Wakimoto H, et al. Oncolytic virus therapy of multiple tumors in the brain requires suppression of innate and elicited antiviral responses. Nat Med 1999;5:881–887.
51. Jorgensen TJ, Katz S, Wittmack EK, et al. Ionizing radiation does not alter the antitumor activity of herpes simplex virus vector G207 in subcutaneous tumor models of human and murine prostate cancer. Neoplasia 2001;3:451–456.
52. Khodarev NN, Beckett M, Labay E, Darga T, Roizman B, Weichselbaum RR. STAT1 is overexpressed in tumors selected for radioresistance and confers protection from radiation in transduced sensitive cells. Proc Natl Acad Sci U S A 2003;101:1714–1719.
53. Chase M, Chung RY, Chiocca EA. An oncolytic viral mutant that delivers the CYP2B1 transgene and augments cyclophosphamide chemotherapy. Nat Biotech 1998;16:444–448.
54. Nakamura H et. al. Multimodality therapy with a replication – conditional herpes simplex virus 1 mutant that expresses yeast cytosine deaminase for intratumoral conversion of 5-fluorocytosine to 5-fluorouracil. Cancer Res 2001;61:5447–5452.
55. Mohr I, Sternberg D, Ward S, Leib D, Mulvey M, Gluzman Y. A herpes simplex virus type 1 gamma34.5 second-site suppressor mutant that exhibits enhanced growth in cultured glioblastoma cells is severely attenuated in animals. J Virol 2001;75:5189–5196.
56. Taneja S, Macgregor J, Markus S, Ha S, Mohr I. Enhanced antitumor efficacy of a herpes simplex virus mutant isolated by genetic selection in cancer cells. Proc Natl Acad Sci U S A 2001;98:8804–8808.
57. Todo T, Martuza Rl, Rabkin SD, Johnson PA. Oncolytic herpes simplex virus vector with enhanced MHC class I presentation and tumor cell killing. Proc Natl Acad Sci U S A 2001;98:6396–6401.
58. Liu BL, Robinson M, Han Z-Q, et al. ICP34.5 deleted herpes simplex virus with enhanced oncolytic, immune stimulating, and anti-tumour properties. Gene Therapy 2003;10:292–303.

59. Chung RY, Saeki Y, Chiocca EA. B-myb promoter retargeting of herpes simplex virus gamma34.5 gene-mediated virulence toward tumor and cycling cells. J Virol 1999;73:7556–7564.
60. Nakamura H, Kasuya H, Mullen JT, et al. Regulation of herpes simplex virus gamma (1) 34.5 expression and oncolysis of diffuse liver metastases by Myb34.5. J Clin Invest 2002;109: 871–882.
61. Meignier B, Longnecker R, Roizman B. In vivo behavior of genetically engineered herpes simplex viruses R7017 and R7020: construction and evaluation in rodents. J Infect Dis 1988;158:602–614.
62. Meignier B, Martin B, Whitley RJ, Roizman B. In vivo behavior of genetically engineered herpes simplex viruses R7017 and R7020. II. Studies in immunocompetent and immunosuppressed owl monkeys (Aotus trivirgatus). J Infect Dis 1990;162:313–321.
63. Advani SJ, Chung SM, Yan SY, et al. Replication-competent, nonneuroinvasive genetically engineered herpes virus is highly effective in the treatment of therapy-resistant experimental human tumors. Cancer Res 1999;59:2055–2058.
64. Todo T, Martuza RL, Dallman MJ, Rabkin SD. In situ expression of soluble B7-1 in the context of oncolytic herpes virus induces potent antitumor immunity. Cancer Res 2001;61: 153–161.
65. Parker JN, Gillespie GY, Love CE, Randall S, Whitley RJ, Markert JM. Engineered herpes simplex virus expressing IL-12 in the treatment of experimental murine brain tumors. Proc Natl Acad Sci U S A 2000;97:2208–2213.
66. Wong RJ, Patel SG, Kim S-H, et al. Cytokine gene transfer enhances herpes oncolytic therapy in murine squamous cell carcinoma. Hum Gene Ther 2001;12:253–265.
67. Walker JR, McGeagh KG, Sundaresan P, Jorgensen TJ, Rabkin SD, Martuza RL. Local and systemic therapy of human prostate adenocarcinoma with the conditionally replicating herpes simplex virus vector G207. Hum Gene Ther 1999;10:2237–2243.
68. Yu YA, Shabahang S, Timiryasova TM, et al. Visualization of tumors and metastases in live animals with bacteria and vaccinia virusencoding light-emitting proteins. Nat Biotech 2004;22:313–320.
69. Keda K, Wakimoto H, Ichikawa T, et al. Complement depletion facilitates the infection of multiple brain tumors by an intravascular, replication-conditional herpes simplex virus mutant. J Virol 2000; 74:4765–4775.
70. Wong RJ, Joe JK, Kim SH, Shah JP, Horsburgh B, Fong Y. Oncolytic herpesvirus effectively treats murine squamous cell carcinoma and spreads by natural lymphatics to treat sites of lymphatic metastases. Hum Gene Ther 2002;13:1213–1223.
71. Herrlinger U, Kramm CM, Aboody-Guterman KS, et al. Pre-existing herpes simplex virus 1 (HSV-1) immunity decreases, but does not abolish gene transfer to experimental braintumors by a HSV-1 vector. Gene Ther 1998;5:809–819.
72. Chahlavi A, Rabkin S, Todo T, Sundaresan P, Martuza R. Effect of prior exposure to herpes simplex virus 1 on viral vector-mediated tumor therapy in immunocompetent mice. Gene Ther 1999;6:1751–1758.
73. Delman KA, Bennett JJ, Zager JS, et al. Effects of preexisting immunity on the response to herpes simplex-based oncolytic viral therapy. Hum Gene Ther 2000;11:2465–2472.
74. Toda M, Rabkin SD, Kojima H, Martuza RL. Herpes simplex virus as an in situ cancer vaccine for the induction of specific anti-tumor immunity. Hum Gene Ther 1999;10:385–393.
75. Todo T, Rabkin SD, Sundaresan P, et al. Systemic antitumor immunity in experimental brain tumor therapy using a multimutated, replication-competent herpes simplex virus. Hum Gene Ther 1999; 10:2741–2755.
76. Wong RJ, Chan M-K, Yu Z, et al. Effective intravenous therapy of murine pulmonary metastases with an oncolytic herpes virus expressing Interleukin 12. Clin Cancer Res 2004;10:251–259.
77. Shah AC, Benos D, Gillespie GY, Markert JM. Oncolytic viruses: clinical applications as vectors for the treatment of malignant gliomas. J Neuro-Oncol 2003;65:203–226.
78. Papanastassiou V, Rampling R, Fraser M, et al. The potential for efficacy of the modified (ICP 34.5(-)) herpes simplex virus HSV1716 following intratumoural injection into human malignant glioma: a proof of principle study. Gene Ther 2002;9:398–406.
79. Mackie RM, Stewart B, Brown SM. Intralesional injection of herpes simplex virus 1716 in metastatic melanoma. Lancet 2001;357:525–526.
80. Wang Y, Hallden G, Hill R, et al. E3 gene manipulations affect oncolytic adenovirus activity in immunocompetent tumor models. Nat Biotech 2003;21:1328–1335.
81. Cassady KA, Gross M, Gillespie GY, Roizman B. Second-site mutation outside of the Us10-12 domain of delta gamma (1) 34.5 herpes simplex virus 1 recombinant blocks the shutoff of protein synthesis induced by avtivated protein kinase R and partially restores neurovirulence. J. Virol 2002; 76:942–990.

82. York IA, Roop C, Andrews DW, Riddell SR, Graham FL, Johnson DC. A cytosolic herpes simplex virus protein inhibits antigen presentation to CD8+ T lymphocytes. Cell 1994;77:525–535.
83. Hill A, Jugovic P, York I, et al. Herpes simplex virus turns off the TAP to evade host immunity. Nature 1995;375:411–415.
84. Goldsmith K, Chen W, Johnson DC, Hendricks RL. Infected cell protein (ICP)47 enhances herpes simplex virus neurovirulence by blocking the CD8+ T cell response. J Exp Med 1998;187:341–348.
85. Ahn K, Meyer TH, Uebel S, et al. Molecular mechanism and species specificity of TAP inhibition by herpes simplex virus ICP47. EMBO J 1996;15:3247–3255.
86. Spear PG, Eisenberg RJ, Cohen GH. Three classes of cell surface receptors for alphaherpesvirus entry. Virology 2000;275:1–8.
87. Zhou G, Ye G-J, Debinski W, Roizman B. Engineered herpes simplex virus 1 is dependent on IL13Rα2 receptor for cell entry and independent of glycoprotein D receptor interaction. Proc Natl Acad Sci U S A 2002;99:15,124–15,129.

6 Alphavirus Vectors for Gene Therapy Applications

Kenneth Lundstrom, PhD

CONTENTS

Summary

Alphavirus vectors can infect a broad range of mammalian cells both in cell cultures and in vivo. The presence of the RNA replicon generates extreme RNA levels in infected cells, which is the basis for the very high levels of heterologous gene expression. Application of replication-deficient vectors leads to short-term expression, which makes these vectors highly attractive for cancer gene therapy. Alphaviruses can be used as vaccine vectors for both prophylactic and therapeutic applications. In this context, the P185 tumor antigen and human papilloma virus gene E7, when administered in mice, resulted in protection against tumor challenge and tumor regression in animals with pre-existing tumors. Alphavirus vectors carrying therapeutic or toxic genes used for intratumoral injections have demonstrated efficient tumor regression. For systemic delivery, expression targeting has been obtained by the introduction of targeting sequences in the envelope structure of the virus. Alternatively, alphavirus particles have been encapsulated in liposome, which can target tumor cells.

Key Words: Alphavirus vectors; cancer vaccines; intratumoral injection; tumor targeting.

1. INTRODUCTION

Alphaviruses belong to the Togaviruses and harbor a single-stranded RNA genome surrounded by a capsid structure and envelope spike proteins embedded in a lipid bilayer *(1)*. The genome consists of four nonstructural genes (nsP1–4) and the capsid protein and two or three envelope proteins (E1–E3). The function of nsP1 is to initiate the minus-strand RNA synthesis and capping of viral RNAs, whereas nsP2 possesses protease and helicase activities and nsP4 contains the catalytic subunit of viral RNA polymerase *(1)*. Although the precise function of nsP3 is not known, it is described to

From: *Cancer Drug Discovery and Development: Gene Therapy for Cancer*
Edited by: K. K. Hunt, S. A. Vorburger, and S. G. Swisher © Humana Press Inc., Totowa, NJ

be a phosphoprotein involved in RNA replication *(2)*. The host range for alphaviruses is broad and includes insect, amphibian, reptile, avian, and mammalian cells. The infection occurs through the recognition of cell-surface receptors and, although these have not been definitely identified for all alphaviruses, it is suggested that common receptors for many cell types, such as laminin receptors, are the targets for alphaviruses *(3)*. After the initial cell recognition step, the virus particles are brought into the cytoplasm either through fusion of the viral envelope structures to the host cell or by endocytosis depending on the cell type. Next a minus-strand copy is generated from the plus-strand genome as a template for generation of extreme numbers of new plus strand copies. Both full-length 42S RNA and the subgenomic 26S RNA encoding the structural genes are synthesized in the cells. The capsid protein forms the nucleocapsid structure together with the single-stranded viral RNA and nucleocapsids are transported to the plasma membrane. Simultaneously, the envelope proteins are processed through the rough endoplasmatic reticulum and Golgi to the plasma membrane encapsulating the nucleocapsid, which results in release of mature virus particles by budding. The process is highly efficient generating virus particles with titers of 10^9–10^{10} particles/mL within 24 h.

To apply alphaviruses for heterologous gene expression, basically three types of vectors have been engineered (*see* Fig. 1).

1. Replication-deficient vectors. For this application, the alphavirus nonstructural and structural genes have been split on separate plasmid vectors. The nonstructural genes and the subgenomic 26S promoter followed by a multilinker cloning region have been introduced into the expression vector downstream of a prokaryotic T7 or SP6 RNA polymerase promoter for in vitro transcription of RNA *(4)*. Likewise the structural genes are transcribed from helper vectors *in trans* as a safety precautious to prevent the generation of replication competent particles. Furthermore, to eliminate homologous recombination between RNA generated from expression and helper vectors, the capsid and envelope genes have been split on separate helper vectors *(5)*. Once RNA molecules have been transcribed from the two vectors, these are introduced into BHK-21 (baby hamster kidney) cells by either electroporation or applying transfection reagents. Rapid RNA replication generates up to 200,000 RNA copies/cell, which results in efficient production of recombinant virus particles. As the packaging signal is located on the recombinant RNA only, this species of RNA will be packaged into the nucleocapsid leading to generation of replication-deficient particles. However, these particles can be applied for only one round of infection of various host cells to generate high transient expression levels of recombinant proteins as described below.
2. Replication-competent vectors. Especially for in vivo applications, where an extended expression pattern and spread of infection is advantageous, vectors with ability to replicate could be attractive. In this context, a second subgenomic promoter with a down stream multilinker cloning region was engineered into vectors with a full-length alphavirus genome *(6)*. Although different constructs have been engineered the most common site for the insertion of the second subgenomic promoter has been downstream of the E1 gene in the 3′ nontranslated region *(6)*. Generally, the replication-competent vectors have been less frequently used than the replication-deficient ones.
3. DNA-based vectors. Replacement of the T7 or SP6 RNA polymerase promoter with a cytomegalo virus (CMV) or RSV promoter has allowed the use of alphavirus vectors directly in the form of plasmid DNA *(7)*. In this form, plasmid DNA can conveniently be directly introduced into mammalian cells for transient heterologous gene expression. However, using this approach the advantage of the broad range of alphavirus

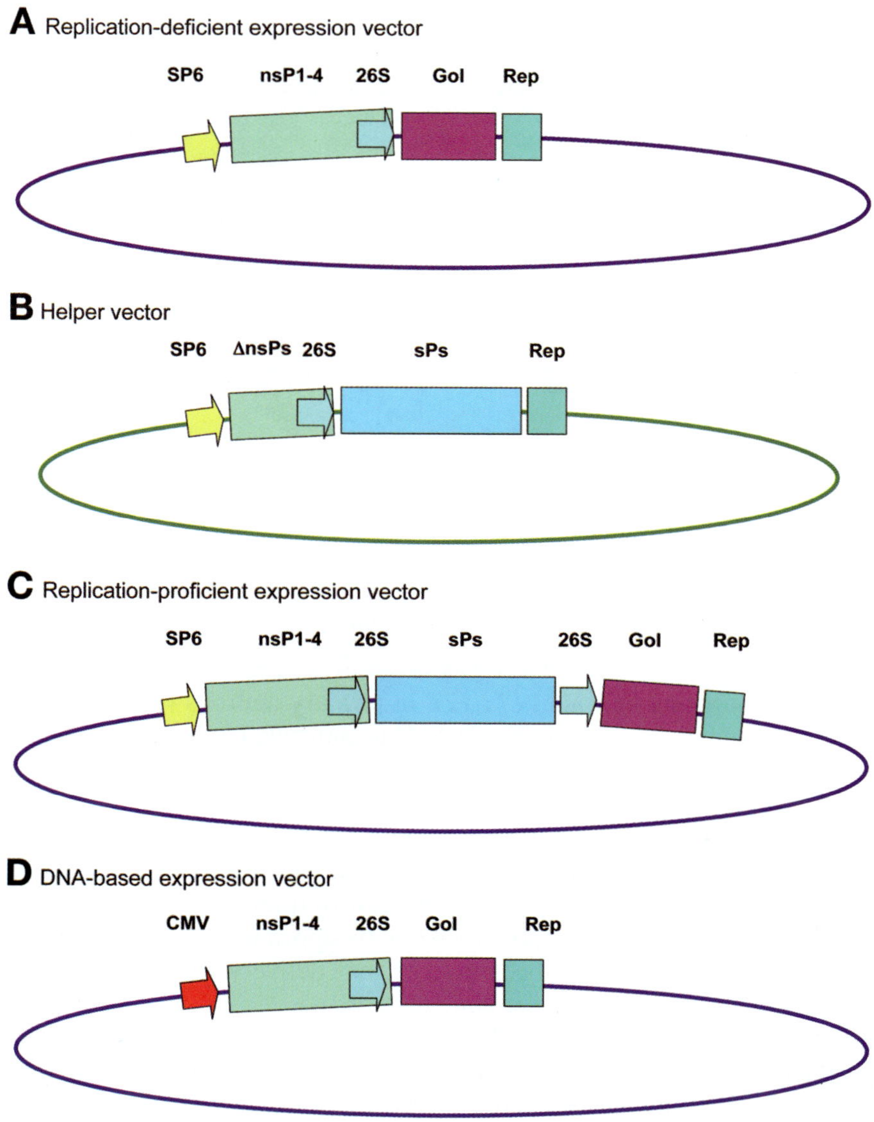

Fig. 1. Schematic presentation of alphavirus vectors. (**A**) Replication-deficient RNA-based expression vector. (**B**) RNA-based helper vector. (**C**) Replication-proficient RNA-based expression vector. (**D**) DNA-based expression vector. GoI, Gene of interest; Rep, Replicase signal.

infection is lost as the gene delivery success relies on DNA transfection methods. Introduction of a type II promoter in the helper vector, DNA-based vectors have also been applied for virus production although the titers have generally been 100-1000 fold lower than observed from RNA-based vectors *(8)*.

Several alphaviruses have been subjected to vector development. The most frequently used alphaviruses are Semliki Forest virus (SFV) *(4)*, Sindbis virus (SIN) *(9)*, and Venezuelan equine encephalitis virus (VEE) *(10)*. SFV, SIN, and VEE have shown very similar features concerning host range, cytotoxic effect on infected host cells and transgene expression. Both SFV and SIN have been frequently used for recombinant protein

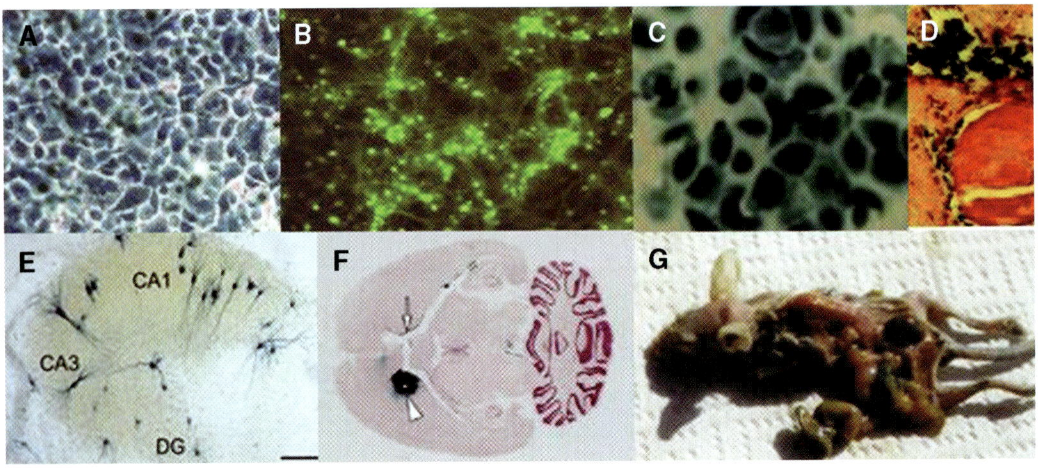

Fig. 2. Broad host range of alphaviruses. (**A**) SFV-LacZ infection of BHK cells. (**B**) SFV-GFP infection of rat primary hippocampal neurons. (**C**) SFV-LacZ infection of human prostate tumor cell line DU-145. (**D**) Ex vivo SFV-LacZ infection of prostate biopsy. (**E**) SFV-LacZ infection of rat hippocampal slice culture. (**F**) Stereotactic injection of SFV-LacZ virus into rat brain. (**G**) Systemic delivery of liposome-encapsulated SFV-LacZ virus in SCID mice with human LnCaP xenografts.

expression in mammalian cell lines *(11,12)*, in primary neurons *(13)*, in hippocampal slice cultures *(14)*, and in vivo *(15,16)* (Fig 2). SFV in particular has been applied for successful high-level expression of integral membrane proteins such as G protein-coupled receptors and ligand-gated ion channels, generally known to be difficult to express *(17)*. This has allowed studies on pharmacology and cell biology of many therapeutically important receptors and has provided material for drug screening programs and structural biology. Alphavirus vectors have been frequently used for expression of tumor antigens *(18)* and viral antigens *(19)* in approaches to develop vaccines. Moreover, alphavirus vectors have been used as gene delivery tools in neuroscience and also as vectors in experimental cancer gene therapy.

In this chapter, the applications of alphavirus vectors for cancer vaccines and also as delivery vehicles for therapeutic genes in cancer are described. Much attention is paid to vector development to improve the expression properties treatment and to modify the toxicity of the alphaviruses themselves. Safety issues related to the use of viral vectors are also discussed. Finally, the possibility of targeting systemic delivery of alphaviruses is presented.

2. ALPHAVIRUS USED IN CANCER VACCINES

Alphavirus vectors have frequently been applied for vaccine production. In this context, recombinant particles as well as naked nucleic acids have been applied. The proof of concept was originally demonstrated for viral surface proteins known for their potential immunogenicity and capability to induce cytotoxic T-cell (CTL) responses and protection against challenges with lethal viruses *(20)*. Moreover, immunization against tumor challenges has resulted in some promising observations (Table 1). For instance, injection of RNA from an SFV vector expressing bacterial β-galactosidase into mice provided protection against tumor challenges *(21)*. Administration of recombinant SFV particles expressing the P1A gene resulted in protection against P185 tumor challenges in mice *(22)*. The human papilloma virus (HPV) E6 and E7 oncoproteins have been

Table 1
Application of Alphavirus Vectors for Tumor Vaccinations

Vector	*Gene target*	*Vehicle*	*Animal model*	*Response*	*Ref.*
SFV	IL-12	Particles	Mouse	Immunogenicity	*(27)*
	IL-18	Particles	Mouse	Tumor protection	*(28)*
	HPV E6-7	Particles	Mouse	Tumor protection	*(24)*
	B16	Particles	Mouse	Tumor protection	*(26)*
	203	Particles	Mouse	Tumor protection	*(26)*
	β-galactosidase	RNA	Mouse	Tumor protections	*(21)*
	MHC Class II	Particles/DNA	Mouse	Immunogenicity	*(57)*
	P185	Particles	Mouse	CTL, tumor protection	*(33)*
SIN	HPV E7-VP22	Particles	Mouse	CD^{8+} T-cell response	*(25)*
	tyr-related prot 1	DNA	Mouse	Antitumor activity	*(58)*
VEE	HPV E7	Particles	Mouse	Tumor protection	*(23)*

expressed from various alphavirus vectors *(23,24)*. For instance, when mice were vaccinated with VEE vectors expressing the HPV type 16 E7 gene, protection against new tumor development could be established *(25)*. Expression of the E6 and E7 genes as a fusion protein from SFV vectors led to a strong and long-lasting CTL response *(24)*. Furthermore, the tumor growth was prevented in animals with xenografts and new tumor generation did not occur in vaccinated animals. In another study, SIN particles with the herpes simplex virus type 1 VP22 protein fused to HPV E7 demonstrated an antitumor response in vaccinated C57BL/6 mice *(25)*. Comparative studies with DNA vectors, RNA replicons and viral particles indicated that the best therapeutic effect was achieved by particle administrations.

In another approach, dendritic cells were isolated from mouse bone marrow and subjected to ex vivo infection with SFV particles expressing B16 and 203 antigens. Immunization of mice with these cells gave protection against challenges with B16 and 203 gliomas *(26)*. Tumor-bearing animals also showed prolonged survival after vaccination. A similar approach was taken for SFV vectors expressing interleukin 12 (IL-12), which demonstrated that a therapeutic immunization with dendritic cells (DCs) pulsed with SFV-IL-12 prolonged the survival of mice with established tumors *(27)*. In another study, DCs infected with SFV-IL-18 and/or systemic administration of IL-12 were injected into mice with B16 brain tumors, which resulted in enhanced T-helper type 1 response from tumor-specific $CD4^+$ and $CD8^+$ T-cells and in antitumor immunity *(28)*.

3. ALPHAVIRUS FOR THE TRANSFECTION OF TUMOR CELL LINES

The broad host range of alphaviruses has made it possible to obtain transgene expression in various cell lines including human tumor cell lines. Using the SFV-LacZ virus for the expression of the β-galactosidase reporter gene, it was demonstrated that human prostate tumor cell lines such as JCA-1, PPC-1, TSU-PR1, ALVA-1, PC-3, DU-145 and LnCaP could not only be efficiently infected, but that SFV also induced an apoptotic response *(29)*. Moreover, the same apoptotic response has been observed in prostate biopsies from patients transduced ex vivo with SFV-LacZ. In another study, tumor cell lines were infected with SFV vectors carrying a fusion construct of the green fluorescence protein (GFP) and herpes simplex virus thymidine kinase (HSV-*tk*) gene, which allowed parallel monitoring of the infection efficency by fluorescence (GFP) and tumor killing (HSV-*tk*) after ganciclovir (GCV) administration *(30)*. To simulate in vivo conditions, only low multiplicity of infection (MOI) was applied, which resulted in fairly modest GFP expression. However, the tumor killing was much better than anticipated because of the by-stander effect previously observed for HSV-*tk* treatment *(31)*. These studies, however, made it clear that the delivery of the therapeutic gene is essential and approaches such as intratumoral injections or improved targeting for systemic delivery are essential.

4. INTRATUMORAL GENE DELIVERY BY ALPHAVIRUS

Alphavirus vectors have been applied for several studies in tumor animal models. In this context, SFV particles expressing the p40 and p35 subunits of the murine interleukin-12 (IL-12) gene were injected into mice bearing B16 melanoma tumors *(32)*. The tumor development was followed by Doppler ultrasonography and demonstrated a significant tumor regression as well as inhibition of tumor blood vessel formation. It was also shown, that repeated injections improved the tumor regression efficacy. In another study, significant regression of P185A tumor growth was achieved after intratumoral injections with SFV-IL-12 vectors *(33)*. The size of the tumor played an important role in relation to efficacy as treatment of large tumors was less successful. The intratumoral injections also presented prophylactic efficacy, as long-term immunity and absence of reoccurrence of tumors were achieved.

The capacity of SFV particles to induce apoptosis in infected cells has allowed tumor regression responses also after intratumoral expression of reporter genes only. For instance, intratumoral delivery of SFV-GFP particles into human lung tumor xenografts in nude mice showed a rapid regression of tumor volumes *(34)*. The best efficacy was achieved after three injections on consecutive days followed by three additional injections 1 wk later. Expression of proapoptotic genes such as Bax from SFV vectors increased cell death in BHK-21 cells and also in AT3, a rat prostate cancer cell line, where the antiapoptotic gene Bcl-2 was overexpressed *(35)*. However, the production of SFV-Bax virus was problematic as the proapoptic Bax gene killed the cells needed for amplification of the virus, resulting in very low virus titers. Reduction of the growth temperature to 33°C improved to some extent the virus production. Applying SFV-Bax particles to nude mice with implanted AT3-Neo and AT3-Bcl-2 tumors resulted in reduction of tumor growth.

Intraperitoneal administration of SFV particles was studied with luciferase as a reporter gene, which demonstrated high-level expression in the peritoneal lining and in tumor cells in the peritoneal cavity *(36)*. Despite intraperitoneal injections the spread into other organs such as the liver, spleen, and lungs was low. The introduction of the granulocyte-macrophage colony-stimulating factor (GM-CSF) in the SFV vectors to therapeutically activate tumor cell killing by macrophages resulted in tumor growth inhibition, but not in prolongation of the survival of animals with implanted tumors.

5. TUMOR TARGETING OF ALPHAVIRUS VECTORS

The broad host range of alphaviruses, and particularly their strong preference for neuronal cells, has made cell/tissue specific targeting an especially important issue.

One approach to obtain targeting for SIN has been to introduce IgG binding domains of protein A in the envelope proteins of SIN *(37)*. The study demonstrated that inserts could be introduced in a specific region in the envelope protein E2, which did not affect the viability and infectivity of generated SIN particles. The chimeric SIN particles showed a significantly reduced infectivity could be established through the protein A domain by treatment of cells with a monoclonal antibody against a cell surface protein. In another study, it was demonstrated that a single point mutation in one of the SIN envelope proteins resulted in preferential infection of DCs *(38)*. A recent approach has included the engineering of a fusion between avidin and the low-density lipoprotein (LDL) receptor for targeting biotinylated molecules to desired tissues *(39)*. Studies in vivo demonstrated that malignant rat glioma tumors were transduced by SFV containing such avidin fusion proteins.

Yet another approach to obtain tumor selective transfection was attained by encapsulation of recombinant SFV particles in liposomes *(40)*. By this procedure, targeted gene delivery to human LnCaP prostate tumors implanted in severe combined immunodeficiency (SCID) mice was achieved after systemic delivery of encapsulated SFV-LacZ particles. Systemic administration of encapsulated SFV particles expressing the p40 and p35 subunits of IL-12 to SCID mice with human Panc-1 pancreatic tumors resulted in statistically significant reduction in tumor growth after a single injection *(41)*. Furthermore, an initial phase I study on advanced melanoma and kidney carcinoma patients demonstrated the safe use of this SFV vector in humans. In this study the maximum tolerated dose (MTD) for encapsulated SFV-IL-12 particles was 3×10^9 particles/m^2, which might seem relatively low compared with doses for other viruses, usually administered in the range of 10^{11} particles. However, in this case the dose is mainly dictated by the fever response observed in patients after high IL-12 expression. The IL-12 expression in patients was transient and the IL-12 levels returned to normal levels after 5 to 7 d. Re-administration of encapsulated SFV particles did not induce any immune response, another indication of safe use in humans.

A recent study on the systemic delivery of SIN vectors has generated some unexpected and controversial results *(42)*. Without engineering any targeting sequences on the SIN vectors it was demonstrated that they efficiently homed to tumor cells; intraperitoneal injection of SIN-LacZ virus led to specific expression in implanted BHK tumors. Moreover, strong bioluminescence was observed in animals with BHK tumors, but not in control mice. SIN vectors were also able to target human micrometastatic ES-2 ovarian cancer cells. Stable overexpression of luciferase in ES-2 cells (ES-2/luc) permitted microscopic monitoring of tumor growth. Subcutaneous daily injections of SIN-IL12 virus led to a tumor load of 6.2% of that observed from control animals. Probably the most astonishing example came from studies on spontaneous fibrosarcomas in the mouse tail. Intraperitoneal injections of SIN-luc virus resulted in tumor targeted expression. This tropism to tumor tissue of SIN virus, however, has not yet been studied in full details and it will need additional research of the mechanisms behind it to eventually apply it in clinical settings.

6. PRODUCTION OF RETROVIRUS-LIKE PARTICLES BY ALPHAVIRUS

Retrovirus vectors integrate into genomic DNA and, thus, have proven useful for long-term transgene expression. However, the production of high-titer retrovirus stock has been problematic. Because alphavirus vectors express heterologous genes at high levels they can be used in the production of retrovirus-like particles. One approach has been to express the *gag-pol*, *env* genes and the genome (LTR-ψ^+-*neo*-LTR) from the Moloney murine leukemia virus (MMLV) from three individual SFV vectors in BHK cells *(43)*. This procedure generated retrovirus-like particles at relatively high titers (4×10^6 colony forming units/mL). These particles showed similar properties to retroviruses and possessed reverse transcriptase activity. Additionally, it was possible to package intron-containing sequences in these retrovirus-like particles with the aid of SFV vectors *(44)*.

A second approach has been to in vitro transcribe retrovirus RNA from the 26S subgenomic promoter and then electroporate the RNA into a retrovirus packaging cell line *(45)*. The produced retrovirus particles transduced target cells, showed reverse transcriptase activity and could integrate into the host cell genome. Hybrid SFV-retrovirus vectors have also been applied for minigene-containing constructs, which resulted in stable minigene transfer and Factor IX expression *(46)*. Engineering of chimeric vectors where the SFV envelope protein genes were replaced with the murine leukemia virus (MuLV) *env* gene allowed packaging of chimeric particles for specific infection of cells with MuLV receptors *(47)*.

7. SAFETY OF ALPHAVIRUS VECTORS

The pathogenicity of the alphavirus family varies significantly, but the three most commonly used vectors, SFV, SIN, and VEE, are considered only mild pathogens *(1)*. There are descriptions of some SFV-related epidemics of febrile illnesses in the Central Republic of Africa *(48)*. The typical symptoms of the infected individuals were fever and persistent headache. Some SIN and SFV strains have additionally showed strong neurovirulence and pathogenicity in young mice.

However, most of the alphavirus vectors used so far are replication-deficient, which generates one cycle of infection and no further virus progeny production. Additional safety has been achieved by using attenuated alphavirus strains with a reduced virulence as the basis for vector construction. As homolog sequences are present in alphavirus expression and helper vectors, there is a slight chance of generating replication competent particles through homologous recombination. To prevent any amplification and spread of these particles, conditionally infectious particles can be produced from second generation helper vectors with point mutations *(49)*. Applying a split-helper vector approach with separate helper vectors carrying the capsid and envelope protein genes has further enhanced the safety *(50)*. For large-scale virus production and future good manufacturing practice (GMP) grade material for clinical trials the use of packaging cell lines developed for SFV and SIN vectors is highly recommended *(51)*.

8. VECTOR DEVELOPMENT

The basic alphavirus vectors have shown features that under some circumstances and for certain applications are less favorable. For instance, alphavirus vectors demonstrate a strong cytotoxicity on infected cells by two main mechanisms. They induce apoptosis through activation of caspases and they shut down the endogenous host cell protein synthesis. Obviously, these features are of advantage in cancer therapy, where the goal is to kill tumor cells. However, many applications would gain from less toxic vectors and prolonged survival of host cells, like in antitumor therapy with cytokine genes such as IL-12, where it might be preferential to achieve extended secretion of interleukins. This is why novel SFV and SIN vectors with reduced cytotoxicity have been engineered; point mutations in the nsP2 and nsP4 genes, for example, resulted in temperature-sensitive SIN vectors with lower cytotoxicity *(52,53)*. Similarly, SFV vectors with point mutations in their nonstructural genes exhibited reduced cytotoxicity *(54,55)*. Another vector, the SFV-PD vector, which has two point mutations in S259P and R650D displayed enhanced protein expression, substantially higher endogenous gene expression, reduced host cell cytotoxicty and resulted in prolonged survival of host cells. Alphaviruses are generally highly transient by nature and even for mutant vectors extension of expression for more than 7 d is rare. However, point mutation L713P in nsP2 of SFV resulted in a replication-persistent phenotype *(56)*. The introduction of the nsP2-L713P mutation in the SFV-PD vector led to a low-toxicity vector with relatively long-term expression (for 20 d) *(55)*.

9. CONCLUSIONS AND FUTURE PROSPECTS

Alphavirus vectors have been used for a wide range of applications including recombinant protein expression in cell lines, primary cell cultures and in vivo.

Vaccination against tumor challenges has also been frequently explored. Therapeutic effects have been seen after intratumoral injections in various animal models. The recent description of SIN vectors homing naturally to tumor tissue is a new and intriguing finding. This tumor targeting capability can be achieved in alphavirus vectors by introduction of target sequences into envelope genes or by the inclusion of virus particles into liposomes. This liposomal protection, furthermore, avoids host immune responses and, therefore, allows repeated vector applications. Engineering of novel, less cytotoxic vectors that lead to prolonged host cell survival will be beneficial for gene therapeutic approaches that base on the expression of immunostimulatory proteins. The current challenge of alphavirus vector production for future clinical trials is the development of vectors, host cell lines and technologies compatible with GMP standards.

REFERENCES

1. Strauss JH, Strauss EG. The alphaviruses: gene expression, replication and evolution. Microbiol Rev 1994;58:491–562.
2. Peränen J, Takkinen K, Kalkkinen N, Kääriäinen L. Semliki Forest virus-specific non-structural protein nsP3 is a phosphoprotein. J Gen Virol 1998;69:2165–2178.
3. Wang KS, Kuhn RJ, Strauss EG, Ou S, Strauss JH. High-affinity laminin receptor is a receptor for Sindbis virus in mammalian cells. J Virol 1992;66:4992–5001.
4. Liljeström P, Garoff H. A new generation of animal cell expression vectors based on the Semliki Forest virus replicon. Bio/Technology 1991;9:1356–1361.
5. Smerdou C, Liljeström P. Two-helper RNA system for production of recombinant Semliki Forest virus particles. J Virol 1999;73:1092–1098.
6. Vaha-Koskela MJ, Tuittila MT, Nygardas PT, et al. A novel neurotropic expression vector based on the avirulent A7(74) strain of Semliki Forest virus. J Neurovirol 2003;9:1–15.
7. Berglund P, Smerdou C, Fleeton MN, Tubulekas I, Liljestrom P. Enhancing immune responses using suicidal DNA vaccines. Nat Biotechnol 1998;16:562–565.
8. DiCiommo DP, Bremner R. Rapid, high level protein production using DNA-based Semliki Forest virus vectors. J Biol Chem 1998;273:18,060–18,066.
9. Xiong C, Levis R, Shen P, et al. Sindbis virus: an efficient broad host range vector for gene expression in animal cells. Science 1989;243:1188–1191.
10. Davis NL, Brown KW, Johnston RE. In vitro synthesis of infectious Venezuelan equine encephalitis virus RNA from a cDNA clone: Analysis of a viable deletion mutant. Virology 1989;171:189–204.
11. Lundstrom K, Schweitzer C, Rotmann D, Hermann D, Schneider EM, Ehrengruber MU. Semliki Forest virus vectors: efficient vehicles for in vitro and in vivo gene delivery. FEBS Lett 2001;504: 99–103.

12. Schlesinger S. Alphavirus vectors: development and potential therapeutic applications. Expert Opin Biol Ther 2001;1:177–191.
13. Olkkonen VM, Liljestrom P, Garoff H, Simons K, Dotti CG. Expression of heterologous proteins in cultured rat hippocampal neurons using the Semliki Forest virus vector. J Neurosci Res 1993;35:445–451.
14. Ehrengruber MU, Lundstrom K, Schweizer C, et al. Recombinant Semliki Forest virus and Sindbis virus efficiently infect neurons in hippocampal slice cultures. Proc Natl Acad Sci U S A 1999;96:7041–7046.
15. Lundstrom K, Richards JG, Pink JR, Jenck F. Efficient in vivo expression of a reporter gene in rat brain after injection of replication-deficient Semliki Forest virus. Gene Ther Mol Biol 1999;3:15–23.
16. Gwag BJ, Kim EY, Ryu BR, et al. A neuron-specific gene transfer by a recombinant defective Sindbis virus. Brain Res Mol Brain Res 1998;63:53–61.
17. Lundstrom K. Semliki Forest virus vectors for rapid and high-level expression of integral membrane proteins. Biochim Biophys Acta 2003;1610:90–96.
18. Lundstrom K. Alphavirus vectors for vaccine production and gene therapy. Expert Rev Vaccines 2003;2:447–459.
19. Zhou X, Berglund P, Zhao H, Liljestrom P, Jondal M. Generation of cytotoxic and humoral immune responses by nonreplicative recombinant Semliki Forest virus. Proc Natl Acad Sci U S A 1995;92: 3009–3013.
20. Lundstrom K. Alphavirus vectors for vaccine production and gene therapy. Exp Rev Vaccines 2003;2:447–459.
21. Ying H, Zaks TZ, Wang RF, et al. Cancer therapy using a self-replicating RNA vaccine. Nat Med 1999;5:823–827.
22. Colmenero P, Liljestrom P, Jondal M. Induction of P815 tumor immunity by recombinant Semliki Forest virus expressing the P1A gene. Gene Ther 1999;6:1728–1733.
23. Velders MP, McElhiney S, Cassetti MC, et al. Eradication of established tumors by vaccination with Venezuelan equine encephalitis virus replicon particles delivering human papillomavirus 16 E7 RNA. Cancer Res 2001;61:7861–7867.
24. Daemen T, Regts J, Holtrop M, Wilschut J. Immunization strategy against cervical cancer involving an alphavirus vector expressing high levels of a stable fusion protein of human papillomavirus 16 E6 and E7. Gene Ther 2002;9:85–94.
25. Cheng WF, Hung CF, Hsu KF, et al. Cancer immunotherapy using Sindbis virus replicon particles encoding a VP22-antigen fusion. Hum Gene Ther 2002;13:553–568.
26. Yamanaka R, Zullo SA, Tanaka R, Blaese M, Xanthopoulos KG. Enhancement of antitumor immune response in glioma models in mice by genetically modified dendritic cells pulsed with Semliki forest virus-mediated complementary DNA. J Neurosurg 2001;94:474–481.
27. Yamanaka R, Zullo SA, Ramsey J, et al. Marked enhancement of antitumor immune responses in mouse brain tumor models by genetically modified dendritic cells producing Semliki Forest virus-mediated interleukin-12 J Neurosurg 2002;97:611–618.
28. Yamanaka R, Tsuchiya N, Yajima N, et al. Induction of an antitumor immunological response by an intratumoral injection of dendritic cells pulsed with genetically engineered Semliki Forest virus to produce interleukin-18 combined with the systemic administration of interleukin-12. J Neurosurg 2003;99:746–753.
29. Hardy PA, Mazzini MJ, Schweitzer C, Lundstrom K, Glode LM. Recombinant Semliki forest virus infects and kills human prostate cancer cell lines and prostatic duct epithelial cells ex vivo. Int J Mol Med 2000;5:241–245.
30. Loimas S, Toppinen MR, Visakorpi T, Janne J, Wahlfors J. Human prostate carcinoma cells as targets for herpes simplex virus thymidine kinase-mediated suicide gene therapy. Cancer Gene Ther 2001;8: 137–144.
31. Culver KW, Ram Z, Wallbridge S, Ishii H, Oldfield EH, Blaese RM. In vivo gene transfer with retroviral vector-producer cells for treatment of experimental brain tumors. Science 1992;256:1550–1552.
32. Asselin-Paturel C, Lassau N, Guinebretiere JM, et al. Transfer of the murine interleukin-12 gene in vivo by a Semliki Forest virus vector induces B16 tumor regression through inhibition of tumor blood vessel formation monitored by Doppler ultrasonography. Gene Ther 1999;6:606–615.
33. Colmenero P, Chen M, Castanos-Velez E, Liljestrom P, Jondal M. Immunotherapy with recombinant SFV-replicons expressing the P815A tumor antigen or IL-12 induces tumor regression. Int J Cancer 2002;98:554–560.
34. Murphy AM, Morris-Downes MM, Sheahan BJ, Atkins GJ. Inhibition of human lung carcinoma cell growth by apoptosis induction using Semliki Forest virus recombinant particles. Gene Ther 2000; 7:1477–1482.

35. Murphy AM, Sheahan BJ, Atkins GJ. Induction of apoptosis in BCL-2-expressing rat prostate cancer cells using the Semliki Forest virus vector. Int J Cancer 2001;94:572–578.
36. Klimp AH, van der Vaart E, Lansink PO, et al. Activation of peritoneal cells upon in vivo transfection with a recombinant alphavirus expressing GM-CSF. Gene Ther 2001;8:300–307.
37. Ohno K, Sawai K, Iijima Y, Levin B, Meruelo D. Cell-specific targeting of Sindbis virus vectors displaying IgG-binding domains of protein A. Nat Biotechnol 1997;15:763–767.
38. Gardner JP, Frolov I, Perri S, et al. Infection of human dendritic cells by a sindbis virus replicon vector is determined by a single amino acid substitution in the E2 glycoprotein. J Virol 2000;74: 11,849–11,857.
39. Lehtolainen P, Wirth T, Taskinen AK, et al. Targeting of biotinylated compounds to its target tissue using a low-density lipoprotein receptor-avidin fusion protein. Gene Ther 2003;10:2090–2097.
40. Lundstrom K, Boulikas T. Viral and non-viral vectors in gene therapy: technology development and clinical trials. Technol Cancer Res Treat 2003;2:471–486.
41. Ren H, Boulikas T, Lundstrom K, Soling A, Warnke PC, Rainov NG. Immunogene therapy of recurrent glioblastoma multiforme with a liposomally encapsulated replication-incompetent Semliki forest virus vector carrying the human interleukin-12 gene—a phase I/II clinical protocol. Neurooncol 2003;64:147–154.
42. Tseng JC, Levin B, Hurtado A, et al. Systemic tumor targeting and killing by Sindbis viral vectors. Nat Biotechnol 2004;22:70–77.
43. Li KJ, Garoff H. Production of infectious recombinant Moloney murine leukemia virus particles in BHK cells using Semliki Forest virus-derived RNA expression vectors. Proc Natl Acad Sci U S A 1996;93:11,658–11,663.
44. Li KJ, Garoff H. Packaging of intron-containing genes into retrovirus vectors by alphavirus vectors. Proc Natl Acad Sci U S A 1998;9:3650–3654.
45. Wahlfors JJ, Xanthopoulos KG, Morgan RA. Semliki Forest virus-mediated production of retroviral vector RNA in retroviral packaging cells. Hum Gene Ther 1997;8:2031–2041.
46. Wahlfors JJ, Morgan RA. Production of minigene-containing retroviral vectors using an alphavirus/retrovirus hybrid vector system. Hum Gene Ther 1999;10:1197–1206.
47. Lebedeva I, Fujita K, Nihrane A, Silver J. Infectious particles derived from Semliki Forest virus vectors encoding murine leukemia virus envelopes. J Virol 1997;71:7061–7067.
48. Mathiot CC, Grimaud G, Garry P, et al. An outbreak of human Semliki Forest virus infections in Central African Republic. Am J Trop Med Hyg 1990;42:386–393.
49. Berglund P, Sjoberg M, Garoff H, Atkins GJ, Sheahan BJ, Liljestrom P. Semliki Forest virus expression system: production of conditionally infectious recombinant particles. Biotechnology (NY) 1993;11:916–920.
50. Smerdou C, Liljestrom P. Two-helper RNA system for production of recombinant Semliki forest virus particles. J Virol 1999;73:1092–1098.
51. Polo JM, Belli BA, Driver DA, et al. Stable alphavirus packaging cell lines for Sindbis virus and Semliki Forest virus-derived vectors. Proc Natl Acad Sci U S A 1999;96:4598–4603.
52. Agapov EV, Frolov I, Lindenbach BD, Pragai BM, Schlesinger S, Rice CM. Noncytopathic Sindbis virus RNA vectors for heterologous gene expression.Proc Natl Acad Sci U S A 1998;95:12,989–12,994.
53. Boorsma M, Nieba L, Koller D, Bachmann MF, Bailey JE, Renner WA. A temperature-regulated replicon-based DNA expression system. Nat Biotechnol 2000;18:429–432.
54. Lundstrom K, Rotmann D, Hermann D, Schneider EM, Ehrengruber MU. Novel mutant Semliki Forest virus vectors: gene expression and localization studies in neuronal cells. Histochem Cell Biol 2001;115:83–91.
55. Lundstrom K, Abenavoli A, Malgaroli A, Ehrengruber MU. Novel Semliki Forest virus vectors with reduced cytotoxicity and temperature sensitivity for long-term enhancement of transgene expression. Mol Ther 2003;7:202–209.
56. Perri S, Driver DA, Gardner JP, et al. Replicon vectors derived from Sindbis virus and Semliki forest virus that establish persistent replication in host cells. J Virol 2000;74:9802–9807.
57. Ying H, Zeng G, Black KL. Innovative cancer vaccine strategies based on the identification of tumour-associated antigens. BioDrugs 2001;15:819–831.
58. Leitner WW, Hwang LN, deVeer MJ, et al. Alphavirus-based DNA vaccine breaks immunological tolerance by activating innate antiviral pathways. Nat Med 2003;9:33–39.

7 Vesicular Stomatitis Virus and RNA Viruses as Gene Therapy Vectors

Glen N. Barber, PhD

CONTENTS

Summary

The ability of RNA viruses to efficiently reproduce in transformed cells was first recognized nearly 100 yr ago. However, it wasn't until the late 1990s that a resurrection of the interest in the ability of certain viruses to preferentially replicate in malignant cells and less so in normal cells occurred, the curiosity being to evaluate whether these agents could be useful in cancer therapy regimes. It was following these reports, demonstrating that DNA viruses such as adenovirus and herpes simplex virus (HSV) could act as antineoplastic agents, that similar encouraging investigations were conducted using RNA viruses such as reovirus and Newcastle Disease virus, vesicular stomatitis Virus (VSV), and measles virus (MV). Here we will review the use of RNA viruses as oncolytic agents in the treatment of malignant disease, focusing on the negative-stranded RNA virus, VSV. The general mechanisms by which oncolytic viruses such as VSV achieve their antitumor effectiveness and specificity are discussed, including the role of the innate immune system involving the interferon response.

Key Words: VSV; oncolytic virus; interferon; PKR; virotherapy.

1. INTRODUCTION

The ability of particular viruses to preferentially replicate in tumor cells compared with normal cells, first documented nearly 100 yr ago, has provided an opportunity to develop new therapies for the treatment of malignant disease. However, it wasn't until recently that selected viruses such as adenovirus and herpesviruses were seriously evaluated in strategies designed to make use of their potentially valuable properties *(1–5)*. To date, replication-competent as well as incompetent DNA viruses have been demonstrated to exhibit preferential growth properties in tumor cells. Some of these viral therapies involve exploiting defects in the p53 pathway, prevalent in many tumor cells, or in targeting the retinoblastoma (Rb) pathway *(6–8)*. In addition, tissue or tumor specific targeting has been achieved using DNA viruses whose gene

From: *Cancer Drug Discovery and Development: Gene Therapy for Cancer*
Edited by: K. K. Hunt, S. A. Vorburger, and S. G. Swisher © Humana Press Inc., Totowa, NJ

expression is under control of tissue specific promoters such as the prostate specific antigen (PSA) *(9)*. Other strategies developed to better target virus replication to certain tumors types involve genetically engineering tumor-tissue specific ligands on the surface of viruses *(10,11)*. Moreover, to increase the tumor killing process, viral vectors have been modified to contain and deliver foreign genes, such as a tumor suppressor genes that can cause cell-cycle arrest and/or apoptosis *(2,12,13)*. The delivery of suicide genes to cancer cells has also been utilized in cancer gene therapy approaches, with herpes simplex virus (HSV) thymidine kinase (TK) being most widely used *(14,15)*. This approach makes use of an induced bystander effect which may avoid the viral vector having to target all cells within a tumor to induce death. Finally, the delivery of immunomodulatory genes such as cytokines to tumor cells has been considered and tested in many gene therapy methodologies, the strategy being to enhance an immune response to the tumor cells to facilitate their eradication *(4,5,16,17)*.

However, DNA viruses are not the only category of viruses that have exhibited considerable potential in oncolytic studies or for use in the development of gene therapy vectors. It had been previously documented that Newcastle Disease Virus (NDV), influenza viruses (INV), and rabies viruses are also able to exert tumor cell killing properties and later studies indicated that reovirus, measles, and vesicular stomatitis virus (VSV) shared similar traits *(2,18–20)*. Comparable with the situation with replication-competent oncolytic DNA viruses, the mechanisms of preferential viral replication in tumor cells remains to be fully clarified. Nevertheless, at least with selected RNA viruses some insight has recently been shed on the reasons behind their intrinsic oncolytic activity in tumors *(21,22)*. For example, studies with reovirus and VSV indicated that defects in innate immune defenses may be prevalent in malignant cells and largely responsible for facilitating the observed preferential virus replication, which eventually leads to tumor cell lysis *(23,24)*. This chapter focuses on the recent developments in the utilization of VSV and other RNA viruses as potential antitumor agents and gene therapy vectors, as well as discuss some of the mechanisms that may explain their selective oncolytic activity.

2. VESICULAR STOMATITIS VIRUS

Vesicular stomatitis virus (VSV) is member of the Rhabdoviridae family, which are negative-stranded viruses that replicate in the cytoplasm *(25,26)*. There are five genera within the Rhabdoviruses family; namely Vesiculoviruses, Lyssaviruses, and Ephemeroviruses which infect animals (including insects), and Cytorhabdoviruses and Nucleorhabdoviruses which infect plants. The prototype of the family and perhaps its best known member is the rabies virus, which is an associate of the Lyssavirus genus, whereas VSV is classified into the Vesiculovirus genus. Rhabdoviruses are bullet shaped in structure and approx 100 to 400 nm long and 45 to 100 nm in diameter *(26)*. The genome of VSV consists of an 11-kilobase (kb) negative sense, single-standed RNA that is responsible for encoding five proteins referred to as the nucleocapsid (N), polymerase proteins, (L) and (P), surface glycoprotein (G), and a peripheral matrix protein (M) *(25–27)*. Similar to many other RNA viruses, Rhabdoviruses are enveloped viruses covered with peplomers consisting of trimers of the virus G protein, a type I membrane glycoprotein. G is responsible for binding to cell-surface receptors and initiating the infectious process *(28,29)*. In addition, G is the major antigen responsible for type

Table 1
In Vivo Targeting of Tumors by VSV

	Tumor tissue	*Ref.*
Nonrecombinant VSV		
WtVSV	Glioblastoma	*(21,34,59,104)*
	Sarcoma	*(59)*
	Transformed fibroblast	*(59)*
	Melanoma	*(34)*
VSV-AV1 and -AV2	Colon carcinoma	*(102)*
	Ovarian carcinoma	*(102)*
Recombinant oncolytic VSV		
VSV-GFP	Colon carcinoma	*(108)*
	Hepatocellular carcinoma	*(105)*
VSVΔ51M	Colon carcinoma	*(102)*
VSV expressing immunomodulatory genes		
VSV-IL-4	Mammary adenocarcinoma	*(70)*
	Melanoma	*(70)*
VSV-IFN-β	Renal carcinoma	*(71)*
	Mammary carcinoma	*(71)*
VSV expressing suicide genes		
VSV-TK	Mammary adenocarcinoma	*(70,103)*
	Melanoma	*(70)*
	B-cell lymphoma	*(103)*
VSV-CD/UPRT	Mammary adenocarcinoma	*(103)*
	B-cell lymphoma	*(103)*

specificity and key target for neutralizing antibody *(30)*. The genome of VSV is tightly encased in nucleocapsid (N) protein although some polymerase proteins (L) and (P) are also present. The matrix (M) protein binds to the RNA genome/nucleocapsid core (RNP) and also to the glycosylated (G) protein and is responsible for inhibiting host cell mRNA export from the nucleus in an attempt to prevent antiviral gene expression *(31–33)*.

2.1. Cycle of Infection

Following infection of the host, the virus (G) protein binds to a cellular receptor, which has yet to be specifically identified, and penetrates the cell membrane to release the RNP particles *(28)*. VSV is known to infect a wide range of cell types including many transformed cells, indicating that receptor target(s) for G are commonly expressed molecules *(21,34)*. This property is obviously advantageous when considering VSV as a treatment for malignant disease, because the agent can be potentially used against different tumor types. Phosphatidylserine (PS) on the cell membrane is thought to be involved in binding to G and assisting with VSV endocytosis *(26,28)*. A reduction in pH within the endosome then induces membrane fusion, which liberates the viral cores into the cytoplasm. Some free polymerase protein, which is carried into the cell by VSV, binds to the 3′-end of the genome and starts to sequentially synthesize the individual

Table 2
In Vivo Tumor Models of Oncolytic RNA Viruses other than Rhabdoviridae

	Tumor tissue	Ref.
Paramyxoviridae		
Newcastle Disease virus	Glioblastoma	*(132,133)*
	Colon cancer	*(131,132)*
	Breast cancer	*(131,132)*
	Pancreatic cancer	*(131)*
	Lung carcinoma	*(131,132)*
	Renal carcinoma	*(131)*
	Prostate cancer	*(132)*
	Epidermoid cancer	*(132)*
Measles Virus	Glioblastoma	*(123)*
	Ovarian cancer	*(121)*
	Myeloma, lymphoma	*(127)*
	Fibrosarcoma	*(125)*
Reoviridae		
Reovirus	Glioblastoma	*(24,117)*
	Medulloblastoma	*(118)*
	Myeloma, lymphoma	*(114)*
	Breast adenocarcinoma	*(111)*
	Ovarian cancer	*(116)*
	Colon cancer	*(116)*
	Pancreatic cancer	*(115)*
Orthomyxoviridae		
Influenza Virus	Melanoma	*(135,136)*
Picornoviridae		
Poliovirus	Glioblastoma	*(139,140)*
Togaviridae		
Alphavirus	Colon carcinoma	*(143)*

mRNAs encoding N, P, M, G, and L *(27,28)*. The five individual mRNAs are capped and polyadenylated. The polymerase recognizes viral nucleotide sequences at the 3′-end of the genome and initiates transcription. Termination probably occurs after polyadenylation whereupon the polymerase is freed to reinitiate transcription of the next gene product *(26)*. The mechanism that allows the polymerase to switch from transcription to replication has not been entirely clarified, although following mRNA and viral protein synthesis, negative-sense progeny genomes are generated in high quantities. The newly synthesized N, P, and L proteins associate in the cytoplasm and form RNP cores, which bind to regions of the plasma membrane now rich in both M and G proteins. VSV particles form and budding/release of progeny virus occurs followed by cellular lysis *(26,35)*.

2.2. Pathogenesis and Immunity

VSV does not undergo genetic recombination, exhibits no resortment activity, has no known transforming potential, and does not integrate any part of its genome into the host *(21)*. Importantly, VSV is not known to cause any disease in humans, though in rare circumstances where infection has occurred, the outcome has been reported as essentially asymptomatic *(25)*. Seroprevalence in the human population is generally estimated to be low. However, VSV can cause vesicular lesions in the mucous membranes of the mouth and nose of horses, cattle, and pigs *(26)*. Although the infections are rarely fatal, major epizootics have occurred in the United States *(36,37)*. Serologic evaluation studies indicate a low ratio of prior exposure to VSV in animals in the United States(two serotypes are common, Indiana and New Jersey strain). For example, in Colorado, the prevalence of antibody against VSV was estimated at approx 1% in cattle and horses *(36)*. VSV can cause neuropathy in mice, following intranasal infection *(38,39)*. Olfactory receptor neurons are highly tropic for VSV and once infected the virus can travel down the nerve to replicate in cells of the central nervous system (CNS) *(39,40)*. Hence, lethal encephalitis can occur when administered in high doses, but most often, the virus can also be cleared through activation of both the innate and adaptive immune responses *(38)*. In animal models, primary infection with VSV results in a humoral immune response developing within 1 wk after exposure *(30)*. Antibodies generated during the humoral response are directed towards the N and G protein. However, it is the latter antigen that is targeted by neutralizing antibodies, which are largely responsible for effectively eradicating disease *(30)*. The N and G proteins also appear to be the major antigens that mediate the cytotoxic T-lymphocyte (CTL) response. Not surprisingly, data indicates that B-cell deficient mice are extremely sensitive to VSV and such animals die from encephalitis within 9 d *(41)*. However, T-cells are required for long-term survival as well, as T-cell deficient mice also succumb to lethal VSV infection after 30 d *(41)*.

In addition to the adaptive immune response it is also clear that the innate immune response also comprises a major component of immunity to VSV infection. Without a functional innate immune response, VSV rapidly replicates to lethal levels prior to the development of the adaptive immune response, which includes the neutralizing antibody directed against the G protein *(41,42)*. As described below, we suggest that innate host defense systems that normally constrain VSV following infection are likely defective in transformed cells *(21)*. Thus, malignant cells are devoid of critical antiviral responses that would usually impede virus infection. It is these properties that allowed VSV to be considered an interesting cytotoxic agent specific for cancer cells.

2.3. Mechanisms of Selectively Targeting Tumor Cells: The Interferon System

The basis for using VSV as an antitumor agent arose through studies that we were conducting on evaluating the importance of the dsRNA-dependent protein kinase, PKR, in innate immunity. It has recently been demonstrated that embryonic fibroblasts and mice lacking PKR are extremely susceptible to VSV infection *(21,34)*. PKR is an interferon (IFN)-inducible serine threonine protein kinase that undergoes autophosphorylation following interaction with dsRNA species *(43)*. Following activation, PKR is able to catalyze the phosphorylation of cellular substrates, the most important being the α subunit of eukaryotic initiation factor 2 (elF2α). This translation initiation factor forms part of the ternary complex (elF-2/GTP/Met-tRNA) that is responsible for transferring initiator Met-tRNA to 40S ribosomal subunits prior to the binding of mRNA *(44)*. Phosphorylated eIF2α effectively sequesters eIF2B (also known as the guanine nucleotide exchange factors [GEF]), a rate-limiting component in the protein synthesis of the cell, and subsequently causes a dramatic inhibition in the initiation of translation *(45)*. Thus, in normal cells, activation of PKR inhibits viral protein synthesis *(45,46)*. In PKR null cells, however, we noticed that virus replication proceeded at high levels *(47)*. Further, PKR deficient animals were extremely susceptible to intranasal infection with VSV *(47–49)*. This data confirmed that PKR is an essential and nonredundant component of antiviral host defense. However, PKR alone is not sufficient to thwart virus infection. Presumably, PKR inhibits virus replication by inhibiting translation until other innate immune components can be galvanized in order to fortify the antiviral state. One of these key components that needs time to become activated is the IFN system *(47)*.

Indeed, it is now clear that the IFN-inducible genes are very important in preventing VSV-mediating cytolysis *(50)*. The IFNs are a family of cytokines produced in response to infection, which act by inducing the expression of many cellular genes. The IFNs comprise two main families, referred to as type I (α/β) and type II (γ) *(51)*. Type I IFNs, induced by most cell types, are clustered on the short arm of chromosome 9 and consist of several α genes and pseudogenes, and one β gene *(50,52)*. In contrast, type II IFN consists of a single gene on chromosome 12 that is mainly secreted by Th-1 lymphocytes and natural killer (NK) cells. The IFNs can be induced by a number of stimuli, including viruses, dsRNA, growth factors and cytokines and are known to exert potent antitumor, antiviral, and immunomodulatory activities *(53)*. PKR likely affords a first line of defense, to buy time for IFN to be induced (transcribed and translated). The importance of IFN in innate immunity to VSV infection has been demonstrated in studies with mice rendered defective in type I IFN signaling (such as lacking STAT1 or the type I IFN receptor, IFNAR). Such animals are also remarkably susceptible to lethal infection by VSV, regardless of whether they have functional adaptive immunity *(54–56)*. Collectively, data indicates that a functional IFN system is required to induce powerful antiviral genes responsible for inhibiting virus replication. However, similar to PKR, the IFN system alone is not sufficient to repel VSV infection and essentially only slows the infection process down until components of the adaptive immune response are galvanized *(47)*.

In the last few years, the molecular mechanisms responsible for initially recognizing viral infection and triggering the innate and adaptive immune response have been identified. These processes involve the Toll receptor pathway, and the toll-like receptor (TLR)-3, which recognizes exogenous dsRNA species generated as a consequence of virus replication *(22,57,58)*. This event leads to the activation of NF-κB (NF-κB), interferon-regulatory factor-3 (IRF-3), and perhaps elements of the JNK2 pathway *(50,57)*. Activation of these signaling components by virus leads to the potent transcriptional induction of IFN-β, which is secreted and functions, in a paracrine or autocrine manner, as a ligand by binding to species-specific cellular receptors (INFARs). The binding of IFN-β to its receptor causes activation of the Jak/STAT pathway (a complex consisting of Jak1/STAT1 and 2 with IRF9) and to the induction of numerous genes (in the hundreds) in the cell. IFN-induced genes are known to include the multiple histocompatibility complex (MHC) family, proapoptotic tumor necrosis factor related apoptosis-inducing ligand (TRAIL), heat shock proteins, and transcription factors that lead to the further activation of IFN-α *(50)*. In addition, IFN is able to potently activate NK cells and facilitate dendritic cells (DC) maturation *(52)*. Because it was well known that VSV replicated very well in nearly all tissue cultured cell-lines so far examined, many of which were transformed or malignant, we surmised that the innate immune pathways might be defective in VSV susceptible cells. We thus started to examine the use of VSV as an oncolytic vector.

3. VSV AS A THERAPY AGAINST CANCER

Our studies indicate that VSV can infect many types of tumor cells, almost certainly a result of the widely tropic nature of the VSV G protein *(21)*. Whereas the infected tumor cells rapidly die, normal cells are much more resistant to VSV-mediated cytoloysis. Importantly, the oncolytic effect of VSV does not appear to be restricted to tumor cells with specific genetic aberrancies. For example, VSV can destroy cells carrying defective *Myc* or *p53*, cells with activated *Ras*, and even cells overexpressing *Bcl*-2 *(59)*. The involvement of one or more of these oncogenes in promoting transformation of the cell has been documented in nearly all tumors so far analyzed. The mechanism of VSV oncolysis involves the induction of apoptosis by as yet undetermined mechanisms, though it predominantly utilizes the caspase-9 pathway *(59,60)*.

Our data, as well as that of others, also indicated that whereas normal cells treated with IFN were protected from VSV infection, transformed cells were much less protected *(21,34)*. Even many types of IFN-treated tumor cells eventually succumbed to virus infection, speculatively inferring a common defect in innate immune responses *(61,62)*. Given our above data, we naturally examined the status of PKR in VSV-susceptible tumor cells. For example, it was plausible that PKR could be defective in cells sensitive to VSV. However, our data indicated that PKR was functional in many cases and remained able to phosphorylate eIF2α *(23)*. We subsequently noted that a key translation factor that recognized phosphorylated eIF2α and slowed protein synthesis, referred to as eIF2B, was frequently defective *(23)*. The consequences of this were that phosphorylated eIF2α did not impede translation rates. This may assist viral translation and allow VSV to replicate faster than an antiviral state involving IFN induction can be established. The role of translation regulation (or rather dysregulation) in tumorigenesis still remains an extremely complex issue but may play a key role in mediating VSV-mediated oncolysis. Certainly, all viruses require host-protein synthesis machinery to facilitate their replication. Collectively, defects in the innate immune responses, including translational regulation could commonly occur in cancer *(63–69)*.

3.1. VSV Targeting Tumors In Vivo

Given that VSV seemed to target tumor cells very efficiently, we next started to evaluate whether VSV may be useful as an in vivo antineoplastic therapeutic agent. Our early studies clearly indicated robust oncolytic ability against tumors in athymic nude mice as well as in syngeneic tumors in immunocompetent animals *(21,59,70,71)*. Preliminary studies also indicated that VSV treated mice exhibited no detectable virus in the lung, brain, kidney, spleen, or liver of mice 3 wk after treatment, presumably because the majority of virus has been eliminated by the innate immune response and by neutralizing antibody *(70)*. VSV has also been shown capable of exerting its antitumor effects when inoculated at sites distant from the tumor *(59)*. Importantly, when introduced intravenously, VSV has been demonstrated to repress the growth of metastatic breast adenocarcinoma in syngeneic animal models *(70,71)*. Following intravenous inoculation, VSV plausibly infects a number of the animal's normal cells as well as tumor cells. In this situation, the IFN system would doubtlessly be activated within the normal cells and virus replication thwarted. Secreted IFN from innocuously targeted cells, including high-level IFN-producing plasmacytoid DCs would activate antiviral pathways in surrounding uninfected normal cells, causing them, and the animal in general, to become resistant to VSV infection. In contrast, tumor cells would allow the replication of VSV to proceed, because these cells harbor defects in innate immune responses and would become lysed. Progeny viruses would, in turn, infect surrounding tumor cells. Eventually, neutralizing antibody would be generated toward the virus and the infection eliminated. Collectively, these results generated significant enthusiasm for further development and evaluation of VSV as an oncolytic therapy. Further projects included the attempt to improve VSVs oncolytic capabilities while simultaneoulsy trying to create a virus more specifically lytic for tumor cells. Both of these requirements may be realistic options because of the genetic malleability of this virus, as discussed in Section 4.1.

4. GENETICALLY ENGINEERING RNA VIRUSES AND VSV

The advent of genetic engineering facilitated the manipulation of DNA viruses such as phage viruses, insect viruses, and then mammalian viruses including vaccinia virus and adenovirus *(2–4,72)*. This allowed virus genetics to be performed and even new vaccine and gene therapy concepts to be developed. In the mid 1990s it was reported that adenovirus lacking the E1B-55k gene could replicate in tumor cells lacking functional *p53 (6)*. This event has encouraged a number of studies aimed at improving the oncolytic activity of a variety of DNA viruses through genetic engineering *(10,14)*. However, the ability to genetically manipulate RNA viruses proved a little more difficult because a DNA copy of the entire RNA genome was first required. The development of retroviruses as gene therapy vectors then progressed. Retroviruses are single-stranded RNA viruses that contain a core structural protein (gag) an RNA-dependent RNA polymerase (pol), and viral envelope (env) *(73)*. Usually, some of these genes are replaced with a therapeutic gene, such as a suicide gene, to prevent virus replication. One of the most frequently used retrovirus is the Moloney murine leukemia virus (MMLV). Retroviruses, which predominantly infect dividing cells, have also been psuedotyped (for example, using VSV G) to broaden their host range and have been used in a variety of clinical trials to combat cancer *(74)*. It was then discovered that the genomic RNA of positive stranded viruses, such as poliovirus, could directly function as an mRNA when transfected into recipient cells *(75)*. These genomes became translated to give rise to progeny virions. Further, plasmid DNA versions of the positive stranded viruses could also give rise to infectious virions following transfection of the cell. Despite this progress, a problem with generating recombinant negative-stranded viruses, such as VSV, was apparent because their genomic RNAs or their antigenome complements could serve as mRNAs and so neither could be used directly to recover infectious virus *(76)*. The minimal infectious unit for these viruses is the genome complexed with nucleocapsid and RNA-dependent RNA polymerase proteins in a ribonucleoprotein complex. It was subsequently found that the segmented negative-stranded RNA influenza virus, which has eight small genomes, could be assembled with RNPs in vitro and used to transfect cells that were already infected with influenza virus *(77,78)*. Some of these progeny viruses acquired a cloned gene through resortment and could be isolated and studied. Whiereas such approaches were useful for influenza virus analysis, it proved difficult to assemble the 11-kb genome of viruses such as VSV, into RNPs in vitro as a result of their large size. A breakthrough was then made on recovering infectious, cloned rabies virus, the prototype of the rhabdovirus family and relative of VSV *(79)*. This was achieved by placing a cDNA version of the entire rabies genome under control of a vaccinia encoded T7 polymerase. The cDNA was transfected into cells along with vaccinia virus to generate a supply of T7, and the full length antigenomic RNA (positive strand) was generated, along with the subgenomic mRNAs encoding the viral proteins, which in turn further assist replication. This system was subsequently found to work well with VSV and has now been used to recover infectious segmented negative-stranded RNA viruses such as Bunyamwera *(80–82)*. In addition, other oncolytic RNA viruses are now able to be cloned through similar "reverse genetic" approaches. Example include the paramyxoviruses NDV and measles *(83,84)*.

Recovering infectious cloned VSV was first reported from the laboratories of John Rose and Gail Wertz *(81,85)*. A T7 promoter directed synthesis of the full-length negative-stranded RNA and the polymerase was generated from vaccinia virus infection. However, infectious virus was not recoverable from this strategy, possibly because the subgenomic mRNAs generated from this strand hybridized with its parental genomic negative sense partner. Thus, constructs were redesigned to express the antigenomic RNA of VSV and the L, N, and P mRNAs (which were also transfected into cells to supply L, N, and P protein and help replication) were not able to hybridize to the encoded genomic template. Thus infectious VSV could be recovered from DNA and amplified for analysis *(81,85)*.

It was then demonstrated that new transcription units could be inserted into the VSV genome, between established genes (such as the G and L gene products) *(86)*. Nucleotide sequence analysis indicated a conserved 11-23 nucleotide motif present at the beginning and end of each gene. Insertion or addition of the conserved sequence in the 3′-noncoding region of a heterologous gene was found to be sufficient to terminate transcription of the preceding viral gene and promote transcription of the foreign gene. In preliminary studies using the chloramphenicol acetyltransferase (CAT) gene, high-level expression of the foreign gene was reported *(86)*. Of further importance was that the recombinant viruses were quite stable, and did not rapidly "lose" the gene. It was rapidly noticed in subsequent studies that recombinant VSV designed to express large gene inserts could be potentially created where such limitations associated with other viruses are evident *(87)*. Indeed, VSV was found to increase its length to accommodate extension of its genome. Later studies indicated that recombinant VSV could be generated to contain more than one foreign gene and to increase its genome length to greater than 40% *(88)*.

4.1. VSV, Gene Therapy and Vaccines

The generally low seroprevalence of VSV antibodies in the general population and genetic malleability indicated that VSV could be an attractive vector to develop new vaccines *(26)*. VSV elicits strong humoral and cellular immune responses in vivo and naturally infects at mucosal surfaces *(89–91)*. As mentioned, a major observation also included that VSV were found to accommodate large gene inserts and multiple genes in their genomes *(88)*. Thus, it wasn't long before a variety of foreign viral glycoproteins were cloned into VSV vectors for the purpose of developing novel vaccines *(89,92,93)*. Early studies involved placing the hemagglutinin (HA) or neuraminidase (NA) of influenza virus into VSV as extra genes. High-level expression of the heterologous products were obtained and animals inoculated with these VSV vectors were protected against lethal doses of influenza virus *(88,89)*. Substitution of the VSV G protein with influenza virus HA was also found to function well and to exhibit similar protective efficacy *(88)*. VSV vectors have subsequently been shown to be effective in vaccine studies designed to protect against respiratory syncytial virus (RSV), human papillomavirus (HPV), and viruses associated with acquired immunodeficiency syndrome (AIDS), amongst others *(88–91,93–96)*. In addition, new generations of attenuated, nonpropagating viruses are being developed where the VSV G protein has been deleted. These nonpropagating viruses (ΔG) lacking G, which is essential for infectivity, are generated via helper-cells that supply the VSV G glycoprotein in *trans (29,88,97)*. Budding viruses incorporate the G protein on their surface and are released. Such viruses can infect cells through the highly tropic G protein and commence replication. However, ΔG progeny viruses, when released from their primary targets, cannot infect other cells because they lack the G protein gene product. In vaccine studies, such viruses have been shown to retain their protective efficacy compared with their wild-type, replication competent counterparts, yet are considerably attenuated *(88,97)*. Other studies have shown that the parts of the membrane-proximal stem region of VSV G can be fused to foreign genes with the result that the heterologous product substitutes for the G protein *(97)*. Thus, these new recombinant viruses harbor new proteins on their surface, instead of G. Such strategies may be useful for developing recombinant VSVs that target specific cell types *(93,98)*. For example, a recent study indicated that VSV expressing a chimeric Sindbis glycoprotein containing the Fc-binding domain of *Staphylococcus aureus* protein A, conjugated to an antibody to Her2/neu could target cancer cells overexpressing the Her2/neu receptor *(99)*. Further, the ability to develop a variety of VSVs all with different sets of surface proteins is feasible and may prove useful in vaccines studies where sequential deliveries are required. Such viruses would avoid immune responses, such as neutralizing antibody, that would be generated by their predecessors and thus may exert significantly greater immunogenic/gene therapeutic activity *(93)*. Similar strategies may be useful in oncolysis studies where delivery of the first viral treatment generates significant immune responses, effectively eliminating the effectiveness of a second similar dose. Indeed, the genetic malleability of VSV is one of the attractive incentives for further evaluating VSV as an anticancer agent.

4.2. VSV, Recombinants, and Stability

There are no genetic resortment, significant gene loss, integration or transforming properties associated with VSV *(25,26)*. However, polymerase errors can be encountered during the replication of RNA viruses, the result of a lack of robust proofreading capacity *(87,100)*. Neutral mutation frequencies in VSV have been estimated at 1 in 10^3 to 10^4 for specific nucleotides in the genome. However, the mutation rate of VSV is so low that it does not present a problem when the virus is used to express foreign genes, even during extensive packaging. A single overnight passage on 10^7 BHK cells from a single plaque (approx 10^5 infectious particles) can be amplified to approximately 10^{11} infectious particles, corresponding to over 200ug of virus protein *(87)* . Thus a single passage of 10^6-fold amplification would produce 200g of virus. Experiments using VSV expressing the CAT gene indicated stable expression over 15 passages with nearly 2% of the total cellular protein comprising the foreign insert. Sequencing CAT mRNAs from several cloned viruses after 15 passages revealed only 2 base changes out of 2400 nucleotides. Further, recombinant VSV expressing other foreign genes have been shown to be stable over 26 passages, with similar low-mutation rates *(88)*. However, some rare instances of elimination of foreign gene expression have been documented (measles virus F protein) as results of mutations occurring in the transcription termination site *(87)*. This probably occurred because of the severe toxicity of the protein that may have effected the virus life cycle.

The ability of VSV to mutate was recently exploited in strategies designed to develop VSV vectors that were more attenuated in normal cells yet retained oncolytic activity. For example, variants of VSV (referred to as AV1 and AV2, with mutations in the M protein; M51R and V221F/S226R, respectively) were found to induce considerable amounts of IFN-α and thus replicate inefficiently in normal cells. However, these viruses remained highly lytic in 80% of human tumor cell lines tested and exerted oncolytic activity in immunocompetent animals harboring metastatic colon cancer *(101,102)*. One of the many functions of the M protein involves its ability to block host mRNA export through association with nuclear pore proteins such as Nup 98, which are IFN-inducible. Following infection, VSV activates the IFN pathway. However, following induction, IFN mRNA needs to be exported out of the nucleus for translation, a requirement the M protein prevents. The AV variants do not potently inhibit host mRNA export because the mutant M proteins may not interact efficiently with the Nup 98 complex to prevent their host mRNA export function *(31,33)*. Thus, virus induced antiviral gene expression in normal cells is not prevented and virus replication is impeded. In cancer cells, the IFN pathway or induced genes may not work properly anyway, so virus replication proceeds unchecked. This work illustrates again how taking advantage of defects in the innate immune system can be used to generate new oncolytic agents.

4.3. Genetically Engineered VSV as a Gene Therapy Tool Against Cancer

Oncolytic studies indicated that wild type VSV exhibited considerable potential as an anticancer agent. However, the ability to modify VSV through genetic engineering obviously affords the prospect of creating new generations of custom-made VSV vectors that contain immunomodulatory and/or suicide cassettes designed to increase their antitumor activity. In order to begin evaluating whether genetically engineered VSV carrying tumor-killing cassettes could be created and whether such viruses were more efficacious in tumor therapy than the wild-type VSV, we developed VSV vectors carrying, as models, the herpesvirus TK suicide cassette or the cytokine gene interleukin-4 (IL-4). The foreign genes were cloned as additional transcription units between the VSV G and L genes and all viruses were grown to exceptionally high titers *(71,103)*. TK protein was synthesized to extremely high levels and was functional, being able to phosphorylate ganciclovirs (GCV). Recombinant viruses also retained oncolytic activity against melanoma and adenocarcinoma tumors and were effective at eliminating the growth of metastatic disease. Importantly such viruses generated antitumor T-cell responses and were, in general, superior to that of VSV alone *(71)*. Given these data, we sought to exploit the discovery that innate immunity to VSV in normal cells is mediated primarily through PKR-mediated translation control and the IFN-β-induced antiviral state. We therefore constructed novel recombinant VSV expressing the murine or human IFN-β gene (VSV-IFN-β) *(71)*. We hypothesized that, because many transformed cells are defective in IFN signaling, VSV expressing IFN would rapidly replicate to induce cytolysis. However, such viruses would be unable to destroy normal cells, because the IFN-β produced by this virus would act in an autocrine and paracrine manner to bolster protection. Thus, VSV-IFN-β would need to be a more attenuated and a more specifically oncolytic agent designed to speifically exploit defects in the IFN system that appear common in malignant cells. In addition, the production of recombinant IFN by VSV-IFN-β might stimulate antitumor host defenses as well as the adaptive immune responses. Thus VSV-IFN-β might be a safer, more specific, and yet more potent oncolytic agent. Because we knew from our murine in vivo studies that VSV did not appear lethal to mice unless the IFN system was defective, we hypothesized that tumors grown in vivo would be susceptible to VSV-induced cytolysis and not the mice themselves. Indeed, preliminary data indicated that that VSV- expressing IFN-β were significantly attenuated when used to infect normal cells and mice, yet retained considerable oncolytic activity against metastatic disease *(71)*. These studies indicated that new generations of VSV, designed to be more specific for tumor cells and yet safer toward normal cells and tissue, could be generated. These new generations of VSV could conceivably target tumor cells and tissue for destruction as well as increase the immune response against such malignant cells through expression of immunomodulatory genes.

In summary, VSV has now been shown to be efficacious against malignant glioma, melanoma, hepatocellular carcinoma, breast adenocarcinoma, selected leukemias, and prostate cancer based tumors *(21,23,31,34,59,70,97,103–108)*. Genetically engineered VSVs have also now been generated with the intention of making these agents more specific, safer, and effective. Such viruses will be geared toward enhancing the immune system against the tumors and will take advantage of what we know about defects in the innate immune system. The evident ability of VSV to be manipulated clearly creates the possibility of generating many new vectors and strategies to combat cancer. However, VSV is not the only RNA virus to be evaluated as an anticancer agent. The next section briefly summarizes the potential utilization of other RNA viruses as gene therapy vectors for use against malignant disease.

5. OTHER ONCOLYTIC RNA VIRUSES

5.1. Reovirus

Reovirus (respiratory, enteric, orphan virus) is a nonenveloped member of the Reoviridae family, not associated with any disease, that comprises 10 segments of dsRNA, surrounded by 2 concentric, icosahedral protein capsids *(109,110)*. The 10 genome segment encodes 8 structural proteins and 3 nonstructural proteins not present in the mature virion. Reovirus was reported at the end of the 1990s to exert significant oncolytic ability in cells defective in the Ras pathway *(24)*. The molecular mechanisms have recently been reported to involve Ras regulation of Ral/GEF/p38 signaling *(111,112)*. In part, an over-activated Ras pathway may cause the inhibition of the antiviral protein PKR, by unknown mechanisms, allowing viral protein synthesis to ensue and cell lysis to occur *(24,113)*. Interestingly, Ras deregulation may also play a role in dictating the permissiveness of cancer cells to HSV 1. Reovirus uses junctional adhesion molecule 1 (JAM1) as a serotype independent cellular receptor, a broadly expressed immunoglobulin superfamily protein member *(109)*. Antitumor studies has revealed that reovirus exerts oncolytic activity in vitro, and in vivo in animal models against glioma, medulloblatoma, breast, ovarian, pancreatic, and lymphoid related malignancies *(107,111,114–118)*. In addition, reovirus has been shown to exhibit significant activity in purging strategies for autologous stem cell transplantation *(119)*. Unfortunately, unlike other RNA viruses, reovirus cannot yet be genetically modified because it's genome consists of dsRNA. Nevertheless, this virus may be significantly useful in therapeutic strategies against cancers harboring defects in the Ras pathway and is in clinical trails.

5.2. Paramyxoviruses: Measles virus and Newcastle Disease Virus

Measles virus (MV) and Newcastle Disease virus (NDV) are members of the negative single-stranded RNA paramyxoviridae family *(120)*. MV is a member of genus Morbillivirus whereas NDV is a member of the Rubulovirus genus that comprises mumps virus. These family members encode 6 to 7 covalently linked genes from a 15- to 16-kb genome and are enveloped viruses *(83)*. In the case of MV, the hemagglutinin (H) attachment protein binds to one of two cellular receptors, CD46 or the signaling activation molecule. CD46 is frequently overexpressed on cancer cells *(20)*. Given that other replicating RNA viruses were becoming noted for their oncolytic effects, it was decided to evaluate whether derivatives of the Edmonston-B-strain of measles virus (MV-Ed), which are live attenuated vaccines that have been effectively used for over 30 yr, exhibited similar properties. Indeed, intratumoral and intravenous inoculation of MV-Ed was found to induce the regression of human lymphoma in xenographed models *(18,121)*. Further, using reverse genetic techniques, MV has now been genetically modified to express reporter genes and soluble marker peptides such as CEA, and have retained oncolytic activity against ovarian tumor cells *(84,121–124)*. MV, which has the H envelope protein replaced by single chain anti-CD20 antibody was effectively able to target CD20 expressing cells *(125)*. Similar strategies have been used to target plasma cells expressing CD38, indicating that these viruses can be modified to target different tumor types and avoid the limitation of only targeting CD46 expressing cells (many normal cells also express CD46) *(126)*. The mechanisms underlying MVs tumor selectivity remains unknown, although it could involve defects in the innate immune signaling pathways described earlier *(127,128)*.

NDV and even mumps virus was first noted to replicate in selected tumors in the 1950s. NDV, which binds to sialic acid containing glycoconjugates whose exact identification remain to be elucidated, has been found to exhibit oncolytic effects against human neuroblastoma, fibrosarcoma, colon, breast, and prostate xenografts in nude mice *(129)*. Based on these studies, a replication-competent strain of NDV, referred to as PV701 has been examined in phase I studies on a variety of advanced solid tumors, that were unresponsive to standard therapy *(100)*. Approximately 10% tumor responses were reported using PV701 and phase II trials are now in progress *(130–132)*. In addition to this study, another live attenuated NDV strain, referred to as MTH-68/H was used in patients with glioblastoma multiforme *(133)*. Although a small study, four cases of advanced high grade glioma that had failed standard therapies responded well to the treatment with survival rates of 5 to 9 yr (as opposed to 6 mo using standard treatments) being stated. NDV has been reported to be genetically manipulative, but few studies are presently available on these types of study.

5.3. Orthomyxoviruses: Influenza Virus

Early recognized oncolytic viruses also included influenza A virus *(134)*. Influenza virus (INV) is a negative-stranded enveloped virus comprising 8 gene segments that replicates in the nucleus of infected cells. Cells are targeted by INV through their surface haemagglutinins (H) attaching to widely expressed sialyloligosaccharide moieties of cellular glycoconjugates. A genetically engineered INV that lacks a nonstructural protein (NS1) that has been reported to inhibit the antiviral protein PKR have similarly been used in anticancer strategies *(135)*. Similar to the situation with VSV (and perhaps reovirus), such mutant viruses cannot replicate in normal cells because the innate immune system involving PKR prevents their replication. However, because this innate pathway is defective in cancer cells, such NS1 lacking viruses replicate to induce specific cytolysis. Thus, these viruses may be safe to normal cells but not to cancer cells. Interestingly, INV as well as NDV and VSV were also used many years ago in viral oncolysate studies designed to stimulate an immune response to selected cancers *(134,137)*. It is not yet clear how viral-infected cell lysates promote antitumor activity, but the mechanisms could involve dsRNA stimulation of the innate immune system, which triggers robust adaptive immune responses. Future oncolytic studies using genetically engineered INV may provide more insight into the use of such vectors in the treatment of cancer.

5.4. Picornaviruses, Poliovirus

Poliovirus (PV) is a nonenveloped, positive-stranded RNA virus, which is responsible for causing poliomyelitis. PV RNA is composed of a 5′-nontranslated region that contains an internal ribosomal entry site (IRES) which directs the synthesis of a single polypeptide that is subsequently processed by viral proteases into structural and nonstructural proteins *(75)*. Polioviruses tropism is restricted to cells expressing CD155, a member of the Ig superfamily, which is prevalent on lower motor neurons resident within the spinal cord and brainstem *(138)*. The IRES elements encode strong cell-type specific restrictions and probably play a key role in the neurovirulent behavior of the virus. It subsequently became apparent, that other viruses, such as hepatitis C virus (HCV) or rhinoviruses also contain IRES elements. Experiments into the importance of the IRES elements lead to creation of a poliovirus chimera (referred to as PV1) *(139)*, which contained the human rhinovirus type 2 IRES element. PV1 was noted to be avirulent and generally nonpathogenic, even in primates. However PV1 was noted to grow well in tissue cultured cells derived from malignant gliomas, for reasons that remain unknown, but could speculatively involve defects in the innate immune responses or an upregulation of translation rates *(139)*. PV1 showed oncolytic potential in experimentally induced gliomas in athymic nude mice and may thus be useful for the treatment of cancers expressing CD155, which, may include other tumors in addition to those of brain cancer origin *(140)*. Subsequent studies have also demonstrated that live attenuated poliovirus exhibits oncolytic activity against neuroblastoma, in vitro and in vivo and other picornoviruses such as bovine enterovirus (BEV) may share similar traits *(141)*.

5.5. Togaviruses and Replicons

In an effort to improve the immunogenicity of nucleic acid vaccines, plasmid DNA vectors were developed that contained replicons derived from Alphaviruses such as Sindbis Virus (SV) and Semliki Forest Virus (SFV), which are enveloped positive strand RNA viruses of the Togavirus family *(142,143)*. When introduced into cells or animals the plasmids initiate a self-replicating RNA vector referred to as a replicon, which in turn directs the expression of a model tumor antigen. The vectors have been found to be extremely immunogenic, when compared with normal plasmid based vectors. The original goal was to produce more antigen, but the mechanism of the observed increased immunogenicity appears to involve activating dsRNA-dependent "stress-response" pathways which potentially activate innate immune pathways and eventually induce cell death, which presumably facilitates antigen uptake by DCs *(143)*. It is not yet clear if such replicons could be targeted to tumor cells to facilitate their apoptosis. Nevertheless, such approaches may be useful in generating immune response against tumor specific antigens, which may facilitate cancer rejection.

6. CONCLUSIONS

A number of different types of RNA viruses have now been observed to exert preferential growth in tumor cells, which ultimately leads to their apoptosis. The mechanisms of oncolysis in many instances may involve flaws in the innate immune response of transformed cells which are effectively exploited by the virus. For example, defects in the IFN system render cells extremely susceptible to many types of virus infection. In transformed cells, the IFN system does not seem to be fully functional, an observation that may speculatively mean that defects in this pathway may be a prerequisite for the cell to become fully malignant. All the RNA viruses highlighted above generate dsRNA-species, which are able to activate the IFN pathway. In normal cells these dsRNA signaling pathways are sufficient in many instances to initiate IFN production and IFN-induced genes to prevent virus infection. Whereas some RNA viruses still being evaluated for their potential use as anticancer agents, reasons for pursuing VSV may include: (1) VSV is a relatively safe, well characterized virus with little apparent disease documented in humans; (2) VSV is a simple RNA virus, with only 5 genes; (3) VSV has no genetic transforming properties; (4) VSV has no genetic reassortment properties; (5) VSV has no genetic integration properties; (6) the mechanisms of oncolytic activity are considerably better characterized; (7) VSV has high tropism for tumor cells; (8) VSV is genetically malleable, making the future creation of safer, more specific, and more effective vectors a realistic prospect; and (9) VSV lyses tumor cells regardless of the oncogenic events contributing to tumorigenesis (eg., it will kill cells harboring defects in the p53, ras or myc, or BCL-2 pathways). Collectively, the use of DNA and RNA viruses to treat malignant disease will escalate as mechanisms of oncolysis and knowledge of the enhancement of the immune system become apparent.

REFERENCES

1. Martuza RL, Malick A, Markert, JM, Ruffner KL, Coen DM. Experimental therapy of human glioma by means of a genetically engineered virus mutant. Science 1991;252:854–856.
2. Ring CJ. Cytolytic viruses as potential anti-cancer agents. J Gen Virol 83:491–502.
3. Stanziale SF, Fong Y. Novel approaches to cancer therapy using oncolytic viruses. 2002; Curr Mol Med 3:61–71.
4. Steele TA. Recent developments in the virus therapy of cancer. Proc Soc Exp Biol Med 2000;223: 118–127.
5. Zwiebel JA. Cancer gene and oncolytic virus therapy. Semin Oncol 2001;28:336–343.
6. Bischoff JR, Kirn DH, Williams A, et al. An adenovirus mutant that replicates selectively in p53-deficient human tumor cells. Science 1996;274:373–376.
7. Parr MJ, Manome Y, Tanaka T, Wen P, Kufe DW, Kaelin WG, Jr, Fine HA. Tumor-selective transgene expression in vivo mediated by an E2F-responsive adenoviral vector. Nat Med 1997;3:1145–1149.
8. Riley DJ, Nikitin AY, Lee WH. Adenovirus-mediated retinoblastoma gene therapy suppresses spontaneous pituitary melanotroph tumors in Rb+/- mice. Nat Med 1996;2:1316–1321.
9. Latham JP, Searle PF, Mautner V, James ND. Prostate-specific antigen promoter/enhancer driven gene therapy for prostate cancer: construction and testing of a tissue-specific adenovirus vector. Cancer Res 2000;60:334–341.
10. Alemany R, Balague C, Curiel DT. Replicative adenoviruses for cancer therapy. Nat Biotechnol 2000;18:723–727.
11. Kanerva A, Hemminki A. Modified adenoviruses for cancer gene therapy. Int J Cancer 2004;110:475–480.
12. Jiang H, Su ZZ, Lin JJ, Goldstein NI, Young CS, Fisher PB. The melanoma differentiation associated gene mda-7 suppresses cancer cell growth. Proc Natl Acad Sci U S A 1996;93:9160–9165.
13. Kirn D, Martuza RL, Zwiebel J. Replication-selective virotherapy for cancer: Biological principles, risk management and future directions. Nat Med 7:781–787.
14. Boviatsis EJ, Chase M, Wei MX, et al. Gene transfer into experimental brain tumors mediated by adenovirus, herpes simplex virus, and retrovirus vectors. Hum Gene Ther 2001;5:183–191.

15. McCormick F. Cancer gene therapy: fringe or cutting edge? Nat Rev Cancer 2001;1:130–141.
16. Leimig T, Brenner M, Ramsey J, Vanin E, Blaese M, Dilloo D. High-efficiency transduction of freshly isolated human tumor cells using adenoviral interleukin-2 vectors. Hum Gene Ther 1996;7:1233–1239.
17. Paillard F. The search for the "best" cytokine to induce antitumor immunity. Hum Gene Ther 1998;9:2457–2458.
18. Bluming AZ, Ziegler JL. Regression of Burkitt's lymphoma in association with measles infection. Lancet 1971;2:105–106.
19. Hammon WM, Yohn DS, Casto BC, Atchison RW. Oncolytic Potentials of Nonhuman Viruses for Human Cancer. I. Effects of Twenty-Four Viruses on Human Cancer Cell Lines. J Natl Cancer Inst 1963;31:329–345.
20. Russell SJ. RNA viruses as virotherapy agents. Cancer Gene Ther 2002;9:961–996.
21. Balachandran S, Barber GN. Vesicular stomatitis virus (VSV) therapy of tumors. IUBMB Life 2000;50:135–138.
22. Boehme KW, Compton T. Innate sensing of viruses by toll-like receptors. J Virol 2004;78:7867–7873.
23. Balachandran S, Barber GN. Defective translational control facilitates vesicular stomatitis virus oncolysis. Cancer Cell 2004;5:51–65.
24. Coffey MC, Strong JE, Forsyth PA, Lee PW. Reovirus therapy of tumors with activated Ras pathway. Science 1998;282:1332–1334.
25. Dietzschold B, Rupprecht CE, Fu AF, Koprowski H. Rhabdoviruses. In:. Fields Virology, 3rd ed., Howley, et al., eds. Philadelphia: Lippincott-Raven Publishers, 1996; pp. 1137–1159.
26. Wagner RR. a. R., J.K. Rhabdoviridae: The Viruses and Their Replication, p. 1121–1135. In Fields Virology, 3rd ed., D. M. K. B.N. Fields, P.M. Howley, et al., eds. Philadelphia: Lipincott-Raven Publishers, 1996; pp. 1121–1135.
27. Ball LA, Pringle CR, Flanagan B, Perepelitsa VP, Wertz GW. Phenotypic consequences of rearranging the P, M, and G genes of vesicular stomatitis virus. J Virol 1999;73:4705–4712.
28. Carneiro FA, Bianconi ML, Weissmuller G, Stauffer F, Da Poian AT. Membrane recognition by vesicular stomatitis virus involves enthalpy-driven protein-lipid interactions. J Virol 2002;76:3756–3764.
29. Jeetendra E, Robison CS, Albritton LM, Whitt MA. The membrane-proximal domain of vesicular stomatitis virus G protein functions as a membrane fusion potentiator and can induce hemifusion. J Virol 2002;76:12,300–12,311.
30. Ochsenbein AF, Fehr T, Lutz C, Suter M, Brombacher F, Hengartner H, Zinkernagel RM. Control of early viral and bacterial distribution and disease by natural antibodies. Science 1999;286:2156–2159.
31. Enninga J, Levy DE, Blobel G, Fontoura BM. Role of nucleoporin induction in releasing an mRNA nuclear export block. Science 2002;295:1523–1525.
32. Petersen JM, Her LS, Varvel V, Lund E, Dahlberg JE. The matrix protein of vesicular stomatitis virus inhibits nucleocytoplasmic transport when it is in the nucleus and associated with nuclear pore complexes. Mol Cell Biol 2000;20:8590–8601.
33. von Kobbe C, van Deursen JM, Rodrigues JP, et al. Vesicular stomatitis virus matrix protein inhibits host cell gene expression by targeting the nucleoporin Nup98. Mol Cell 2000;6:1243–1252.
34. Stojdl DF, Lichty B, Knowles S, et al. Exploiting tumor-specific defects in the interferon pathway with a previously unknown oncolytic virus. Nat Med 2000;6:821–825.
35. Pattnaik AK, Ball LA, LeGrone AW, Wertz GW. Infectious defective interfering particles of VSV from transcripts of a cDNA clone. Cell 1992;69:1011–1020.
36. Kim L, Morley PS, McCluskey BJ, Mumford EL, Swenson SL, Salman MD. Oral vesicular lesions in horses without evidence of vesicular stomatitis virus infection. J Am Vet Med Assoc 2000;216:1399–1404.
37. Mumford EL, McCluskey BJ, Traub-Dargatz JL, Schmitt BJ, Salman MD. Public veterinary medicine: public health. Serologic evaluation of vesicular stomatitis virus exposure in horses and cattle in 1996. J Am Vet Med Assoc 1996;213:1265–1269.
38. Bi Z, Barna M, Komatsu T, Reiss CS. Vesicular stomatitis virus infection of the central nervous system activates both innate and acquired immunity. J Virol 1995;69:6466–6472.
39. Plakhov IV, Arlund EE, Aoki S, Reiss CS. The earliest events in vesicular stomatitis virus infection of the murine olfactory neuroepithelium and entry of the central nervous system. Virology 1995;209:257–262.
40. van den Pol AN, Dalton KP, Rose JK. Relative neurotropism of a recombinant rhabdovirus expressing a green fluorescent envelope glycoprotein. J Virol 2002;76:1309–1327.
41. Thomsen AR, Nansen A, Andersen S, Johansen J, Marker O, Christensen JP. Cooperation of B cells and T cells is required for survival of mice infected with vesicular stomatitis virus. Int Immunol 1997;9:1757–1766.

42. Gresser I, Tovey MG, Bourali-Maury C. Efficacy of exogenous interferon treatment initiated after onset of multiplication of vesicular stomatitis virus in the brains of mice. J Gen Virol 1975;27:395–398.
43. Meurs E, Chong K, Galabru J, et al. Molecular cloning and characterization of the human double-stranded RNA-activated protein kinase induced by interferon. Cell 1990;62:379–390.
44. Hershey JW. Translational control in mammalian cells. Annu Rev Biochem 1991;60:717–755.
45. Kimball SR. Eukaryotic initiation factor eIF2. Int J Biochem Cell Biol 1999;31:25–29.
46. Perkins DJ, Barber GN. Defects in translational regulation mediated by the alpha subunit of eukaryotic initiation factor 2 inhibit antiviral activity and facilitate the malignant transformation of human fibroblasts. Mol Cell Biol 2004;24:2025–2040.
47. Balachandran S, Roberts PC, Brown LE, et al. Essential role for the dsRNA-dependent protein kinase PKR in innate immunity to viral infection. Immunity 2000;13:129–141.
48. Abraham N, Stojdl DF, Duncan PI, et al. Characterization of transgenic mice with targeted disruption of the catalytic domain of the double-stranded RNA-dependent protein kinase, PKR. J Biol Chem 1999;274:5953–5962.
49. Stojdl DF, Abraham N, Knowles S, et al. The murine double-stranded RNA-dependent protein kinase PKR is required for resistance to vesicular stomatitis virus. J Virol 2000;74:9580–9585.
50. Stark GR, Kerr IM, Williams BR, Silverman RH, Schreiber RD. How cells respond to interferons. Annu Rev Biochem 1998;67:227–264.
51. Chadha KC, Ambrus JL, Jr, Dembinski W, Ambrus JL, Sr. Interferons and interferon inhibitory activity in disease and therapy. Exp Biol Med (Maywood) 2004;229:285–290.
52. Tough DF. Type I interferon as a link between innate and adaptive immunity through dendritic cell stimulation. Leuk Lymphoma 2004;45:257–264.
53. Malmgaard L. Induction and regulation of IFNs during viral infections. J Interferon Cytokine Res 2004;24:439–454.
54. Durbin JE, Hackenmiller T, Simon MC, Levy DE. Targeted disruption of the mouse Stat1 gene results in compromised innate immunity to viral disease. Cell 1996;84:443–450.
55. Meraz MA, White JM, Sheehan KC, et al. Targeted disruption of the Stat1 gene in mice reveals unexpected physiologic specificity in the JAK-STAT signaling pathway. Cell 1996;84:431–442.
56. Muller U, Steinhoff U, Reis LF, et al. Functional role of type I and type II interferons in antiviral defense. Science 1994;264:1918–1921.
57. Akira S, Takeda K. Toll-like receptor signalling. Nat Rev Immunol 4:499-511.
58. Pasare C, Medzhitov R. Toll-like receptors: balancing host resistance with immune tolerance. Curr Opin Immunol 2003;15:677–682.
59. Balachandran S, Porosnicu M, Barber GN. Oncolytic activity of vesicular stomatitis virus is effective against tumors exhibiting aberrant p53, Ras, or myc function and involves the induction of apoptosis. J Virol 2001;75:3474–3479.
60. Balachandran S, Roberts PC, Kipperman T, et al. Alpha/beta interferons potentiate virus-induced apoptosis through activation of the FADD/Caspase-8 death signaling pathway. J Virol 2000;74:1513–1523.
61. Dovhey SE, Ghosh NS, Wright KL. Loss of interferon-gamma inducibility of TAP1 and LMP2 in a renal cell carcinoma cell line. Cancer Res 2000;60:5789–5796.
62. Dunn GP, Bruce AT, Ikeda H, Old LJ, Schreiber RD. Cancer immunoediting: from immunosurveillance to tumor escape. Nat Immunol 2002;3:991–998.
63. Kovarik J, Boudny V, Kocak I, Lauerova L, Fait V, Vagundova M. Malignant melanoma associates with deficient IFN-induced STAT 1 phosphorylation. Int J Mol Med 2003;12:335–340.
64. Linge C, Gewert S, Rossmann S, Bishop JA, Crowe JS. Interferon system defects in human malignant melanoma. Cancer Res 1995;55:4099–4104.
65. Matin SF, Rackley RR, Sadhukhan PC, et al. Impaired alpha-interferon signaling in transitional cell carcinoma: lack of p48 expression in 5637 cells. Cancer Res 2001;61:2261–2266.
66. Persing DH, Prendergast FG. Infection, immunity, and cancer. Arch Pathol Lab Med 1999;123: 1015–1022.
67. Sun WH, Pabon C, Alsayed Y, et al. Interferon-alpha resistance in a cutaneous T-cell lymphoma cell line is associated with lack of STAT1 expression. Blood 1998;91:570–576.
68. Suriawinata A, Xu R. An update on the molecular genetics of hepatocellular carcinoma. Semin Liver Dis 2004;24:77–88.
69. Wong LH, Krauer KG, Hatzinisiriou I, et al. Interferon-resistant human melanoma cells are deficient in ISGF3 components, STAT1, STAT2, and p48-ISGF3gamma. J Biol Chem 1997;272:28,779–28,785.
70. Fernandez M, Porosnicu M, Markovic D, Barber GN. Genetically engineered vesicular stomatitis virus in gene therapy: application for treatment of malignant disease. J Virol 2002;76:895–904.

71. Obuchi M, Fernandez M, Barber GN. Development of recombinant vesicular stomatitis viruses that exploit defects in host defense to augment specific oncolytic activity. J Virol 2003;77:8843–8856.
72. Bonnet MC, Tartaglia J, Verdier F, et al. Recombinant viruses as a tool for therapeutic vaccination against human cancers. Immunol Lett 2000;74:11–25.
73. Dornburg R. The history and principles of retroviral vectors. Front Biosci 2003;8:d818–d835.
74. Yee JK, Friedmann T, Burns JC. Generation of high-titer pseudotyped retroviral vectors with very broad host range. Methods Cell Biol 1994;43 Pt A:99–112.
75. Golini F, Semler BL, Dorner AJ, Wimmer E. Protein-linked RNA of poliovirus is competent to form an initiation complex of translation in vitro. Nature 1980;287:600–603.
76. Rose JK. Positive strands to the rescue again: a segmented negative-strand RNA virus derived from cloned cDNAs. Proc Natl Acad Sci U S A 1996;93:14,998–15,000.
77. Luytjes W, Krystal M, Enami M, Pavin JD, Palese P. Amplification, expression, and packaging of foreign gene by influenza virus. Cell 1989;59:1107–1113.
78. Neumann G, Brownlee GG, Fodor E, Kawaoka Y. Orthomyxovirus replication, transcription, and polyadenylation. Curr Top Microbiol Immunol 2004;283:121–143.
79. Schnell MJ, Mebatsion T, Conzelmann KK. Infectious rabies viruses from cloned cDNA. Embo J 1994;13:4195–4203.
80. Bridgen A, Elliott RM. Rescue of a segmented negative-strand RNA virus entirely from cloned complementary DNAs. Proc Natl Acad Sci U S A 1996;93:15,400–15,404.
81. Lawson ND, Stillman EA, Whitt MA, Rose JK. Recombinant vesicular stomatitis viruses from DNA. Proc Natl Acad Sci U S A 1995;92:4477–4481.
82. Peeters BP, de Leeuw OS, Koch G, Gielkens AL. Rescue of Newcastle disease virus from cloned cDNA: evidence that cleavability of the fusion protein is a major determinant for virulence. J Virol 1999;73:5001–5009.
83. Nagai Y. Paramyxovirus replication and pathogenesis. Reverse genetics transforms understanding. Rev Med Virol 1999;9:83–99.
84. Radecke F, Spielhofer P, Schneider H, et al. Rescue of measles viruses from cloned DNA. EMBO J 1995;14:5773–5784.
85. Whelan SP, Ball LA, Barr JN, Wertz GT. Efficient recovery of infectious vesicular stomatitis virus entirely from cDNA clones. Proc Natl Acad Sci U S A 1995;92:8388–8392.
86. Schnell MJ, Buonocore L, Whitt MA, Rose JK. The minimal conserved transcription stop-start signal promotes stable expression of a foreign gene in vesicular stomatitis virus. J Virol 1996;70: 2318–2323.
87. Quinones-Kochs MI, Schnell MJ, Buonocore L, Rose JK. Mechanisms of loss of foreign gene expression in recombinant vesicular stomatitis viruses. Virology 2001;287:427–435.
88. Roberts A, Buonocore L, Price R, Forman J, Rose JK. Attenuated vesicular stomatitis viruses as vaccine vectors. J Virol 1999;73:3723–3732.
89. Roberts A, Kretzschmar E, Perkins AS, et al. Vaccination with a recombinant vesicular stomatitis virus expressing an influenza virus hemagglutinin provides complete protection from influenza virus challenge. J Virol 1998;72:4704–4711.
90. Roberts A, Reuter JD, Wilson JH, Baldwin S, Rose JK. Complete protection from papillomavirus challenge after a single vaccination with a vesicular stomatitis virus vector expressing high levels of L1 protein. J Virol 2004;78:3196–3199.
91. Rose NF, Marx PA, Luckay A, et al. An effective AIDS vaccine based on live attenuated vesicular stomatitis virus recombinants. Cell 2001;106:539–549.
92. Buonocore L, Blight KJ, Rice CM, Rose JK. Characterization of vesicular stomatitis virus recombinants that express and incorporate high levels of hepatitis C virus glycoproteins. J Virol 2002;76:6865–6872.
93. Rose NF, Roberts A, Buonocore L, Rose JK. Glycoprotein exchange vectors based on vesicular stomatitis virus allow effective boosting and generation of neutralizing antibodies to a primary isolate of human immunodeficiency virus type 1. J Virol 2000;74:10,903–10,910.
94. Kahn JS, Roberts A, Weibel A, Buonocore L, Rose JK. Replication-competent or attenuated, nonpropagating vesicular stomatitis viruses expressing respiratory syncytial virus (RSV) antigens protect mice against RSV challenge. J Virol 2001;75:11,079–11,087.
95. Ramsburg E, Rose NF, Marx PA, et al. Highly effective control of an AIDS virus challenge in macaques by using vesicular stomatitis virus and modified vaccinia virus Ankara vaccine vectors in a single-boost protocol. J Virol 2004;78:3930–3940.
96. Schnell MJ, Johnson JE, Buonocore L, Rose JK. Construction of a novel virus that targets HIV-1-infected cells and controls HIV-1 infection. Cell 1997;90:849–857.

97. Duntsch CD, Zhou Q, Jayakar HR, et al. Recombinant vesicular stomatitis virus vectors as oncolytic agents in the treatment of high-grade gliomas in an organotypic brain tissue slice-glioma coculture model. J Neurosurg 2004;100:1049–1059.
98. Kretzschmar E, Buonocore L, Schnell MJ, Rose JK. High-efficiency incorporation of functional influenza virus glycoproteins into recombinant vesicular stomatitis viruses. J Virol 1997;71: 5982–5989.
99. Bergman I, Whitaker-Dowling P, Gao Y, Griffin JA, Watkins SC. Vesicular stomatitis virus expressing a chimeric Sindbis glycoprotein containing an Fc antibody binding domain targets to Her2/neu overexpressing breast cancer cells. Virology 2003;316:337–347.
100. Huang Z, Elankumaran S, Panda A, Samal SK. Recombinant Newcastle disease virus as a vaccine vector. Poult Sci 2003;82:899–906.
101. Desforges M, Charron J, Berard S, et al. Different host-cell shutoff strategies related to the matrix protein lead to persistence of vesicular stomatitis virus mutants on fibroblast cells. Virus Res 2001;76:87–102.
102. Stojdl DF. Lichty BD, tenOever BR, et al. VSV strains with defects in their ability to shutdown innate immunity are potent systemic anti-cancer agents. Cancer Cell 2003;4:263–275.
103. Porosnicu M, Mian A, Barber GN. The oncolytic effect of recombinant vesicular stomatitis virus is enhanced by expression of the fusion cytosine deaminase/uracil phosphoribosyltransferase suicide gene. Cancer Res 2003;63:8366–8376.
104. Connor JH, Naczki C, Koumenis C, Lyles DS. Replication and cytopathic effect of oncolytic vesicular stomatitis virus in hypoxic tumor cells in vitro and in vivo. J Virol 2004;78:8960–8970.
105. Ebert O, Shinozaki K, Huang TG, Savontaus MJ, Garcia-Sastre A, Woo SL. Oncolytic vesicular stomatitis virus for treatment of orthotopic hepatocellular carcinoma in immune-competent rats. Cancer Res 2003;63:3605–3611.
106. Ebert O, Shinozaki K, Kournioti C, Park MS, Garcia-Sastre A, Woo SL. Syncytia induction enhances the oncolytic potential of vesicular stomatitis virus in virotherapy for cancer. Cancer Res 2004;64: 3265–3270.
107. Hirasawa K, Nishikawa SG, Norman KL, et al. Systemic reovirus therapy of metastatic cancer in immune-competent mice. Cancer Res 2003;63:348–353.
108. Huang TG, Ebert O, Shinozaki K, Garcia-Sastre A, Woo SL. Oncolysis of hepatic metastasis of colorectal cancer by recombinant vesicular stomatitis virus in immune-competent mice. Mol Ther 2003;8:434–440.
109. Forrest JC, Dermody TS. Reovirus receptors and pathogenesis. J Virol 2003;77:9109–9115.
110. Tyler KL, Clarke P, DeBiasi RL, Kominsky D, Poggioli GJ. Reoviruses and the host cell. Trends Microbiol 2001;9:560–564.
111. Norman KL, Coffey MC, Hirasawa K, et al. Reovirus oncolysis of human breast cancer. Hum Gene Ther 2002;13:641–652.
112. Norman KL, Hirasawa K, Yang AD, Shields MA, Lee PW. Reovirus oncolysis: the Ras/RalGEF/p38 pathway dictates host cell permissiveness to reovirus infection. Proc Natl Acad Sci U S A 2004;101: 11,099–11,104.
113. Strong JE, Coffey MC, Tang S, Sabinin P, Lee PW. The molecular basis of viral oncolysis: usurpation of the Ras signaling pathway by reovirus. EMBO J 1998;17:3351–3362.
114. Alain T, Hirasawa K, Pon KJ, et al. Reovirus therapy of lymphoid malignancies. Blood 2002;100: 4146–4153.
115. Etoh T, Himeno Y, Matsumoto T, et al. Oncolytic viral therapy for human pancreatic cancer cells by reovirus. Clin Cancer Res 2003;9:1218–1223.
116. Hirasawa K, Nishikawa SG, Norman KL, Alain T, Kossakowska A, Lee PW. Oncolytic reovirus against ovarian and colon cancer. Cancer Res 2002;62:1696–1701.
117. Wilcox ME, Yang W, Senger S, et al. Reovirus as an oncolytic agent against experimental human malignant gliomas. J Natl Cancer Inst 2001;93:903–912.
118. Yang WQ, Senger S, Muzik H, et al. Reovirus prolongs survival and reduces the frequency of spinal and leptomeningeal metastases from medulloblastoma. Cancer Res 2003;63:3162–3172.
119. Thirukkumaran CM, Luider JM, Stewart DA, et al. Reovirus oncolysis as a novel purging strategy for autologous stem cell transplantation. Blood 2003;102:377–387.
120. Curran J, Kolakofsky D. Replication of paramyxoviruses. Adv Virus Res 1999;54:403–422.
121. Peng KW, TenEyck CJ, Galanis E, Kalli KT, Hartmann LC, Russell SJ. Intraperitoneal therapy of ovarian cancer using an engineered measles virus. Cancer Res 2002;62:4656–4662.
122. Peng KW, Frenzke M, Myers R, et al. Biodistribution of oncolytic measles virus after intraperitoneal administration into Ifnar-CD46Ge transgenic mice. Hum Gene Ther 2003;14:1565–1577.

123. Phuong LK, Allen C, Peng KW, et al. Use of a vaccine strain of measles virus genetically engineered to produce carcinoembryonic antigen as a novel therapeutic agent against glioblastoma multiforme. Cancer Res 2003;63:2462–2469.
124. Plumb J, Duprex WP, Cameron CH, Richter-Landsberg C, Talbot P, McQuaid S. Infection of human oligodendroglioma cells by a recombinant measles virus expressing enhanced green fluorescent protein. J Neurovirol 2002;8:24–34.
125. Bucheit AD, Kumar S, Grote DM, et al. An oncolytic measles virus engineered to enter cells through the CD20 antigen. Mol Ther 2003;7:62–72.
126. Peng KW, Donovan KA, Schneider U, Cattaneo R, Lust JA, Russell SJ. Oncolytic measles viruses displaying a single-chain antibody against CD38, a myeloma cell marker. Blood 2003;101:2557–2562.
127. Grote D, Russell SJ, Cornu TI, et al. Live attenuated measles virus induces regression of human lymphoma xenografts in immunodeficient mice. Blood 2001;97: 3746–3754.
128. Peng KW, Facteau S, Wegman T, DO'Kane, Russell SJ. Non-invasive in vivo monitoring of trackable viruses expressing soluble marker peptides. Nat Med 2002;8:527–531.
129. Nakaya T, Cros J, Park MS, et al. Recombinant Newcastle disease virus as a vaccine vector. J Virol 2001;75:11,868–11,873.
130. Lorence RM, Pecora AL, Major PP, et al. Overview of phase I studies of intravenous administration of PV701, an oncolytic virus. Curr Opin Mol Ther 2003;5:618–624.
131. Pecora AL, Rizvi N, Cohen GI, et al. Phase I trial of intravenous administration of PV701, an oncolytic virus, in patients with advanced solid cancers. J Clin Oncol 2002;20:2251–2266.
132. Phuangsab A, Lorence RM, Reichard KW, Peeples ME, Walter RJ. Newcastle disease virus therapy of human tumor xenografts: antitumor effects of local or systemic administration. Cancer Lett 2001;172:27–36.
133. Csatary LK, Gosztonyi G, Szeberenyi J, et al. MTH-68/H oncolytic viral treatment in human high-grade gliomas. J Neurooncol 2004;67:83–93.
134. Sinkovics JG, Horvath JC. Newcastle disease virus (NDV): brief history of its oncolytic strains. J Clin Virol 2000;16:1–15.
135. Muster T, Rajtarova J, Sachet M, et al. Interferon resistance promotes oncolysis by influenza virus NS1-deletion mutants. Int J Cancer 2004;110:15–21.
136. Bergmann M, Romirer I, Sachet M, et al. A genetically engineered influenza A virus with ras-dependent oncolytic properties. Cancer Res 2001;61:8188–8193.
137. Livingston PO, Albino AP, Chung TJ, et al. Serological response of melanoma patients to vaccines prepared from VSV lysates of autologous and allogeneic cultured melanoma cells. Cancer 1985;55: 713–720.
138. Shah AC, Benos D, Gillespie GY, Markert JM. Oncolytic viruses: clinical applications as vectors for the treatment of malignant gliomas. J Neurooncol 2003;65:203–226.
139. Gromeier M, Lachmann S, Rosenfeld MR, Gutin PH, Wimmer E. Intergeneric poliovirus recombinants for the treatment of malignant glioma. Proc Natl Acad Sci U S A 2000;97:6803–6808.
140. Ansardi DC, Porter DC, Jackson CA, Gillespie GY, Morrow CD. RNA replicons derived from poliovirus are directly oncolytic for human tumor cells of diverse origins. Cancer Res 2001;61:8470–8479.
141. Smyth M, Symonds A, Brazinova S, Martin J. Bovine enterovirus as an oncolytic virus: foetal calf serum facilitates its infection of human cells. Int J Mol Med 2002;10:49–53.
142. Yamanaka R. Alphavirus vectors for cancer gene therapy (review). Int J Oncol 2004;24:919–923.
143. Ying H, Zaks TZ, Wang RF, et al. Cancer therapy using a self-replicating RNA vaccine. Nat Med 1999;5:823–827.

8 Parvovirus Vectors

Selvarangan Ponnazhagan, PhD

CONTENTS

Summary

Parvoviruses are among the smallest of eukaryotic viruses. The association of parvovirus with cancer has been reported much before realizing the potential application of parvovirus-based vectors in cancer gene therapy. Unique characteristics of paroviruses such as nonpathogenicity, antioncogenicity, and methods of efficient recombinant vector production have drawn more attention toward utilizing parvovirus-based vectors in cancer gene therapy. Although more than 30 different parvoviruses have been identified thus far, recombinant vectors derived from adeno-associated virus (AAV), minute virus of mice (MVM), LuIII and parvovirus H1 have been successfully tested in many preclinical models of human diseases including cancer. This chapter focuses on the potential of nonreplicating and autonomously replicating parvoviral vectors in cancer gene therapy including strategies that target tumor cells directly or indirectly.

Key Words: Parvovirus; adeno-associated virus; minute virus of mice; LuIII; parvovirus H1.

1. INTRODUCTION

Parvoviruses are among the smallest eukaryotic viruses, which were initially discovered in 1960s *(1)*. Parvoviruses are subdivided into three major groups namely densoviruses, autonomous parvoviruses (APV), and dependoviruses *(2)*. Whereas densoviruses

From: *Cancer Drug Discovery and Development: Gene Therapy for Cancer*
Edited by: K. K. Hunt, S. A. Vorburger, and S. G. Swisher © Humana Press Inc., Totowa, NJ

infect only insects, APV and dependoviruses infect vertebrate animals. The autonomous parvoviruses replicate in proliferating target cells without the need of helper viruses but dependoviruses require helper virus functions for replication. The simple organization of parvoviral genome and life cycle originally attracted investigators towards understanding the molecular basis of viral replication and biology of virus–host cell interaction. Further, the advent of gene therapy approaches has drawn enormous interest in the potential use of parvoviruses in general and the adeno-associated virus (AAV) in particular. Although initial studies on gene therapy using parvoviruses have concentrated on the phenotypic correction of genetic metabolic defects owing to the ability of long-term expression of AAV-based vectors, increased understanding on many aspects of parvovirus biology and molecular pathology of cancer has led to the realization of utilizing parvovirus-based vectors for cancer gene therapy.

2. MOLECULAR ORGANIZATION OF PARVOVIRUSES

The genome of parvoviruses consist of approx a 5-kilobase (kb) linear, monopartite, single-stranded DNA *(3–5)*. At both the ends of the genome are sequences known as terminal palindromes, which do not encode any protein. The parvoviral genome consists of only two overlapping genes that encode two types of proteins. The genetic map of parvoviruses can be broadly divided into left- and right-halves that encode regulatory and capsid proteins respectively. The regulatory protein involved in replication is known as Rep or NS (for nonstructural protein) and the structural capsid protein is referred to as VP. There are two major promoters in the viral genome that express the rep/NS and VP proteins. In addition, AAV genome also contains a third promoter, which transcribes smaller rep proteins. By alternate splicing, the proteins are generated in different molecular sizes. Nonetheless, the isotypes of rep/NS and VP share same C-terminal amino acid sequences. A fully assembled parvovirus capsid forms an icosahedral structure of approx 20 to 25 nm. Electron micrographs have shown icosahedral particles made up of multiple capsomeres, which are easily distinguished from those of most other virus groups by their smaller size. Recent studies on AAV capsids have indicated that in a fully assembled capsid, about 60 individual protein molecules are present *(6)*. A prototypic parvoviral structure and genome is shown in Fig. 1.

3. HISTORY OF PARVOVIRUS AND CANCER

Since the discovery of parvoviruses, there has been significant advance on the relationship between parvoviruses and cancer. Epidemiological surveys in humans have revealed a correlation between serological evidence of parvoviral infection and lower incidence of certain human cancers *(7,8)*. In vivo studies have demonstrated that animals infected with parvoviruses exhibited increased protection against chemical carcinogen- and virus-induced tumorigenesis *(9)*. Several in vitro studies have also reported inhibition of cellular transformation by parvoviruses and interestingly, preferential killing of established tumor cell lines by parvovirus infection compared with normal cells *(9)*. Results of these studies have led to the belief of possible interference with the induction of malignant transformation as well as survival and proliferation of tumor cells. Subsequent studies have provided molecular evidence on the role of NS proteins of parvoviruses in oncosuppression *(10–12)*. More recently, it has also been shown with AAV that the nature of single-stranded genomic structure itself triggers cellular events in p53 mutant tumor cells leading to apoptosis *(13)*.

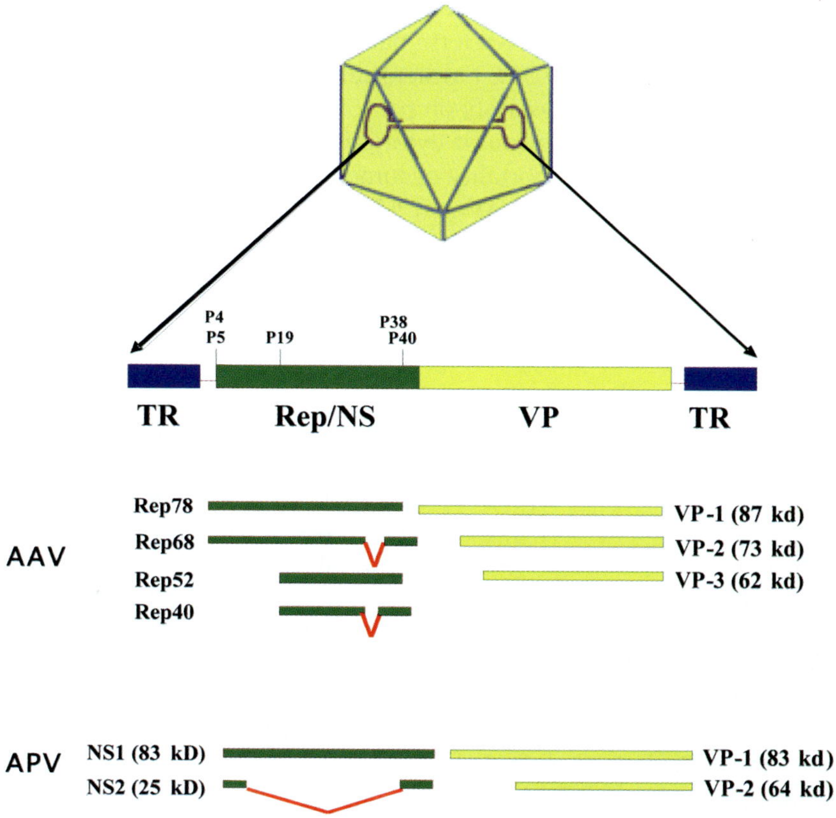

Fig. 1. Genomic organization of prototypic parvovirus. The genome of parvoviruses comprise of approx a 5-kb single-stranded DNA packaged within a icosahedral capsid of 25 to 30 nm. The major promoter near the 5′-end encodes NS or Rep proteins as in APV and AAV respectively. The capsid proteins are derived from the VP gene situated at the right half of the genome and expressed by a promoter situated immediately upstream of the gene in the middle of the vector genome. Relative map units of the location of respective promoters are given above. P5, P19, and P40 represent promoters of AAV and P4 and P38 are corresponding promoters in APV. The size of alternately spliced NS/Rep and VP are indicated in parenthesis. TR represents the palindromic terminal repeat sequences.

4. ANTIONCOGENIC PROPERTIES OF APV

Parvovirus related anticancer effect was first discovered in 1967. Hamsters persistently infected with H viruses developed 5 to 25 fewer spontaneous tumors than control animals *(1)*. Subsequent studies showed that parvoviral surveillance could also affect various types of tumors induced experimentally in rodents and chicken by means of oncogenic viruses or a chemical carcinogen *(14,15)*. Following these observations, several possible mechanisms for APV-mediated killing of tumor cells have been postulated. Direct effects on cell metabolism were attributed to the terminal sequences of the viral DNA as well as the regulatory NS proteins. Analysis of defective particles also suggested that the noncoding hairpin ends of the parvoviral genome, which contained replication and transcription control sequences contributed to the inhibition of a response frequently associated with malignant transformation such as DNA amplification *(16)*. Evidence for a role of parvovirus NS protein in the inhibition of cellular events was provided by studies in which expression of NS protein was driven by heterologous promoters *(17–20)*. Mutation studies on NS proteins of MVM have determined that domains near the amino- and carboxy-terminal regions of the NS proteins are important for host cell cytotoxicity *(10,21)*. Further, transregulation of APV NS proteins has been reported to exert an effect not only on parvoviral promoters but also heterologous promoters *(22)*. Thus, a combination of cytotoxicity and transregulation of APV NS proteins appears to increase the mortality of tumor cells.

More preclinical evaluations of AAV and APV and improvements in the production of APV should result in the application of parvovirus-based vectors in clinical gene therapy trials.

5. PRODUCTION OF RECOMBINANT PARVOVIRUSES

Despite the antioncogenic properties of parvoviruses and absence of disease pathogenesis with the exception of parvovirus B19, utilization of wild-type parvoviruses in cancer gene therapy is highly unlikely. Thus, major efforts centered on the advancements in the production of recombinant parvoviral vectors for their potential gene therapy applications in vivo *(5,44,45)*. Elucidation of the genomic organization, sequence determination of parvoviruses and cloning of parvovirus genome in plasmid vectors has led to the development of methods to produce recombinant parvoviral vectors *(44,45)*. In a typical methodology, a gene of interest is cloned between the terminal repeat sequences of parvoviral genome in a plasmid. Genes encoding NS/Rep or VP of the wild type virus and that of required helper viral proteins are provided in *trans*, also from nonreplicating helper plasmids. Whereas the helper-dependent parvoviruses require the functions of helper virus proteins for a productive life cycle, the APV do not require helper functions from other viruses. However, both dependoviruses and APV require host cell machinery for the replication of viral genome. In the production of recombinant parvoviruses, a combination of the packaging and helper plasmid DNA is transfected into packaging cells *(45–48)*. Approximately 48 to 72 h after the transfection, the cells are lysed and extract containing recombinant parvoviruses subjected to gradient centrifugation or affinity/ion exchange chromatography to purify the virions. Methods such as infectious center assay, genomic slot blot, and real-time PCR are routinely used to determine the titer of the purified recombinant virus.

6. RECOMBINANT APV FOR CANCER GENE THERAPY

Although more than 30 different APV have been identified so far, most of the work has focused on vectors that can infect human cells namely LuIII, minute virus of mice (MVM), and parvovirus H1, which are members of rodent group of parvoviruses. Following the development of recombinant vectors based on AAV packaging by transcomplementing the vector proteins, similar strategies have been successfully tested with the APV including MVM, LuIII, and H1. MVM, one of the first parvoviruses to be described, is closely related to LuIII although there is significant difference that exists in the capsid sequence. Parvovirus H1 is less closely related to MVM and LuIII. The use of MVM as a vector was first reported in 1992 *(45)*. These studies demonstrated transduction of interleukin (IL)-2 and IL-4 from cDNA substituted for capsid sequences in an infectious clone of the viral genome. Subsequent development of MVM and H1 vectors was pursued by many investigators, which reported increase in viral titers, vector purification, and development of stable packaging cell lines *(48–51)*. Most of these methods have adapted strategies to replace the capsid gene with a transgene and not the entire genome of the wild-type virus. Unlike AAV-based recombinant vectors, which are replication incompetent, replacement of only a portion of the vector genome of APV encountered the problem of generating replication-competent virus *(51,52)*.

Despite certain limitations in the production of recombinant APV, recent reports indicated successful production and transduction in vivo leading to therapeutic efficacy against tumors in preclinical animal models. Recombinant H1 encoding either IL-2 or monocyte chemotactic protein (MCP-1) replacing the capsid gene was found to reduce the growth of transduced HeLa cells as xenograft in nude mice *(53)*. Recombinant MVM encoding an antiangiogenic chemokine IP-10 significantly retarded the growth of syngeneic tumors in immunocompetent mouse model of Kaposi's sarcoma *(54)*. The concept of utilizing replicating APV in cancer gene therapy has been recently published using a colon cancer cell line constitutively overexpressing a gene of the wnt signaling pathway *(55)*. In these studies, the expression from P4 promoter of MVM was modified to include binding sites for the heterodimeric β-catenin/Tcf transcription factor. The mutant virus not only rendered susceptibility for lysis of Tcf-overexpressing colon cancer cells as a result of viral replication but also showed a 1000-fold reduction in the viral load of Tcf-negative cells, indicating that such modifications in the regulatory elements of APV genome might be beneficial in cancer therapy *(55)*.

So far, the only human parvovirus that has been associated with pathogenicity is the human parvovirus B19, which is also an autonomously replicating parvovirus. B19 infection has been primarily associated with cells of erythroid lineage in the human hematopoietic system *(56)*. The reasons for the erythroid-specificity of B19 infection are still elusive although studies indicate the roles of primary receptor and coreceptor *(57–59)* and erythroid-specific expression of the B19 promoter *(60)*. Recent studies in the production of B19-based vectors demonstrated that it is not only possible to make a recombinant parvovirus vector by cross-packaging genomic structure of rAAV inside B19 capsids but also that such a virus selectively transduced only cells of the human erythroid lineage *(61)*. Although the titers of recombinant B19 vectors were several logs less than that of rAAV, the possibility of packaging rAAV genome within B19 capsids may lead to further development of such a vector system, which can be used for targeting cancers of human erythroid lineage. However, greater advancements need to be made in the production efficiency and pathogenicity of such a hybrid vector before attempting in clinical settings for cancers of the human erythroid lineage.

7. ADENO-ASSOCIATED VIRUS FOR CANCER GENE THERAPY

Similar to the APV, wild-type AAV has also been identified to possess antioncogenic properties *(62,63)*. Although rAAV vectors are relatively less studied in cancer gene therapy, those reported so far indicate their future potential. In addition, whereas most of the cancer gene therapy strategies target tumor cells directly for increasing therapeutic benefit, targeting normal cells that regulate key events conducive for tumor growth is becoming a promising alternative for cancer therapy. For direct targeting of tumor cells, although long-term expression is not required, this may be beneficial in strategies aimed at targeting normal cells, such as tumor endothelium, that exert a sustained control over tumor growth. In this regard, AAV remains a promising vector for cancer gene therapy. The last few years have also seen increased application of AAV serotypes other than the widely used serotype 2-based vectors *(64–68)*. Variations in the amino acid sequences of capsid protein between different serotype vectors has also correlated on the nature of receptor proteins on cell surface *(69)*, which increases the possibility of using different serotype vectors according to the type of target cell/tissue. A description of the biology and potential of rAAV as applied to direct and indirect cancer gene therapy approaches is described in the following sections.

8. ANTIONCOGENIC PROPERTIES OF AAV

The antitumor effects of AAV had been initially reported within a few years of identification of the virus itself when it was identified that infection of herpes simplex virus (HSV)-transformed hamster tumor cells with AAV delayed the appearance of palpable tumors and increased the survival time of the animals *(70)*. Since then, several reports have confirmed the inhibition of viral oncogenesis by a variety of DNA viruses, including bovine papillomavirus-1 *(71)*, human papillomavirus (HPV)-16 *(72–74)*, and Epstein-Barr virus *(75)*. Evidence from several reports also suggested that AAV infection might protect against human cervical cancer, in part, by interfering with HPV-induced tumorigenesis *(76)* although studies of Stickler et al. reported a lack of correlation of between AAV infection and cervical tumorigenesis in a Jamaican population *(77)*.

Elucidation of the molecular mechanisms directing the antitumor properties of AAV identified a role for Rep78 in the inhibition of oncogenic transformation, specifically the downregulation of human c-*fos* and c-*myc* proto-oncogene promoters by Rep78 *(78)*. Inhibition of HPV-16 P97 promoter activity *(76)* may partially account for the tumor inhibitory property of Rep78 in cervical cancer cells. A recent study reported that whereas Rep78 and Rep68 inhibited the growth of primary, immortalized, and transformed cells, Rep52 and Rep40 did not *(79)*. Further Rep68 induced cell-cycle arrest in G_1 and G_2 with elevated cyclin dependent kinase inhibitor p21 and reduced cyclin E-, A- and B1-associated kinase activities. Rep78 was also found to arrest the cell cycle, preventing S-phase progression by binding to the hypophosphorylated retinoblastoma protein *(79)*. The regulatory differences between Rep78 and Rep68 have now been mapped to the C-terminal zinc finger domain of Rep78. These studies indicate that Rep proteins exert heterologous control at both the molecular and cellular levels in inhibiting tumor growth. Despite the significance of Rep78 and Rep68 in tumor-suppression, potential utilization of Rep as a therapeutic molecule is limited by its toxicity *(80)*. Thus, further advancements in highly tumor cell-specific delivery and/or expression of Rep gene is required before Rep can be used as a therapeutic molecule. Current advances in technology to identify both tissue-specific regulatory elements, and candidate ligands/molecules for receptors that are overexpressed in tumor cells should lead to the development of transductional and transcriptional targeting of rAAV vectors encoding Rep as a therapeutic molecule in future.

9. MOLECULAR CHEMOTHERAPY WITH rAAV

Delivery of a gene-encoded toxin into cancer cells to achieve tumor eradication is usually performed by indirect killing through activation by a prodrug. This approach has focused mainly on delivery of the herpes simplex virus thymidine kinase (HSV-*tk*) gene. Expression of HSV-*tk* results in replicating tumor cells having enhanced sensitivity to nucleoside analogs, such as ganciclovir (GCV) or acyclovir. GCV is phosphorylated initially by TK and subsequently by cellular factors to a triphosphate form that becomes incorporated into cellular DNA *(81)*. This inhibits both DNA synthesis and RNA polymerase activity resulting in cell death *(81)*.

Although a majority of both preclinical and clinical gene therapy studies using molecular chemotherapy approaches have been conducted with recombinant adenoviral vectors, AAV-mediated in vivo studies have also indicated therapeutic benefits for tumor regression. Selective killing of α fetoprotein (AFP)-positive hepatocellular carcinoma cells by AAV-mediated gene transfer of HSV-*tk* gene was reported in a mouse model using an albumin promoter and an AFP enhancer *(82)*. Further work by the same group also reported therapeutic efficacy and a bystander effect of AAV-mediated intratumoral delivery of the HSV-*tk* gene followed with treatment using GCV *(83)*. Interestingly, in additional experiments, the same group also reported an enhancement of tumor cell killing with a rAAV containing the HSV-*tk* gene along with IL-2 gene compared with transduction of vector containing only the HSV-*tk* gene *(84)*. Thus, it is possible to enhance antitumor effects by delivering two different therapeutic genes in the same vector. Although there is a size constraint in the packaging of foreign genes in rAAV, most of the therapeutic genes in the context of cancer therapy are well within the packaging limits of rAAV either alone or in tandem. Similar in vivo therapeutic effects of AAV-mediated delivery of the HSV-*tk* gene have also been reported in an experimental glioma model *(85)*.

Consideration of molecular chemotherapy strategies for selective killing of tumor cells suggests that long-term expression of transgenes is not an imminent requirement; hence, AAV-based vectors are less preferred over adenoviral vectors. Further, the efficacy of adenoviral infection in different tumor cells has been reported to be significantly higher than many other available gene therapy vectors. However, it has recently been reported that the efficiency of rAAV transduction of primary tumor material, derived from malignant melanoma and ovarian carcinoma, is significantly higher (>90%) than that seen in established tumor cells of the same derivation in culture *(86)*. This observation suggests that it is possible to utilize rAAV in direct targeting of tumor cells for an effective killing by approaches such as molecular chemotherapy, cytokine gene transfer, and inactivation of protooncogene expression. In addition, studies by Su et al. using an AAV-TK-IL-2 vector reported disappearance of the rAAV genome following GCV treatment and regression of the transduced hepatocellular carcinoma *(84)*. Although a proportion of rAAV integrates into the host genome, unlike transgene expression, integration of the vector does not occur immediately following transduction. Hence, GCV treatment following vector administration at an early time point should still achieve therapeutic benefit minimizing long-term retention of the transgene. Identification of tumor cell-specific ligands and use of tissue-specific promoters may also allow transduction and transcriptional targeting of rAAV intratumorally. Possible correction of malignant phenotype by rAAV-mediated p53 gene transfer has been reported recently *(87)* suggesting the efficacy of rAAV-mediated phenotypic correction at a molecular level.

10. ADENO-ASSOCIATED VIRUS-MEDIATED LONG-TERM EXPRESSION FOR CANCER THERAPY

It is now well established that tumor growth and metastasis are dependent upon recruitment of a functional blood supply by a process known as tumor angiogenesis and the angiogenic phenotype has been shown to correlate with poor prognosis in many human tumors *(88,89)*. The establishment of an angiogenic requirement for tumor growth led to the identification of several antiangiogenic molecules that potentially inhibit growth of tumor neovasculature *(90)*. Antiangiogenic therapies devised so far target different steps of the angiogenic process, ranging from inhibition of expression of angiogenic molecules, through overexpression of antiangiogenic factors, to direct targeting of tumor endothelial cells using endogenous angiogenic inhibitors or artificially constructed targeting ligands *(91)*.

Although majorities of preclinical and clinical antiangiogenic therapies to date have been conducted with purified antiangiogenic factors *(92)*, gene therapy appears to be more powerful than other forms of antiangiogenic therapy. Potential advantages of antiangiogenic gene therapy are sustained expression of the antiangiogenic factors and highly localized delivery *(91)*. Adenoviruses are again the most commonly used vectors for this strategy and have shown promise in several preclinical studies *(93–97)*. Nonetheless, stable expression of antiangiogenic factors mediated by adenovirus-based vectors is limited by an effective host immune response and also secondary to the episomal nature of the vector.

The advantages of rAAV over other vectors for antiangiogenic gene therapy are multifold. First, AAV is a nonpathogenic vector with a very limited host immune response. Second, sustained expression of AAV transgenes will lead to long-term expression of antiangiogenic factors in vivo. Third, most of the antiangiogenic genes have the capacity to be cloned in AAV either independently or in tandem. Provision of two different antiangiogenic genes from the same vector may yield added therapeutic benefits because different antiangiogenic factors may work through different metabolic pathways. Further, undiminished long-term persistent expression of rAAV-encoded proteins have been reported in a variety of studies *(98,99)*. Reports also indicated that efficacy of rAAV transduction to primary tumor cells is significantly higher when compared with cell lines although this phenomenon may not apply for all tumor types *(100)*. Advances in the development of targeted-AAV for cell-specific delivery may well be employed in future AAV-mediated antiangiogenic gene therapy applications which target tumor cells directly in vivo to enhance locoregional delivery and effective suppression of tumor growth.

A recent study on the potential use of rAAV encoding sFlt1 in ovarian cancer reported that transduction of a human ovarian cancer cell line RMG-1 with AAV-sFlt1 in vitro followed by intraperitoneal administration in nude mice resulted in a decrease in proliferative and metastatic indices suggesting the feasibility of localized AAV-sFlt1 antiangiogenic gene therapy *(101)*. However, a major limitation of intratumoral delivery of rAAV is the inefficient rate of transduction and limited dispersion of the vector in tumor cells. Also, unlike genetic metabolic diseases, which require only partial amounts of the deficient protein/enzyme for phenotypic correction of the disease, tumor therapy requires inhibition of the tumor growth in toto. Antiangiogenic therapy, in particular, requires a constant level of the inhibitory factor(s) for sustained therapeutic effect. Recent studies with rAAV encoding antiangiogenic factors angiostatin and endostatin have also shown in vivo antitumor efficacy *(102–105)*. In our own studies evaluating the efficacy of angiostatin and endostatin in xenograft models by intramuscular delivery of rAAV encoding the antiangiogenic factors as secretory protein, we found that angiostatin gene transfer was superior over endostatin gene therapy *(104)*. Interestingly, when a rAAV encoding both angiostatin and endostatin was used there was a total protection against the growth of implanted tumor growth indicating synergy of combining more than one factor *(106)*. Studies on combining AAV-mediated antiangiogenic gene therapy with other therapies such as radiation therapy *(104)* and chemotherapy may have high translational utility. Recently, it has been demonstrated that AAV-mediated endostatin therapy increases radiation sensitivity of tumor cells indicating the potential of such a combination *(107)*.

11. ADENO-ASSOCIATED VIRUS FOR IMMUNOTHERAPY

The potential of AAV vectors for cancer immunotherapy is evident from recent studies using cytokine gene transfer and in vivo immunization approaches *(108–110)*. Active immunization with tumor cells transduced with rAAV encoding cytokines either by a plasmid based-delivery system or by a recombinant virus-mediated infection has resulted in regression of tumor growth upon further challenge. In a separate study, high-level IFN-γ and elevated major histocompatibility complex (MHC) class I expression was observed following transfer of D122 gene-modified murine lung cancer cells that significantly delayed tumor development *(111)*. Similar findings of antitumor immunity following transfer of cytokine-encoding AAV DNA in a rat prostatic tumor model *(112)* were reported. Enhancements in antitumor T-cell response was observed in vitro by AAV-mediated transduction of B7.1 and B7.2 genes in a human multiple myeloma cell line *(113)*. In a vaccination scheme, Liu et al. have recently shown that intramuscular administration of a rAAV encoding a dominant HPV16-E7 CTL epitope and a heat shock protein, delivered as a fusion protein, elicited a potent antitumor response against challenge with an E-7 expressing syngeneic cell line in immunocompetent mice *(114)*. In vitro analysis also indicated both CD4- and CD8-dependent cytolytic activity in these studies.

AAV-based vectors have been shown to be less immunogenic when compared with other commonly used viral vectors for gene therapy. Although one of the reasons for this is the absence of vector genes in the rAAV constructs, in studies based on intramuscular administration of the vector, it had been reported initially by Jooss et al. in a mouse model that rAAV delivered by this route failed to transduce dendritic cells (DCs), the most potent antigen-presenting cells *(115)*. Reports by Brockstedt et al. however, indicated generation of antibody-mediated and T-cell-mediated immunity against rAAV-encoded ovalbumin delivered intramuscularly and intraperitoneally *(116)*. Further studies by Zhang et al. reported that although mature murine DCs are refractory to AAV transduction, immature DCs are still transducible and that the transduction yields are lower in the absence of adenovirus coinfection *(117)*.

Although these characteristics may limit one's ability to test rAAV in an ex vivo immunotherapy strategy in a murine system by genetic transfer of a potent tumor antigen gene into DCs, it may indeed be possible to evaluate the efficacy of this approach by transducing the cells prior to differentiation. This may in fact provide additional benefits such as stable expression of the AAV-transgene over time. The potential of such a strategy has been recently reported utilizing human DCs in vitro. In these studies, transfer of the IL-4 gene into human peripheral blood monocytes and culturing of these cells with granulocyte macrophage-colony stimulating factor (GM-CSF) resulted in their differentiating into potent DCs *(118)*. We have recently determined that transfer of a rAAV encoding the firefly luciferase in monocytes, following differentiation with IL-4 and GM-CSF, resulted in a robust increase in transgene expression in differentiated DCs *(119)*. Using fluorescent *in situ* hybridization analysis, we were also able to identify the transgene in potent DCs 10 d after transduction *(119)*. Similar to our earlier findings in human bone marrow-derived $CD34^+$ cells *(120)*, we also observed differences in AAV transduction of DCs obtained from different individuals *(119)*. Application of AAV vectors capable of packaging the recombinant genome as a self-complementary double strand *(121,122)* may prove useful in this context to achieve gene expression earlier.

12. RECOMBINANT AAV-MEDIATED CANCER GENE THERAPY AS ADJUVANT THERAPY

Based on several studies over the last decade, it is becoming increasingly clear that gene therapy includes a repertoire of cancer treatment paradigms. At the same time, limitations in both target definition and vector efficacy need to be overcome to utilize this as an exclusive therapeutic modality. However, important to this discussion is the realization that gene therapy can be combined with other traditional treatments as an adjuvant therapy. For many of the solid tumors, surgery, chemotherapy, radiation therapy, and hormonal therapy constitute the major therapeutic measures. Despite advances in early detection and successful initial control, many tumors recur yielding a much more ominous prognosis. In these situations, it may be more appropriate to advance our ability to effectively utilize gene therapy to prevent such recurrences. These adjunct therapies may well be targeted toward secondary cellular events such as antiangiogenesis or toward elicitation of host immunity for a greater control over local tumor recurrence or metastasis. For these strategies, rAAV remains a promising vector because of its low immunogenicity and stable expression. Improvements in the efficacy of chemotherapy following AAV2 infection was also reported indicating the potential of AAV gene therapy for enhancing sensitivity of chemotherapy *(123,124)*. Preclinical studies also indicate the feasibility of regulated expression of rAAV-transgenes in vivo in murine and nonhuman primate models *(125–127)* and it will be a next logical step to utilize this strategy to not only achieve high-level expression of therapeutic genes but also to do so under highly controlled conditions.

13. CONCLUSION

Based on several reports, it is becoming increasingly clear that parvovirus vectors are potential alternatives to other vectors for cancer gene therapy. It is also becoming apparent that for genetic therapy of cancer to be successful, a better understanding of target molecules and cancer types is necessary prior to the application of this technology. The unique diversity of parvoviral vectors with innate antioncogenic properties, autonomous replication, ease of recombinant vector production and stable transgene expression in target cells should provide more versatility to develop effective cancer gene therapy protocols in future. A significant preclinical evaluation of the parvovirus vectors needs should lead to their application in future clinical cancer gene therapy trials.

ACKNOWLEDGMENTS

Financial support from National Institutes of Health grants R01CA90850, and R01CA98817, United States Army Department of Defense grants BC04440, PC020372, PC050949, and Susan G. Komen Breast Cancer Foundation grant BCTR0504027 is gratefully acknowledged.

REFERENCES

1. Toolan HW, Ledinko N. Growth and cytopathogenecity of H-viruses in human and simian cell cultures. Nature 1965;208:812–813.
2. Siegl G, Bates RC, Berns KI, et al. Characteristics and taxonomy of parvoviridae. Intervirol 1987;23: 61–73.
3. Berns KI, Bohenzky RA. Adeno-associated viruses: an update. Adv Virus Res 1987;32:243–307.
4. Comtore SF, Tatersall P. The autonomously replicating parvoviruses of vertebrates. Adv Virus Res 1987;33:91–169.
5. Berns KI, Labow MA. Parvovirus gene regulation. J Gen Virol 1987;68:601–614.

6. Xie Q, Bu W, Bhatias, et al. The atomic structure of adeno-associated virus (AAV-2;vector for human gene therapy. Proc Natl Acad Sci U S A 2002;99:10,405–10,410.
7. Sprecher-Goldberger S, THiry L, Lefebvre N, Dekegel D, De Halleux F. Complement-fixation antibodies to adenovirus associated virus, adenoviruses, cytomegaloviruses and herpes simplex viruses in patients with tumors and in control individuals. Amer J Epidemiol 1971;94:351–358.
8. George-Fries B, Biederlack S, Wolf J, Xur Hausen H. Analysis of proteins, helper dependence and sero-epidemiology of a new human parvovirus. Virology 1984;134:64–71.
9. Rommelaere J, Cornelis JJ. Anti-neoplastic activity of parvoviruses. J.Virol Meth 1991;33:233–251.
10. Laegendre D, Rommelaere J. Terminal regions of the NS-1 protein of the parvovirus minute virus if mice are involved in cytotoxicity and promoter trans inhibition. J Virol 1992;66:5705–5713.
11. Van Pachterbeke C, Tuynder M, Cosyn JP, Lespagnard D, Rommelaere JJ. Parvovirus H-1 inhibits growth of short-term tumor-derived but not normal mammary tissue cultures. Int J Cancer 1993; 55:672–677.
12. Legrand C, Rommelaere J, Caillet-Fauquet PMVM(p) NS-2 protein expression is required with NS-1 for maximal cytotoxicity in human transformed cells. Virol 1993;195:149–155.
13. Raj K, Ogston P, Beard P. Virus-mediated killing of cells that lack p53 activity. Nature 2001;412:914–917.
14. Toolan HW, Ledinko N. inhibition by H-1 virus of the incidence of tumors produced by adenovirus 12 in hamsters. Virol 1968;35:475–478.
15. Bergs VV. Rat virus-mediated suppression of leukemia induction by Moloney virus in rats. Cancer Res 1969;29:1669–1673.
16. Bantel-Schaal U, Zur Housen HH. Adeno-associated viruses inhibit SV40-transformed cells. Virology 1988;164:64–74.
17. Labow MA, Graf LH, Berns KI. Adeno-associated virus gene expression inhibits cellular transformation by heterologous genes. Mol Cell Biol 1987;7:1320–1325.
18. Rhode SL, Richard SM. Characterization of the trans-activation-responsive element of the parvovirus H-1 P38 promoter. J Virol 1987;61:2807–2815.
19. Bradenburger A, Legendre D, Avalosse B, Rommelaere J. NS-1 and NS-2 proteins may act synergistically in the cytopathogenecity of parvovirus MVMp. Virol 1990;174:576–584.
20. Antoni BA, Rabson AB, Miller IL, Trempe PJ, Chejanovski N, Careter BJ. Adeno-associated virus rep protein inhibits human immunodeficiency virus type 1 production in human cells. J Virol 1990;65:396–404.
21. Skiadopoulos MH, Faust EA. Mutational analysis of conserved tyrosines in the NS-1 protein of the parvovirus minute virus of mice. Virology 1993;194:509–517.
22. Vanacker JM, Laudet V, Adelmant G, Stehelin D, Rommelaere J. Interconnection between thyroid hormone signaling pathways and parvovirus cytotoxic functions. J Virol 1993;67:7668–7672.
23. Roth JA, Cristiano RJ. Gene Therapy for cancer: what have we done and where are we going? J. Natl Cancer Inst 1997;89:21–39.
24. Tepper RI, Mule JJ. Experimental and clinical studies of cytokine gene-modified tumor cells. Hum Gene Ther 1994;5:153–164.
25. Pardoll DM. Paracrine cytokine adjuvants in cancer immunotherapy. Ann Rev Immunol 1995;13:399–415.
26. Jaffee EM. Immunotherapy of cancer. Ann NY Acad Sci 1991;886:67–72.
27. Tagawa M. Cytokine therapy for cancer. Curr Pharm Des 2000;6:681–699.
28. Tüting T, Storkus WJ, Lotze MT. Gene-based strategies for the immunotherapy of cancer. J Mol Med 1997;75:478–491.
29. Boczkowski D, Nair SK, Snyder D, Gilboa E. Dendritic cells pulsed with RNA are potent antigen-presenting cells in vitro and in vivo. J Exp Med 1996;184:465–472.
30. Nair SK, Boczkowski D, Morse M, Cumming RI, Lyerly HK, Gilboa E. Induction of primary carcinoembryonic antigen (CEA)-specific cytotoxic T lymphocytes in vitro using human dendritic cells transfected with RNA. Nat Biotechnol 1998;16:364–369.
31. De Veerman M, Heirman C, Van Meirvenne S. et al. Retrovirally transduced bone marrow-derived dendritic cells require CD4+ T cell help to elicit protective and therapeutic antitumor immunity. J Immunol 1999;162:144–151.
32. Brossart P, Goldrath AW, Butz EA, Martin S, Bevan MJ. Virus-mediated delivery of antigenic epitopes into dendritic cells as a means to induce CTL. J Immunol 1997;158:3270–3276.
33. Tillman BW, deGruijl TD, Luykx-de Bakker SZ, et al. Maturation of dendritic cells accompanies high-efficiency gene transfer by a CD40-targeted adenoviral vector. J Immunol 1999;162:6378–6383.

34. Tillman BW, Hayes TL, de Gruijl TD, Douglas JT, Curiel DT. Adenoviral vectors targeted to CD40 enhance the efficacy of dendritic cell-based vaccination against human papillomavirus 16-induced tumor cells in a murine model. Cancer Res 2000;60:5456–5463.
35. van Gool SW, Barcy S, Devos S. CD80 (B7-1) and CD86 (B7-2): potential targets for immunotherapy? Res Immunol 1995;146:183–196.
36. Hwu P, Yannelli J, Kriegler M, et al. Functional and molecular characterization of tumor-infiltrating lymphocytes transduced with tumor necrosis factor-alpha cDNA for the gene therapy of cancers in humans. J Immunol 1993;150:4104–4115.
37. Dranoff G, Mulligan R. Gene transfer as cancer therapy. Adv Immunol 1995;58:417–454.
38. Wwasha PD, Zielske SP, Roth JC, Ballas CB, Bowman JE, Gerson SL. Cancer gene therapy: scientific basis. Ann Rev Med 2002;53:437–452.
39. Reid T, Galanis E, Abbruzzese J, et al. Intra-arterial administration of a replication-selective adenovirus (dl1520) in patients with colorectal carcinoma metastatic to the liver: a phase I trial. Gene Ther 2001;8:1618–1626.
40. Habib N, Salama H, Abd El, et al. Clinical trial of E1B-deleted adenovirus (dl1520) gene therapy for hepatocellular carcinoma. Cancer Gene Ther 2002;9:254–259.
41. Reid T, Warren R, Kirn D. Intravascular adenoviral agents in cancer patients: lessons from clinical trials. Cancer Gene Ther 2002;9:979–986.
42. Kubo H, Gardner TA, Wada Y, et al. Phase I dose escalation clinical trial of adenovirus vector carrying osteocalcin promoter-driven herpes simplex virus thymidine kinase in localized and metastatic hormone-refractory prostate cancer. Human Gene Ther 2003;14:227–241.
43. Savontaus MJ, Sauter BV, Huang TG, Woo SL. Transcriptional targeting of conditionally replicating adenovirus to dividing endothelial cells. Gene Ther 2002;9:972–979.
44. Samulski RJ, Berns KI, Tan M, Muzyczka N. Cloning of adeno-associated virus into pBR322: rescue of intact virus from the recombinant plasmid in human cells. Proc Natl Acad Sci U S A 1982;79:2077–2081.
45. Samulski RJ, Chang LS, Shenk T. Helper-free stocks of recombinant adeno-associated viruses: normal integration does not require viral gene expression. J Virol 1989;63:3822–3838.
46. Maxwell IH, Terrell KL, Maxwell F. Autonomous parvovirus vectors. Methods 2002;28:168–181.
47. Russell SJ, Brandenburger A, Flemming CL, Collins MK, Rommelaere J. Transformation-dependent expression of interleukin genes delivered by a recombinant parvovirus. J Virol 1992;66:2821–2828.
48. Kestler J, Neeb B, Struyf S. et al. cis requirements for the efficient production of recombinant DNA vectors based on autonomous parvoviruses. Human Gene Ther 1999;10:1619–1632.
49. Brandenburger A, Russell S. A novel packaging system for the generation of helper-free oncolytic MVM vector stocks. Gene Ther 1996;3:927–931.
50. El Bakkouri K, Clement N, Velu A, Bradenburger A. Amplification of MVM(p) vectors through serial infection of a new packaging cell line. Tumor Targeting 1999;4:210–217.
51. Clement N, Velu T, Brandenburger A. Construction and production of oncotropic vectors, derived from MVM(p), that share reduced sequence homology with helper plasmids. Cancer Gene Ther 2002;9:762–770.
52. Clement N, Avalosse B, El Bakkouri K, Velu T, Brandenburger A. Cloning and sequencing of defective particles derived from the autonomous parvovirus minute virus of mice for the construction of vectors with minimal cis-acting sequences. J Virol 2001;75:1284–1293.
53. Hagg A, Menten P, Van Damme J, Dinsart C, Rommelaere J, Cornelius JJ. Highly efficient transduction and expression of cytokine genes is human tumor cells by means of autonomous parvovirus vectors: generation of antitumor response in mice. Hum Gene Ther 2000;11:597–609.
54. Geise NA, Raykov Z, Demartino L, et al. Suppression of metastatic hemangiosarcoma by a parvovirus MVMp vector transducing the IP-10 chemokine in immunocompetent mice. Cancer Gene Ther 2002;9:432–442.
55. Malerba M, Daeffler L, Rommelaere J, Iggo RD. Replicating parvoviruses that target colon cancer cells. J Virol 2003;77:6683–6691.
56. Ozawak K, Kurtzman G, Young NS. Replication of the B19 parvovirus in human bone marrow cell cultures. Science 1986;233:883–886.
57. Brown KE, Anderson SM, Young NS. Erythrocyte P antigen: cellular receptor for parvovirus B19. Science 1993;262:114–117.
58. Weigel-Kelly KA, Yoder MC, Srivastave A. Recombinant human parvovirus B19 vectors: Erythrocyte P antigen is necessary but not sufficient for successful transduction of human hematopoietic cells. J Virol 2001;75:4110–4116.

59. Wiegel-Kelly KA, Yoder MC, Srivastava A. α5β1 integrin as a cellular co-receptor for human parvovirus B19: requirement of functional activation of β1 integrin for viral entry. Blood 2003;102:3927–3933.
60. Wang X-S, Yodr MC, Zhou SZ, Srivastava A. Parvovirus B19 promoter at map unit 6 confers autonomous replication competence and erythroid specificity to adeno-associated virus 2 in primary human hematopoietic progenitor cells. Proc Natl Acad Sci U S A 1995;92:12,416–12,420.
61. Ponnashagan S, Weigel KA, Raikwar SP, Mukherjee P, Yoder MC, Srivastava A. Recombinant human B19 vectors: erythroid cell-specific delivery and expression of transduced genes. J Virol 1998;75:5224–5230.
62. Blacklow NR. In: Parvoviruses and Human Disease, CRC Press, Boca Raton, FL, 1988.
63. De la Maza LM, Carter BJ. Inhibition of adenovirus oncogenicity in hamsters by adeno-associated virus DNA. J Natl Cancer Inst 1981;67:1323–1326.
64. Zabner J, Seiler M, Walters R, et al. Adeno-associated virus type 5 (AAV5) but not AAV2 binds to the apical surfaces of airway epithelia and facilitates gene transfer. J Virol 2000;74:3852–3858.
65. Chao H, Liu Y, Rabinowitz J, Li C, Samulski RJ, Walsh CE. Several log increase in therapeutic transgene delivery by distinct adeno-associated viral serotype vectors. Mol Ther 2000;2:619–623.
66. Gao GP, Alvira MR, Wang L, Calcedo R, Johnston J, Wilson JM. Novel adeno-associated viruses from rhesus monkeys as vectors for human gene therapy. Proc Natl Acad Sci U S A 2002; 99:11,854–11,859.
67. Passini MA, Watson DJ, Vite CH, Landsburg DJ, Feigenbaum AL, Wolfe JH. Intraventricular brain injection of adeno-associated virus type 1 (AAV1) in neonatal mice results in complementary patterns of neuronal transduction to AAV2 and total long-term correction of storage lesions in the brains of beta-glucuronidase-deficient mice. J Virol 2003;77:7034–7040.
68. Sarkar R, Tetreault R, Gao G, et al. Total correction of hemophilia A mice with canine FVIII using an AAV8 serotype. Blood 2004;103:1253–1260.
69. Grimm D, Kay MA. From virus evolution to vector revolution: use of naturally occurring serotypes of adeno-associated virus (AAV) as novel vectors for human gene therapy. Current Gene Ther 2003;3:281–304.
70. Cukor G, Blacklow NR, Kibrick S, Swan IC. Effect of adeno-associated virus on cancer expression by herpesvirus-transformed hamster cells. J Natl Cancer Inst 1975;55:957–959.
71. Hermonat PL, Meyers C, Parham GP, Santin, AD. Inhibition/stimulation of bovine papillomavirus by adeno-associated virus is time as well as multiplicity dependent. Virology 1998;247:240–250.
72. Hermonat PL. Adeno-associated virus inhibits human papillomavirus type 16: a viral interaction implicated in cervical cancer. Cancer Res 1994;54:2278–2281.
73. Horer M, Weger S, Butz K, Hoppe-Seyler F, Geisen C, Kleinschmidt JA. Mutational analysis of adeno-associated virus Rep protein-mediated inhibition of heterologous and homologous promoters. J Virol 1995;69:5485–5496.
74. Hermonat PL, Plott RT, Santin AD, Parham GP, Flick JT. Adeno-associated virus Rep78 inhibits oncogenic transformation of primary human keratinocytes by a human papillomavirus type 16-ras chimeric. Gynecol Oncol 1997;66:487–494.
75. Wu FY, Wu CY, Lin CH, Wu CH. Suppression of tumorigenicity in cervical carcinoma HeLa cells by an episomal form of adeno-associated virus. Int J Oncol 1999;15:101–106.
76. Zhan D, Santin AD, Liu Y, Parham GP, Li C, Meyers C, Hermonat PL. Binding of the human papillomavirus type 16 p97 promoter by the adeno-associated virus Rep78 major regulatory protein correlates with inhibition. J Biol Chem 1999;274:31,619–31,624.
77. Strickler HD, Viscidi R, Escoffery C, et al. Adeno-associated virus and development of cervical neoplasia. J Med Virol 1999;59:60–65.
78. Hermonat PL. Down-regulation of the human c-fos and c-myc proto-oncogene promoters by adeno-associated virus Rep78. Cancer Lett 1994;81:129–136.
79. Sauden P, Vlach J, Beard P. Inhibition of S-phase progression by adeno-associated virus Rep78 protein is mediated by hypophosphorylated pRb. EMBO J 2000;19:4351–4361.
80. Schmidt M, Afione S, Kotin RM. Adeno-associated virus type 2 Rep78 induces apoptosis through caspase activation independently of p53. J Virol 2000;74:9441–9450.
81. Furman P, McGujirt P, Keller P, Fyfe J, Elion G. Inhibition by acyclovir of cell growth and DNA synthesis of cells biochemically transformed with herpes virus genetic information. Virology 1980;102:420–430.
82. Su H, Chang JC, Xu SM, Kan YW. Selective killing of AFP-positive hepatocellular carcinoma cells by adeno-associated virus transfer of the herpes simplex virus thymidine kinase gene. Hum Gene Ther 1996;7:463–470.

83. Su H, Lu R, Chang JC, Kan JW. Tissue-specific expression of herpes simplex virus thymidine kinase gene delivered by adeno-associated virus inhibits the growth of human hepatocellular carcinoma in athymic mice. Proc Natl Acad Sci U S A 1997;94:13,891–13,896.
84. Su H, Lu R, Ding R, Kan YW. Adeno-associated viral-mediated gene transfer to hepatoma: thymidine kinase/interleukin 2 is more effective in tumor killing in a non-ganciclovir (GCV)-treated than in GCV-treated animals. Mol Ther 2000;1:509–525.
85. Mizuno M, Yoshida J, Colosi P, Kurtzman G. Adeno-associated virus vector containing thymidine kinase gene causes complete regression of intracerebrally implanted human gliomas in mice, in conjunction with ganciclovir administration. Jpn J Cancer Res 1998;89:76–80.
86. Maass G, Bogedain C, Scheer U, et al. Recombinant adeno-associated virus for the generation of autologous, gene-modified tumor vaccines: evidence for high transduction efficiency into primary epithelial cancer cells. Hum Gene Ther 1998;9:1049–1059.
87. Qazilbash MH, Xiao X, Seth P, Cowan KH, Walsh CE. Cancer gene therapy using a novel adeno-associated virus vector expressing human wild-type p53. Gene Ther 1997;4:675–682.
88. Folkman J, Cole P, Zimmerman S. Tumor behavior in isolated perfused organs: in vitro growth and metastases of biopsy material in rabbit thyroid and canine intestinal segment. Ann Surg 1996;164:491–502.
89. Folkman J. Tumor angiogenesis: therapeutic implications. N Engl J Med 1971;285:1182–1186.
90. Gasparini G. The rationale and future potential of angiogenesis inhibitors in neoplasia. Drugs 1999;58:17–38.
91. Feldman AL, Libutti SK. Progress in antiangiogenic gene therapy of cancer. Cancer 2000;89: 1181–1194.
92. Malonne H, Langer I, Kiss R, Atassi G. Mechanisms of tumor angiogenesis and therapeutic implications: angiogenesis inhibitors. Clin Exp Metastasis 1999;17:1–14.
93. Sauter BV, Martinet O, Zhang WJ, Mandeli J, Woo SL. Adenovirus-mediated gene transfer of endostatin in vivo results in high level of transgene expression and inhibition of tumor growth and metastases. Proc Natl Acad Sci U S A 2000;97:4802–4807.
94. Feldman AL, Restifo NP, Alexander HR, et al. Antiangiogenic gene therapy of cancer utilizing a recombinant adenovirus to elevate systemic endostatin levels in mice. Cancer Res 2000;60:1503–1506.
95. Chen CT, Lin J, Li Q, et al. Antiangiogenic gene therapy for cancer via systemic administration of adenoviral vectors expressing secretable endostatin. Hum Gene Ther 2000;11:1983–1996.
96. Goldman CK, Kendall RL, Cabrera G, et al. Paracrine expression of a native soluble vascular endothelial growth factor receptor inhibits tumor growth, metastasis, and mortality rate. Proc Natl Acad Sci U S A 1998;95:8795–8800.
97. Regulier E, Paul S, Marigliano M, et al. Adenovirus-mediated delivery of antiangiogenic genes as an antitumor approach. Cancer Gene Ther 2001;8:45–54.
98. Schimmenti S, Boesen J, Claassen EA, Valerio D, Einerhand MP. Long-term genetic modification of rhesus monkey hematopoietic cells following transplantation of adenoassociated virus vector-transduced CD34+ cells. Hum Gene Ther 1998;9:2727–2734.
99. Kay MA, Manno CS, Ragni MV, et al. Evidence for gene transfer and expression of factor IX in haemophilia B patients treated with an AAV vector. Nat Genet 2000;24:257–261.
100. Maass G, Bogedain C, Scheer U, et al. Recombinant adeno-associated virus for the generation of autologous, gene-modified tumor vaccines: evidence for a high transduction efficiency into primary epithelial cancer cells. Hum Gene Ther 1998;9:1049–1059.
101. Hasumi Y, Mizukami H, Urabe M, et al. Soluble FLT-1 expression suppresses carcinomatous ascites in nude mice bearing ovarian cancer. Cancer Res 2002;62:2019–2023.
102. Shi W, Teschendorf C, Muzyczka N, Sieman DW. Adeno-associated virus-mediated gene transfer of endostatin inhibits angiogenesis and tumor growth in vivo. Can Gene Ther 2002;9:513–521.
103. Ma HI, Lin SZ, Chiang YH, et al. Intratumoral gene therapy of malignant brain tumor in a rat model with angiostatin delivered by adeno-associated viral (AAV) vector. Gene Ther 2002;9:2–11.
104. Lalani AS, Chang B, Lin J, et al. Anti-tumor efficacy of human angiostatin using liver-mediated adeno-associated virus gene therapy. Mol Ther 2004;9:56–66.
105. Ponnazhagan S, Mahendra G, Kumar S, et al. Adeno-associated virus 2-mediated antiangiogenic cancer gene therapy: long-term efficacy of a vector encoding angiostatin and endostatin over vectors encoding a single factor. Cancer Res 2004;64:1781–1787.
106. Boehm T, Folkman J, Browder T, Reilly MO. Antiangiogenic therapy of experimental cancer does not induce acquired drug resistance. Nature 1997;390:404–407.

107. Shi W, Teschendorf C, Muzyczka N, Siemann DW. Gene therapy delivery of endostatin enhances the treatment efficacy of radiation. Radiother Oncol 2003;66:1–9.
108. Wendtner CM, Nolte A, Mangold E, et al. Gene transfer of the costimulatory molecules B7-1 and B7-2 into human multiple myeloma cells by recombinant adeno-associated virus enhances the cytolytic T cell response. Gene Ther 1997;4:726–735.
109. Anderson R, Macdonald I, Corbett T, Hacking G, Lowdell MW, Prentice HG. Construction and biological characterization of an interleukin-12 fusion protein (Flexi-12): delivery to acute myeloid leukemic blasts using adeno-associated virus. Hum Gene Ther 1997;8:1125–1135.
110. Manning WC, Paliard X, Zhou S, et al. Genetic immunization with adeno-associated virus vectors expressing herpes simplex virus type 2 glycoproteins B and D. J Virol 1997;71:7960–7962.
111. Clary BM, Coveney EC, Blazer DG, et al. Active immunization with tumor cells transduced by a novel AAV plasmid-based gene delivery system. J Immunother 1997;20:26–37.
112. Vieweg J, Boczkowski D, Roberson KM, et al. Efficient gene transfer with adeno-associated virus-based plasmids complexed to cationic liposomes for gene therapy of human prostate cancer. Cancer Res 1995;55:2366–2372.
113. Chiorini JA, Wendtner CM, Urcelay E, Safer B, Hallek M, Kotin RM. High-efficiency transfer of the T cell co-stimulatory molecule B7-2 to lymphoid cells using high-titer recombinant adeno-associated virus vectors. Hum Gene Ther 1995;6:1531–1541.
114. Liu DW, Tsao YP, Kung JT, et al. Recombinant adeno-associated virus expressing human papillomavirus type 16 E7 peptide DNA fused with heat shock protein DNA as a potential vaccine for cervical cancer. J Virol 2000;74:2888–2894.
115. Jooss K, Yang Y, Fisher KJ, Wilson JM. Transduction of dendritic cells by DNA viral vectors directs the immune response to transgene products in muscle fibers. J Virol 1998;5:4212–4223.
116. Brockstedt DG, Podsakoff GM, Fong L, Kurtzman G, Mueller-Ruchholtz W, Engleman EG. Induction of immunity to antigens expressed by recombinant adeno-associated virus depends on the route of administration. Clin Immunol 1999;92:67–75.
117. Zhang Y, Chirmule N, Gao GP, Wilson J. CD40 ligand-dependent activation of cytotoxic T lymphocytes by adeno-associated virus vectors in vivo: role of immature dendritic cells. J Virol 2000;74:8003–8010.
118. Liu Y, Santin AD, Mane M, Chiriva-Internati M, Parham GP, Ravaggi A, Hermonat PL. Transduction and utility of the granulocyte-macrophage colony-stimulating factor gene into monocytes and dendritic cells by adeno-associated virus. J Interferon Cytokine Res 2000;20:21–30.
119. Ponnazhagan S, Mahendra G, Curiel DT, Shaw DR. Adeno-associated virus type 2-mediated transduction of human monocyte-derived dendritic cells: implications for ex vivo immunotherapy. J Virol 2001;75:9493–9501.
120. Ponnazhagan S, Mukherjee P, Wang X-S, et al. Adeno-associated virus 2-mediated transduction of primary human bone marrow derived CD34+ hematopoietic progenitor cells: Donor variation and correlation of expression with cellular differentiation. J Virol 1997;71:8262–8267.
121. McCarty DM, Monahan PE, Samulski RJ. Self-complementary recombinant adeno-associated virus (scAAV) vectors promote efficient transduction independently of DNA synthesis. Gene Ther 2001;8:1248–1254.
122. Wang Z, Ma HI, Li J, Sun L, Zhang J, Xiao X. Rapid and highly efficient transduction by double-stranded adeno-associated virus vectors in vitro and in vivo. Gene Ther 2003;10:2105–2111.
123. Klein-Bauernschmitt P, Von Knebel Doeberitz M, Ehrbar M, Geletneky K, Kleinschmidt J. Improved efficacy of chemotherapy by parvovirus-mediated sensitization of human tumor cells. Applied Tumor Virol 1996;32A:1774–1780.
124. Duverger V, Sartorius U, Klein-Bauernschmitt P, Krammer PH, Schlehofer Jr. Enhancement of cisplatin-induced apoptosis by infection with adeno-associated virus type 2. Cancer 2002;97:706–712.
125. Rendahl KG, Leff SE, Otten GR, et al. Regulation of gene expression in vivo following transduction by two separate rAAV vectors. Nat Biotechnol 1999;16:757–761.
126. Ye X, Rivera VM, Zoltick P, et al. Regulated delivery of therapeutic proteins after in vivo somatic cell gene transfer. Science 1999;283:88–91.
127. Rivera VM, Ye X, Courage NL, et al. Long-term regulated expression of growth hormone in mice after intramuscular gene transfer. Proc Natl Acad Sci U S A 1999;15:8657–8662.

9 Nonviral Vector Systems

Pui-yan Lee, PhD *and Leaf Huang,* PhD

CONTENTS

Summary

Gene therapy requires efficient vectors for delivering therapeutic genes. Advances in developments of nonviral vectors have been established for improving the efficiency of gene delivery. This chapter describes different nonviral methods as well as their applications. Some new directions in developing nonviral vectors are also discussed.

Key Words: Nonviral vectors; gene delivery; liposome; naked DNA; polyplex.

1. INTRODUCTION

The success of gene therapy depends highly on an efficient means of delivering genes into target cells with minimal toxicity. Various viral vectors have proven to be effective in transducing cells. However, immunogenicity is the major safety concern associated with viral vectors. Viral vectors accompanied with their viral components cause inflammation. In therapeutic applications, the vector should be stable and should not elicit any significant immune response.

Nonviral vectors are favorable alternatives because of their ease of preparation and reduced immunogenicity and toxicity. Indeed, naked DNA and other nonviral vectors have been used in one-quarter of the clinical trials. Several major nonviral methods have been developed for delivering genes to eukaryotic cells: (1) naked DNA, (2) DNA/liposome complex (lipoplex), (3) polymer/DNA complex (polyplex), and

From: *Cancer Drug Discovery and Development: Gene Therapy for Cancer*
Edited by: K. K. Hunt, S. A. Vorburger, and S. G. Swisher © Humana Press Inc., Totowa, NJ

Table 1
Nonviral Vectors

Naked DNA
Direct injection
Electroporation
Gene gun
Jet injection
DNA/liposome (lipoplex)
DNA/polymer complex (polyplex)
DNA/peptide complex

(4) DNA/peptide complex (Table 1). Side effects are rare and mostly mild in all of these studies. Expression of the transgene has been demonstrated in the treated patients.

This chapter highlights many successes as well as challenges of these different approaches. Future directions of these approaches will also be discussed.

2. NAKED DNA

The simplest approach to nonviral vectors is direct injection of naked DNA. The promise of direct injection of naked DNA was initiated in Wolff's study *(1)* on the expression of a reporter gene following direct intramuscular injection of DNA. The study revealed that the reporter gene delivered with the naked DNA could lead to a long-term expression of the gene in the muscle. Shortly after, several experiments have were performed to introduce naked DNA into skin by direct injection *(2–4)*. Injection of plasmids encoding the β-galactosidase (*LacZ*) reporter gene into the superficial dermis of porcine skin resulted in a visible expression of the encoded protein. The expression of the reporter gene lasted for 3 d, whereas the expression of the encoded protein was visualized for up to 3 wk *(2)*. Compared with gene expression in the muscle tissue, gene expression in the skin is relatively short-lived. Therefore, genetic immunization was initiated with the intramuscular injection of viral antigens to provoke cellular and humoral immune responses in animal models *(5,6)*. However, it was later demonstrated that direct injection of DNA encoding a viral antigen into the skin elicited a comparable immune response as the intramuscular injection. The immune response lasted up to 68 to 70 wk after vaccination *(7)*. Since then, a tremendous interest has emerged in the genetic immunization using naked DNA. Because immune cells (dendritic cells [DCs], macrophages, lymphocytes), skin cells (fibroblasts and keratinocytes), and tumor cells are all transfectable by naked DNA, this gives rise to the vastly appealing idea of "tumor vaccination" that is to activate immunity against tumors by injecting DNA. Toxicity studies revealed that delivery of plasmid DNA was safe. When different routes of local tissue injection and systemic injection (intramuscular, intradermal, intravenous, and intratumoral injection) were compared, no significant pathological or histological toxicity was observed *(1,8–13)*. In the case of intratumoral injection, a toxicity study showed that it did not cause cytoxicity in major organs and found that DNA predominantly localized to the injected tumor and was occasionally found in heart, kidney, lung and spleen *(14)*.

Without the protection of vectors, however, the efficiency of gene transfer is low under most circumstances.

2.1. Hydrodynamic-Based Intravenous Injection (High-Pressure DNA-Transfer)

It was found that hydrodynamic pressure induces gene delivery in the liver. Hydrodynamic pressure by rapidly injecting a large volume of DNA solutions through the tail vein (so called hydrodynamics-based intravenous injection, or high-pressure method) induced gene expression in the kidney, spleen, and heart but the primary effect was observed in the liver *(15)*. Such pressure resulting from the rapid injection induces transient formation of pores on the hepatocyte membrane to allow effective DNA entry and gene expression *(16)*. Hydrodynamic-based injection of interferon (IFN) plasmid DNA exhibits a significant increase in interferon gene expression, resulting in a visible decrease in liver metastatic growth *(17)*. Although this method is relatively harsh and cannot be directly applied to humans, it nevertheless serves as a useful tool for gene transfer in the mouse liver. Recently, a much milder although less effective method has been developed. A few minutes after intravenous injection of naked DNA, repeated mechanical massages of the mouse abdomen under normal pressure resulted in a significantly elevated gene transfer in the liver *(18)*.

In addition to hydrodynamic pressure, several other physical approaches have been developed to increase gene transfer efficiency. Jet injection of a low volume of DNA solution in pressurized air was employed as the driving force for efficient gene transfer in tumor *(19)*.

2.2. Electroporation

Electroporation that is one of the most common techniques used in laboratory is another approach. Electroporation uses brief electric pulses to induce the formation of transient pores in the membrane of the host cell *(20)*. Such pores appear to act as passageways through which the naked DNA can enter the host cell *(20,21)*. Enhancement of gene transfer using electroporation is generally about 100- to 1000-fold greater than the delivery of naked DNA alone. Optimization of electrical parameters such as voltage, duration, and number of pulses, for in vivo electroporation are important to gene delivery. Voltage that is optimal in one tissue may not be optimal in another. For example, an electric voltage of 200V in tumor was used to enhance 100-fold gene expression whereas 100V was necessary in muscle *(22)*. Besides voltages, duration and number of pulses are also necessary for optimization because intense application of electric pulses causes local inflammation and tissue damage.

2.3. Gene Gun

Gene gun is another physical approach to enhance the gene delivery. Gene gun uses particle bombardment to shoot DNA-coated microscopic pellets through the cell membrane *(21)*. Compared with the performance of electroporation in gene delivery, the application of gene gun has been limited to superficial tissues as a result of the short penetration depth (<0.5mm in murine muscle) into tissue *(23)*. Until recently, a significant improvement in tissue penetration had been achieved using a new design of the gene gun by Dileo et al. The gene gun which delivers DNA-coated gold beads at a high pressure allows the transgene access to subcutaneous tissues, such as muscle or tumor, and consequently achieved longer-term gene expression *(24)*.

2.4. Polymer-Based Delivery

Another concern with the delivery of naked DNA is its short duration of gene expression. Because of the rapid clearance of the naked DNA, the DNA expression is transient. To this end, episomal plasmids have been developed to prolong the stability of the plasmid *(25)*. Recently, biodegradable polymer-based delivery has been developed to increase the gene transfer efficiency of naked DNA. The polymers, such as hyaluronan matrix, polyvinylpyrrolidone (PVP) and poly [α-(4-aminobutyl)-L-glycolic acid] (PAGA) act as release carriers of DNA and provide protection of DNA from damage or enzyme degradation. So far, a prolonged lifespan of DNA using these polymers has been reported in vitro *(26)* and in *vivo (27,28)*. Recently, our lab developed a copolymer, poly(D,L-lactide-co-4-hydroxy-l-proline) (PLHP). Microspheres containing PLHP and plasmid DNA induce long lasting gene expression in the transfected cells *(29)*. Polymer-mediated delivery demonstrated promising results in therapeutic applications against tumors. The laboratory of Kim discovered polymer entrapped cytokine gene increased cytokine gene expression, resulting in an improved inhibition of tumor growth *(30–32)*.

Unfortunately, under most circumstances, it is known that gene transfer with naked DNA is not as efficient as DNA delivered by vectors. However, in certain tissues, such as the wounded skin where DNA can be freely transported, naked DNA can be effective and is preferred over other vectors *(33,34)*. We have shown that naked DNA encoding transforming growth factor (TGF)-β1 mixed in a thermosensitive PEG-PLGA-PEG hydrogel can effectively enhance the healing of skin wound in a diabetic mouse model *(35)*. Overall, to improve naked DNA delivery, a better understanding of the naked DNA uptake mechanism is the crucial step.

3. LIPOSOME/DNA COMPLEX (LIPOPLEX)

Whereas researchers have put efforts on improving the gene transfer using naked DNA, many efforts were also placed on lipid development in gene delivery. Because the initial formulation of liposomes by Bangham's group for the study of the membrane diffusion of electrolyte *(36)*, liposomes have come a long way to become a vehicle for gene delivery. There are three kinds of liposomes: anionic, neutral, and cationic. Liposomes were initially used in drug delivery, which was successfully achieved using anionic and neutral liposomes. However, not much attention was paid to cationic liposome because this type of liposome was best known as a toxic chemical *(37)*. Whereas anionic and neutral liposomes were commonly used in drug delivery, contribution to gene delivery was low resulting from the difficulty of entrapping sufficient amount of DNA into these vesicles. A major breakthrough in lipidic gene delivery was the report by Felgner et al. that the cationic liposome could enhance DNA transfection in vitro *(38)*. Since then, cationic lipids have been commonly used to introduce DNA into the cell.

3.1. Cationic Liposomes

Cationic liposomes can be formed from a variety of cationic lipids. The best known cationic lipids are the DOTMA (Lipofectin, *N*(1-2,3-dioleyloxypropyl)-*N*, *N*, *N*-triethylammonium chloride), DOTAP (*N*-(1-2,3-dioleyloxypropyl)-*N*, *N*,*N*-triethylammoniumethyl sulfate) and DC-chol (3β[-*N*-*N′*-*N′*-dimethylaminoethane) carbamoyl]

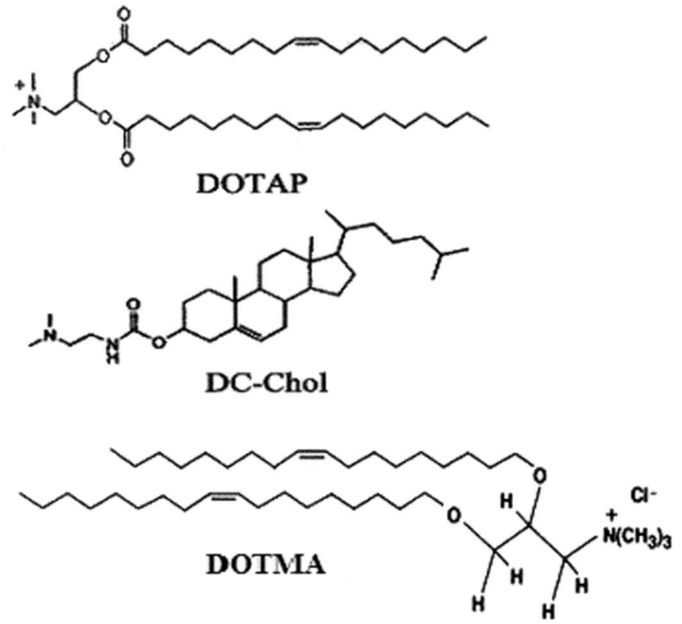

Fig. 1. Structure of cationic lipids.

cholesterol) (*see* Fig. 1). They are all characterized with amine groups which give the lipid positive charge. Unlike neutral or anionic liposomes, which require entrapment of DNA inside the vesicles, cationic lipid forms a complex with DNA. The addition of cationic liposome to DNA decreases its negative charge and reduces the repulsion between cell surfaces and DNA. Thus, cationic lipid is important to facilitate DNA binding to cell membranes for internalization. In addition to the DNA uptake, DNA intracellular trafficking is relatively inefficient without lipids. To design of an efficient lipoplex, it is important to understand and deal with a multitude of cellular barriers.

4. INTRACELLULAR TRAFFICKING OF LIPOPLEX

The intracellular trafficking of lipoplex consists of a series of steps, including the initial binding, endocytotic internalizaiton, trafficking in the endosome/lysosome compartment, escape from the endosome/lysosome compartment, and transport to the nucleus (*see* Fig. 2). Fusion of the lipid and membrane (mainly plasma membrane) was initially believed as the essential step for lipoplex uptake *(39)*. Later on, studies found that lipoplexes are taken up primarily via endocytosis *(40)* (*see* Fig. 2). Zhou and Huang have studied the intracellular trafficking of DNA complexed with cationic liposomes, which are made of lipopolylysine and DOPE (**dioleoylphosphatidylethanolamine**). In the study, it was observed that DOPE formed an inverted hexagonal phase in the cell. Because this form of lipid polymorphism is involved in membrane fusion, it was hypothesized that DOPE in the liposome promoted membrane fusion or destabilization *(40)*. DOPE and other neutral lipids (such as cholesterol), which have been called "helper lipids," are believed to facilitate the release of DNA by disrupting endosomal or lysosomal membrane upon endocytosis. Besides the presence of a helper lipid, a high charge ratio (+/–) is also favorable for the intracellular trafficking of the

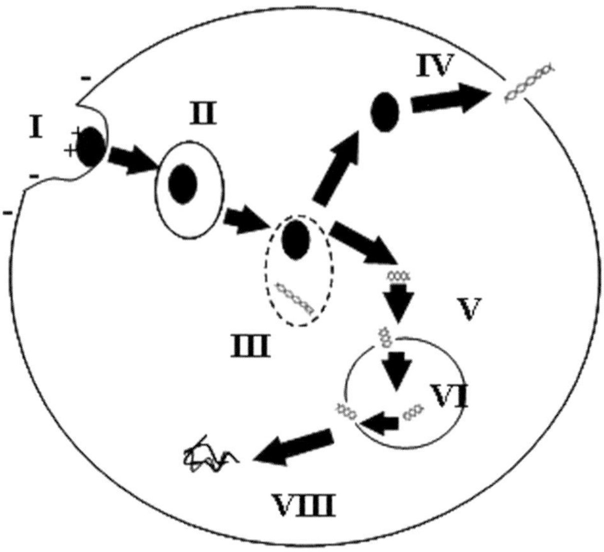

Fig. 2. Internalization pathway and fate of cationic liposome-DNA complexes. (1) Binding of cationic lipoplexes to cell surface by charge interaction. (II) Transport from plasma membrane to endosome. (III) Lysosome becomes endosome by maturation and a release of lipoplex to cytosol. (IV) DNA moves to exterior of the cell. (V) DNA moves toward nucleus. (VI) Transcription of DNA to mRNA. (VII) Transcripted mRNA exported to cytoplasm. (VIII) Translation of mRNA to protein.

lipoplex *(41)*. Sakuri et al. formed a complex with different ratio of plasmid DNA (labeled with fluorescein isothiocyanate [FITC]) to cationic liposomes. At higher charge ratios, a higher intensity of the green fluorescence was observed in the endosomes/lysosomes, indicating more lipoplexes had moved into these compartments. Thus, the efficiency of gene transfer is highly dependent on the charge ratio between the cationic liposome and DNA.

However, the drawback of a high charge ratio is, that it results in an increased serum sensitivity. Serum proteins cause aggregation of the positively charged lipoplex, as well as a decrease of the positive charge of the complex and its interaction with the cell membrane. Thus, serum induced aggregation compromises gene transfection efficency *(42,43)*. Another concern is that cationic liposome formulations interact nonspecifically with the majority of negatively charged glycoproteins on the cell surface. To resolve this issue, a lipoplex formulation has been developed using anionic liposomes *(44)*. However, the lipoplex gene transfection activity observed was lower than with cationic liposomes. It was proposed that the reason for this less effective transfection resulted from the degradation of anionic lipoplex formulations in the lysosomes, whereas cationic liposomes can bypass this endosomal–lysosomal route and escape early degradation in these compartments.

To reduce this lysosomal–endosomal degradation of transgenes, Yang and Huang developed a pH-sensitive anionic liposome formulation. This pH-sensitive liposome was stable in physiological pH, but became destabilized in an acidic environment. Typically, these liposomes were prepared at pH 8.0. Under the acidic environment in the endosomes (~ pH 5.0), the pH-sensitive liposomes were protonated and destabilized, resulting in the release of DNA. A subsequent study hasshown that a pH-sensitive liposome formulation perform DNA release prior to the endosomal–lysosomal degradation, actually, suggesting that the pH-sensitive liposome could also bypasse the endosome-lysosome route *(45)*.

5. POLYMER/DNA COMPLEX (POLYPLEX)

Besides liposomes, cationic polymers have been used to promote the entry of DNA into cells. The complex of the polymer with DNA is termed polyplexes. Polycations include natural DNA binding proteins such as histones, the synthetic amino acid polymers, polylysine, polyethyleneimine (PEI), cationic dendrimers, or carbohydrate-based polymer chitosan. Generally, a cationic polymer performs multiple tasks, including compacting DNA to improve the migration toward and into cells, protecting DNA from degradation and enhancing cell binding or intracellular delivery into the cytoplasm and the nucleus. For example, polylysine was used to protect DNA, condense DNA, and deliver DNA into cells through its positive charge interaction with the cell surface. On the other hand, PEI and cationic dendrimers, which vary the degree of protonation corresponding to the surrounding pH, contribute to the endosomal release of DNA. At low pH (i.e., in endosomes), an increased protonation is assumed to trigger the endosomal release by osmotic imbalance. This effect is called the "proton sponge" effect *(46)*.

Polyplex show high activity in cell culture transfection. However, gene transfection in vivo was not as successful, as exampled by PEI *(47,48)*. Additionally, the high positive charge that is effective in gene transfer is associated with high serum sensitivity as explained in the previous section.

6. LIPOSOME/POLYMER/DNA COMPLEX (LIPOPOLYPLEX)

Similar to polyplex, the incorporation of polymers in the formation of liposome-DNA complex is developed to facilitate gene transfection. Addition of a cationic polymer, such as poly-L-lysine (PLL), is used to condense DNA and reduce the possibility of aggregation and enzyme degradation. The resulting ternary complex containing liposome, polycation and DNA is called LPD *(49,50)*.

Initially, cationic liposome was used to synthesize LPD and the resulting purified complex is called LPD-I. The biodistribution of LPD-I following systemic administration is more controllable compared with the lipoplex formulations. Furthermore, LPD-I are smaller and more stable than the lipoplex. The resulting size is reduced to less than 100 nm whereas the complex formed between DNA and DC-chol/DOPE had an average diameter of 1.2 μm. The reduced size favors endocytosis, which is the major pathway for DNA entry *(51)*.

Furthermore, LPD-I show a higher transfection activity than the corresponding lipoplex in vivo *(52)*. The improved transfection resulted partly from the enhanced condensation of DNA within the polymer. The enhanced transfection is also associated with the quenching ability of the polycationic polymer. Multiple protonable groups on the polymer act as a buffer to quench lysosomal acidification and impede DNA degradation. Additionally, because of the increased osmolarity of the endosomes containing LPD-I their membrane rupture and release of the entrapped DNA into the cytoplasm (i.e., the proton sponge effect) *(46)*.

In addition to these biochemical properties of LPD-I, their lipid structure and composition also affect the transfection efficiency. So far, it is known that cholesterol-anchored cationic lipids are less efficient than the double-chain hydrocarbon anchored lipids for intravenous delivery *(53)*. On the other hand, the choice of the helper lipid greatly affects the transfection efficiency. For example, DOPE as a helper lipid decreases in vivo transfection activity of LPD-I while cholesterol significantly enhances in vivo transfection activity *(52)*. This is probably related to the fact that some amphipathic proteins in the blood inhibit the formation of the inverted hexagonal phase of DOPE *(54,55)*.

Because of the high sensitivity of LPD-I to serum proteins, the transfection efficiency of LPD-I in systemic applications site is low. That is why a new lipidic vector has been developed by Lee and Huang *(56)*, called LPD-II. The structure of LPD-II is similar to that of the LPD-I, but it is composed of anionic liposome instead, which renders LPD-II more compatible with biological fluids. Furthermore, the design of LPD-II particles eliminated potential problems associated with the traditional anionic liposomal DNA vectors, such as low encapsulation efficiency and generation of excessive empty liposomes *(56)*. To increase cell-specific transfection (targeting) Lee et al. used a folate ligand that was covalently attached to the surface of the LPD-II particles *(56)*. Folate was chosen as a targeting ligand because many human tumors, especially ovarian carcinoma, overexpress folate binding protein or folate receptor *(57)*. Another targeting LPD-II was developed by mixing cationic PLL/DNA complex with anionic liposome containing the ligand transferrin. Transferrin-targeted LPD-II was shown to selectively deliver a reporter gene to myogenic cells *(58)*. However, serum sensitivity is still an existing problem with LPD-II.

7. PEPTIDE–DNA COMPLEX

In addition to cationic polymers and lipids, cationic peptides were used to enhance gene transfection. The primary role of the cationic peptide is to condense DNA. For example, Huang and colleagues *(59)* have combined a Food and Drug Administration (FDA)-approved polycationic peptide, protamine sulfate, with cationic liposomes to enhance DNA delivery in vitro. Protamine sulfate as a condensing agent was superior to polylysine as well as to various other types of protamine *(59)*.

Similarly, Schwartz and colleagues *(60)* have synthesized short peptides derived from human histones or protamine and formed peptide-DNA-lipid complexes that enhanced DNA delivery both in vitro and in vivo. More recently, McKenzie et al. developed a peptide containing a cysteine residue, Cyc-Trp-Lys. In addition to DNA condensation, the thiol group in the peptide, which is spontaneously oxidized to form interpeptide disulfide bonds, resulted in a highly stable complex in vitro. In addition to the stabilization of the complex, the increased gene expression observed might also result from the reduction of the disulfide bonds that trigger the intracellular DNA release *(61)*. In 2003, Lee and his colleagues conjugated Listeriolysin O (LLO, a sulfhydryl-activated pore-forming protein from *Listeria monocytogenes*) to polycationic peptide protamine (PN) through a reversible, endosome-labile disulfide bond and formed a LLO-s-s-PN complex. The LLO-s-s-PN incorporating the condensed PN/pDNA complex resulted in approximately three orders of magnitude higher luciferase gene expression compared to PN/pDNA in vitro *(62)*.

8. STRATEGIES USING NONVIRAL VECTORS IN CANCER GENE THERAPY

Various nonviral vector systems have been used to deliver DNA into cancer cells to induce an antitumor effect. Naked DNA encoding genes ranging from cytokine genes to tumor antigen genes have been delivered alone *(63)*, by gene gun *(64,65)*, or by electroporation *(66,67)*, resulting in significantly induced cytokine levels or specific antigen expression. Electroporation has also been used to introduce plasmids that encode antisense RNA against E6 and E7 mRNA to human papilloma virus (HPV) expressing cancer cells, which resulted in a significant inhibition of tumor growth *(68)*. Another approach involved gene gun-mediated delivery of heat-shock protein 70 (Hsp70) linked to the HPV16 E7 tumor antigen gene into antigen presenting cells (APCs). It led to an enhanced E7-specific immune response of lymphocytes after exposure to these transfected APCs *(69)*.

Lipoplex has been shown to greatly enhance the efficiency of gene transfer in the spinal cord *(70)*, lungs *(71)*, and tumors *(72)*, both, by intratumoral injection and intravenous injection. That delivery of cationic liposomes is safe in humans, even with the high charge ratio of cationic liposome to DNA, was shown early in gene therapy trials *(41,73)*. This was in contrast to the previous understanding that the positive charge of cationic liposomes led to potential harmfull aggregations with serum proteins that could impede blood circulation and hemostasis. In clinical studies, complex of DNA and cationic liposomes induces gene expression resulting in reduction of tumor size *(74)*. That repeated administration of lipoplex is feasible and well supported was made evident in a recent clinical study in patients with cystic fibrosis *(75)*. In that study, repeated administration of the cystic fibrosis transmembrane regulator (CFTR) cDNA in DC-Chol/DOPE cationic liposomes resulted in continued expression of CFTR in the airway epithelium.

LPD also plays an increasingly important role in antitumor gene therapy. An interesting method is to deliver a plasmid containing an unmethylated CpG motif flanked by two 5′-purines and two 3′-pyrimidines in the form of LPD. This approach induced proinflammatory cytokine levels leading to a nonspecific immune response and it showed a remarkable decrease of tumor burden in lung cancers *(76)*. In order to enhance a specific immune response against tumor antigens, such as a peptide epitope of the HPV16 E7 protein expressed by cervix cancer cells, entrapping of the epitope peptide in LPDs was tested. With this approach, specific immunity was induced and complete tumor regression was observed in all tumor-bearing mice treated with LPD/E7 nanoparticles *(63)*.

9. LIMITATIONS AND POSSIBLE SOLUTIONS IN DNA TRANSPORT AND UPTAKE IN VIVO

Despite encouraging results in the use of nonviral vectors for cancer therapy, it became evident that solutions to overcome various intracellular and extracellular obstacles were necessary in order to improve the performance of nonviral tumor gene transfer. Intracellular uptake and transport is greatly dependent on the size of the DNA and/or the DNA combined with its vector. Usually, the size of liposomes varies from 80 to 100 μm. The most efficient and useful liposomes for the delivery of therapeutic genes, peptides or drugs are 80 to 200 nm in diameter. Considering the transport of macromolecules in tissue, small size should be more favorable for diffusion in the matrix and uptake by cells. For the application to tumors, however, large lipoplex (400 nm–1.4 μm in diameter) could be more favorable *(77,78)* because large lipoplex tends to be retained in the capillary bed within the tumor. In contrast, small lipoplex (200–400 nm) tends to be taken up by the organs of the reticuloendithelial system (RES) *(79)*. Theoretically, the transport of large lipoplex is feasible in tumor. The vasculature is extensive in most tumors but because of its "immature" endothelium the permeability of these tumor vessels is greater than that in tissues with a mature vascular bed *(80)*. This increased permeability may facilitate the extravasation of lipoplex in the tumor. However, in reality, the high interstitial pressure within the tumor tissue is one of the major barriers for the transport of macromolecules into cancer cells *(79)*. Unlike endothelial cells, tumor cells are not readily accessible and extravasation across the blood vessel is necessary to reach the tumor cells. The high pressure prohibits convective extravasation of molecules into the tumor tissue. This is the reason, why, in vivo, lipoplex molecules greater than 400 nm in diameter may not be able to extravasate and penetrate the tumor tissue *(81)*. Additional hindrance of transtumoral vector transportation results from the viscous extracellular matrix in the tumor. In a solid tumor, tumor cells occupy less than 50% of the total volume whereas from 1 to 10% of the volume is occupied by the vasculature *(80)*. The rest of the tumor consists of a collagen-rich extracellular matrix. Therefore, to transfect cancer cells efficiently in vivo, DNA has to travel through the endothelial barrier and the interstitial matrix to access tumor cells.

One way to increase transendothelial and transinterstitial transfer of DNA to the target cell might be by hydrodynamics-based gene delivery via the local tumor circulation. Because the hydrodynamic pressure should counter the high interstitial pressure of the tumor, this way of application could, if applied locally, be an alternative strategy. However, to date little is known about the transport mechanism of macromolecules through the tumor interstitium, and research focusing on the understanding of macromolecular transport will be vital to overcome these barriers.

10. FUTURE DIRECTIONS

The ultimate goal of nonviral gene therapy is to cure genetic diseases, such as cancer, with minimal toxicity. Over the past decades, it has been encouraging to see significant progress and improvements in the design of nonviral vectors. This chapter attempted to highlight some major achievements of nonviral gene therapy in antitumor strategies. However, several challenges still must be addressed and overcome.

First, the performance of nonviral vectors in gene transfer still remains to be improved. The transfection efficiency achieved by cationic liposomes is still a few orders of magnitude lower than viral vectors. As the transfer of a therapeutic gene is not trivial, different and specific steps in the DNA internalization need to be elucidated. Furthermore, a better understanding of the viral vector internalization mechanism may facilitate improvement in the design of the nonviral vectors.

Another concern is the safety of nonviral vectors. Although nonviral vectors are less immunogenic as compared with viral vectors, they nonetheless induce an inflammatory response in the host. This ris the result of immune stimulation of unmethylated CpG motifs of the plasmid, which could enhance antitumor effects but concurrently it has the potential to induce inflammatory responses in untargeted tissues, leading to unwanted toxicity. After intratumoral injection or other local administrations most of the DNA accumulates in or near the injections site, facilitating local antitumor therapies. However, systemic administration, especially hydrodynamic-based injection via the tail vein can cause extensive biodistribution of the gene to locations including spleen and kidney *(82)*. This increases the possibility of an inflammatory response in untargeted tissue. Researchers tried to overcome this problem with the coapplication of immunosuppressant agents and more efforts have been placed on the modification of plasmid DNA by mutating the CpG motifs *(83–85)*. We, in our laboratory have chosen to explore the potential of sequential injection of cationic liposome followed by DNA in reducing unwanted inflammatory response in non/target tissues. We found that the sequential injection could avoid serious systemic inflammation without sacrificing transfection efficiency in the lung *(86)*. Whether these approaches will be applicable in humans will have to be tested in the near future.

Overall, nonviral gene therapy is potentially favorable for cancer treatments because of its flexiblility in design and reduced immunogenicity and toxicity. A nonviral vector with increasing gene expression and minimal toxicity is anticipated in the future if the previously discussed challenges could be overcome.

ACKNOWLEDGMENT

The original work performed in this lab was supported by NIH grants, AR 45925, AI 48851, DK 068556.

REFERENCES

1. Wolff JA, Malone RW, Williams P, et al. Direct gene transfer into mouse muscle in vivo. Science 1990;247(4949 Pt 1):1465–1468.
2. Hengge UR, Chan EF, Foster RA, Walker PS, Vogel JC. Cytokine gene expression in epidermis with biological effects following injection of naked DNA. Nat Genet 1995;10(2):161–166.
3. Ciernik IF, Krayenbuhl BH, Carbone DP. Puncture-mediated gene transfer to the skin. Hum Gene Ther 1996;7(8):893–899.
4. Eriksson E, Yao F, Svensjo T, et al. In vivo gene transfer to skin and wound by microseeding. J Surg Res 1998;78(2):85–91.
5. Ulmer JB, Donnelly JJ, Parker SE, et al. Heterologous protection against influenza by injection of DNA encoding a viral protein Science 1993;259(5102):1745–1749.
6. Wang B, Boyer J, Srikantan V, et al. DNA inoculation induces neutralizing immune responses against human immunodeficiency virus type 1 in mice and nonhuman primates. DNA Cell Biol 1993;12(9): 799–805.
7. Raz E, Carson DA, Parker SE, et al. Intradermal gene immunization: the possible role of DNA uptake in the induction of cellular immunity to viruses. Proc Natl Acad Sci U S A1994;91(20):9519–9523.
8. Davis HL, Jasmin BJ. Direct gene transfer into mouse diaphragm. FEBS Lett 1993;333(1-2):146–150.
9. Parker SE, Vahlsing HL, Serfilippi LM, et al. Cancer gene therapy using plasmid DNA: safety evaluation in rodents and non-human primates. Hum Gene Ther 1995;6(5):575–590.
10. Hartikka J, Sawdey M, Cornefert-Jensen F, et al. An improved plasmid DNA expression vector for direct injection into skeletal muscle. Hum Gene Ther 1996;7(10):1205–1217.
11. Winegar RA, Monforte JA, Suing KD, O'Loughlin KG, Rudd CJ, Macgregor JT. Determination of tissue distribution of an intramuscular plasmid vaccine using PCR and in situ DNA hybridization. Hum Gene Ther 1996;7(17):2185–2194.
12. Torres CA, Iwasaki A, Barber BH, Robinson HL. Differential dependence on target site tissue for gene gun and intramuscular DNA immunizations. J Immunol 1997;158(10):4529–4532.
13. Ferlinz K, Hurwitz R, Vielhaber G, Suzuki K, Sandhoff K. Occurrence of two molecular forms of human acid sphingomyelinase. Biochem J 1994;301 (Pt 3):855–862.
14. Stewart MJ, Plautz GE, Del Buono L, Yang ZY, Xu L, Gao X, Huang L, Nabel EG, Nabel GJ. Gene transfer in vivo with DNA-liposome complexes: safety and acute toxicity in mice. Hum Gene Ther 1992;3(3):267–275.
15. Liu F, Song Y, Liu D. Hydrodynamics-based transfection in animals by systemic administration of plasmid DNA. Gene Ther 1999;6(7):1258–1266.
16. Zhang G, Gao X, Song YK, Vollmer R, Stolz DB, Gasiorowski JZ, Dean DA, Liu D. Hydroporation as the mechanism of hydrodynamic delivery. Gene Ther 2004;11(8): 675–682.
17. Kobayashi N, Kuramoto T, Chen S, Watanabe Y, Takakura Y. Therapeutic effect of intravenous interferon gene delivery with naked plasmid DNA in murine metastasis models. Mol Ther 2002;6:737–744.
18. Liu F, Huang L. Noninvasive gene delivery to the liver by mechanical massage. Hepatology 2002;35(6):1314–1319.
19. Walther W, Stein U, Fichtner I, Voss C, Schmidt T, Schleef M, Nellessen T, Schlag PM. Intratumoral low-volume jet-injection for efficient nonviral gene transfer. Mol Biotechnol 2002;21(2):105–115.

20. Neumann E, Kakorin S, Toensing K. Fundamentals of electroporative delivery of drugs and genes. Bioelectrochem Bioenerg 1999;48(1):3–16.
21. Nishikawa M, Huang L. Nonviral vectors in the new millennium: delivery barriers in gene transfer. Hum Gene Ther 2001;12(8):861–870.
22. Cichon T, Jamrozy L, Glogowska J, Missol-Kolka E, Szala S. Electrotransfer of gene encoding endostatin into normal and neoplastic mouse tissues: inhibition of primary tumor growth and metastatic spread. Cancer Gene Ther 2002;9(9):771–777.
23. Zelenin AV, Kolesnikov VA, Tarasenko OA, et al. Bacterial beta-galactosidase and human dystrophin genes are expressed in mouse skeletal muscle fibers after ballistic transfection. FEBS Lett 1997; 414(2):319–322.
24. Dileo J, Miller Jr TE, Chesnoy S, Huang L. Gene transfer to subdermal tissues via a new gene gun design. Hum Gene Ther 2003;14:79–87.
25. Cui FD, Kishida T, Ohashi S, et al. Highly efficient gene transfer into murine liver achieved by intravenous administration of naked Epstein-Barr virus (EBV)-based plasmid vectors. Gene Ther 2001; 8(19):1508–1513.
26. Kim A, Checkla DM, Dehazya P, Chen W. Characterization of DNA-hyaluronan matrix for sustained gene transfer. J Control Release 2003;90(1):81–95.
27. Anwer K, Earle KA, Shi M, et al. Synergistic effect of formulated plasmid and needle-free injection for genetic vaccines. Pharm Res 1999;16(6):889–895.
28. Yun YH, Goetz DJ, Yellen P, Chen W. Hyaluronan microspheres for sustained gene delivery and site-specific targeting. Biomaterials 2004;25(1):147–157.
29. Li Z, Huang L. Sustained delivery and expression of plasmid DNA based on biodegradable polyester, poly(d,l-lactide-co-4-hydroxy-l-proline). J Control Release 2004;98(3):437–446.
30. Mahato RI, Lee M, Han S, Maheshwari A, Kim SW. Intratumoral delivery of p2CMVmIL-12 using water-soluble lipopolymers. Mol Ther 2001;4(2):130–138.
31. Maheshwari A, Han S, Mahato RI, Kim SW. Biodegradable polymer-based interleukin-12 gene delivery: role of induced cytokines, tumor infiltrating cells and nitric oxide in anti-tumor activity. Gene Ther 2002;9(16):1075–1084.
32. Maheshwari A, Mahato RI, McGregor J, et al. Soluble biodegradable polymer-based cytokine gene delivery for cancer treatment. Mol Ther 2000;2(2):121–130.
33. Udvardi A, Kufferath I, Grutsch H, Zatloukal K, Volc-Platzer B. Uptake of exogenous DNA via the skin. J Mol Med 1999;77(10):744–750.
34. Meuli M, Liu Y, Liggitt D, et al. Efficient gene expression in skin wound sites following local plasmid injection. J Invest Dermatol 2001;116(1):131–135.
35. Lee PY, Li Z, Huang L. Thermosensitive hydrogel as a Tgf-beta1 gene delivery vehicle enhances diabetic wound healing. Pharm Res 2003;20(12):1995–2000.
36. Cohen BE, Bangham AD. Diffusion of small non-electrolytes across liposome membranes. Nature 1972;236(5343):173–174.
37. Fraley R, Papahadjopoulos D. Liposomes: the development of a new carrier system for introducing nucleic acid into plant and animal cells. Curr Top Microbiol Immunol 1982;96:171–191.
38. Felgner PL, Gadek TR, Holm M, et al. Lipofection: a highly efficient, lipid-mediated DNA-transfection procedure. Proc Natl Acad Sci U S A 1987;84(21):7413–7417.
39. Almofti MR, Harashima H, Shinohara Y, Almofti A, Baba Y, Kiwada H. Cationic liposome-mediated gene delivery: biophysical study and mechanism of internalization. Arch Biochem Biophys 2003; 410(2): 246–253.
40. Zhou X, Huang L. DNA transfection mediated by cationic liposomes containing lipopolylysine: characterization and mechanism of action. Biochim Biophys Acta 1994;1189(2):195–203.
41. Sakurai F, Inoue R, Nishino Y, et al. Effect of DNA/liposome mixing ratio on the physicochemical characteristics, cellular uptake and intracellular trafficking of plasmid DNA/cationic liposome complexes and subsequent gene expression. J Control Release 2000;66(2-3):255–269.
42. Yang JP, Huang L. Overcoming the inhibitory effect of serum on lipofection by increasing the charge ratio of cationic liposome to DNA. Gene Ther 1997;4(9):950–960.
43. Yang JP, Huang L. Time-dependent maturation of cationic liposome-DNA complex for serum resistance. Gene Ther 1998;5(3):380–387.
44. El Ouahabi A, Thiry M, Pector V, Fuks R, Ruysschaert JM, Vandenbranden M. The role of endosome destabilizing activity in the gene transfer process mediated by cationic lipids. FEBS Lett 1997;414(2):187–192.
45. Budker V, Gurevich V, Hagstrom JE, Bortzov F, Wolff JA. pH-sensitive, cationic liposomes: a new synthetic virus-like vector. Nat Biotechnol 1996;14(6):760–764.

46. Boussif O, Lezoualc'h F, Zanta MA, et al. A versatile vector for gene and oligonucleotide transfer into cells in culture and in vivo: polyethylenimine. Proc Natl Acad Sci U S A 1995;92(16):7297–7301.
47. Fischer D, Bieber T, Li Y, Elsasser HP, Kissel TA. novel non-viral vector for DNA delivery based on low molecular weight, branched polyethylenimine: effect of molecular weight on transfection efficiency and cytotoxicity. Pharm Res 1999;16(8):1273–1279.
48. Morimoto K, Nishikawa M, Kawakami S, et al. Molecular weight-dependent gene transfection activity of unmodified and galactosylated polyethyleneimine on hepatoma cells and mouse liver. Mol Ther 2003;7(2):254–261.
49. Gao X, Huang LA. Novel cationic liposome reagent for efficient transfection of mammalian cells. Biochem Biophys Res Commun 1991;179:280–285.
50. Gao X, Huang L. Potentiation of cationic liposome-mediated gene delivery by polycations. Biochemistry 1996;35(3):1027–1036.
51. Matsui H, Johnson LG, Randell SH, Boucher RC. Loss of binding and entry of liposome-DNA complexes decreases transfection efficiency in differentiated airway epithelial cells. J Biol Chem 1997;272(2):1117–1126.
52. Li S, Rizzo MA, Bhattacharya S, Huang L. Characterization of cationic lipid-protamine-DNA (LPD) complexes for intravenous gene delivery. Gene Ther 5(7):930–937.
53. Armeanu S, Pelisek J, Krausz E, et al. Optimization of nonviral gene transfer of vascular smooth muscle cells in vitro and in vivo. Mol Ther 2000;1(4):366–375.
54. Zuhorn IS, Hoekstra D. On the mechanism of cationic amphiphile-mediated transfection. To fuse or not to fuse: is that the question? J Membr Biol 2002;189(3):167–179.
55. Zuhorn IS, Visser WH, Bakowsky U, Engberts JB, Hoekstra D. Interference of serum with lipoplex-cell interaction: modulation of intracellular processing. Biochim Biophys Acta 2002;1560(1-2): 25–36.
56. Lee RJ, Huang L. Folate-targeted, anionic liposome-entrapped polylysine-condensed DNA for tumor cell-specific gene transfer. J Biol Chem 1996;271(14):8481–8487.
57. Weitman SD, Lark RH, Coney LR, et al. Distribution of the folate receptor GP38 in normal and malignant cell lines and tissues. Cancer Res 1992;52:3396–3401.
58. Feero WG, Li S, Rosenblatt JD, et al. Selection and use of ligands for receptor-mediated gene delivery to myogenic cells. Gene Ther 1997;4(7):664–674.
59. Sorgi FL, Bhattacharya S, Huang L. Protamine sulfate enhances lipid-mediated gene transfer. Gene Ther 1997;4:961–968.
60. Schwartz B, Ivanov MA, Pitard B, et al. Synthetic DNA-compacting peptides derived from human sequence enhance cationic lipid-mediated gene transfer in vitro and in vivo. Gene Ther 1999;6(2):282–292.
61. McKenzie DL, Kwok KY, Rice KG. A potent new class of reductively activated peptide gene delivery agents. J Biol Chem 2000;275(14):9970–9977.
62. Saito G, Amidon GL, Lee KD. Enhanced cytosolic delivery of plasmid DNA by a sulfhydryl-activatable listeriolysin O/protamine conjugate utilizing cellular reducing potential. Gene Ther 2003;10(1):72–83.
63. Dileo J, Banerjee R, Whitmore M, Nayak JV, Falo LD Jr, Huang L. Lipid-protamine-DNA-mediated antigen delivery to antigen-presenting cells results in enhanced anti-tumor immune responses. Mol Ther 2003;7(5 Pt 1):640–648.
64. Oshikawa K, Shi F, Rakhmilevich AL, Sondel PM, Mahvi DM, Yang NS. Synergistic inhibition of tumor growth in a murine mammary adenocarcinoma model by combinational gene therapy using IL-12, pro-IL-18, and IL-1beta converting enzyme cDNA. Proc Natl Acad Sci U S A 1999;96(23):13,351–13,356.
65. Tuting T, Gambotto A, DeLeo A, Lotze MT, Robbins PD, Storkus WJ. Induction of tumor antigen-specific immunity using plasmid DNA immunization in mice. Cancer Gene Ther 1999;6(1):73–80.
66. Lucas ML, Heller L, Coppola D, Heller R. IL-12 plasmid delivery by in vivo electroporation for the successful treatment of established subcutaneous B16.F10 melanoma. Mol Ther 2002;5(6):668–675.
67. Yu DS, Lee CF, Hsieh DS, Chang SY. Antitumor effects of recombinant BCG and interleukin-12 DNA vaccines on xenografted murine bladder cancer. Urology 2004;63(3):596–601.
68. Steele C, Sacks PG, Adler-Storthz K, Shillitoe EJ. Effect on cancer cells of plasmids that express antisense RNA of human papillomavirus type 18. Cancer Res 1992;52(17):4706–4711.
69. Chen CH, Ji H, Suh KW, Choti MA, Pardoll DM, Wu TC. Gene gun-mediated DNA vaccination induces antitumor immunity against human papillomavirus type 16 E7-expressing murine tumor metastases in the liver and lungs. Gene Ther 1999;6(12):1972–1981.
70. Yang K, Mu XS, Hayes RL, et al. Neuroreport 1997;8(9-10):2355–2358.
71. Hazinski TA, Ladd PA, DeMatteo CA. Localization and induced expression of fusion genes in the rat lung. Am J Respir Cell Mol Biol 1991;4(3):206–209.

72. Hengge UR, Chan EF, Foster RA, Walker PS, Vogel JC. Cytokine gene expression in epidermis with biological effects following injection of naked DNA. Nat Genet 1995;10(2):161–166.
73. Reynier P, Briane D, Cao A, et al. In vitro and in vivo transfection of melanoma cells B16-F10 mediated by cholesterol-based cationic liposomes. J Drug Target 2002;10(7):557–566.
74. Nabel GJ, Nabel EG, Yang ZY, et al. Direct gene transfer with DNA-liposome complexes in melanoma: expression, biologic activity, and lack of toxicity in humans. Proc Natl Acad Sci U S A 1991;90(23): 11,307–11,311.
75. Nabel EG, Yang Z, Muller D, et al. Safety and toxicity of catheter gene delivery to the pulmonary vasculature in a patient with metastatic melanoma. Hum Gene Ther 1994;5(9):1089–1094.
76. Hyde SC, Southern KW, Gileadi U, et al. Repeat administration of DNA/liposomes to the nasal epithelium of patients with cystic fibrosis. Gene Ther 2000;7(13):1156–1165.
77. Whitmore MM, Li S, Falo L Jr, Huang L. Systemic administration of LPD prepared with CpG oligonucleotides inhibits the growth of established pulmonary metastases by stimulating innate and acquired antitumor immune responses. Cancer Immunol Immunother 2001;50(10):503–514.
78. Kawaura A, Tanida N, Nishikawa M, et al. Inhibitory effect of 1alpha-hydroxyvitamin D3 on N-methyl-N′-nitro-N-nitrosoguanidine-induced gastrointestinal carcinogenesis in Wistar rats. Cancer Lett 1998;122(1-2):227–230.
79. Ross PC, Hui SW. Lipoplex size is a major determinant of in vitro lipofection efficiency. Gene Ther 1999;6(4):651–659.
80. Dass CR. Biochemical and biophysical characteristics of lipoplexes pertinent to solid tumour gene therapy. Int J Pharm 2002;241(1):1-25.
81. Jain RK. Normalizing tumor vasculature with anti-angiogenic therapy: a new paradigm for combination therapy. Nat Med 2001;7(9):987–989.
82. Kong G, Braun RD, Dewhirst MW. Hyperthermia enables tumor-specific nanoparticle delivery: effect of particle size. Cancer Res 2000;60(16):4440–4445.
83. Kunath K, von Harpe A, Fischer D, et al. Low-molecular-weight polyethylenimine as a non-viral vector for DNA delivery: comparison of physicochemical properties, transfection efficiency and in vivo distribution with high-molecular-weight polyethylenimine. J Control Release 2003;89(1):113–125.
84. Redford TW, Yi AK, Ward CT, Krieg AM. Cyclosporin A enhances IL-12 production by CpG motifs in bacterial DNA and synthetic oligodeoxynucleotides. J Immunol 1998;161(8):3930–3935.
85. Tan Y, Li S, Pitt BR, Huang L. The inhibitory role of CpG immunostimulatory motifs in cationic lipid vector-mediated transgene expression in vivo. Hum Gene Ther 1999;10(13):2153–2161.
86. Yew NS, Zhao H, Wu IH, Song A, Tousignant JD, Przybylska M, Cheng SH. Reduced inflammatory response to plasmid DNA vectors by elimination and inhibition of immunostimulatory CpG motifs. Mol Ther 2000;1(3):255–262.
87. Tan Y, Liu F, Li Z, Li S, Huang L. Sequential injection of cationic liposome and plasmid DNA effectively transfects the lung with minimal inflammatory toxicity. Mol Ther 3(5 Pt 1):2001;673–682.

II Gene Therapy Approaches

10 Oncogenes, Tumor Suppressor Genes and Apoptosis-Inducing Genes Utilized in Cancer Gene Therapy

Lidong Zhang, MD, PhD
and Bingliang Fang, MD, PhD

CONTENTS

Summary

Oncogenes, tumor suppressor genes, and apoptosis-inducing genes play critical roles in cell proliferation, differentiation, and death. Their expressions are frequently altered in cancer cells by gene mutation, deletion, rearrangement, inactivation, or overexpression. Some of these alterations are directly related to the development and maintenance of malignant phenotypes; others relate to the response of cancer cells to various anticancer therapies. Both preclinical and clinical studies have indicated that restoring the normal function of these genes may be an effective means of cancer therapy although full realization of any anticancer benefit will depend on effective delivery of these genes to cancer cells.

Key Words: Gene therapy; neoplasia; apoptosis; oncogene; tumor suppressor gene; adenovirus.

1. INTRODUCTION

A fundamental feature of cancer is the loss of normal cell behavior (i.e., cell proliferation, differentiation, and death), resulting in the unlimited and continuous growth of cancer cells. Because this malignant phenotype can be inherited by the offspring of cancer cells, it is widely considered that cancer is a genetic disease of somatic cells and that genes which regulate cell growth, cycling, differentiation, and death are frequently altered or mutated *(1,2)*.

Stepwise development of malignant phenotype is another well-recognized feature of cancer *(2)*. Premalignant lesions have been observed for several types of cancer. For example, in the familial adenomatous polyposis (FAP) syndrome, a large number of precancerous colonic polyps may develop in affected individuals between 7 and 36 yr of age,

From: *Cancer Drug Discovery and Development: Gene Therapy for Cancer*
Edited by: K. K. Hunt, S. A. Vorburger, and S. G. Swisher © Humana Press Inc., Totowa, NJ

and without colectomy, will inevitably lead to colon cancer *(3)*. Another example is myelodysplasia syndromes (MDS), which are clonal stem cell disorders characterized by progressive cytopenia and the presence of multilineage dysplasia in bone marrow. It is estimated that between 20 and 40% of adults with MDS will develop acute leukemia *(4)*.

Because cancer is considered a genetic disease, its stepwise development must involve distinct gene alterations in at each step of cancer development *(1,2)*. Moreover, it has long been realized that in normal situation, cell growth is under control of two distinct groups of signals. Oncogenes normally encode positive signals that promote cell growth and division. Tumor suppressor genes normally encode negative signals that inhibit cell growth and division and induce cell-cycle arrest or initiate apoptotic programs. Apoptosis-related genes encode a variety of gene products that promote either cell survival (antiapoptotic) or cell death (proapoptotic). The resulting progrowth and antigrowth and proapoptotic and antiapoptotic functions collectively determine the cell's fate to grow or not to grow, to die or not to die. Any dysfunction or imbalance of these signals may lead to abnormal cell behavior and malignant transformation *(7,8)*.

2. ONCOGENES

2.1. Viral Oncogenes

The concept of oncogenes initially came from studies of neoplastic transformation by tumor-producing viruses. As early as the 1960s, it was noticed that some DNA or RNA viruses could induce tumor formation either in their natural hosts or in heterologous species *(9,10)*. Among the RNA viruses, only retroviruses can induce neoplastic transformation. Some retroviruses, such as the avian leucosis virus (ALV), can induce tumor formation only after long incubation periods, usually lasting more than several months. Other retroviruses, such as the Rous sarcoma virus (RSV), can induce tumor formation very rapidly in infected chickens, usually within 1 to 2 wk, and are thus named acute transforming viruses. Comparison of the genome of acute transforming virus RSV with that of nonacute transforming virus ALV resulted in the discovery of the first viral oncogene (*src*), consisting of an extra gene sequence on the 3′-end between the *env* gene and 3′-long terminal repeats (LTRs) *(11)*. Gene transfer experiments demonstrated that this additional gene could induce neoplastic transformation in chickens. Since then, more than 20 viral oncogenes have been identified and isolated from acute transforming retroviruses *(12)*.

2.2. Proto-Oncogenes and Cellular Oncogenes

Although viral oncogenes can induce neoplastic transformation in animals, their mechanisms for doing so do not involve viral replication. This suggests that viral oncogenes are not necessary for viral life cycles and that they derive from other species. In fact, some early researchers observed that animals occasionally developed tumors very rapidly when they were infected with nonacute transforming retroviruses such as ALV. These nonacute transforming retroviruses were then isolated from the tumor sites and were subsequently shown not to be novel retroviruses but rather contained additional gene sequences in the genome. This finding strongly indicated that viral oncogenes derived from hosts that the viruses had infected. Direct evidence in support of this hypothesis came from DNA hybridization experiments. Isotope-labeled viral oncogenes, such as *src*, hybridized to DNA samples from a broad range of species including chicken, dog, and human.

Currently, normal cellular genes from which viral oncogenes or cellular oncogenes are derived are defined as proto-oncogenes *(11,12)*. Nevertheless, there are fundamental differences between proto-oncogenes and oncogenes. Proto-oncogenes are functionally normal cellular genes that are regulated by normal molecular mechanisms, whereas oncogenes are functionally abnormal genes that are deregulated by abnormal molecular mechanisms. However, proto-oncogenes may induce neoplastic transformation when gene mutations or abnormal transcriptional activation cause them to function abnormally and behave like viral oncogenes. In these situations, the abnormally functioning proto-oncogenes are called cellular oncogenes. Gene transfer assays can detect the presence of cellular oncogenes *(11,12)*. For example, when transfected with the DNA of chemically transformed cells, cells from an immortalized but nontransformed mouse cell line designated NIH3T3 can develop tumor clones very efficiently. In contrast, NIH 3T3 cells transfected with normal DNA do not develop tumor clones efficiently. This suggests that normal cellular proto-oncogenes might be abnormally activated to function oncogenically by causing the neoplastic transformation of normal cells *(5,13)*.

2.3. Classification of Proto-Oncogenes

By using different approaches such as neoplastic transformation assays, karyotypic analysis, and oncogenic virus studies, more than 100 human genes have been identified as proto-oncogenes *(5)*. These can be classified into three categories according to the cellular levels they act on. The first class includes growth factors and growth factor receptors such as platelet-derived growth factors (PDGF), fibroblast growth factors, epidermal growth factor receptors (EGFR), the stem cell factor (SCF) receptor kinase c-kit, and the angiotensin receptor mas. The second class of proto-oncogenes acts on cellular cytoplasm and includes tyrosine and serine/threonine kinases (e.g., c-src, c-abl, c-fps, c-raf, and c-mos), several guanosine binding proteins (e.g., ras and gsp/gip), and other signaling cytoplasmic proteins (e.g., crk and vav). The third class includes nuclear transcription factors of the NF-κB family (e.g., c-rel), the leucine zipper family (e.g., c-fos and c-jun), and the HLH family (e.g., c-myc) *(5,14)*. Upon phosphorylation, these transcription factors can bind to specific DNA sequences on target genes to induce transcriptional activation.

2.4. Molecular Mechanisms of Oncogenes in Carcinogenesis

2.4.1. Platelet-Derived Growth Factor and Its Receptors

So far, four PDGF polypeptide chains have been identified and designated A, B, C, and D. Formed from these chains are five dimeric PDGF isoforms (PDGF-AA, -AB, -BB, -CC, and -DD), which exert their cellular effects through two tyrosine kinase receptors (i.e., PDGF-α and PDGF-β). Interaction of PDGF ligands with PDGF receptors leads to receptor dimerization, autophosphorylation, and further receptor activation. The activated PDGF receptors then recruit SH2 domain-containing signaling molecules (e.g., c-Src, phospholipase PLC-γ, PI3K, and Grb2/Sos complex) to activate a number of signaling pathways, including c-Src-c-myc, PLC-γ-PKC-Raf1-MEK-ERK, PI3K-PDK1-AKT, and Grb2-Sos1-Ras-Raf1-MEK-ERK. Activation of these pathways ultimately induces various cellular processes including division, cell proliferation, and migration *(15,16)*.

In certain malignancies, PDGF receptor signaling is constitutively activated by the genetic alteration of either PDGF or PDGF receptors. In dermatofibrosarcoma protuberans (DFSP), for example, chromosomal translocation creates a fusion gene composed of collagen 1A1 and the PDGF B chain whose expression results in persistent activation the of PDGF-BB gene *(17)*. In patients with high-grade gliomas or gastrointestinal stromal tumors (GIST), amplification, activating point mutations, and small deletions in the PDGF-α receptor have been reported *(18,19)*. Constitutive activation of the PDGF-β receptor has also been described in chronic myelomonocytic leukemia (CMML) *(20)*.

2.4.2. Epidermal Growth Factor Receptors

The EGFR family contains a series of structurally and functionally related receptors: EGF receptor (EGFR, or ErbR-1/HER1), ErB-2/neμ/HER2, ErbB-3/HER3, and ErbB-4/HER4. All EGF receptors are transmembrane glycoproteins and have tyrosine kinase activity in their intracellular regions. However, the extracellular regions of the different receptors selectively bind to specific EGF-like growth factors. As for the PDGF receptors, the binding of EGF receptors to their ligands leads to dimerization and autophosphorylation of tyrosine residues on the receptors, and finally activation. The activated receptors then activate two important intracellular kinase pathways (Ras-Raf-MEK-ERK and PI3K-PDK1-AKT), which in turn activate related transcription factors in the nucleus, resulting in cell proliferation, differentiation, migration, and adhesion *(21,22)*.

EGF receptors are commonly overexpressed in a number of epithelial malignancies and are often associated with an aggressive phenotype. They are overexpressed in over 50% of non-small-cell lung cancers (NSCLC), head and neck squamous cell carcinoma (HNSCC), and colon cancers, along with overexpression of one or more other EGFR family members *(21,23,24)*.

2.4.3. ras Oncogenes

The ras oncogene family consists of three members: K-ras, H-ras, and N-ras. An estimated 10 to 50% of acute leukemias, 50% of colon carcinomas, and 90% of pancreatic carcinomas have activating mutations in different ras oncogenes. Evidence suggests that *ras* gene products have GTPase activity. When bound to GTP, ras proteins are in their active state. However, when GTP converts to GDP, ras proteins return to an inactive GDP-binding state. A single amino acid substitution at ras codon 12, 13, or 61 affects the GTPase activity, resulting in the accumulation of the ras-GTP binding isoform and the constitutive activation of downstream pathways, such as Ras-Raf-MEK-ERK, PI3K-PDK1-AKT, Tiam1-Rac, and Ral GEF-Ral. Activation of these pathways leads to transformation, invasion, and metastasis *(26,27)*.

2.4.4. c-abl Oncogene

Karyotypic abnormalities, including the translocation, duplication deletion, and loss of chromosomes, have long been recognized. Most chromosomal abnormalities do not correlate with cancer types, suggesting that these abnormalities are likely secondary events and reflecting the inherent genetic instability of cancer cells. In contrast, some types of malignancies consistently undergo certain chromosomal changes. For example, a reciprocal translocation between chromosomes 9 and 22 occurs in the leukemia cells of more than 90% of patients with chronic myelogenous leukemia (CML) *(28)*. As a result of this translocation, the abl proto-oncogene, on the long arm of chromosome 9 is translocated to chromosome 22. The translocation breakpoints on chromosome 9 occur either upstream or downstream of *abl* exon 1A. The translation breakpoints on chromosome 22 occur near the middle of a region encoding the functional *bcr* gene. The translocation thus produces a fusion gene comprising the half of the *bcr* gene and all of the *abl* gene except for its small 5′-end. Like the viral *abl* oncogene, this *bcr/abl* fusion protein has an enhanced tyrosine kinase activity that may cause CML *(29)*. Two strong lines of evidence support this hypothesis. First, the *bcr/abl* fusion protein is capable of inducing the neoplastic transformation of hematopoietic cells in culture. Second, specific tyrosine kinase inhibitors of the *bcr/abl* fusion protein can induce and sustain clinical remission in CML patients *(30)*. The key pathways of *bcr/abl* may involve c-myc, PI3K-PDK1-AKT, and Ras-Raf1-MEK-ERK *(16)*.

3. TUMOR SUPPRESSOR GENES

3.1. The Concept of Tumor Suppressor Genes

Whereas oncogenes promote oncogenesis and regulate cell growth in a dominant positive fashion, tumor suppressor genes regulate cell growth in a dominant negative fashion. Thus, their loss of function correlates with tumor development *(31)*. Cell fusion experiments provided the first insights into this concept of tumor suppressor genes. In such studies, somatic cell hybrids resulting from the fusion of normal cells with tumor cells lost their tumorigenicity, thus strongly suggesting the existence of one or more tumor suppressor genes in the normal cells. Further experiments showed that the tumorigenicity of the tumor cells could be restored when the cell hybrids lost some chromosomes specific to the normal cells *(32)*. For example, loss of chromosome 11 from normal cells led to recovery of the tumorigenic phenotype in a hybrid formed by the fusion of normal human fibroblasts and cervical carcinoma (HeLa) cells. This finding suggested that normal tumor suppressor genes in normal cells can compensate for the inactivation of tumor suppressor genes in tumor cells and thus reverse the tumorigenic phenotype *(33)*.

3.2. Identification of the Retinoblastoma (Rb)*—The First Tumor Suppressor Gene*

Retinoblastoma is a malignant tumor arising in the retina of the eye. Inherited retinoblastoma, as opposed to sporadic form, is characterized by a single autosomal dominant inheritance that results in the early onset of multiple tumors in both retinas. In patients with inherited retinoblastoma, every retinal cell inherits the retinoblastoma susceptibility gene (*Rb*), but only a very few develop retinoblastoma. This suggests that the development of retinoblastoma requires not only the susceptibility gene but also at least one other molecular event *(34)*. This is so-called "two-hit" hypothesis, originally proposed by Alfred Knudson, is in agreement with that retinoblastoma is caused by two mutations. In inherited retinoblastoma, the first mutation occurs in germ-line cells, and the second mutation occurs in somatic cells. In sporadic retinoblastoma, both mutations occur in somatic cells. Further evidence in support of this hypothesis is the fact that the two mutations required for retinoblastoma occur on two alleles of the same tumor suppressor gene, which results in inactivation of the gene. The Rb tumor suppressor gene, which maps to chromosome 13q14, is about 200-kb long and consists of 27 exons. Its protein product is composed of 928 amino acids and has a molecular mass of 110 kDa *(34–36)*.

3.3. Classification of Tumor Suppressor Genes

Tumor suppressor genes can be classified according to their function as gatekeepers, caretakers, or landscapers *(6)*. Gatekeepers are rate-limiting tumor suppressor genes involved in tumor initiation and progression or metastasis. For example, mutations of the adenomatous polyposis coli (*APC*) gatekeeper gene are key molecular events in the development of FAP; mutations of p53 or K-ras alone are not sufficient to lead to tumorigenesis if the APC gene product is functionally normal. Other gatekeeper genes besides *APC* are *PTEN*, *p53*, *p73*, *Fhit*, *Rb*, von Hippel-Lindau, and neurofibromatosis type 1. In contrast, caretakers suppress cell growth by ensuring the fidelity of DNA through the repair of DNA damage or the prevention of genomic instability. The caretaker genes include *ATM* (ataxia telangiectasia mutated), *ATR* (ATM and Rad3-related), *BRCA1*, *BRCA2,* and mismatch-repair genes. The inactivation of caretaker genes leads to genetic instabilities that promote the mutation of all genes, including gatekeepers. Landscaper genes are genes that lead to the abnormal proliferation of normal cells. For example, mutation of a landscaper gene in patients with juvenile polyposis syndromes leads to the abnormal proliferation of stromal cells instead of tumor cells. As a result of this abnormal microenvironment, the epithelial cells associated with the polyps are more likely to undergo neoplastic transformation *(6,37)*.

Genes such as *p53* can function as both gatekeepers and caretakers. As a gatekeeper, *p53* protein downregulates the expression of Bcl-2 and directly activates the expression of *Bax*, Noxa, *p53*-regulated apoptosis-inducing protein 1 (*p53*AIP1), *p53*-upregulated modulator of apoptosis (PUMA), Fas, and death receptor killer/DR5, thus initiating both mitochondria- and membrane-mediated apoptotic pathways. As a caretaker, *p53* transactivates genes that mediate G_1 and G_2 arrest so as to prevent replication of damaged DNA or prevent transmission of damaged DNA to the next generation *(6,37)*.

3.4. Interaction of Oncogenes and Tumor Suppressor Genes in Human Carcinogenesis

Humans are the highest class of organism on earth, likewise, human carcinogenesis is more complicated than carcinogenesis in any other organisms. For example, a single activated oncogene can cause neoplastic transformation in avians and rodents. In humans, however, expression of a single oncogene such as *myc* or *ras* in normal human cells induces only apoptosis or senescence *(31)*. This has led to the widely accepted concept of multistep carcinogenesis involving the activation of multiple cellular oncogenes and the inactivation of tumor suppressor genes. Often, several tumor suppressor genes form pathways with other tumor suppressor genes or with oncogenes that govern cell growth, apoptosis, differentiation, and genome integrity *(31)*.

A good example is the *Rb* pathway. In its nonphosphorylated form, *Rb* inhibits the cell cycle by blocking DNA synthesis (S-phase). It does so by binding to proteins of the E2F family of transcriptional factors and inhibiting their functions as transcriptional activator. On the other hand, phosphorylated Rb catalyzes the release of E2F proteins, which then function as transcriptional activators. It is important to note that most of the genes targeted by E2F proteins play important roles in cellular DNA synthesis and DNA replication *(38)*. *Rb* itself is the main substrate for cdk4, cdk6, and cyclin D complexes, all three of which are drivers of the cell cycle and can phosphorylate Rb. The INK4 family of proteins that includes the tumor suppressor p16, can inhibit the activity of the cdk4 and cdk6 kinases. Like other members of the INK family, p16 can be transcriptionally upregulated in response to senescence and oncogenic stress. Therefore, upregulation of p16 is a major inhibitor of Rb phosphorylation in stressed normal cells. In cancerous cells, the Rb pathway is deregulated by loss of p16 or Rb or by activation of oncogenes such as cdk4 or cyclin D1 *(31,38)*.

Another example is the p53 pathway. DNA damage or oncogene activation can activate p53, which in turn induces cell-growth arrest or apoptosis. The ability of p53 to induce cell-growth arrest is mediated by the cdk inhibitor p21. Interestingly, p21 activity is also involved in the Rb pathway. The pathway of p53-induced apoptosis is mediated mainly by a group of BH3 domain-containing proteins, that includes bax, NOXA, and PUMA *(38,39)*.

4. APOPTOSIS-INDUCING GENES

Apoptosis is an evolutionarily conserved mechanism for eliminating unwanted cells not only during development but also during a variety of physiological and pathologic processes. Unlike necrosis, apoptosis is an active form of cell death that is tightly and precisely regulated by molecular machinery in cells. Although apoptosis can be triggered by diverse stimuli, it is usually initiated through two major cell-intrinsic pathways, the mitochondrial pathway and the membrane pathway. Apoptosis is characterized by characteristic morphological changes that include cell shrinkage, chromatin condensation, membrane blebbing, internucleosomal DNA degradation, and fragmentation of cells into apoptotic bodies. A variety of genes, some of them proapoptotic and some of them antiapoptotic are involved in these two pathways. The relative balance of these competing activities determines whether a cell will live or die *(7,40)*.

4.1. Bcl-2 Family Genes

Bcl-2 family genes are involved in the so-called mitochondrial pathway of apoptosis. When stimulated by apoptotic signals including DNA damage, hypoxia, withdrawal of cell growth factors, some Bcl-2 genes exert a proapoptotic function whereas others exert an antiapoptotic function *(41)*. At least 15 Bcl-2 family members have been identified *(8)*. The proapoptotic genes Bax, Bak, and Bok genes contain BH1, BH2, and BH3 domains. The proapoptotic genes Bik, Blk, Bim, Bad, Bid, Hrk, BNIP3, EGL-1, Rad-9, and PUMA contain only the BH3 domain. The antiapoptotic genes Bcl-2 and Bcl-X_L inhibit apoptosis.

The proapoptotic protein Bax responds to apoptotic signals by accumulating in mitochondria, which results in the release of two key apoptogenic factors-cytochrome *c* and SMAC/DIABLO from mitochrondria into the cytosol *(7,41–43)*. There, cytochrome *c* binds to APAF1 and then recruits and activates caspase-9, which can then activate executioner proteases caspase-3 and caspase-7 *(44)*. Once released into the cytosol, SMAC/DIABLO can bind inhibitors of apoptosis (IAPs), thus blocking their inhibitory effects on executioner caspases *(42,43)*. Most of the proapoptotic genes in the Bcl-2 family induce a very strong cell-killing effect when overexpressed *(8,45,46)*. In the mitochondrial death pathway, the ratio of proapoptotic and antiapoptotic Bcl-2 family proteins ultimately determines whether a cell lives or dies *(8,47,48)*.

4.2. Tumor Necrosis Factor Family

The tumor necrosis factor (TNF) family contains at least three proteins-TNF-α, FasL, and TNF-related apoptosis-inducing ligand (TRAIL)-that are known to promote cell death by activating a death receptor pathway *(49)*. The interaction of these ligands with their death receptors is the initial step in the pathway. In brief, ligand binding leads to trimerization and activation of the death receptors, which in turn recruit and activate two adaptor proteins known as Fas-associated death domain protein (FADD) and TNF receptor-associated death domain protein (TRADD). FADD and TRADD in turn activate the caspases that ultimately trigger apoptosis *(50,51)*.

4.3. Caspases

Caspases are a family of cysteine proteases that play critical roles in apoptosis signaling pathways. For example, activation of executive caspases caspase-3 and -7 functions in both the mitochondrial and death-receptor apoptosis pathways, whereas caspase-8 activation is usually an essential step in the death-receptor apoptosis pathway *(41,42,52,53)*. Caspases normally exist in their inactive precursor forms as zymogens, which become activated during apoptosis through proteolysis at internal aspartic acid residues *(54)*. Mutation or malfunction of some caspases may render cancer cells resistant to conventional anticancer therapy *(55,56)*.

5. ONCOGENES, TUMOR SUPPRESSOR GENES, AND APOPTOSIS-INDUCING GENES IN CANCER GENE THERAPY

Recent advances in molecular biology and biotechnology have led to the development of nucleic acid–based medicines that directly target the genetic alterations or molecular mechanisms required for tumorigenesis or for maintenance of the malignant phenotype. The rationale is that local intratumoral expression of the desired therapeutic proteins may exert a constant therapeutic effect at the cancer site without causing substantial systemic toxicity. A growing body of evidence indicates that enforced overexpression or downregulation of various genetically encoded functions can directly or indirectly exert a therapeutic benefit by augmenting the response to conventional therapeutics *(37)*.

5.1. Overexpression of Tumor Suppressor Genes and Apoptosis-Inducing Genes

The fact that overexpression of tumor suppressor genes and apoptosis-inducing genes can induce cell-cycle arrest or apoptosis has led to numerous experimental and clinical investigations into their use as anticancer therapeutics *(37,40)*. Transfer of various tumor suppressor genes directly into cancer cells has been demonstrated to suppress tumor growth by inducing apoptosis and cell-cycle arrest while also exerting lethal bystander effects. Adenovirus-mediated p53 gene therapy has produced promising results in lung cancer and head and neck cancer, among cancers. Combination of tumor suppressor gene therapy with conventional anticancer therapy has been shown to yield synergistic therapeutic benefits. In clinical trials, tumor suppressor genes, especially the *p53* gene, have been well tolerated and produced favorable clinical responses, including pathologically complete responses, in subsets of patients with advanced disease or cancers resistant to conventional therapy *(37)*.

In preclinical studies, the intratumoral injection and ectopic overexpression of adenoviral proapoptotic genes (e.g., Bax, Bak, Bik, Bid, TNF, FasL, TRAIL) and constitutively active genes (e.g., caspase-3 and caspase-6) induced apoptosis and suppressed tumor growth *(57–65)*. Adenovirus-mediated Bax or Bak gene therapy has been especially effective both in vitro and in vivo *(57,58)*. On the other hand, soluble TRAIL protein can induce apoptosis in a wide range of cancer cell lines including leukemia and solid tumors. Injection of soluble TRAIL into subcutaneous tumors of nude mice results in tumor growth suppression without systemic toxicity *(40)*. Nevertheless, the therapeutic benefit of recombinant TRAIL protein is frequently attenuated by weak antitumor activity and resistance. Interestingly, however, cancer cells resistant to TRAIL protein can be effectively killed by the TRAIL gene *(66–68)*, as has been found in certain breast cancer cell line *(66)*, prostate cancers *(67)*, and hepatomas *(68)*. Because most of the proapoptotic genes mentioned above induce apoptosis regardless of a cell's p53 status, they are effective in both p53-sensitive and p53-resistant cancer cells *(69)*.

5.2. Downregulation of Oncogenes and Antiapoptotic Genes

Because cell growth and cell death are determined by a balance between oncogene and tumor suppressor gene and antiapoptotic and proapoptotic gene function, it is conceivable that downregulation of oncogene or antiapoptotic gene function, or both, can also change the balance of signals for growth or death in cancer cells, resulting in suppression of growth or apoptosis. Downregulating the function of oncogenes or antiapoptotic genes can be achieved in a variety of ways, including the use of ribozymes *(70)*, dominant-negative mutants *(71)*, intracellular single-chain antibodies *(72)*, antisense oligonucleotides *(73)*, and small interfering RNA (siRNA) *(74)*. siRNA is comprised of small, double-stranded RNAs that can induce the intracellular degradation of specific mRNAs. For instance, efficient apoptosis has been observed in HeLa cells, transiently transfected with a siRNA expression vector specific for Bcl-2 and subsequently treated with doxorubicin *(75)*. We also found that transfection of siRNA specific for Bcl-xL can by itself lead to cell death in some colon cancer cell lines.

Recently, more attention has been paid to the therapeutic potential of small molecules that can interact with and inhibit, or downregulate oncogene and antiapoptotic gene products. This has been shown to occur in patients with CML who achieved clinical remission after treatment with Imatinab (Glivec). Because activation of the single *bcr/abl* oncogene as a result pf translocation is sufficient to initiate tumorigenesis, Imatinab treatment is a good model of targeted therapy *(76)*.

5.3. Targeted Gene Therapy

Although overexpression of some tumor suppressor genes such as p53 does not necessarily cause damage to normal cells, overexpression of apoptotic genes or down regulation of antiapoptotic genes may do so. For example, systemic administration of the Bax-expressing adenovector causes massive cell death in the mouse liver *(57,77)*. Similarly, overexpression of the full-length TRAIL protein in normal human primary hepatocytes leads to widespread apoptosis *(63)*. Thus, any successful clinical application of these agents will have to include efforts to limit their cytotoxic/oncolytic effects to cancer cells. Strategies for achieving this have so far fallen into two categories: specific transduction of cancer cells with targeted vectors (targeted transduction) and control of transgene expression with tumor-specific promoters (nonspecific transduction). These two strategies are discussed in more detail in Chapter 1.

ACKNOWLEDGMENTS

We thank Jude Richard for editorial review and Alma Vega for assistance in preparing this chapter. This work was supported in part by grants from the National Cancer Institute and the National Institutes of Health (RO1 CA 092487-01A1and RO1 CA 098582-01A1).

REFERENCES

1. Knudson AG. Two genetic hits (more or less) to cancer. Nature Reviews Cancer, 2001;1:157–162.
2. Yokota J. Tumor progression and metastasis. Carcinogenesis, 2000;21:497–503.
3. Fearnhead NS, Wilding JL, Bodmer WF. Genetics of colorectal cancer: hereditary aspects and overview of colorectal tumorigenesis. Br Med Bull 2002;64:27–43.
4. Parker JE, Mufti GJ. The Myelodysplastic syndromes: A matter of life or death. Acta Haematol 2003;111:78–99.
5. Urbain JL. Oncogenes, cancer and imaging. J Nucl Med 1999;40:498–504.
6. Macleod K. Tumor suppressor genes. Curr Opin Genet Dev 2000;10:81–93.
7. Daniel PT, Wieder T, Sturm I, Schulze-Osthoff K. The kiss of death: promises and failures of death receptors and ligands in cancer therapy. Leukemia 2001;15:1022–1032.
8. Adams JM, Cory S. The Bcl-2 protein family: Arbiters of cell survival. Science 1998;281:1322–1326.
9. Colledge WH, Richardson WD, Edge MD, Smith AE. Extensive Mutagenesis of the Nuclear Location Signal of Simian Virus-40 Large-T Antigen. Mol Cell Biol 1986;6:4136–4139.
10. Varmus HE. Form and Function of Retroviral Proviruses. Science 1982;216:812–820.
11. Stehelin D, Varmus HE, Bishop JM, Vogt PK. Dna Related to Transforming Gene(S) of Avian-Sarcoma Viruses Is Present in Normal Avian Dna. Nature 1976;260:170–173.
12. Rhim JS. Viruses, Oncogenes, and Cancer. Cencer Detect Prev 1988;11:139–149.
13. Perucho M, Goldfarb M, Shimizu K, Lama C, Fogh J, Wigler M. Human-Tumor-Derived Cell-Lines Contain Common and Different Transforming Genes. Cell 1981;27:467–476.
14. Bell JC. Oncogenes. Cancer Lett 1988;40:1–5.
15. Pietras K, Sjoblom T, Rubin K, Heldin CH, Ostman A. PDGF receptors as cancer drug targets. Cancer Cell 2003;3:439–443.
16. Mechtersheimer G, Egerer G, Hensel M, et al. Gastrointestinal stromal tumours and their response to treatment with the tyrosine kinase inhibitor imatinib. Virchows Archiv 2004;444:108–118.
17. Shimizu A, O'Brien KP, Sjoblom T, et al. The dermatofibrosarcoma protuberans-associated collagen type I alpha 1/platelet-derived growth factor (PDGF) B-chain fusion gene generates a transforming protein that is processed to functional PDGF-BB. Cancer Res 1999;59:3719–3723.
18. Fleming TP, Saxena A, Clark WC, et al. Amplification and Or Overexpression of Platelet-Derived Growth-Factor Receptors and Epidermal Growth-Factor Receptor in Human Glial Tumors. Cancer Res 1992;52:4550–4553.
19. Heinrich MC, Corless CL, Duensing A, et al. PDGFRA activating mutations in gastrointestinal stromal tumors. Science 2003;299:708–710.
20. Golub TR, Barker GF, Lovett M, Gilliland DG. Fusion of Pdgf Receptor-Beta to A Novel Ets-Like Gene, Tel, in Chronic Myelomonocytic Leukemia with T(512) Chromosomal Translocation. Cell 1994;77:307–316.
21. Ciardiello F, De Vita F, Orditura M, Tortora G. The role of EGFR inhibitors in nonsmall cell lung cancer. Curr Opin Oncol, 2004;16:130–135.
22. Yano S, Kondo K, Yamaguchi M, et al. Distribution and function of EGFR in human tissue and the effect of EGFR tyrosine kinase inhibition. Anticancer Res 2003;23:3639–3650.
23. Hirsch FR, Varella-Garcia M, Bunn PA, et al. Epidermal growth factor receptor in non-small-cell lung carcinomas: Correlation between gene copy number and protein expression and impact on prognosis. J Clin Oncol 2003;21:3798–3807.
24. Vlahovic G, Crawford J. Activation of tyrosine kinases in cancer. Oncologist 2003;8:531–538.
25. Bos JL. Genetic Mechanisms in Tumor Initiation and Progression .10. the Ras Gene Family and Human Carcinogenesis. Mutation Res 1988;195:255–271.
26. Campbell PM, Der CJ. Oncogenic Ras and its role in tumor cell invasion and metastasis. Sem Cancer Biol 2004;14:105–114.
27. Osada H, Takahashi T. Genetic alterations of multiple tumor suppressors and oncogenes in the carcinogenesis and progression of lung cancer. Oncogene 2002;21:7421–7434.
28. Sandberg AA. Chromosomes and Causation of Human Cancer and Leukemia - 40 the Ph1 and Other Translocations in Cml. Cancer 1980;46:2221–2226.
29. Deklein A, Vankessel AG, Grosveld G, et al. A Cellular Oncogene Is Translocated to the Philadelphia-Chromosome in Chronic Myelocytic-Leukemia. Nature 1982;300:764–767.
30. Apperley JF, Gardembas M, Melo JV, et al. Response to imatinib mesylate in patients with chronic myeloproliferative diseases with rearrangements of the platelet-derived growth factor receptor beta. New Engl J Med 2002;347:481–487.

31. Munger K. Disruption of oncogene/tumor suppressor networks during human carcinogenesis. Cancer Invest 2002;20:71–81.
32. Stanbridge EJ. Genetic-Analysis of Human Malignancy Using Somatic-Cell Hybrids and Monochromosome Transfer. Cancer Surv 1988;7:317–324.
33. Misra BC, Srivatsan ES. Localization of Hela-Cell Tumor-Suppressor Gene to the Long Arm of Chromosome-Ii. Am J Hum Genet 1989;45:565–577.
34. Goodrich DW, Lee WH. The Molecular-Genetics of Retinoblastoma. Cancer Surv 1990;9:529–554.
35. Lee WH, Bookstein R, Hong F, et al. Human Retinoblastoma Susceptibility Gene - Cloning, Identification, and Sequence. Science 1987;235:1394–1399.
36. Bookstein R, Lee EYHP, To H, et al. Human Retinoblastoma Susceptibility Gene - Genomic Organization and Analysis of Heterozygous Intragenic Deletion Mutants. Proc Natl Acad Sci U S A 1988;85:2210–2214.
37. Fang B, Roth JA. Tumor-suppressing gene therapy. Cancer Biol Ther 2003;2:S115–S121.
38. Bringold F, Serrano M. Tumor suppressors and oncogenes in cellular senescence. Exper Gerontol 2000;35:317–329.
39. Lowe SW. Activation of p53 by oncogenes. Endocrine-Related Cancer 1999;6:45–48.
40. Bhojani MS, Rossu BD, Rehemtulla A. TRAIL and anti-tumor responses. Cancer Biol Ther 2003;2:S71–S78.
41. Green DR, Reed JC. Mitochondria and apoptosis. Science 1998;281:1309–1312.
42. Verhagen AM, Ekert PG, Pakusch M, et al. Identification of DIABLO, a mammalian protein that promotes apoptosis by binding to and antagonizing IAP proteins. Cell 2000;102:43–53.
43. Du CY, Fang M, Li YC, Li L, Wang XD. Smac, a mitochondrial protein that promotes cytochrome c-dependent caspase activation by eliminating IAP inhibition. Cell 2000;102:33–42.
44. Zou H, Li YC, Liu HS, Wang XD. An APAF-1 center dot cytochrome c multimeric complex is a functional apoptosome that activates procaspase-9. J Biol Chem1999;274:11,549–11,556.
45. Komatsu K, Miyashita T, Hang HY, et al. Human homologue of S-pombe Rad9 interacts with BCL-2/BCL-x(L) and promotes apoptosis. Nat Cell Biol 2000;2:1–6.
46. Nakano K, Vousden K. H. PUMA, a novel proapoptotic gene, is induced by p53. Mol Cell 7: 683–694.
47. Liu XS, Kim CN, Yang J, Jemmerson R, Wang XD. Induction of apoptotic program in cell-free extracts: Requirement for dATP and cytochrome c. Cell 1996;86:147–157.
48. Kluck RM, BossyWetzel E, Green DR, Newmeyer DD. The release of cytochrome c from mitochondria: A primary site for Bcl-2 regulation of apoptosis. Science 1997;275:1132–1136.
49. Bodmer JL, Schneider P, Tschopp J. The molecular architecture of the TNF superfamily. Trend Biochem Sci 2002;27:19–26.
50. Locksley RM, Killeen N, Lenardo MJ. The TNF and TNF receptor superfamilies: Integrating mammalian biology. Cell 2001;104:487–501.
51. Chen GQ, Goeddel DV. TNF-R1 signaling: A beautiful pathway. Science 2002;296:1634–1635.
52. Seol DW, Li JR, Seol MH, et al. Signaling events triggered by tumor necrosis factor-related apoptosis-inducing ligand (TRAIL): Caspase-8 is required for TRAIL-induced apoptosis. Cancer Res 2001;61:1138–1143.
53. Sprick MR, Rieser E, Stahl H, Grosse-Wilde A, Weigand MA, Walczak H. Caspase-10 is recruited to and activated at the native TRAIL and CD95 death-inducing signalling complexes in a FADD-dependent manner but can not functionally substitute caspase-8. EmMBO J 2002;21:4520–4530.
54. Reed JC. Apoptosis-based therapies for neoplastic diseases. International J Hematol 2002;76:261.
55. Bian X, Giordano TD, Lin HJ, Solomon G, Castle VP, Opipari AW. Chemotherapy-induced apoptosis of S-type neuroblastoma cells requires caspase-9 and is augmented by CD95/Fas stimulation. J Biol Chem 2004;279:4663–4669.
56. Yang XH, Sladek TL, Liu XS, Butler BR, Froelich CJ, Thor AD. Reconstitution of caspase 3 sensitizes MCF-7 breast cancer cells to doxorubicin- and etoposide-induced apoptosis. Cancer Res 2001;61:348–354.
57. Gu J, Kagawa S, Takakura M, et al. Tumor-specific transgene expression from the human telomerase reverse transcriptase promoter enables targeting of the therapeutic effects of the Bax gene to cancers. Cancer Res 2000;60:5359–5364.
58. Pataer A, Smythe WR, Yu R, et al. Adenovirus-mediated Bak gene transfer induces apoptosis in mesothelioma cell lines. J Thor Cardiovasc Surg 2001;121:61–67.
59. Naumann U, Schmidt F, Wick W, et al. Adenoviral natural born killer gene therapy for malignant glioma. Hum Gene Ther 2003;14:1235–1246.

60. Fukazawa T, Walter B, Owen-Schaub LB. Adenoviral bid overexpression induces caspase-dependent cleavage of truncated bid and p53-independent apoptosis in human non-small cell lung cancers. J Biol Chem 2003;278:25,428–25,434.
61. Ehtesham M. Samoto K, Kabos P, et al. Treatment of intracranial glioma with *in situ* interferon-gamma and tumor necrosis factor-alpha gene transfer. Cancer Gene Ther 2002;9:925–934.
62. Shinoura N, Yamamoto N, Asai A, Kirino T, Hamada H. Adenovirus-mediated transfer of Fas ligand gene augments radiation-induced apoptosis in U-373MG glioma cells. Jap J Cancer Res 2000; 91:1044–1050.
63. Lin TY, Gu J, Zhang LD, et al. Targeted expression of green fluorescent protein/tumor necrosis factor-related apoptosis-inducing ligand fusion protein from human telomerase reverse transcriptase promoter elicits antitumor activity without toxic effects on primary human hepatocytes. Cancer Res 2002;62:3620–3625.
64. Yamabe K, Shimizu S, Ito T, et al. Cancer gene therapy using a pro-apoptotic gene, caspase-3. Gene Ther 1999;6:1952–1959.
65. Marcelli M, Cunningham GR, Walkup M, et al. Signaling pathway activated during apoptosis of the prostate cancer cell line LNCaP: Overexpression of caspase-7 as a new gene therapy strategy for prostate cancer. Cancer Res 1999;59:382–390.
66. Lin TY, Huang XF, Gu J, et al. Long-term tumor-free survival from treatment with the GFP-TRAIL fusion gene expressed from the hTERT promoter in breast cancer cells. Oncogene 2002;21: 8020–8028.
67. Voelkel-Johnson C, King DL, Norris JS. Resistance of prostate cancer cells to soluble TNF-related apoptosis-inducing ligand (TRAIL/Apo2L) can be overcome by doxorubicin or adenoviral delivery of full-length TRAIL. Cancer Gene Ther 2002;9:164–172.
68. Armeanu S, Lauer UM, Smirnow I, et al. Adenoviral gene transfer of tumor necrosis factor-related apoptosis-inducing ligand overcomes an impaired response of hepatoma cells but causes severe apoptosis in primary human hepatocytes. Cancer Res 2003;63:2369–2372.
69. Kagawa S, Gu J, Swisher SG, et al. Antitumor effect of adenovirus-mediated Bax gene transfer on p53-sensitive and p53-resistant cancer lines. Cancer Res 2000;60:1157–1161.
70. Khan AU, Lal SK. Ribozymes: A modern tool in medicine. J Biomed Sci 2003;10:457–467.
71. Yi HK, Nam SY, Kim JC, Kim JS, Lee DY, Hwang PH. Induction of apoptosis in K562 cells by dominant negative c-myb. Exper Hematol 2002;30:1139–1146.
72. Rousselet N, Mills L, Jean D, Tellez C, Bar-Eli M, Frade R. Inhibition of tumorigenicity and metastasis of human melanoma cells by anti-cathepsin L single chain variable fragment. Cancer Res 2004;64:146–151.
73. Duggan BJ, Maxwell P, Kelly JD, et al. The effect of antisense Bcl-2 oligonucleotides on Bcl-2 protein expression and apoptosis in human bladder transitional cell carcinoma. J Urol 2001;166: 1098–1105.
74. Dillin A. The specifics of small interfering RNA specificity. Proc Natl Acad Sci U S A 2003;100: 6289–6291.
75. Futami T, Miyagishi M, Seki M, Taira K. Induction of apoptosis in HeLa cells with siRNA expression vector targeted against bcl-2. Nucleic Acids Res Suppl, 2002;251–252.
76. Ross DM, Hughes TP. Cancer treatment with kinase inhibitors: what have we learnt from imatinib? Br J Cancer 2004;90:12–19.
77. Kagawa S, Pearson SA, Ji L, et al. A binary adenoviral vector system for expressing high levels of the proapoptotic gene bax. Gene Ther 2000;7:75–79.

11 Gene Silencing Therapy Against Cancer

Chao-Zhong Song, MD, PhD

CONTENTS

Summary

Over the past 25 yr, gene silencing therapy derived from nucleic acid-based molecules has evolved from bench research to clinical therapy. The recent discovery of RNA interference (RNAi), a mechanism by which double stranded RNAs mediate sequence-specific gene silencing, provided a new tool in the fight against cancer. The application of RNAi technology in basic cancer research will facilitate the identification and validation of potential therapeutic targets for cancer, and the elucidation of the molecular pathways governing cancer growth and development. RNAi technology could be further developed into therapeutics for cancer by selectively silencing aberrantly activated oncogenes. However, major challenges of delivery, specificity and efficacy need to be overcome before siRNAs can be used as therapeutic agents.

Key Words: Gene silencing; cancer therapy; RNA interference (RNAi); small interfering RNA (siRNA); short hairpin RNA (shRNA).

1. MAJOR APPROACHES TO SEQUENCE-SPECIFIC GENE SILENCING

Tumorigenesis in humans is the consequence of multiple genetic and epigenetic events that lead to uncontrollable cell proliferation *(1)*. Aberrant activation of many genes as a result of overexpression or oncogenic mutations is often associated with oncogenic phenotypes of human cancers. The determination of whether their aberrant activation is the cause or merely a consequence of tumorigenesis will identify the real targets for effective anticancer therapy. Because silencing of cancer-causing genes should cure the disease at its genetic root, the development of agents that are able to specifically silence target genes has been a rational strategy for cancer therapy.

Over the past two decades, nucleic-acid-based gene inhibition has been one of the major approaches to the development of gene-silencing therapeutics. Several types of nucleic acid molecules which are capable of sequence-specific inhibition of gene expression have been developed as therapeutics for many disorders such as viral infections and cancer *(2–5)*. The three major nucleic-acid-based gene-silencing molecules

From: *Cancer Drug Discovery and Development: Gene Therapy for Cancer*
Edited by: K. K. Hunt, S. A. Vorburger, and S. G. Swisher © Humana Press Inc., Totowa, NJ

are chemically modified antisense oligonucleotides (ODNs), ribozymes, and small interfering RNAs (siRNAs). Although they are all antisense-guided sequence-specific gene silencing molecules, the mechanisms and potency of gene silencing by the three types of molecules are significantly different.

1.1. ODNs and Ribozymes

ODNs act by hybridizing to target mRNA. Depending on the backbone modifications, ODNs can block target gene function through two different mechanisms. Negatively charged ODNs form RNA–DNA duplexes to produce a substrate for ribonuclease H (RNAse H), which specifically cleaves the target mRNA. ODNs with other backbone modifications do not recruit RNAse H. These ODNs act by steric hindrance to block the splicing of heteronuclear RNA into mature mRNA, nuclear-cytoplasmic transport or translation of mRNA. The mechanisms and application of ODNs have been the subject of several comprehensive reviews *(2,3,6,7)*. Ribozymes are RNA molecules that have intrinsic catalytic activity. Ribozymes bind to substrate RNAs through Watson-Crick base pairing and cleave target RNAs by catalyzing the hydrolysis of the phosphodiester backbone *(2,3)*. At least six classes of ribozymes have been described. The hammerhead ribozyme is the most extensively studied. The catalytic motif within the ribozyme is flanked by sequences that are complementary to sequences surrounding the target RNA cleavage site and serve as guides of ribozymes to its mRNA targets.

1.2. RNAi

RNAi is a relatively new and rapidly developing technology for sequence-specific gene silencing *(8–13)*. Studies have shown that siRNAs are more potent in gene silencing than different types of ODNs *(14–19)* and ribozymes *(20–22)*. RNAi is a cellular mechanism by which double-stranded RNAs (dsRNAs) trigger the silencing of the corresponding gene that was first observed in the nematode worm, *Caenorhabditi selegans* *(23)*, and plants *(24)*. It is now known that RNAi is an evolutionarily conserved mechanism of dsRNA-mediated gene silencing in diverse species. siRNAs found in nature are derived from long dsRNAs that are expressed from viruses, transposons, experimentally introduced transgenes or endogenous genes. In plants, the RNAi pathway is used as a natural defense mechanism against viral infection. In mammalian cells, however, dsRNAs longer than 30 nucleotides will provoke the activation of dsRNA-activated protein kinase (PKR), which causes nonspecific inhibition of protein translation and cell death *(25,26)*. A major breakthrough in the application of RNAi technology in mammalian cells came from the observation that synthetic siRNAs of 21 nucleotides in length that mimic Dicer cleavage products efficiently induced sequence-specific gene silencing when transiently transfected into mammalian cells *(27,28)*. However, one drawback of transient transfected synthetic siRNAs is that their effects are transient, as mammals apparently lack the mechanisms that amplify silencing in worms and plants *(11)*. Therefore, this approach is not suitable for studies that require long-term gene silencing in mammalian cells. Another important technical advance came from the demonstration that dsRNAs of 19–29 nucleotides that are expressed endogenously using RNA polymerase III promoters, either as short hairpin RNAs (shRNAs) or as separate complementary RNAs, efficiently induced target gene silencing in mammalian cells *(21,29–35)*. The endogenous expression of siRNAs from DNA templates has several advantages over the exogenous delivery of synthetic siRNAs *(36,37)*. For example, it allows stable gene silencing both in vitro in cultured cells and in vivo in animals

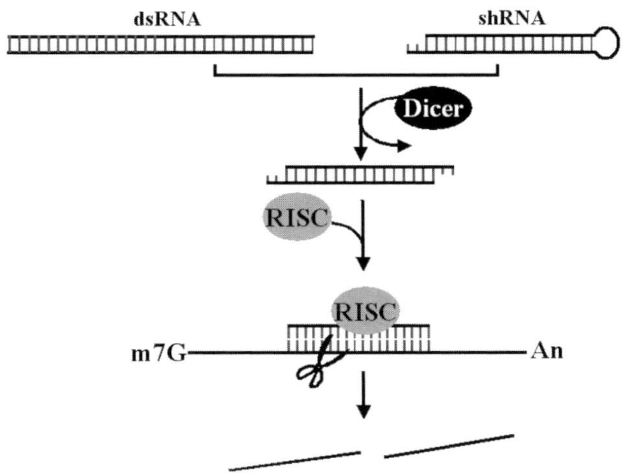

Fig. 1. The RNAi pathway. Double-stranded RNA (dsRNA) or short-hairpin RNA (shRNA) is processed into small interfering RNA (siRNA) by Dicer inside the cell. One of the strands of the siRNA is incorporated into RISC and guides the specific degradation of homologous mRNA.

(32,38–42). More recently, it was demonstrated that transgenic mice expressing shRNA can pass the RNAi to the next generation *(43,44)*.

The long dsRNA or shRNA silencing triggers are cleaved to produce siRNAs by Dicer, which is a member of the RNase-III family of dsRNA-specific endonucleases *(45)*. Dicer cleaves long dsRNA or shRNA into 21- to 28- nucleotide siRNA duplexes that contain 2-nucleotide 3′-overhangs with 5′-phosphate and 3′-hydroxyl termini *(46,47)* (*see* Fig. 1). This configuration is functionally important for siRNA incorporation into the RNA-induced silencing complex (RISC) *(47,48)*. Components of the RNAi machinery specifically recognize the siRNA duplex and incorporate a single siRNA strand into RISC *(49)*. The antisense strand of the siRNA in the RISC complex functions as a guide for target mRNA degradation *(49,50)* (*see* Fig. 1). Cleavage of target mRNA by RISC complex is endonucleolytic. RISC cleaves mRNAs containing perfectly complementary sequences, 10 nucleotides from the 5′-end of the incorporated siRNA strand *(46)*.

2. RNAi IN BASIC CANCER RESEARCH

The release of nearly complete human genome sequences and the identification of a large number of genes whose aberrant expression is associated with a variety of cancers by high-throughput genomic and proteomic approaches have provided both unprecedented opportunities and challenges for the development of new cancer therapeutics. For example, gene expression profiling using DNA microarray technology has identified distinct signatures of cancer gene expression that are associated with metastatic capacity and prognosis of cancer. Although the identification of a large number of genes that are up- or down-regulated in cancer has provided a large amount of information for both basic and clinical cancer research, it provides no information on whether the altered expression of a particular gene is the cause or a consequence of cancer. Because only the tumor-causing genes are the likely druggable targets, functional validation of therapeutic targets among these genes become a major challenge in the development of cancer therapeutics.

Therefore, techniques that permit high-throughput functional validation of this large number of candidate genes are in high demand. The RNAi technology which has the potential ability to silence any genes of interest with high specificity and potency is becoming a promising tool to meet this demand.

Several near-genome-wide RNAi screens have been performed in *C. elegans* and *Drosophila melangogaster (51,52)*. Until recently, most of the functional studies using RNAi in mammalian cells have been performed on a single gene or a limited number of genes in a family or specific pathway. The recent reports using RNAi to target a family of genes *(53,54)* or thousands of genes that are involved in specific pathways and cellular processes demonstrated the utility of RNAi for genome-wide high-throughput functional studies in mammalian systems *(55–57)*. By combining RNAi and microarray technologies, now it is experimentally feasible to functionally establish the causal role of genes in tumorigenesis with high throughput. So far, these large scale applications of RNAi to gene function studies are carried out using the reverse genetic screening approach. Recently, technology of enzymatic production of siRNA has been developed *(58–60)*. This technology enables the generation of shRNAs targeting genes of interest without the requirement of a prior knowledge of their sequence information, thus making it possible to apply RNAi directly in forward genetic screens. For cancer research, the reverse genetic approach using RNAi may have several advantages. First, the sequence information for almost all of the genes in the human genome are available; second, gene expression profiling databases for most types of human malignancies are established and readily accessible; and third, it will allow the scoring of neutral or negative phenotypes such as cell death and growth arrest. By comparing phenotypic readouts such as invasiveness, growth and apoptosis among cancer cells that express shRNAs targeting different genes, reverse cancer genetic screens using RNAi will permit functional validation of genes whose aberrant expression contributes to specific caner phenotypes. On the other hand, the forward genetic approach will allow RNAi libraries to be generated directly from cDNA libraries derived from mRNAs isolated from cancer cells or mRNAs enriched for a specific cancer phenotype. This is especially advantageous for studies involving species from which sequences for most of the genes are not yet readily available. However, this forward genetic approach will not be able to score the neutral and negative phenotypes. This will impose significant limitations on the utility of forward genetic RNAi screen for cancer research unless improved screening strategies are developed that can score negative phenotypes.

The down-regulation of essential cellular genes required for cell growth and survival by RNAi will result in an arrest of cell growth or in cell death, thus imposing significant limitations on the applications of RNAi to long-term studies on the function of these genes in vitro using cultured cells or in vivo using animals. The availability of an inducible RNAi system will overcome this limitation. Therefore, the development of inducible RNAi systems that allow controllable RNAi in vivo and in vitro will significantly increase the utility of RNAi for both basic research and therapeutic applications to cancer *(61–66)*. RNAi can be used to simultaneously target multiple genes in one cell, thus generating multiple knockdowns *(67,68)*. The ability to knockdown more than one gene by simply cointroducing or sequentially introducing siRNAs targeting multiple genes into cells in vitro or in vivo makes it easy to study functional interactions between genes in the control of cancer growth and development. During the short period since its discovery, RNAi technology has been developing at a rapid pace. These technical advances in RNAi have significantly improved the utility of RNAi in both basic and clinical cancer research including target discovery and validation. Thus, RNAi has evolved into a functional genomic tool allowing both forward and reverse genetic screens in cancer research. As discussed below, concerns on RNAi specificity have been raised in recent studies. Therefore, appropriate controls of and alternative approaches to siRNA should be included in studies using RNAi to confirm the results.

3. RNAi IN CLINICAL CANCER THERAPY

In concept, diseases such as cancer, which are characterized by overexpression or aberrant activation of specific oncogenes, are suitable candidates for nucleic acid-based gene-silencing therapies. Several nucleic acid drugs that are based on ODNs were under clinical trials and Vitravene (sodium fomivirsen) has been used for the treatment of cytomegalovirus (CMV) infection of the eye in clinics *(2,3,5)*. Several ribozyme-based phase I/II clinical trials are in early-phase of clinical evaluation for patients with breast cancer, colon cancer, and hepatitis *(3)*. The problems of toxicity and poor clinical efficacy with antisense and ribosome molecules remain to be solved even after more than a decade of drug development attempts. Although the term RNAi was coined just 6 yr ago *(23)* and the application of siRNAs in mammalian cells was started only three years ago *(27,28)*, RNAi is rapidly taking center stage of the development of nucleic acid-based therapeutics. siRNA-based biotechnology companies were established and many companies switched their focus from developing ODNs and ribozyme therapeutics to siRNA therapeutics *(5,69)*. Currently, the enthusiasm toward RNAi therapeutics is high, partly because RNAi is a natural defense mechanism that protects organisms from viral infections, and it is more potent than ODNs and ribozymes in target gene silencing. Because the RNAi field is still young, siRNAs have not yet had the time to enter clinical trials. However, some companies are planning to begin clinical trials in the near future. Animal experiments with RNAi have demonstrated the therapeutic potential of RNAi. For example, siRNAs have been shown to protect mice from hepatitis *(70,71)*, viral infection *(72,73)*, sepsis *(74)*, tumor growth *(75–79)*, and ocular neovascularization causing macular degeneration *(80)*.

In spite of the tremendous promises that RNAi holds as potential therapeutics, many hurdles need to be overcome before it can be used to treat human diseases safely and effectively. High on the list are specificity, potency, and delivery. Gene silencing by RNAi has been demonstrated to be highly specific. For example, even a single nucleotide mismatch between the antisense strand of the siRNA and target mRNA can abolish the RNAi effect *(46,81)*. RNAi specifically targeting the M-BCR/ABL fusion site has been used to kill leukemic cells with such a rearrangement *(82)*. RNAi was used to specifically and stably inhibit the expression of the oncogenic K-RAS^{v12} allele while leaving the wild type K-RAS intact in human tumor cells *(32)*. RNAi was also used for the isoform-specific knockdown of vascular endothelial growth factor (VEGF) *(83)* and destruction of particular splice variants of a gene *(84)*. In addition, gene expression profiling studies also demonstrated that siRNA targeting specific genes showed no nonspecific effects on the global gene expression pattern *(85,86)*.

However, one of the potential problems for nucleic-acid-based gene silencing molecules is the induction of off-target effects by hybridizing to sequences with homology to the intended target. It appears that RNAi is also no exception. In contrast to the aforementioned studies, several recent reports showed the off-target effects of siRNA. Transcript profiles revealed siRNA-specific rather than target-specific signatures, including the direct silencing of nontargeted genes containing as few as eleven contiguous nucleotides of identity to the siRNA *(87)*. It was also indicated that siRNAs have partial complementary sequence matches to off-target genes may result in a microRNA-like inhibition of translation *(88)*. Nonspecific off-target effects were found to be siRNA concentration-dependent *(89)*. These results together demonstrated that siRNAs may crossreact with targets of limited sequence homology under certain conditions. Recent studies also showed that siRNAs or endogenously expressed shRNAs also have the potential to activate the interferon system *(90,91)*. Another recent study, however, showed that siRNAs generated by phage polymerases but not their synthetic counterparts elicited interferon induction *(92)*. The authors concluded that it was the initiating 5′-triphosphate of the siRNA generated by T3, T7, or Sp6 RNA polymerase that induced interferon production. On the basis of these studies, it is apparent that the side effects of RNAi are dependent on several factors including siRNA concentration and sequence, as well as methods of siRNA generation.

These results emphasize the importance of proper RNAi design to minimize side effects. If the sequences of the siRNAs are carefully selected, RNAi can have exquisite specificity. siRNAs are able to discriminate targets from nontargets by a single nucleotide difference *(32,93–95)*. If the most effective sequence for RNAi is identified, it is possible to use the lowest concentration of siRNA to achieve sufficient gene silencing, thus reducing the possibility of eliciting nonspecific side effects. This requires more basic studies towards a better understanding of the molecular basis of the RNAi machinery. The effectiveness of RNAi is determined by several factors. First, some sequences within the mRNA cannot be targeted by RNAi. Although the reason for this is still unclear, it is believed that some regions in the target mRNA are not accessible to siRNA as a result of the formation of secondary or tertiary structures or the binding of RNA interacting proteins. It is difficult to accurately predict which region within an mRNA will serve as an effective siRNA target. A common solution to this problem is to select multiple regions within the target mRNA almost randomly so that at least one of them may be targeted. Secondly, the hairpin loop structure of the endogenously expressed shRNA also influences RNAi potency. Because exactly how shRNA is processed into functional siRNA is largely unknown, it is impossible to make a rational design of an effective hairpin loop. Therefore, a hairpin loop sequence is usually selected through trial and error. Once a working hairpin loop is identified, it will be used in the design of shRNAs for subsequent RNAi studies as it is not feasible to select the most effective hairpin loop for each shRNA. However, different sequences in the stem may require different loops for maximum potency. Third, the length of the stem sequence of the shRNA also affects RNAi potency *(31)*. Fourth, the thermodynamic properties of the sequences within a siRNA duplex also play a critical role in determining RNAi effectiveness. Rules for selecting more efficient siRNA have been proposed *(96–98)*. A key step in RNAi is the assembly of the RISC complex. Effective RNAi requires the incorporation of the antisense strand of the siRNA duplex, which is complementary to the target mRNA, into the activated RISC where it functions as a guide for target mRNA degradation. It was shown that the two strands of a siRNA duplex are not equally incorporated into RISC. Both the absolute and relative stabilities of the base pairs at the 5′-end of the two siRNA strands determine the degree to which each strand participates in the RNAi pathway *(99,100)*. If the siRNA or shRNA is not correctly designed, the sense strand of the siRNA duplex will be preferentially assembled into RISC. This will not only result in ineffective on-target silencing, but will also increase the probability of off-target silencing of genes with homology to the sense strand of the siRNA.

A systematic analysis of 180 siRNAs targeting the mRNAs of two genes identified eight characteristics within the siRNA duplex that are associated with siRNA functionality *(101)*. These characteristics should provide important guides for selecting more effective siRNA sequences. Currently, however, the position at which Dicer cleaves shRNAs that are expressed endogenously from RNA polymerase III promoters is not known. Consequently, the rules for selecting effective siRNA may not be reliably applied to the selection of effective shRNAs. In summary, the effectiveness of RNAi is determined by a combination of multiple of factors. All of them must be take into consideration when developing algorithms for effective RNAi design. At present, screening several different siRNA or shRNAs for every target mRNA remains a common practice for identifying effective and specific siRNA.

More importantly, for siRNAs to work as therapeutic agents, they must be able to reach their target in the cells. Delivery is one of the major obstacles for RNAi therapy. Up to now, in vivo gene silencing by RNAi was very limited in the mammalian system. Practical and efficient methods need be developed to deliver siRNA or shRNA expression vectors into the target cells at the therapeutic level and duration so that it can reverse the disease pathophysiology. The long-term inhibition of target mRNA will probably be required for the treatment of chronic diseases such as cancers. Although the basic RNAi pathway is evolutionarily conserved in diverse species, mammalian RNAi lacks the systemic RNAi *(102)* and transitive RNAi *(103)*, mechanisms that spread and amplify RNAi effect respectively. In *C. elegans* and plants, for example, RNAi-mediated gene silencing can spread to remote regions of the body, thus called systemic RNAi. Amplification of the dsRNA silencing trigger (transitive RNAi) in *C. elegans*, through mechanisms that may involve RNA-dependent RNA polymerases (RdRP), results in a self-propagating silencing effect throughout the organism. Because mammalian cells lack both mechanisms, transient transfection of RNAi triggers of siRNAs or shRNAs in mammalian cells will result in a transient effect, lasting 2 to 7 d *(9)* depending upon the speed of cell division and the half-life of the RNAi triggers. Because of the reversible nature of the post-transcriptional gene silencing by RNAi and the lack of the amplification mechanism in mammalian cells, continuous delivery or expression of siRNAs in the cells is required for sustained target gene silencing.

Chemical modification has been shown to protect siRNA molecules from degradation, thus increasing the duration and potency of the RNAi effect *(104,105)*. By preventing siRNA from degradation, the modified siRNAs could be administrated systemically through blood stream or locally to the tumor. A variety of strategies have been developed for delivery of ODNs and ribozymes in vivo *(5)*. These methods could be adopted for the delivery of siRNA. Currently, shRNAs for RNAi are mostly expressed using H1 (RNase P) or U6 promoter. Both are RNA polymerase III promoters that have all the regulatory elements upstream of the transcription initiation site and produce transcripts without a cap or poly A tail *(106)*. Many viral vectors including adenoviral, adeno-associated viral (AAV), onco-retroviral, and lentiviral vectors have been utilized to deliver RNAi expression cassettes in vitro in cultured cells or in vivo in animals *(5,107)*. Each of these viral vectors has its advantages and disadvantages. Currently, issues such as long-term and therapeutic-level transgene expression in target tissues and safety remain to be solved. Of particularly relevance to cancer therapy is that cancer cells are genetically and functionally heterogeneous. It has been shown that only a small subpopulation of cells, called cancer stem cells, within breast cancer possesses tumor-initiating capability and is responsible for maintaining tumor growth and metastasis *(108)*. Cancer stem cells have a long life and increased proliferation potential and self-renewal ability. Differing from the majority of the fast-proliferating cancer cells, however, cancer stem cells are active at a slow rate or inactive until required in response to environmental stimuli. Delivery of siRNAs to the majority of the rapidly dividing cancer cells will result in initial remission, but cancer will relapse later if the cancer stem cells are not targeted. Therefore, to cure cancer, strategies should be developed to deliver siRNA into the relatively slow-dividing or nondividing cancer stem cells.

4. CONCLUSIONS

RNAi has become a powerful tool in cancer research. The successful application of RNAi technology in studies of cancer gene function at near genome-wide level in combination with other approaches such as gene expression profiling will significantly accelerate the identification and validation of targets for cancer therapy. RNAi has great potential in the development of therapeutics for cancer. However, the challenges of ensuring target specificity and effective delivery remain to be met. These obstacles will be overcome with the development of advanced algorithm for design of highly effective siRNAs, transfection reagents for highly efficient siRNA delivery, modifications for more stable and potent siRNAs, and vectors for therapeutic-level expression of shRNAs in cancer cells. With the abilities to design highly specific and effective siRNAs and to deliver them to the target sites at therapeutic levels, siRNAs could be used as therapeutic molecules for gene silencing therapy against cancer.

REFERENCES

1. Hanahan D, Weinberg RA. The hallmarks of cancer. Cell 2000;100:57–70.
2. Scherer LJ, Rossi JJ. Approaches for the sequence-specific knockdown of mRNA. Nat Biotechnol 2003;21:1457–1465.
3. Opalinska JB, Gewirtz AM. Nucleic-acid therapeutics: basic principles and recent applications. Nat Rev Drug Discov 2002;1:503–514.
4. Opalinska JB, Gewirtz AM. Therapeutic potential of antisense nucleic acid molecules. Sci STKE 2003;2003:pe47.
5. Dorsett Y, Tuschl T. siRNAs: applications in functional genomics and potential as therapeutics. Nat Rev Drug Discov 2004;3:318–329.
6. Kurreck J. Antisense technologies. Improvement through novel chemical modifications. Eur J Biochem 2003;270:1628–1644.
7. Dias N, Stein CA. Antisense oligonucleotides: basic concepts and mechanisms. Mol Cancer Ther 2002;1:347–355.
8. Sharp PA. RNA interference—2001. Genes Dev 2001;15:485–490.
9. Paddison PJ, Hannon GJ. RNA interference: the new somatic cell genetics? Cancer Cell 2002;2: 17–23.
10. Zamore PD. Ancient pathways programmed by small RNAs. Science 2002;296:1265–1269.
11. Hannon GJ. RNA interference. Nature 2002;418:244–251.
12. McManus MT, Sharp PA. Gene silencing in mammals by small interfering RNAs. Nat Rev Genet 2002;3:737–747.
13. Tijsterman M, Ketting RF, Plasterk RH. The genetics of RNA silencing. Annu Rev Genet 2002;36:489–519.
14. Aoki Y, Cioca DP, Oidaira H, Kamiya J, Kiyosawa K. RNA interference may be more potent than antisense RNA in human cancer cell lines. Clin Exp Pharmacol Physiol 2003;30:96–102.
15. Miyagishi M, Hayashi M, Taira K. Comparison of the suppressive effects of antisense oligonucleotides and siRNAs directed against the same targets in mammalian cells. Antisense Nucleic Acid Drug Dev 2003;13:1–7.

16. Grunweller A, Wyszko E, Bieber B, Jahnel R, Erdmann VA, Kurreck J. Comparison of different antisense strategies in mammalian cells using locked nucleic acids, 2′-O-methyl RNA, phosphorothioates and small interfering RNA. Nucleic Acids Res 2003;31:3185–3193.
17. Xu Y, Zhang HY, Thormeyer D, et al. Effective small interfering RNAs and phosphorothioate antisense DNAs have different preferences for target sites in the luciferase mRNAs. Biochem Biophys Res Commun 2003;306:712–717.
18. Kretschmer-Kazemi Far R, Sczakiel G. The activity of siRNA in mammalian cells is related to structural target accessibility: a comparison with antisense oligonucleotides. Nucleic Acids Res 2003;31:4417–4424.
19. Bertrand JR, Pottier M, Vekris A, Opolon P, Maksimenko A, Malvy C. Comparison of antisense oligonucleotides and siRNAs in cell culture and in vivo. Biochem Biophys Res Commun 2002;296:1000–1004.
20. Yokota T, Miyagishi M, Hino T, et al. siRNA-based inhibition specific for mutant SOD1 with single nucleotide alternation in familial ALS, compared with ribozyme and DNA enzyme. Biochem Biophys Res Commun 2004;314:283–291.
21. Lee NS, Dohjima T, Bauer G, et al. Expression of small interfering RNAs targeted against HIV-1 rev transcripts in human cells. Nat Biotechnol 2002;20:500–505.
22. Drew HR, Lewy D, Conaty J, Rand KN, Hendry P, Lockett T. RNA hairpin loops repress protein synthesis more strongly than hammerhead ribozymes. Eur J Biochem 1999;266:260–273.
23. Fire A, Xu S, Montgomery MK, Kostas SA, Driver SE, Mello CC. Potent and specific genetic interference by double-stranded RNA in Caenorhabditis elegans. Nature 1998;391:806–811.
24. Jorgensen RA, Cluster PD, English J, Que Q, Napoli CA. Chalcone synthase cosuppression phenotypes in petunia flowers: comparison of sense vs. antisense constructs and single-copy vs. complex T-DNA sequences. Plant Mol Biol 1996;31:957–973.
25. Williams BR. Role of the double-stranded RNA-activated protein kinase (PKR) in cell regulation. Biochem Soc Trans 1997;25:509–513.
26. Gil J, Esteban M. Induction of apoptosis by the dsRNA-dependent protein kinase (PKR): mechanism of action. Apoptosis 2000;5:107–114.
27. Elbashir SM, Harborth J, Lendeckel W, Yalcin A, Weber K, Tuschl T. Duplexes of 21-nucleotide RNAs mediate RNA interference in cultured mammalian cells. Nature 2001;411:494–498.
28. Caplen NJ, Parrish S, Imani F, Fire A, Morgan RA. Specific inhibition of gene expression by small double-stranded RNAs in invertebrate and vertebrate systems. Proc Natl Acad Sci U S A 2001;98:9742–9747.
29. Paul CP, Good PD, Winer I, Engelke DR. Effective expression of small interfering RNA in human cells. Nat Biotechnol 2002;20:505–508.
30. Sui G, Soohoo C, Affar el B, Gay F, Shi Y, Forrester WC. A DNA vector-based RNAi technology to suppress gene expression in mammalian cells. Proc Natl Acad Sci U S A 2002;99:5515–5520.
31. Paddison PJ, Caudy AA, Bernstein E, Hannon GJ, Conklin DS. Short hairpin RNAs (shRNAs) induce sequence-specific silencing in mammalian cells. Genes Dev 2002;16:948–958.
32. Brummelkamp TR, Bernards R, Agami R. Stable suppression of tumorigenicity by virus-mediated RNA interference. Cancer Cell 2002;2:243–247.
33. Zeng Y, Cullen BR. RNA interference in human cells is restricted to the cytoplasm. RNA 2002;8: 855–860.
34. Yu JY, DeRuiter SL, Turner DL. RNA interference by expression of short-interfering RNAs and hairpin RNAs in mammalian cells. Proc Natl Acad Sci U S A 2002;99:6047–6052.
35. Miyagishi M, Taira K. U6 promoter-driven siRNAs with four uridine 3′ overhangs efficiently suppress targeted gene expression in mammalian cells. Nat Biotechnol 2002;20:497–500.
36. Voorhoeve PM, Agami R. Knockdown stands up. Trends Biotechnol 2003;21:2–4.
37. Tuschl T. Expanding small RNA interference. Nat Biotechnol 2002;20:446–448.
38. McCaffrey AP, Meuse L, Pham TT, Conklin DS, Hannon GJ, Kay MA. RNA interference in adult mice. Nature 2002;418:38–39.
39. Xia H, Mao Q, Paulson HL, Davidson BL. siRNA-mediated gene silencing in vitro and in vivo. Nat Biotechnol 2002;20:1006–1010.
40. Lewis DL, Hagstrom JE, Loomis AG, Wolff JA, Herweijer H. Efficient delivery of siRNA for inhibition of gene expression in postnatal mice. Nat Genet 2002;32:107–108.
41. Hemann MT, Fridman JS, Zilfou JT, et al. An epi-allelic series of p53 hypomorphs created by stable RNAi produces distinct tumor phenotypes in vivo. Nat Genet 2003;33:396–400.
42. Rubinson DA, Dillon CP, Kwiatkowski AV, et al. A lentivirus-based system to functionally silence genes in primary mammalian cells, stem cells and transgenic mice by RNA interference. Nat Genet 2003;33:401–406.

43. Carmell MA, Zhang L, Conklin DS, Hannon GJ, Rosenquist TA. Germline transmission of RNAi in mice. Nat Struct Biol 2003;10:91–92.
44. Tiscornia G, Singer O, Ikawa M, Verma IM. A general method for gene knockdown in mice by using lentiviral vectors expressing small interfering RNA. Proc Natl Acad Sci U S A 2003;100:1844–1848.
45. Bernstein E, Caudy AA, Hammond SM, Hannon GJ. Role for a bidentate ribonuclease in the initiation step of RNA interference. Nature 2001;409:363–366.
46. Elbashir SM, Martinez J, Patkaniowska A, Lendeckel W, Tuschl T. Functional anatomy of siRNAs for mediating efficient RNAi in Drosophila melanogaster embryo lysate. EMBO J 2001;20:6877–6888.
47. Zamore PD, Tuschl T, Sharp PA, Bartel DP. RNAi: double-stranded RNA directs the ATP-dependent cleavage of mRNA at 21 to 23 nucleotide intervals. Cell 2000;101:25–33.
48. Hammond SM, Bernstein E, Beach D, Hannon GJ. An RNA-directed nuclease mediates post-transcriptional gene silencing in Drosophila cells. Nature 2000;404:293–296.
49. Martinez J, Patkaniowska A, Urlaub H, Luhrmann R, Tuschl T. Single-stranded antisense siRNAs guide target RNA cleavage in RNAi. Cell 2002;110:563–574.
50. Schwarz DS, Hutvagner G, Haley B, Zamore PD. Evidence that siRNAs function as guides, not primers, in the Drosophila and human RNAi pathways. Mol Cell 2002;10:537–548.
51. Carpenter AE, Sabatini DM. Systematic genome-wide screens of gene function. Nat Rev Genet 2004;5:11–22.
52. Sugimoto A. High-throughput RNAi in Caenorhabditis elegans: genome-wide screens and functional genomics. Differentiation 2004;72:81–91.
53. Brummelkamp TR, Nijman SM, Dirac AM, Bernards R. Loss of the cylindromatosis tumour suppressor inhibits apoptosis by activating NF-kappaB. Nature 2003;424:797–801.
54. Aza-Blanc P, Cooper CL, Wagner K, Batalov S, Deveraux QL, Cooke MP. Identification of modulators of TRAIL-induced apoptosis via RNAi-based phenotypic screening. Mol Cell 2003;12:627–637.
55. Berns K, Hijmans EM, Mullenders J, et al. A large-scale RNAi screen in human cells identifies new components of the p53 pathway. Nature 2004;428:431–437.
56. Paddison PJ, Silva JM, Conklin DS, et al. A resource for large-scale RNA-interference-based screens in mammals. Nature 2004;428:427–431.
57. Zheng L, Liu J, Batalov S, et al. An approach to genomewide screens of expressed small interfering RNAs in mammalian cells. Proc Natl Acad Sci U S A 2004;101:135–140.
58. Sen G, Wehrman TS, Myers JW, Blau HM. Restriction enzyme-generated siRNA (REGS) vectors and libraries. Nat Genet 2004;36:183–189.
59. Shirane D, Sugao K, Namiki S, Tanabe M, Iino M, Hirose K. Enzymatic production of RNAi libraries from cDNAs. Nat Genet 2004;36:190–196.
60. Luo B, Heard AD, Lodish HF. Small interfering RNA production by enzymatic engineering of DNA (SPEED). Proc Natl Acad Sci U S A 2004;101:5494–5499.
61. Chen Y, Stamatoyannopoulos G, Song CZ. Down-regulation of CXCR4 by inducible small interfering RNA inhibits breast cancer cell invasion in vitro. Cancer Res 2003;63:4801–4804.
62. Wiznerowicz M, Trono D. Conditional suppression of cellular genes: lentivirus vector-mediated drug-inducible RNA interference. J Virol 2003;77:8957–8961.
63. Matsukura S, Jones PA, Takai D. Establishment of conditional vectors for hairpin siRNA knockdowns. Nucleic Acids Res 2003;31:e77.
64. Czauderna F, Santel A, Hinz M, et al. Inducible shRNA expression for application in a prostate cancer mouse model. Nucleic Acids Res 2003;31:e127.
65. van de Wetering M, Oving I, Muncan V, et al. Specific inhibition of gene expression using a stably integrated, inducible small-interfering-RNA vector. EMBO Rep 2003;4:609–615.
66. Gupta S, Schoer RA, Egan JE, Hannon GJ, Mittal V. Inducible, reversible, and stable RNA interference in mammalian cells. Proc Natl Acad Sci U S A 2004;101:1927–1932.
67. Schuck S, Manninen A, Honsho M, Fullekrug J, Simons K. Generation of single and double knockdowns in polarized epithelial cells by retrovirus-mediated RNA interference. Proc Natl Acad Sci U S A 2004;101:4912–4917.
68. Yu JY, Taylor J, DeRuiter SL, Vojtek AB, Turner DL. Simultaneous inhibition of GSK3alpha and GSK3beta using hairpin siRNA expression vectors. Mol Ther 2003;7:228–236.
69. Howard K. Unlocking the money-making potential of RNAi. Nat Biotechnol 2003;21:1441–1446.
70. Song E, Lee SK, Wang J, et al. RNA interference targeting Fas protects mice from fulminant hepatitis. Nat Med 2003;9:347–351.
71. Zender L, Hutker S, Liedtke C, et al. Caspase 8 small interfering RNA prevents acute liver failure in mice. Proc Natl Acad Sci U S A 2003;100:7797–7802.

72. McCaffrey AP, Nakai H, Pandey K, et al. Inhibition of hepatitis B virus in mice by RNA interference. Nat Biotechnol 2003;21:639–644.
73. Song E, Lee SK, Dykxhoorn DM, et al. Sustained small interfering RNA-mediated human immunodeficiency virus type 1 inhibition in primary macrophages. J Virol 2003;77:7174–7181.
74. Sorensen DR, Leirdal M, Sioud M. Gene silencing by systemic delivery of synthetic siRNAs in adult mice. J Mol Biol 2003;327:761–766.
75. Verma UN, Surabhi RM, Schmaltieg A, Becerra C, Gaynor RB. Small interfering RNAs directed against beta-catenin inhibit the in vitro and in vivo growth of colon cancer cells. Clin Cancer Res 2003;9:1291–1300.
76. Li K, Lin SY, Brunicardi FC, Seu P. Use of RNA interference to target cyclin E-overexpressing hepatocellular carcinoma. Cancer Res 2003;63:3593–3597.
77. Filleur S, Courtin A, Ait-Si-Ali S, et al. SiRNA-mediated inhibition of vascular endothelial growth factor severely limits tumor resistance to antiangiogenic thrombospondin-1 and slows tumor vascularization and growth. Cancer Res 2003;63:3919–3922.
78. Yang G, Thompson JA, Fang B, Liu J. Silencing of H-ras gene expression by retrovirus-mediated siRNA decreases transformation efficiency and tumorgrowth in a model of human ovarian cancer. Oncogene 2003;22:5694–5701.
79. Yoshinouchi M, Yamada T, Kizaki M, et al. In vitro and in vivo growth suppression of human papillomavirus 16-positive cervical cancer cells by E6 siRNA. Mol Ther 2003;8:762–768.
80. Reich SJ, Fosnot J, Kuroki A, et al. Small interfering RNA (siRNA) targeting VEGF effectively inhibits ocular neovascularization in a mouse model. Mol Vis 2003;9:210–216.
81. Martinez LA, Naguibneva I, Lehrmann H, et al. Synthetic small inhibiting RNAs: efficient tools to inactivate oncogenic mutations and restore p53 pathways. Proc Natl Acad Sci U S A 2002;99: 14,849–14,854.
82. Wilda M, Fuchs U, Wossmann W, Borkhardt A. Killing of leukemic cells with a BCR/ABL fusion gene by RNA interference (RNAi). Oncogene 2002;21:5716–5724.
83. Zhang L, Yang N, Mohamed-Hadley A, Rubin SC, Coukos G. Vector-based RNAi, a novel tool for isoform-specific knock-down of VEGF and anti-angiogenesis gene therapy of cancer. Biochem Biophys Res Commun 2003;303:1169–1178.
84. Harborth J, Elbashir SM, Vandenburgh K, et al. Sequence, Chemical, and Structural Variation of Small Interfering RNAs and Short Hairpin RNAs and the Effect on Mammalian Gene Silencing. Antisense Nucleic Acid Drug Dev 2003;13:83–105.
85. Semizarov D, Frost L, Sarthy A, Kroeger P, Halbert DN, Fesik SW. Specificity of short interfering RNA determined through gene expression signatures. Proc Natl Acad Sci U S A 2003;100: 6347–6352.
86. Chi JT, Chang HY, Wang NN, Chang DS, Dunphy N, Brown PO. Genomewide view of gene silencing by small interfering RNAs. Proc Natl Acad Sci U S A 2003;100:6343–6346.
87. Jackson AL, Bartz SR, Schelter J, et al. Expression profiling reveals off-target gene regulation by RNAi. Nat Biotechnol 2003;21:635–637.
88. Scacheri PC, Rozenblatt-Rosen O, Caplen NJ, et al. Short interfering RNAs can induce unexpected and divergent changes in the levels of untargeted proteins in mammalian cells. Proc Natl Acad Sci U S A 2004;101:1892–1897.
89. Persengiev SP, Zhu X, Green MR. Nonspecific, concentration-dependent stimulation and repression of mammalian gene expression by small interfering RNAs (siRNAs). RNA 2004;10:12–18.
90. Bridge AJ, Pebernard S, Ducraux A, Nicoulaz AL, Iggo R. Induction of an interferon response by RNAi vectors in mammalian cells. Nat Genet 2003;34:263–264.
91. Sledz CA, Holko M, De Veer MJ, Silverman RH, Williams BR. Activation of the interferon system by short-interfering RNAs. Nat Cell Biol 2003;5:834–839.
92. Kim DH, Longo M, Han Y, Lundberg P, Cantin E, Rossi JJ. Interferon induction by siRNAs and ssRNAs synthesized by phage polymerase. Nat Biotechnol 2004;22:321–325.
93. Abdelgany A, Wood M, Beeson D. Allele-specific silencing of a pathogenic mutant acetylcholine receptor subunit by RNA interference. Hum Mol Genet 2003;12:2637–2644.
94. Ding H, Schwarz DS, Keene A, et al. Selective silencing by RNAi of a dominant allele that causes amyotrophic lateral sclerosis. Aging Cell 2003;2:209–217.
95. Harborth J, Elbashir SM, Bechert K, Tuschl T, Weber K. Identification of essential genes in cultured mammalian cells using small interfering RNAs. J Cell Sci 2001;114:4557–4565.
96. Elbashir SM, Harborth J, Weber K, Tuschl T. Analysis of gene function in somatic mammalian cells using small interfering RNAs. Methods 2002;26:199–213.

97. Hsieh AC, Bo R, Manola J, et al. A library of siRNA duplexes targeting the phosphoinositide 3-kinase pathway: determinants of gene silencing for use in cell-based screens. Nucleic Acids Res 2004;32:893–901.
98. Ui-Tei K, Naito Y, Takahashi F, et al. Guidelines for the selection of highly effective siRNA sequences for mammalian and chick RNA interference. Nucleic Acids Res 2004;32:936–948.
99. Khvorova A, Reynolds A, Jayasena SD. Functional siRNAs and miRNAs exhibit strand bias. Cell 2003;115:209–216.
100. Schwarz DS, Hutvagner G, Du T, Xu Z, Aronin N, Zamore PD. Asymmetry in the assembly of the RNAi enzyme complex. Cell 2003;115:199–208.
101. Reynolds A, Leake D, Boese Q, Scaringe S, Marshall WS, Khvorova A. Rational siRNA design for RNA interference. Nat Biotechnol 2004;22:326–330.
102. Winston WM, Molodowitch C, Hunter CP. Systemic RNAi in C. elegans requires the putative transmembrane protein SID-1. Science 2002;295:2456–2459.
103. Sijen T, Fleenor J, Simmer F, et al. On the role of RNA amplification in dsRNA-triggered gene silencing. Cell 2001;107:465–476.
104. Czauderna F, Fechtner M, Dames S, et al. Structural variations and stabilising modifications of synthetic siRNAs in mammalian cells. Nucleic Acids Res 2003;31:2705–2716.
105. Amarzguioui M, Holen T, Babaie E, Prydz H. Tolerance for mutations and chemical modifications in a siRNA. Nucleic Acids Res 2003;31:589–595.
106. Paule MR, White RJ. Survey and summary: transcription by RNA polymerases I and III. Nucleic Acids Res 2000;28:1283–1298.
107. Rutz S, Scheffold A. Towards in vivo application of RNA interference - new toys, old problems. Arthritis Res Ther 2004;6:78–85.
108. Al-Hajj M, Wicha MS, Benito-Hernandez A, Morrison SJ, Clarke MF. Prospective identification of tumorigenic breast cancer cells. Proc Natl Acad Sci U S A 2003;100:3983–3988.

12 Tumor Targeting–Retargeted Adenovirus

Masato Yamamoto, MD, PhD
and David T. Curiel, MD, PhD

CONTENTS

Summary

Adenovirus (Ad) has been applied for gene therapy in various applications. The current Ad vector system has two critical problems; low transduction of the target cancer cells and high transduction of nontarget normal organs. To address these issues, we have been working on "retargeting" of Ad vectors via transductional or transcriptional targeting. Transductional targeting has been achieved with application of various bridging moieties, genetical modification of vector capsid, or chemically coating viral particles. On the other hand, transcriptional targeting has been performed by employing natural or artificial transcriptional control elements with desired selectivity profile. In the field of cancer gene therapy, such retargeting has achieved augmented infectivity in the cancers that have been difficult to transduce with conventional Ad vector, as well as cancer specific transgene expression for avoiding toxicity. Success in cancer gene therapy requires vector design reflecting the pathological/physiological profile of the target disease, such as conditionally replicative adenovirus with combined retargeting mechanisms incorporated. In addition, we must continue to seek new targeting modalities because different tumor context always imposes unique challenges with respect to disease targeting. While reliable preclinical/clinical studies are necessary to establish a legitimate role of adenoviral retargeting in the field of cancer gene therapy, it is obvious that better vector targeting should leads to more potent and safe adenovirus based cancer therapeutics.

Key Words: Adenovirus; retargeting; selectivity; infectivity.

From: *Cancer Drug Discovery and Development: Gene Therapy for Cancer*
Edited by: K. K. Hunt, S. A. Vorburger, and S. G. Swisher © Humana Press Inc., Totowa, NJ

1. THE NECESSITY OF ADENOVIRUS RETARGETING

Adenovirus (Ad) has been applied for gene therapy in various applications, taking advantage of its high transduction efficiency in vivo *(1)*. However, commonly used vectors based on Ad serotype 5 and 2 require the primary adenoviral receptor, the coxsackie adenovirus receptor (CAR), for efficient infection and, hence, show tropism determined by the tissue distribution of the CAR expression *(2–5)*. This characteristic of the current adenoviral vector system leads to two fundamental problems; high transduction of nontarget cells and low transduction of the target cells.

The first issue is transduction of unwanted cell subsets. In vivo, systemically administered adenovirus vectors (or those released from local injection sites) predominantly accumulate in the liver as a result of both CAR-dependent and -independent mechanisms, leading to strong expression of the payload gene *(4–9)*. For some diseases like hemophilia, the expression of the transgene in the liver is desirable, because the predominant, natural production site of those proteins is the liver *(10,11)*. However, for many diseases, which require transgene expression in target cells other than the hepatocyte, vector absorption by the liver and the possible toxicity resulting from ectopic expression of the transgene hampers the systemic application of adenoviral vectors. This is typically the case for cancer gene therapy. If nonselective vectors are employed, for example, for systemic suicide gene therapy, the expression of the activator enzyme in the liver would lead to severe adverse effects as a result of nontarget activation of the prodrug *(6,12–14)*. Hence, a strategy to target cytotoxic transgene expression is required.

The second problem of the current adenoviral vectors is poor transduction efficiency in the cells with low-CAR expression. In many tumors, such as in pancreatic cancers *(15,18)*, esophageal adenocarcinoma *(16,17,19)* as well as gastric *(20)*, gall bladder *(21)*, and bile duct cancers the cells express CAR on the surface at low levels only. As a result, transduction efficiency of those cells is extremely poor with vectors that display the native tropism of wild type Ad 2 or 5. To realize the therapeutic potential of Ad vectors in these CAR-deficient tumors, the development of a retargeted vector system with a CAR-independent infection machinery is mandatory.

These limitations spur the effort to develop retargeted adenoviral vectors in order to fully take advantage of the possibilities of adenoviral vector-based gene therapies.

2. ADENOVIRAL INFECTION

The knowledge of adenovirus infection provides the basics for the development of adenoviral retargeting strategies. The native adenoviral infection pathway starts with the adherence of the virus to the cell surface for which two cellular receptors are responsible. As shown in Fig. 1, the initial binding of the subtype C adenoviruses, like Ad type 5/2, on the cell is mediated by attachment of the adenoviral fiber-knob region (the distal tip of each fiber monomer) onto CAR *(2,3)*. This cell surface protein has two immunoglobulin-like domains in its extracellular region *(22)*. It, thus, has been suggested that it plays a role in cell-cell junction *(23,24)*, but its complete function has not been fully elucidated yet. After binding to the cell surface via CAR, receptor-mediated endocytosis of the virion requires a second step that involves the interaction of Arg-Gly-Asp (RGD) motifs in the penton base with the surface integrins $\alpha v\beta 3$ or $\alpha v\beta 5$[25]. The viral entry is followed by a stepwise disassembly of the virus in the endosome and the consecutive endosomal lysis, which is mediated by the penton base and low

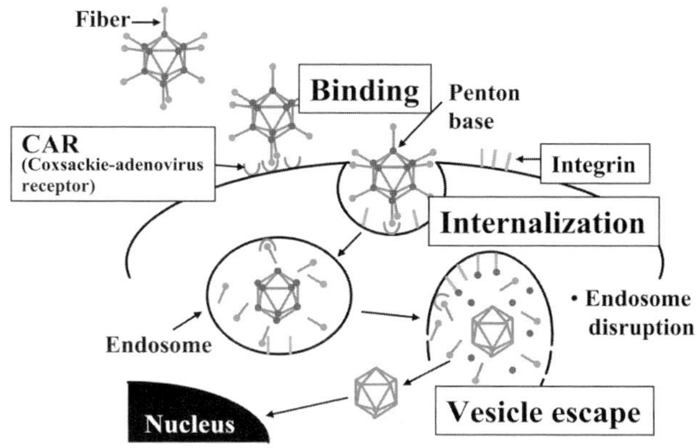

Fig. 1. Mechanism of adenoviral infection. Initial binding of adenovirus to cells is mainly mediated by the interaction between the adenoviral fiber-knob region and the CAR on the surface of the cells. Subsequently, the RGD motif in the viral penton base region binds to integrins on the cell, inducing internalization of the virus. Stepwise disassembly in the endosome, and then endosomal lysis mediated by the penton base and low endosomal pH release the capsid into the cytosol, followed by transportation to the nucleus and finally viral DNA release.

intraendosomal pH. After the release of the capsid into the cytosol, it is transported to the cell nucleus where theviral DNA is released *(26)*. Because viral entry and endosomal escape are independent phenomena, modification of the viral binding capability would not compromise downstream events.

3. BASIC STRATEGIES FOR ADENOVIRUS RETARGETING

The general categorization of adenovirus retargeting is based on whether the retargeting happens prior to or after entry into cells. Strategies redirecting binding and entry are grouped into "transductional targeting" methods controlling the expression of the transgene after vector entry (post-transductional targeting) mostly employ promoters and are called "transcriptional targeting." With respect to transductional targeting, adenovirus is amenable to these strategies because this virus does not have a lipid envelope, but instead relies on protein–protein interaction for cell entry *(26)*. Thus, protein-based modification by both genetic and nongenetic means may be exploited to achieve altered tropism with relative ease compared with enveloped viruses *(27)*. Indeed, elucidation of Ad infection and replication machinery provides a firm foundation for designing targeting strategies *(26)*. Major approaches for transductional targeting are shown in Fig. 2.

3.1. Transductional Targeting

One method of adenoviral retargeting employs antibody conjugates whereby an antibody (Ab) component binds to adenovirus and is cross-linking to a targeting moiety facilitating the binding to an alternative receptor *(27)*. An Ab directed against the fiber-knob region has been used because it not only binds to the virus but also eliminates the undesired adenovirus native tropism by masking the region required for CAR affinity. A conjugate consisting of an anti-knob antibody combined with folate enabled retargeting of adenovirus to folate receptor positive malignancies *(28)*. Along the same lines, adenovirus with a FLAG epitope insertion in the penton base region was retargeted to $\alpha v\beta 5$ integrin of endothelial and smooth muscle cells by using a bispecific conjugate

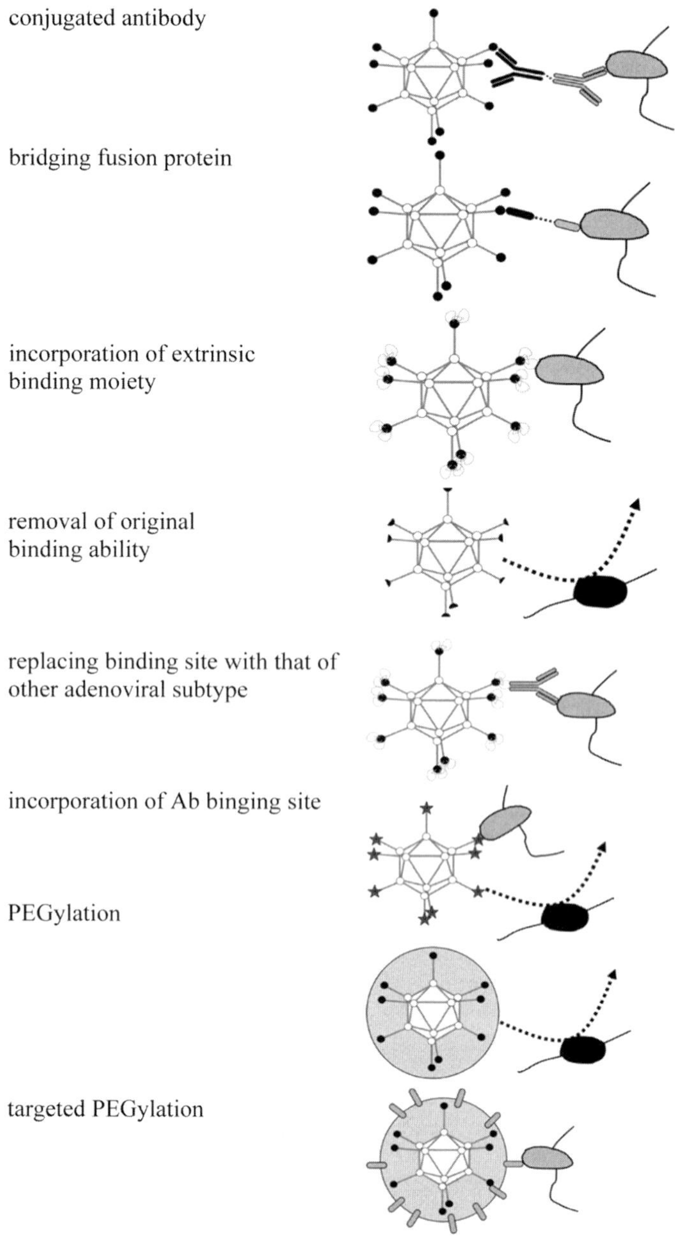

Fig. 2. Methods for transductional retargeting of adenovirus.

with anti-$\alpha v\beta 5$ integrin Ab and anti-FLAG Ab *(29)*[29]. Further Ab conjugate-based retargeting strategies using Abs of receptor ligands combined with an anti-knob Ab have been reported for various cell surface targets. These Abs targeted the fibroblast growth factor (FGF) receptor *(30)*, epidermal growth factor (EGF) receptor *(31)*, and angiotensin-converting enzyme (ACE) *(32)*. Interestingly, the anti-ACE Ab achieved suitable in vivo targeting for the pulmonary vasculature when combined with transcriptional targeting *(32)*. These data indicate that antibody-based targeting can confer CAR-independent infection, infectivity enhancement, and targeting.

Although these approaches validated the concept of adenoviral retargeting using large ligands, antibody-based conjugates encounter production problem. It is rather difficult to maintain structural and functional consistency of the crosslinked bispecific conjugate, making mass-production as a drug nonfeasible. To overcome these problems, fusion proteins created by genetic means are developed as an alternative to chemical crosslinking with the advantage of easier mass-production. The initial report in this field applied a fusion protein of anti-knob single-chain antibody (scFv) and EGF *(33)*. This fusion protein successfully enhanced gene delivery to EGF-receptor positive malignancies. A slightly different fusion protein based system for bridging a targeting moiety to adenovirus uses the extracellular domain of CAR, which binds to the Ad5 fiber-knob region. Combined with the EGF ligand for target recognition, this fusion protein expressed in a Baculovirus system successfully retargeted Ad to EGFR positive cells *(34)*. In contrast with these two methods, which employ extrinsic bridging molecules, genetically modified viruses based on alteration of the viral genome offer several distinct benefits. The most obvious advantage is that production of genetically modified viruses is much simpler relative to targeting conjugates because all components are encoded in the viral genome. So far, several targeting moieties have been successfully incorporated into adenoviruses. An integrin-binding motif and polylysine were successfully incorporated in the carboxyl terminus of fiber *(35)*, whereas the FLAG octapeptide *(36)* and RGD-4C integrin-binding peptide *(37)* were placed in the HI-loop of fiber knob region, yielding clear targeting function. On the other hand, there have been many failed attempts in genetic incorporation of targeting motif into Ad. For example, whereas the HI-loop tolerated the vasoactive intestinal peptide (VIP) sequence, the infectivity of this virus did not show augmented transduction in receptor positive cells *(38)*. This may indicate that successful incorporation does not always translate into successful targeting.

Attempts have also been made to genetically incorporate onto the Ad capsid Ab and scFv, which have clear benefits as target moieties as a result of their high specificity. With the range of current genetic approaches, incorporating these targeting moieties while retaining functionality still remains difficult. For example, although a scFv was successfully incorporated into the Ad capsid as a fusion protein with pIX, it did not show its original binding ability (unpublished data). The reason for this discrepancy has not been clearly elucidated although possible explanations include scFv accessibility, alteration of capsid trafficking, and scFv processing. Instead of using either conjugate-based or genetic strategies above, the combination of both strategies may complement their respective shortcomings. An example of such combination was pursued by incorporating the Fc binding domain from protein A or G into adenovirus *(39–41)*. Because these motifs effectively bind to antibodies, this vector structure enables easy incorporation of various kinds of Abs for targeting. Theoretically, this method has large potential benefit since established antibodies with high affinity and selectivity can be easily exploited to achieve the desired targeting.

A completely different strategy for targeting is to complex Ad with polyethylene glycol (PEG). Because the Ad capsid would not be exposed after PEGylation, this method creates a stealth-like As vector to neutralization in the blood and also eliminate undesired binding to non-target tissues/cells *(42,43)*. In addition, PEGylation permits incorporation of extrinsic targeting ligand on the surface of the PEG capsule. For example, RGD peptide and anti-E-selectin Ab incorporated on the surface of PEG successfully allowed selective transduction of αv integrin and E-selectin positive cells, respectively *(44)*.

3.2. Transcriptional Targeting

Another major adenoviral targeting strategy is to control the expression of the therapeutic gene by using transcriptional regulatory elements (*see* Fig. 3). In the human genome, genes are controlled by distinct promoters *(45)*, which are applicable for the control of transgene expression from an adenovirus vector *(46)*.

The most straightforward way is to place the specific promoter in the 5′-upstream region of the transgene placed in the vector. The transcription cassette with the specific promoter is usually placed in the E1-deleted region in both directions *(47)*. Various transgenes can be incorporated, including reporter genes (e.g., luciferase, β-galactosidase, fluorescent proteins), prodrug activating enzyme (e.g., thymidine kinase, cytosine deaminase). If the adenovirus E1 region (required for replication) is placed under the control of any exogenous promoter, the vector can achieve conditional replication depending on the promoter activity *(18,48,49)*. However, many factors (e.g., intrinsic transcription activation activity and enhancer elements of vector backbone, removal of distant control elements during cloning, and absence of histones) may possibly affect promoter profiles after incorporation in an adenoviral vector system. The most important consideration is that not all promoters showing a suitable profile in plasmid-based experiments will maintain the desired selectivity and strength in an adenovirus vector configuration.

A second way of transcriptional targeting is to use artificially modified or structured promoters to achieve the desired control. In general, promoters consists of core promoter elements including transcription initiation sites, and number of enhancer elements in up- or down-stream of the core region. Those enhancer regions may exist far upstream or sometime in the intron of the gene itself. To configure these elements *(50,51)* or to create new promoters with the required transcription selectivity *(52)*, elements from one or multiple promoters may have to be combined into artificial promoters. This method has big potential for the development of custom-designed transcription profiles. On the other hand, because the activity of newly created promoters is not completely predictable, it has the potential risk to lead to aberrant expression (e.g., unexpected high activity in normal organs, leakiness resulting from the removal of unidentified negative control elements, and so forth). The establishment of appropriate promoter design strategies and high efficient methods for screening are necessary to advance the development of this strategy for Ad targeting.

An extension of using promoters for Ad transcriptional targeting is the application of inducible promoters for the regulation of the expression. There are several promoters known to be inducible by an external nontoxic stimuli (e.g., tetracycline *[53]*) or radiation *(54)*. These promoters are useful should post-administrative regulation of transgene expression be necessary. Also, some vectors which encode highly toxic genes may need negative regulation of expression during viral amplification in order to avoid effects on virus replicaiton *(55,56)*.

Another approach in transcriptional targeting is based on a binary system. This system uses a specific promoter to express a triggering protein which binds to a regulatory element that turns on the transcription of an extrinsic gene *(57)*. Similar effect is also achievable by using the bactriophage RNA polymerase and its recognition sequence *(58)* or with CRE recombinase and its recognition sequence (lox-p) *(59)*. This strategy is extremely useful for constructing an expression system to enhance "selective but weak" promoters although the vector structure and regulation mechanism are more complex than the use of conventional strategies *(60)*.

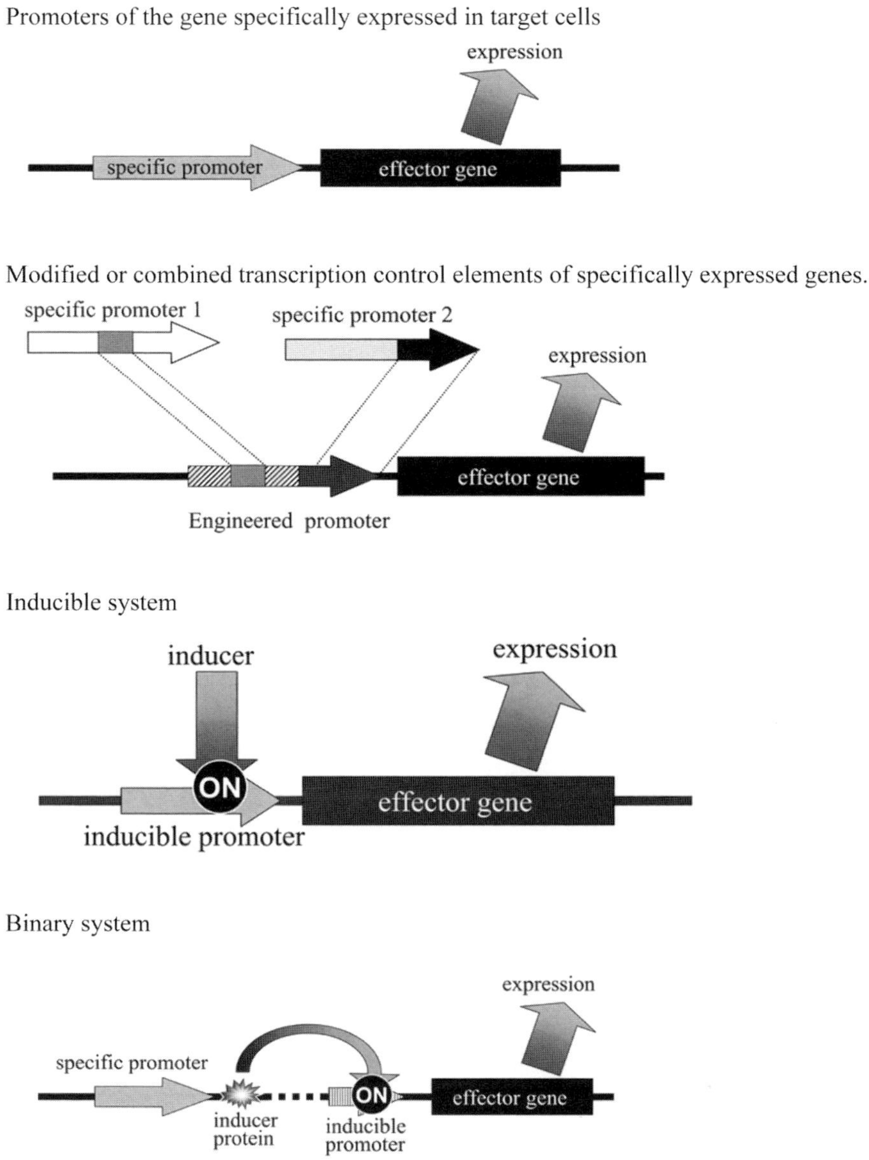

Fig. 3. Methods for transcriptinal retargeting of adenovirus.

4. ADENOVIRAL RETARGETING FOR CANCER GENE THERAPY

A gene therapy for various disease settings requires different selectivity and targeting, highlighting the importance of choosing the right strategy for successful gene therapy. In the field of cancer gene therapy, aggressively proliferating cells need to be killed or suppressed. This unique situation demands multiple levels of function in order to achieve a therapeutic effect. First, virtually all tumor cells must be killed because any remaining viable cancer cells would lead to tumor regrowth. Second, the cytocidal effect needs to be limited to cancer cells, except in limited cases where the payload gene possesses tumor selectivity. In most cases, the transgene used for cancer gene therapy is nonselective. Such nonselectivity indicates that specificity must be achieved at the vector level without impeding killing potency in order to develop clinically usable cancer gene therapy strategies *(6,61)*.

4.1. Augmentation of Infectivity

As mentioned above, augmentation of infectivity in CAR-negative cells is an important issue for adenoviral gene therapy *(62)*. To obtain CAR-independent viral entry, various transductional targeting strategies have been applied. The most frequently used targets are the epidermal growth factor receptor (EGFR) *(33,63)* and the fibroblast growth factor receptor (FGFR) *(30,64)*, which are closely linked to the malignant potential of the tumor cells. Although retargeting to these receptors have been accomplished successfully with conjugate-based systems, consistent manufacturing of uniform bispecific antibody conjugates is considerably difficult. Alternatively, retargeting with fusion proteins against these receptors maybe more advantageous from a pharmaceutical manufacturing standpoint *(34)*.

In comparison with the strategies using targeting conjugates/fusion proteins, genetic modification of the virus has several benefits. The process of vector formulation is much more simple than bridging the virus with an extrinsic moiety because the generated vector would already possess the intended targeting capability. Because upscale production requires high a standard of the stability, this simplicity is a big advantage when considering drug production and clinical application. On the other hand, whereas the genetic incorporation of extrinsic ligands have assisted in efficiently expanding the infection tropism, selectivity has not been high compared with antibodies. Among the various methods, integrin-binding RGD motif incorporation into the HI-loop *(37)* or carboxyl terminus (c-terminus) *(29)* of the fiber, polylysine incorporation into fiber c-terminus *(29)*, and replacement of the Ad5 knob with the other serotypes knob with broader binding tropism (e.g., Ad5/Ad3 chimera) *(65)* have provided dramatic enhancement of infectivity in CAR-negative cancer cells.

Lately, many adenoviruses with tumor-selective replication capability (conditionally replicative adenovirus, CRAd) were developed, and some of them are already in human clinical trials *(48,49,66)*. Although this replicative strategy should overcome poor transduction of the tumor cells, the infectivity of the progeny virus would affect the viral spread during each replication cycle *(62)*. Thus, infectivity enhancement is beneficial in augmenting the therapeutic effect of these viruses *(62)*. We have developed promoter driven CRAds with RGD modified and 5/3 chimera fibers *(18,19,67)*. Both versions, especially the Ad5/Ad3 chimera, showed dramatically enhanced cytocidal effect in vitro and in vivo. Some of these vectors are in preclinical toxicological studies with the goal of reaching clinical trials (RGD CRAdcox2F, Ad5-Δ24RGD).

4.2. Configuration of Selectivity

Selectivity in the context of cancer gene therapy involves two aspects: tumor vs normal cell selectivity in the tumor locale and systemic organ selectivity. Both levels of selectivity have been sought either by transductional or transcriptional means.

Tumor vs normal cell selectivity is achievable by using the cell-surface protein profile as a target for transductional targeting or by employing a promoter with the required activity profile. As targets in transductional targeting, cell-surface proteins with expression profiles that closely correlate with the malignant potential or prognosis (e.g., EGFR for esophageal cancers) are suitable. In addition, promoters of proteins that contribute to malignant potential and/or cancer progression can also be used for targeting (e.g., COX-2 *[6,68]*, Survivin *[69,70]*, CXCR4 *[71,72]*). Promoter-based strategies may provide simple and practical solutions for achieving the required level of selectivity.

For organ selectivity, the biggest issue with adenoviral vectors is transduction of the liver. Liver parenchymal cells express high levels of CAR *(2,73)*, leading to the majority of gene expression observed in the liver from adenovirus administered or released into the systemic circulation *(6,74)*. Thus, in the field of adenoviral vectors, not only tumor retargeting but also liver untargeting should also be implemented *(62)*.

Transductional liver untargeting can be achieved with several different ways. The first is mutation of the CAR binding motif in the fiber-knob region. When combined with mutation of RGD motif of penton base region, this method achieved almost 4 order reduction of liver transduction *(75,76)*. Another way to detarget the liver is removal of the cationic motif in the fiber shaft region (KKTK) *(77)*. However, there is no clear conclusion about the consistency of these methods because the experimental results vary depending on the experimental system *(78)*. One problem associated with deletion of binding regions for untargeting is that the vector production yield drops if the mutation hampers the cell binding required for the production. In this case, addition of another binding motif is required to restore the viral infectivity in the producer cells *(75)*.

Transcriptional liver untargeting can also be achieved by using various promoters with tumor-ON/liver-OFF profiles. For example, the prostate specific antigen (PSA) promoter for prostate cancer *(79)*, cyclooxygenase 2 (cox-2) promoter for gastrointestinal cancers *(6)*, midkine promoter for pediatric malignancies *(61)* have shown high specificity for their respective target tumor context while maintaining low liver activity. Also, some promoters (e.g., tyrosinase promoter *[80]*, cox-2 promoter *[19]*) have shown profitable tumor versus nontumor ratios. The utility of these promoters has been integrated into the concept of suicide gene therapy and displayed the mitigation of toxicity in nontarget cells *(6,61)*. Although various suicide gene therapy protocols have been tested in clinical trials, none of them has shown a remarkable clinical therapeutic effect. However, the combination of transcriptional targeting with the above-mentioned infectivity enhancement strategies may lead to improved clinical efficacy.

5. PROBLEMS ASSOCIATED WITH ADENOVIRAL RETARGETING IN THE FIELD OF CANCER GENE THERAPY AND CURRENT EFFORTS

In 1995, the National Institutes of Health (NIH) director designated a special advisory panel headed by Drs. Orkin and Motulsky which produced a report about the limiting issues in the field of gene therapy and the points in the report are still valid *(81)*. One of the main points was that vector systems still have problems and need to be improved to realize the benefit of gene therapy. Recently there have been several promising reports indicating the clinical benefits of gene therapy in severe combined immunodeficiency mice (SCID) *(82)* and cardiovascular disease *(83,84)*, yet, the realization of the clinical/therapeutic potential of the cancer gene therapy has not been achieved.

Success in gene therapy relies not only on the vector used but also the pathological/physiological profile of the disease as the target. For example, hemophilia has been a candidate target for gene therapy since the research in the field began and is considered to be a relatively simple disease to address because even partial restoration can avoid the severe complications of transgene expression need not be restricted to specific sites *(85)*. However, in the field of cancer, the requirements are totally different and much more stringent. Clinical trial outcomes indicate that current adenoviral therapeutics are well tolerated in the clinical setting but not potent enough to elicit significant and consistent therapeutic effect *(86)*. Thus, augmentation of the antitumor effect of adenoviral vectors is a priority at this time although a higher degree of selectivity needs to be established as potency increases to avoid adverse effects against normal cells *(62)*. To this end, the agent must kill or suppress virtually the whole tumor because even a fraction of residual viable tumor cells can easily lead to the tumor regrowth. Particularly in the case of cancer gene therapy, the situation is further complicated by the inaccessibility of the cancer cells from blood stream. Li et al. reported that tumor vascularity and the amount of extra cellular matrix can determine transduction in a liver metastasis model *(87)*. Whereas target accessibility represents a challenging obstacle, better targeting and infectivity enhancement methods will overcome this issue.

Although there are various candidate targeting strategies as described above, the practicality of clinical grade vector preparation is another determining factor for clinical utility. For example, extensively modified vectors may show lower yield during vector production. These vectors would require a larger preparation to obtain the required titers, and low-yield vectors tend to face contamination issues more frequently because mutants which can propagate with higher yield can easily dominate the batch. Because of the stringent standards of consistency and stability in producing clinical grade agents, this issue should be considered when designing strategies for cancer gene therapy therapeutics.

At the present time, genetic modification of the fiber by using small peptide sequence insertions and subtype switching of the fiber/knob region appear to have the highest practicality for the augmentation of infectivity *(29,37,65)*. These methods can significantly augment vector infectivity via binding to target moieties on the cell surface. Because the modifications are genetically encoded on the viral genome, there are no limiting steps in the production of the targeted vectors after vector production. However, these targeting methods are not highly selective at this time. Adenovirus with Ad5/Ad3 chimeric fiber shows very wide tropism for a variety of normal and cancerous cells of many origins. As a result, combining infectivity enhancement with transcriptional targeting represents a promising approach to obtain both effective gene delivery as well as selectivity of the therapeutic effect.

As an example of this strategy, we employed the combination of fiber modification-based infectivity enhancement and promoter-based selectivity to construct conditionally replicative adenovirus (CRAd) for further improving therapeutic efficacy *(18,19)*. In a CRAd system, selective replication in the target cancer cells results in a cytocidal effect as a result of the lytic nature of the adenovirus, followed by infection of the surrounding cancer cells with the progeny virus *(49)*. We employed an RGD-4C motif insertion into the fiber-knob region (RGD modification) *(18)* or the replacement of the Ad5 knob with the Ad3 knob (Ad5/Ad3 chimeric) *(19)* to enable CAR-independent infection in gastrointestinal cancer target cells which are usually CAR-negative (e.g., pancreatic cancer *[15]*, esophageal adenocarcinoma *[16]*). In parallel, the Cox-2 promoter, which is commonly active in these target cells but inactive in many organs including the liver under normal conditions *(6)*, was employed to achieve replication selectivity. Applying this combination, we successfully constructed GI cancer CRAds which showed strong cytocidal effect in CAR-negative GI cancer cells without hampering the replication selectivity for Cox-2 positive cancers both in vitro and in vivo

(18,19). These CRAds have high potential for the treatment of CAR-negative, Cox-2-positive cancers such as many GI cancers *(62)*.

6. FUTURE DIRECTIONS

Current targeting strategies are not fully adequate for realizing the promise of cancer gene therapy. Combining existing strategies provides a practical solution; however, new targeting modalities should be explored because each tumor context opens unique challenges with respect to disease targeting. The following strategies are promising approached for the development of next-generation targeted adenovirus vectors for cancer gene therapy:

6.1. Infectivity Enhancement Strategies

As mentioned above, the primary problem of current gene therapy is efficacy. To achieve this goal, new infectivity enhancement strategies need to be sought to develop the next generation of vectors.

In the field of adenovirus, interesting direction is exploration of new locales for ligand insertion. We have sought various locales in the capsid which would permit insertion of large motifs for targeting and/or labeling purposes without hampering viral functionality. Protein IX, which exists between the hexon proteins, permits large insertions in the c-terminus of the protein *(88–90)*. Capitalizing the tolerability of this locale, we successfully introduced relatively large proteins, including single chain antibodies (unpublished data), green fluorescent protein *(91)*, and firefly luciferase (unpublished data) into the Ad capsid. Because various ligands have various requirements in terms of placement and the environment of ligand presentation, seeking alternative motif insertion locales need to continue as well.

Another attractive approach is taking advantage of the variable natural tropisms of the adenoviruses of other adenoviral types, including those of other serotypes, xenotypes, and nonadenoviral viruses. Canine, avian, and mice adenovirus fibers have been successfully configured into human Ad based viruses and showed interesting tropism *(92)*. The fiber of reovirus was also recently incorporated into adenoviral capsid *(93,94)*. These efforts will expand the choice of fibers for genetic capsid modification.

6.2. Strategies for Selective Amplification

As briefly mentioned above, conditionally replicative adenoviruses (CRAds) have great potential in the field of cancer gene therapy *(48,49,62)*. Cancer gene therapy requires tumor-wide therapeutic effect in a vast majority of the cancer cells. In this context, infectivity-enhanced CRAds can achieve such wide spread effect by spreading to the surrounding cancer cells via viral progeny infection *(18,19,67)*. Because each tumor type requires different targeting methods, both transductional and transcriptional targeting need to be developed and optimized for each CRAd for each individual disease context.

Another interesting idea is to use CRAds as a modality to support the amplification of E1-deleted vectors in target cells. Alemany et al. showed that a gutless vector conditionally expressing the E1 gene and an E1-deleted vector can trans-complement each other and replicate *(95)*. In another case, an E1B55k-deleted conditionally replicative virus was combined with a replication-incompetent interleukin-12 expression vector, enhanced antitumor effect was observed as a result of dramatically augmented interleukin-12 expression *(96)*. Although precise control of replication of each virus may be difficult, this system is relatively easy to construct and provides large cloning capacity. In this meaning, the versatility of this system may lead to interesting vector systems in the future.

7. CONCLUSION

Although adenovirus retargeting is promising and advancing, no retargeted adenoviral system has been tested in clinical trials yet. Reliable preclinical and subsequent clinical studies are necessary to establish a legitimate role of adenoviral retargeting in the field of cancer gene therapy. However, it is absolutely clear that better vector targeting yielding improved efficiency and selectivity would lead to the development of more potent and safe adenovirus based therapies in the field of cancer.

ACKNOWLEDGMENTS

This work is supported in part by National Institutes of Health grants R01 DK63615, P20CA101955 (project 4), Department of Defense grant DAMD17-03-1-0104 to M.Y., and National Institutes of Health grants R01 CA94084, R01 HL67962, P50 CA89019, RO1 CA86881, R01 AG021875, and R01 CA090547 to D. T. C. We appreciate Dr. Long P. Le for excellent advise and suggestions.

REFERENCES

1. Hallenbeck PL, Chang YN, Hay C, et al. A novel tumor-specific replication-restricted adenoviral vector for gene therapy of hepatocellular carcinoma. Hum Gene Ther 1999;10:1721–1733.
2. Tomko RP, Xu R, Philipson L. HCAR and MCAR: the human and mouse cellular receptors for subgroup C adenoviruses and group B coxsackieviruses. Proc Natl Acad Sci U S A 1997;94:3352–3356.
3. Bergelson JM, Cunningham JA, Droguett G, et al. Isolation of a common receptor for Coxsackie B viruses and adenoviruses 2 and 5. Science 1997;275:1320–1323.
4. Huard J, Lochmuller H, Acsadi G, Jani A, Massie B, Karpati G. The route of administration is a major determinant of the transduction efficiency of rat tissues by adenoviral recombinants. Gene Ther 1995;2:107–115.
5. Reynolds P, Dmitriev I, Curiel D. Insertion of an RGD motif into the HI loop of adenovirus fiber protein alters the distribution of transgene expression of the systemically administered vector. Gene Ther 1999;6:1336–1339.
6. Yamamoto M, Alemany R, Adachi Y, Grizzle WE, Curiel DT. Characterization of the cyclooxygenase-2 promoter in an adenoviral vector and its application for the mitigation of toxicity in suicide gene therapy of gastrointestinal cancers. Mol Ther 2001;3:385–394.
7. Smith T, Idamakanti N, Kylefjord H, et al. In vivo hepatic adenoviral gene delivery occurs independently of the coxsackievirus-adenovirus receptor. Mol Ther 2002;5:770–779.
8. Shayakhmetov DM, Li ZY, Ni S, Lieber A. Analysis of adenovirus sequestration in the liver, transduction of hepatic cells, and innate toxicity after injection of fiber-modified vectors. J Virol 2004;78:5368–5381.
9. Akiyama M, Thorne S, Kirn D, et al. Ablating CAR and integrin binding in adenovirus vectors reduces nontarget organ transduction and permits sustained bloodstream persistence following intraperitoneal administration. Mol Ther 2004;9:218–230.
10. Eisensmith RC, Woo SL. Viral vector-mediated gene therapy for hemophilia B. Thromb Haemost 1997;78:24–30.
11. VandenDriessche T, Collen D, Chuah MK. Viral vector-mediated gene therapy for hemophilia. Curr Gene Ther 2001;1:301–315.
12. Dachs GU, Dougherty GJ, Stratford IJ, Chaplin DJ. Targeting gene therapy to cancer: a review. Oncol Res 1997;9:313–325.
13. van der Eb MM, Cramer SJ, Vergouwe Y, et al. Severe hepatic dysfunction after adenovirus-mediated transfer of the herpes simplex virus thymidine kinase gene and ganciclovir administration. Gene Ther 1998;5:451–458.

14. Bilbao R, Gerolami R, Bralet MP, et al. Transduction efficacy, antitumoral effect, and toxicity of adenovirus- mediated herpes simplex virus thymidine kinase/ganciclovir therapy of hepatocellular carcinoma: the woodchuck animal model. Cancer Gene Ther 2000;7:657–662.
15. Wesseling JG, Bosma PJ, Krasnykh V, et al. Improved gene transfer efficiency to primary and established human pancreatic carcinoma target cells via epidermal growth factor receptor and integrin-targeted adenoviral vectors. Gene Ther 2001;8:969–976.
16. Schrump DS, Chen GA, Consuli U, Jin X, Roth JA. Inhibition of esophageal cancer proliferation by adenovirally mediated delivery of p16INK4. Cancer Gene Ther 1996;3:357–364.
17. Buskens CJ, Marsman WA, Wesseling JG, et al. A genetically retargeted adenoviral vector enhances viral transduction in esophageal carcinoma cell lines and primary cultured esophageal resection specimens. Ann Surg 2003;238:815–824; discussion 825–826.
18. Yamamoto M, Davydova J, Wang M, et al. Infectivity enhanced, cyclooxygenase-2 promoter-based conditionally replicative adenovirus for pancreatic cancer. Gastroenterology 2003;125: 1203–1218.
19. Davydova J, Le L, Gavrikova T, Wang M, Krasnykh V, Yamamoto M. Infectivity-enhanced cyclooxygenase-2-based conditionally replicative adenoviruses for esophageal adenocarcinoma. Cancer Res 2004;64:4319–4327.
20. Ono HA, Davydova JG, Adachi Y, et al. Promoter-controlled infectivity enhanced conditionally replicative adenoviral vectors for the treatment of gastric cancer. J Gastroenterol 2005;40:31–42.
21. Tekant Y, Davydova J, Ramirez PJ, Curiel DT, Vickers SM, Yamamoto M. Oncolytic adenoviral therapy in gallbladder carcinoma. Surgery 2005;137:527–535.
22. Hong SS, Karayan L, Tournier J, Curiel DT, Boulanger PA. Adenovirus type 5 fiber knob binds to MHC class I alpha2 domain at the surface of human epithelial and B lymphoblastoid cells. EMBO J 1997;16:2294–2306.
23. Cohen CJ, Shieh JT, Pickles RJ, Okegawa T, Hsieh JT, Bergelson JM. The coxsackievirus and adenovirus receptor is a transmembrane component of the tight junction. Proc Natl Acad Sci U S A 2001;98:15,191–15,196.
24. Philipson L, Pettersson RF. The coxsackie-adenovirus receptor—a new receptor in the immunoglobulin family involved in cell adhesion. Curr Top Microbiol Immunol 2004;273:87–111.
25. Wickham TJ, Mathias P, Cheresh DA, Nemerow GR. Integrins alpha v beta 3 and alpha v beta 5 promote adenovirus internalization but not virus attachment. Cell 1993;73:309–319.
26. Shenk T. Adenoviridae: The Viruses and Their Replication. In: Virology, vol. 2, Fields B, Knipe D, Howley P, eds. Philadelphia: Lipponcott-Raven,1996;2111–2148.
27. Curiel DT. Strategies to adapt adenoviral vectors for targeted delivery. Ann N Y Acad Sci 1999;886:158–171.
28. Douglas JT, Rogers BE, Rosenfeld ME, Michael SI, Feng M, Curiel DT. Targeted gene delivery by tropism-modified adenoviral vectors. Nat Biotechnol 1996;14:1574–1578.
29. Wickham TJ, Segal DM, Roelvink PW, et al. Targeted adenovirus gene transfer to endothelial and smooth muscle cells by using bispecific antibodies. J Virol 1996;70:6831–6838.
30. Rogers BE, Douglas JT, Ahlem C, Buchsbaum DJ, Frincke J, Curiel DT. Use of a novel cross-linking method to modify adenovirus tropism. Gene Ther 1997;4:1387–1392.
31. MacDonald LR, Patt BE, Iwanczyk JS, Tsui BMW, Wang Y, Frey E, Wessel DE, Acton PD, Kung HF. Pinhole SPECT of mice using the LumaGem Gamma Camera. 2001.
32. Reynolds PN, Nicklin SA, Kaliberova L, et al. Combined transductional and transcriptional targeting improves the specificity of transgene expression in vivo. Nat Biotechnol 2001;19:838–842.
33. Watkins SJ, Mesyanzhinov VV, Kurochkina LP, Hawkins RE. The 'adenobody' approach to viral targeting: specific and enhanced adenoviral gene delivery. Gene Ther 1997;4:1004–1012.
34. Dmitriev I, Kashentseva E, Rogers BE, Krasnykh V, Curiel DT. Ectodomain of coxsackievirus and adenovirus receptor genetically fused to epidermal growth factor mediates adenovirus targeting to epidermal growth factor receptor-positive cells. J Virol 2000;74:6875–6884.
35. Wickham TJ, Tzeng E, Shears LL, 2nd, et al. Increased in vitro and in vivo gene transfer by adenovirus vectors containing chimeric fiber proteins. J Virol 1997;71:8221–8229.
36. Krasnykh V, Dmitriev I, Mikheeva G, Miller CR, Belousova N, Curiel DT. Characterization of an adenovirus vector containing a heterologous peptide epitope in the HI loop of the fiber knob. J Virol 1998;72:1844–1852.
37. Dmitriev I, Krasnykh V, Miller CR, et al. An adenovirus vector with genetically modified fibers demonstrates expanded tropism via utilization of a coxsackievirus and adenovirus receptor-independent cell entry mechanism. J Virol 1998;72:9706–9713.

38. Belousova N, Krendelchtchikova V, Curiel DT, Krasnykh V. Modulation of adenovirus vector tropism via incorporation of polypeptide ligands into the fiber protein. J Virol 2002;76:8621–8631.
39. Korokhov N, Mikheeva G, Krendelshchikov A, et al. Targeting of adenovirus via genetic modification of the viral capsid combined with a protein bridge. J Virol 2003;77:12,931–12,340.
40. Volpers C, Thirion C, Biermann V, et al. Antibody-mediated targeting of an adenovirus vector modified to contain a synthetic immunoglobulin g-binding domain in the capsid. J Virol 2003;77: 2093–2104.
41. Henning P, Magnusson MK, Gunneriusson E, et al. Genetic modification of adenovirus 5 tropism by a novel class of ligands based on a three-helix bundle scaffold derived from staphylococcal protein A. Hum Gene Ther 2002;13:1427–1439.
42. O'Riordan CR, Lachapelle A, Delgado C, et al. PEGylation of adenovirus with retention of infectivity and protection from neutralizing antibody in vitro and in vivo. Hum Gene Ther 1999;10:1349–1358.
43. Chillon M, Lee JH, Fasbender A, Welsh MJ. Adenovirus complexed with polyethylene glycol and cationic lipid is shielded from neutralizing antibodies in vitro. Gene Ther 1998;5:995–1002.
44. Ogawara K-i, Tots MG, Kok RJ, et al. A Novel Strategy to Modify Adenovirus Tropism and Enhance Transgene Delivery to Activated Vascular Endothelial Cells In Vitro and In Vivo. Hum Gene Ther 2004;15:433–443.
45. Lewin B. Genes VII. Oxford, 2000.
46. Galanis E, Vile R, Russell SJ. Delivery systems intended for in vivo gene therapy of cancer: targeting and replication competent viral vectors. Crit Rev Oncol Hematol 2001;38:177–192.
47. Hitt MM, Addison CL, Graham FL. Human adenovirus vectors for gene transfer into mammalian cells. Adv Pharmacol 1997;40:137–206.
48. Curiel DT. The development of conditionally replicative adenoviruses for cancer therapy. Clin Cancer Res 2000;6:3395–3399.
49. Alemany R, Balague C, Curiel DT. Replicative adenoviruses for cancer therapy. Nat Biotechnol 2000;18:723–727.
50. Takahashi M, Sato T, Sagawa T, et al. E1B-55K-deleted adenovirus expressing E1A-13S by AFP-enhancer/promoter is capable of highly specific replication in AFP-producing hepatocellular carcinoma and eradication of established tumor. Mol Ther 2002;5:627–634.
51. Zhang L, Adams JY, Billick E, et al. Molecular engineering of a two-step transcription amplification (TSTA) system for transgene delivery in prostate cancer. Mol Ther 2002;5:223–232.
52. Furuhata S, Ide H, Miura Y, Yoshida T, Aoki K. Development of a prostate-specific promoter for gene therapy against androgen-independent prostate cancer. Mol Ther 2003;7:366–374.
53. Nakagawa S, Massie B, Hawley RG. Tetracycline-regulatable adenovirus vectors: pharmacologic properties and clinical potential. Eur J Pharm Sci 2001;13:53–60.
54. Vereecque R, Saudemont A, Wickham TJ, et al. Gamma-irradiation enhances transgene expression in leukemic cells. Gene Ther 2003;10:227–233.
55. Edholm D, Molin M, Bajak E, Akusjarvi G. Adenovirus vector designed for expression of toxic proteins. J Virol 2001;75:9579–9584.
56. Kagawa S, Pearson SA, Ji L, et al. A binary adenoviral vector system for expressing high levels of the proapoptotic gene bax. Gene Ther 2000;7:75–79.
57. Burcin MM, Schiedner G, Kochanek S, Tsai SY, O'Malley BW. Adenovirus-mediated regulable target gene expression in vivo. Proc Natl Acad Sci U S A 1999;96:355–360.
58. Tomanin R, Bett AJ, Picci L, Scarpa M, Graham FL. Development and characterization of a binary gene expression system based on bacteriophage T7 components in adenovirus vectors. Gene 1997;193:129–140.
59. Sato Y, Tanaka K, Lee G, et al. Enhanced and specific gene expression via tissue-specific production of Cre recombinase using adenovirus vector. Biochem Biophys Res Commun 1998;244:455–462.
60. Koch PE, Guo ZS, Kagawa S, Gu J, Roth JA, Fang B. Augmenting transgene expression from carcinoembryonic antigen (CEA) promoter via a GAL4 gene regulatory system. Mol Ther 2001;3: 278–283.
61. Adachi Y, Raynolds PN, Yamamoto M, et al. Midkine Promoter-Based Adenovirus Vector Gene Delivery for Pediatric Solid Tumors. Cancer Res 2000;60:4305–4310.
62. Yamamoto M. Conditionally replicative adenovirus (CRAd) for gastrointestinal cancers. Expert Opin Biol Ther 2004;4:1241–1250.
63. Miller CR, Buchsbaum DJ, Reynolds PN, et al. Differential susceptibility of primary and established human glioma cells to adenovirus infection: targeting via the epidermal growth factor receptor achieves fiber receptor-independent gene transfer. Cancer Res 1998;58:5738–5748.

64. Gu DL, Gonzalez AM, Printz MA, et al. Fibroblast growth factor 2 retargeted adenovirus has redirected cellular tropism: evidence for reduced toxicity and enhanced antitumor activity in mice. Cancer Res 1999;59:2608–2614.
65. Krasnykh VN, Mikheeva GV, Douglas JT, Curiel DT. Generation of recombinant adenovirus vectors with modified fibers for altering viral tropism. J Virol 1996;70:6839–6846.
66. Kirn D. Replication-selective oncolytic adenoviruses: virotherapy aimed at genetic targets in cancer. Oncogene 2000;19:6660–6669.
67. Suzuki K, Fueyo J, Krasnykh V, Reynolds PN, Curiel DT, Alemany R. A conditionally replicative adenovirus with enhanced infectivity shows improved oncolytic potency. Clin Cancer Res 2001;7:120–126.
68. Godbey WT, Atala A. Directed apoptosis in Cox-2-overexpressing cancer cells through expression-targeted gene delivery. Gene Ther 2003;10:1519–1527.
69. Altieri DC. Survivin, versatile modulation of cell division and apoptosis in cancer. Oncogene 2003;22:8581–8589.
70. Zhu ZB, Makhija SK, Lu B, et al. Transcriptional targeting of tumors with a novel tumor-specific survivin promoter. Cancer Gene Ther 2004;11:256–262.
71. Murphy PM. Chemokines and the molecular basis of cancer metastasis. N Engl J Med 2001;345: 833–835.
72. Zhu ZB, Makhija SK, Lu B, et al. Transcriptional targeting of adenoviral vector through the CXCR4 tumor-specific promoter. Gene Ther 2004;11:645–648.
73. Bergelson JM, Krithivas A, Celi L, et al. The murine CAR homolog is a receptor for coxsackie B viruses and adenoviruses. J Virol 1998;72:415–419.
74. Zinn KR, Douglas JT, Smyth CA, et al. Imaging and tissue biodistribution of 99mTc-labeled adenovirus knob (serotype 5). Gene Ther 1998;5:798–808.
75. Einfeld DA, Schroeder R, Roelvink PW, et al. Reducing the native tropism of adenovirus vectors requires removal of both CAR and integrin interactions. J Virol 2001;75:11,284–11,291.
76. Roelvink PW, Mi L G, Einfeld DA, Kovesdi I, Wickham TJ. Identification of a conserved receptor-binding site on the fiber proteins of CAR-recognizing adenoviridae. Science 1999;286:1568–1571.
77. Smith TA, Idamakanti N, Rollence ML, et al. Adenovirus serotype 5 fiber shaft influences in vivo gene transfer in mice. Hum Gene Ther 2003;14:777–787.
78. Smith TA, Idamakanti N, Marshall-Neff J, et al. Receptor interactions involved in adenoviral-mediated gene delivery after systemic administration in non-human primates. Hum Gene Ther 2003;14:1595–1604.
79. Adams JY, Johnson M, Sato M, et al. Visualization of advanced human prostate cancer lesions in living mice by a targeted gene transfer vector and optical imaging. Nat Med 2002;8:891–897.
80. Nettelbeck DM, Rivera AA, Balague C, Alemany R, Curiel DT. Novel oncolytic adenoviruses targeted to melanoma: specific viral replication and cytolysis by expression of E1A mutants from the tyrosinase enhancer/promoter. Cancer Res 2002;62:4663–4670.
81. Orkin SH, Motulsky AG. Report and recommendation of the panel to assess the NIH invesment in research on gene therapy. National Institutes of Health, 1995.
82. Hacein-Bey-Abina S, Le Deist F, Carlier F, et al. Sustained correction of X-linked severe combined immunodeficiency by ex vivo gene therapy. N Engl J Med 2002;346:1185–1193.
83. Losordo DW, Vale PR, Symes JF, et al. Gene therapy for myocardial angiogenesis: initial clinical results with direct myocardial injection of phVEGF165 as sole therapy for myocardial ischemia. Circulation 1998;98:2800–2804.
84. Losordo DW, Vale PR, Hendel RC, et al. Phase 1/2 placebo-controlled, double-blind, dose-escalating trial of myocardial vascular endothelial growth factor 2 gene transfer by catheter delivery in patients with chronic myocardial ischemia. Circulation 2002;105:2012–2018.
85. Walsh CE. Gene therapy progress and prospects: gene therapy for the hemophilias. Gene Ther 2003;10:999–1003.
86. Hecht JR, Bedford R, Abbruzzese JL, et al. A phase I/II trial of intratumoral endoscopic ultrasound injection of ONYX-015 with intravenous gemcitabine in unresectable pancreatic carcinoma. Clin Cancer Res 2003;9:555–561.
87. Li ZY, Ni S, Yang X, Kiviat N, Lieber A. Xenograft models for liver metastasis: Relationship between tumor morphology and adenovirus vector transduction. Mol Ther 2004;9:650–657.
88. Dmitriev IP, Kashentseva EA, Curiel DT. Engineering of adenovirus vectors containing heterologous peptide sequences in the C terminus of capsid protein IX. J Virol 2002;76:6893–6899.

89. Meulenbroek RA, Sargent KL, Lunde J, Jasmin BJ, Parks RJ. Use of adenovirus protein IX (pIX) to display large polypeptides on the virion—generation of fluorescent virus through the incorporation of pIX-GFP. Mol Ther 2004;9:617–624.
90. Vellinga J, Rabelink MJ, Cramer SJ, et al. Spacers increase the accessibility of peptide ligands linked to the carboxyl terminus of adenovirus minor capsid protein IX. J Virol 2004;78:3470–3479.
91. Le L, Everts M, Dmitriev I, Davydova J, Yamamoto M, Curiel D. Fluorescently labeled adenovirus with pIX-EGFP for vector detection. Mol Imaging 2004;3:105–116.
92. Glasgow JN, Kremer EJ, Hemminki A, Siegal GP, Douglas JT, Curiel DT. An adenovirus vector with a chimeric fiber derived from canine adenovirus type 2 displays novel tropism. Virology 2004;324:103–116.
93. Mercier GT, Campbell JA, Chappell JD, Stehle T, Dermody TS, Barry MA. A chimeric adenovirus vector encoding reovirus attachment protein sigma1 targets cells expressing junctional adhesion molecule 1. Proc Natl Acad Sci U S A 2004;101:6188–6193.
94. Tsuruta Y, Pereboeva L, Glasgow JN, et al. Infectivity Enhemcement of an Adenovirus Vector via Genetic Incorporation of the Reovirus Spike Protein Sigma 1. Mol Ther 2004;9:S50–S51.
95. Alemany R, Lai S, Lou YC, Jan HY, Fang X, Zhang WW. Complementary adenoviral vectors for oncolysis. Cancer Gene Ther 1999;6:21–25.
96. Nagayama Y, Nakao K, Mizuguchi H, Hayakawa T, Niwa M. Enhanced antitumor effect of combined replicative adenovirus and nonreplicative adenovirus expressing interleukin-12 in an immunocompetent mouse model. Gene Ther 2003;10:1400–1403.

13 Oncolytic Herpes Simplex for Gene Therapy in Preclinical and Clinical Trials

Richard H. Pin, MD, *Maura Reinblatt,* MD, *Yuman Fong,* MD, *and William R. Jarnagin,* MD

CONTENTS

Summary

The use of viruses to treat human malignancy is not a new concept but has only recently evolved into a clinically viable therapy. Spurred by advances in molecular biology that have allowed relatively easy manipulation of the viral genome, a number of different viruses have been evaluated and shown to have promise as anticancer agents. Of these, herpes simplex virus (HSV) has been perhaps the most intensively investigated. Several strains of replication competent oncolytic HSV have been developed, some of which have been used in clinical trials. Continuing research efforts are aimed at manipulating the viral genome to more specifically target tumor cells, to further enhance efficacy while maintaining safety, and to assess the role of oncolytic HSV in combination with chemotherapy and radiation therapy.

Key Words: Herpes simplex virus (HSV); oncolytic viral therapy.

1. INTRODUCTION

More than a century has passed since the possibility of using viral pathogens to treat cancer was first recognized. In 1893, remission of leukemia following natural viral infections was reported. Shortly thereafter, Pasteur observed regression of cervical cancer in a patient after vaccination with an attenuated rabies virus *(1)*. Anecdotes of tumor growth inhibition following bouts of severe viral illnesses, such as measles or mumps, were also reported. Initial, sporadic attempts to treat cancer with viruses yielded encouraging results *(2)*; however, the viral treatment for cancer was not pursued further because of fear of uncontrolled viral infection and lack of effective antiviral agents.

From: *Cancer Drug Discovery and Development: Gene Therapy for Cancer*
Edited by: K. K. Hunt, S. A. Vorburger, and S. G. Swisher © Humana Press Inc., Totowa, NJ

With advances in molecular biology, a better understanding of viral pathogenesis and the development of effective antiviral treatments, old notions of employing viruses to treat cancer were revisited. In the early 1990s, genetically engineered attenuated herpes simplex viruses (HSV) were developed and are now under investigation as potential cancer therapies *(3)*. The ability to modify the viral genome to selectively target tumor cells for lysis represented a major advance and has allowed oncolytic viral therapy to emerge as a viable and potentially important cancer therapy. A major focus of investigation in this regard has been the creation of viral strains with mutations or deletions of certain key genes, the protein products of which are expressed at higher levels in tumor cells compared with normal cells, thereby attenuating toxicity to normal tissues. Other efforts have involved the creation of tumor-specific promoters that control viral growth genes and modification of genes encoding viral envelope proteins to restrict viral infection to tumor cells that express specific receptors. Over the past 10 yr, oncolytic HSV have moved from the laboratory bench to patient care. Today, genetically engineered viruses are the most commonly used gene delivery vehicles in clinical trials, with three mutated HSV being tested in phase I studies *(4–6)*.

2. LYTIC CYCLE

HSV are comprised of an outer envelope, tegument, and inner capsid containing the viral genomic DNA (*see* Fig. 1). The virus first attaches to the cell through glycoproteins on the viral envelope that bind to receptors on the cell membrane. Once bound, the viral envelope delivers the tegument and capsid into the cytoplasm where the tegument transfers the capsid to the nucleus. Within the nucleus, the capsid releases the double-stranded viral DNA for replication and transcription (*see* Fig. 2). The viral tegument protein, VP16, initiates the cascade of gene expression. The *immediate-early genes* are the first set of genes transcribed and serve to promote the *early genes* that encode proteins required for viral replication. Once viral replication is initiated, the *late genes* necessary for viral assembly are activated. In this fashion, herpesviruses subvert the cellular machinery for their own replication. The new viral progeny that are produced ultimately lyse the cell and infect and lyse neighboring cells to repeat the replicative cycle. An attractive feature of replication competent HSV and other oncolytic viruses is that a large number of progeny virus arise from relatively few initially infected cells so that injection of a large viral load can be avoided, a feature now being exploited specifically to treat malignant disease.

3. ATTENUATION AND SAFETY

A number of different mutations in the genome of replication-competent viruses attenuate their toxicity to normal cells. The gene $\gamma_1$34.5 exists as two copies in the HSV genome and is largely responsible for neurotoxicity. The $\gamma_1$34.5 gene product prevents the infected host cell from shutting off its cellular machinery, a normal host response to viral infection, and allows ongoing viral replication. A deletion in the $\gamma_1$34.5 gene therefore hinders viral replication, and has been shown to limit viral spread within the central nervous system *(7)*. Another important gene for replication, UL39, encodes the enzyme ribonucleotide reductase (RR). This enzyme is essential for the reduction of ribonucleotides to deoxyribonucleotides, which form the DNA substrate pool *(8)*. Ribonucleotide reductase therefore plays a critical role in viral DNA synthesis, and deletions in RR limit viral replication. Eukaryotic cells also produce a cellular variant

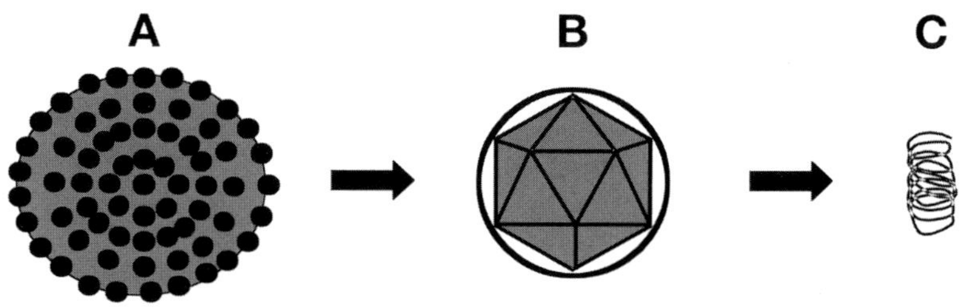

Fig. 1. HSV structure. (**A**) The viral envelope contains membrane-bound glycoproteins that aid in docking the virus and binding to receptors on the tumor cell membrane. (**B**) The proteinaceous tegument is released in the cytoplasm and guides the inner icosahedral capsid to the nucleus. (**C**) The capsid delivers the 152-kb double-stranded DNA viral genome to the nucleus.

of RR during cell division. This cellular RR has significant sequence homology to that of viral RR and can be used to promote viral replication in dividing cells *(9)*. Therefore, HSV with deletions in UL39 can only replicate in rapidly dividing cells, such as some cancer cells, which produce sufficiently high levels of exogenous, cellular RR *(10)*.

Additional mutations in the viral genome allow the host to respond more vigorously to viral infection. The ∀47 gene normally functions to down-regulate MHC class I peptides on the surface of virally infected cells. This cloaks an infected cell from the host's immune system. A mutation in the ∀47 gene enables major histocompatability complex (MHC) class I peptide expression, allowing antigen presentation to $CD8^+$ cells. This interaction improves the hosts ability to identify and destroy infected cells and limits the ability of virus to generate new progeny (Table 1) *(11)*.

Viruses have also been constructed with safety features that prevent undesired infection. A temperature-sensitive mutation in the immediate-early $\alpha 4$ gene leads to inhibition of viral replication at temperatures greater than 39.5°C, thereby offering some protection against a potentially serious viral-mediated illness. Furthermore, an intact thymidine kinase gene confers sensitivity to the antiherpetic drugs acyclovir and gancyclovir. These additional safeguards make attenuated HSV an attractive vector for cancer gene therapy.

4. VIRAL ONCOLYTIC THERAPY

Herpesviruses are effective against a broad spectrum of human tumors. G207 is a mutant HSV with deletions in both copies of $\gamma_1 34.5$, and a mutation in UL39 (Table 1). This attenuated virus was first described in the treatment of malignant gliomas, and further research has demonstrated its efficacy in treating a wide range of tumors types, including breast, bladder, colon, gallbladder, stomach, liver, pancreas, and the orodigestive tract *(10,12–17)*. In these studies, G207 has been able to effectively kill cancer cells in vitro and reduce experimental animal tumor burdens in vivo. Furthermore, G207 has demonstrated preclinical safety in BALB/c mice and Aotus monkeys. In BALB/c mice, doses of 1×10^7 plaque-forming units (pfu) of G207 injected intracerebrally did not produce any adverse effects *(18)*. Likewise, a dose of 1×10^9 pfu in Aotus monkeys did not result in any pathology *(19)*. Clinical safety has been further confirmed in a phase I clinical trial of patients with malignant gliomas resistant to standard therapies subjected to direct intratumoral injections of G207. None of the patients in this study developed serious adverse effects, and eight patients had radiographic reduction in tumor volume (Table 2) *(5)*.

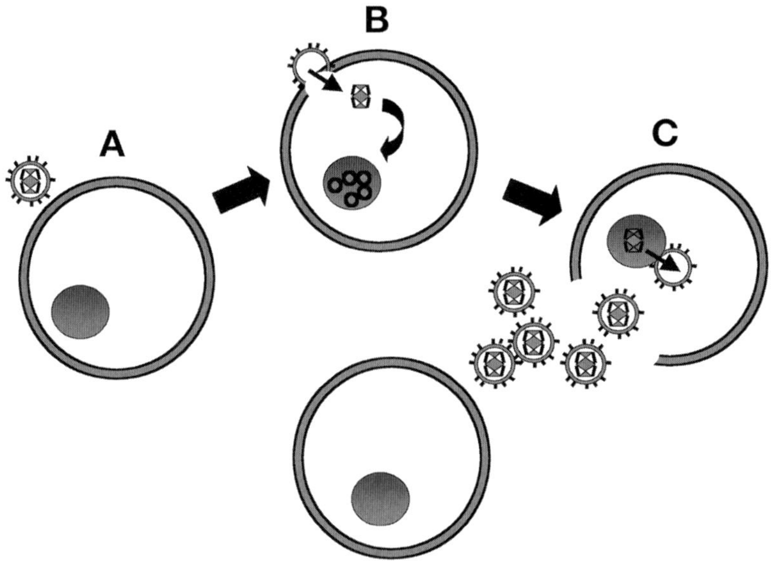

Fig. 2. HSV lytic cycle. (**A**) The herpes virion attaches to the tumor cell membrane. (**B**) After envelope fusion with the cell membrane, the large genome enters the nucleus where viral DNA is replicated and transcribed. A cascade of gene expression ensues which culminates in the production and assembly of new viral particles. (**C**) With viral replication and egress, the tumor cell is lysed and the viral effect amplified. Progeny virions can then infect neighboring tumor cells. The herpes replicative cycle often is completed within 24 h and is the basis of herpes oncolytic viral therapy.

Another widely tested mutant herpes virus is NV1020. Initially failing as a vaccine against HSV-1 and HSV-2, NV1020 subsequently demonstrated potent antitumor properties. This virus differs from G207 in that it contains a deletion in only one copy of $\gamma_1 34.5$, as well as deletions in the viral genes UL24 and UL56 (Table 1) *(20)*. NV1020 has effectively treated a variety of human tumor xenografts including those of the colon, prostate, pancreas, and head and neck. Moreover, NV1020 is being evaluated in a phase I clinical trial for liver metastases from colorectal cancer *(4)*. To date, 9 patients with hepatic metastases have received a maximum dose of 1.3×10^7 pfu of NV1020 delivered through a percutaneous hepatic arterial catheter. No patients suffered severe reactions related to viral inoculation and all patients demonstrated radiographically stable disease and reduced carcinoembryonic antigen (CEA) levels during the, admittedly, very short 28-d observation period. The adverse effects were mild and consisted of fever (7 of 9), nausea (3 of 9), and headache (2 of 9) (Table 2) *(4)*.

Another virus, 1716, has deletions in both copies of the $\gamma_1 34.5$ gene. This virus has been successful in the treatment of a variety of tumors in animal models and has recently completed clinical trials assessing safety (Table 2). In two phase I clinical trials in patients with recurrent gliomas, a maximum dose of 1×10^5 pfu was administered through direct intratumoral injection. No patients suffered adverse effects and viral replication could be demonstrated in resected tumor specimens *(6,21)*. In a third phase I clinical trial involving patients with stage 4 melanoma, 1×10^3 pfu of 1716 was injected into a single nodule. Following treatment, histopathologic necrosis and HSV antigen could be documented in tumor cells *(22)*.

NV1066 is a unique mutant HSV that contains a transgene encoding an enhanced green fluorescent protein (GFP). It is attenuated through a deletion in one copy of

Table 1

Virus	*Mutations*	*Transgene*	*Comments*
G207	UL39 $\gamma_1$34.5 (both copies)	LacZ	Safety confirmed in phase I trial Effective against a broad array of tumors
1716	$\gamma_1$34.5 (both copies)	None	Safety confirmed in phase I trial
NV1020	Joint region ($\gamma g_1$34.5 one copy, UL24, UL56)	HSV-2 segment	Originally developed as an HSV vaccine Ongoing phase I clinical trial
G47Δ	UL39 $\gamma_1$34.5 (both copies) α47	Lac Z	Enhanced antitumor immune response
NV1066	$\gamma_1$34.5 (one copy) α0, α4, TK	GFP	Useful in detecting small tumor deposits Inhibits esophageal tumor xenografts
NV1034	UL56 α47	GM-CSF LacZ	Efficacy demonstrated in SCC xenografts
NV1042	UL56 α47	IL-12 LacZ	Inhibits SCC xenograft growth Elicits memory tumor immunity

HSV, herpes simplex virus; TK, thymidine kinase; GFP, green fluorescent protein; SSC, squamous cell carcinoma.

$\gamma_1$34.5, as well as deletions in the α0 and α4 genes. The α0 and α4 gene products prevent cellular apoptosis and stimulate other viral genes necessary for replication (Table 1). Viral infection can be observed using excitation and emission filters that visualize GFP. In this respect, NV1066 has the potential for effective detection and treatment of cancer. In a murine esophageal cancer model, intraperitoneal metastases less than 2 mm in diameter could be differentiated from normal tissues by fluorescent filtered laparoscopy. Furthermore, tumor burdens were reduced 73% in NV1066-treated animals compared with controls, and 4 of 8 mice treated with NV1066 had no evidence of gross peritoneal disease 4 wkafter infection *(23)*.

5. GENE DELIVERY

Herpesviruses are effective gene transfer agents, and several strains have been developed that contain immunostimulatory or other genes while maintaining replication competence and oncolytic activity. Two such strains are NV1034 and NV1042, which contain the transgenes granulocyte-macrophage colony-stimulating factor (GM-CSF) and interleukin-12 (IL-12), respectively. These viruses are particularly attractive because of their combined immunostimulatory and oncolytic properties, a treatment approach that appears to be more effective than either approach alone. NV1034 and NV1042 have demonstrated efficacy in squamous cell xenograft tumors, with NV1042 specifically eliciting "memory" tumor immunity (Table 1) *(24)*. In addition, a mutant HSV containing a GM-CSF gene insertion has recently entered phase I clinical trial in the United Kingdom. This GM-CSF expressing virus, OncoVEX$^{GM\text{-}CSF}$, contains deletions in the $\gamma_1$34.5 and α4 genes to attenuate its virulence. OncoVEX$^{GM\text{-}CSF}$ is being tested by direct injection into several tumor types including melanoma, breast, head and neck, and

Table 2

Oncolytic virus	*Tumor type*	*Patients*	*Route of delivery*	*Maximum dose (pfu)*	*Findings*
G207	Recurrent glioma	21	Direct injection 1 to 5 injections	3×10^9	G207 well-tolerated and safe No dose-limiting toxicity reached
1716	Recurrent glioma	9	Direct injection	1×10^5	No adverse clinical symptoms No viral shedding or reactivation of latent HSV 4 of 9 patients alive at 14 mo
	Recurrent glioma	12	Direct injection Resection 4 to 9 d later	1×10^5	No toxicity observed HSV DNA detected in 10 of 12 tumors
	Metastatic melanoma	5	Subcutaneous injection 1 to 4 injections	4×10^3	Viral replication confined to tumor No viral toxicity reported Tumor necrosis with ≥2 injections
NV1020	Hepatic colorectal cancer metastases	9 Ongoing	Regional (via percutaneous hepatic artery catheter)	1.3×10^7	No dose-limiting toxicities observed NV1020 confined to tumor cells All patients had a decrease in CEA levels 28 d after surgery
OncoVEX (GM-CSF)	Melanoma Breast Gastrointestinal Head and neck	8 Ongoing	Direct injection	1×10^7	Ongoing trial Doses well-tolerated thus far Necrosis and viral replication detected in tumors

Abbr: HSV, herpes simplex virus; PFU, viral plaque forming units; HAI pump, hepatic arterial infusion pump; CEA, carcinoembryonic antigen.

various gastrointestinal cancers. Thus far, 8 patients have received a maximum dose of 1×10^7 pfu, which was well-tolerated (Table 2) *(25)*.

Herpesviruses may also be used purely as gene delivery vehicles, stripped of their ability to replicate. These replication-incompetent HSV, also known as HSV amplicons, possess the identical envelope, tegument, and capsid as replication-competent viruses and can therefore infect a wide array of tumor types *(26)*. HSV amplicons can infect both dividing and nondividing cells and their genome can accept DNA inserts greater than 100 kilobases (kb) *(27)*. Although they contain less than 2% of the viral genome and lack the ability to replicate, HSV amplicons are capable of utilizing the host cellular machinery to promote specific transgene expression. These replication-incompetent viruses have recently been manufactured using bacterial artificial chromosome technology. With this production method, contamination of amplicon stocks by replication-competent viruses has been nearly eliminated *(28)*.

An HSV amplicon expressing GM-CSF has been used in several studies, one of which reported improved survival of mice with subcutaneous human gliomas from 10% to 60% at 80 d *(29)*. Another GM-CSF-expressing amplicon has been used to treat subcutaneous murine melanomas. The level of tumor inhibition proved to be dose-dependent, and, interestingly, tumoral injection of HSV amplicon reduced tumor growth in both the injected tumors and the noninoculated contralateral tumors *(30)*. In another immunomodulatory approach, HSV amplicons were created to express T-cell costimulating factors, such as ligand B7.1. They were able to cause growth inhibition of established murine lymphomas. Again, direct HSV amplicon injection resulted in the regression of the injected tumor as well as the noninoculated contralateral tumor. Furthermore, mice that demonstrated tumor regression were resistant to further tumor cell injections *(31)*. An HSV amplicon expressing intercellular adhesion molecule-1 (ICAM-1) has been tested in rat hepatocellular and human colorectal cancer cell lines. The transduced tumor cells produced high-level human ICAM-1 surface expression, increased lymphocyte infiltration in vivo, and decreased tumorigenicity *(32)*.

HSV amplicons and replication-competent HSV have also been used in combination. In murine colorectal cancer and rat hepatocellular carcinoma models, low dose regional vascular delivery of G207 along with HSV amplicon expressing the lymphocyte stimulator, IL-2, enhanced reduction of tumor burden in the liver compared with G207 therapy alone was observed. This enhanced antitumor efficacy was abolished when $CD4^+$ and $CD8^+$ lymphocytes were depleted, suggesting that the improved antitumor response was immune-mediated *(33)*.

6. TARGETING

A fundamental problem in anticancer treatment in general, as well as in antitumor gene therapy, is the lack of an agent that specifically targets tumor cells. To overcome this obstacle gene therapy approaches are exploiting certain innate tumor characteristics. For instance, hypoxia is a prevalent condition of many solid tumors. Low tumor oxygen tensions have been correlated with an increased metastatic potential and resistance to standard chemoradiation therapy *(34,35)*. This tumor hypoxia can be utilized to distinguish malignant from normal tissues and may enable the selective targeting of cancer cells in gene therapy *(36)*. Recently, a modified UL39 gene driven by a hypoxia-responsive enhancer was inserted in an oncolytic herpesvirus to treat murine colorectal cancer cells. This hypoxia-inducible UL39 virus showed improved viral susceptibility of hypoxic cancer cells compared with cells transfected with G207, a virus deficient in

UL39. In contrast, no increased viral spread could be noted under normal oxygen concentrations, demonstrating that this approach is specific to hypoxic cancers cells. In a murine liver metastases model, this hypoxia-driven UL39 construct improved G207s baseline reduction of tumor weight and nodule count by 65% *(37)*.

Improved viral targeting may also be achieved by exploiting genes that are expressed at high levels in tumors, such as CEA, α-fetoprotein (AFP), or prostate specific antigen (PSA). These genes are not significantly activated in normal, differentiated tissue but they are found to be overexpressed in a variety of different malignancies (CEA, colorectal, pancreatic, gastric cancer; AFP, hepatocellular carcinoma, testicular cancer; PSA, prostate cancer) *(38,39)*. This tumor-specific expression can be used to target cancer cells by expression of critical viral growth genes from tumor-specific promoters *(40–42)*. Viral proliferation can be thus restricted to cells with high level expression of the tumor-associated gene, an approach that has already been shown effective in HSV and other viral systems *(40,41)*.

The effective entry of viral particles into a cell depends on a sequence of interactions between viral glycoproteins and cell surface receptors. Hence, the modifications of viral envelope glycoproteins is another strategy that may allow for selective targeting of tumors without attenuating viral oncolytic activity. Unlike other mutations which compromise the ability of the virus to replicate or to utilize cellular components, these glycoprotein mutations do not attenuate the viral lytic cycle once the cell is infected. R5111 is a genetically engineered HSV containing IL-13 insertional mutations in key envelope glycoproteins. R5111 has been shown to bind to the IL13Rα2 receptor found on the surface of malignant gliomas only. This particular strain was found to specifically infect and replicate within cells bearing the IL13Rα2 receptor, whereas cells lacking the receptor were not infected. Furthermore, R5111 replication was as robust as wild-type HSV in IL12Rα2 receptor-positive cells *(43)*.

7. CONCLUSIONS

The concept to use herpes virus to kill cancer led to its application that is now advancing from the laboratory the bench to the bedside. In a relatively short period of time, herpesviruses have been characterized, genetically modified, redirected to treat malignant disease, and utilized in numerous preclinical studies. Furthermore, several oncolytic viral mutants have been used in phase I trials that have demonstrated their safety in humans, with sporadic reports of antitumor efficacy. In addition, both replication-competent and replication-incompetent herpesviruses have been utilized for therapeutic transgene expression in the treatment of cancer. Future work must be focused on ways to enhance viral targeting without sacrificing oncolytic activity and to determine how best to combine oncolytic agents with conventional cancer treatments.

REFERENCES

1. De Pace N. Sulla scomparsa di un enorme cancro vegetante del collo dell'utero senza cura chirurgica. Ginecologia 1912;9:82–89.
2. Moss RW. Cancer and microbes. The Cancer Chronicles 1996;7:1–16.
3. Martuza RL, Malick A, Markert JM, Ruffner KL, Coen DM. Experimental therapy of human glioma by means of a genetically engineered virus mutant. Science 1991;252:854–856.
4. Fong Y. Phase I study of a replication-competent herpes simplex oncolytic virus for treatment of hepatic colorectal metastases. Am Soc Clin Oncol Ann Meeting 2002.
5. Markert JM, Medlock MD, Rabkin SD, et al. Conditionally replicating herpes simplex virus mutant, G207 for the treatment of malignant glioma: results of a phase I trial. Gene Ther 2000;7:867–874.

6. Rampling R, Cruickshank G, Papanastassiou V, et al. Toxicity evaluation of replication-competent herpes simplex virus (ICP 34.5 null mutant 1716) in patients with recurrent malignant glioma. Gene Ther 2000;7:859–866.
7. Kesari S, Randazzo BP, Valyi-Nagy T, et al. Therapy of experimental human brain tumors using a neuroattenuated herpes simplex virus mutant. Lab Invest 1995;73:636–648.
8. Thelander L, Reichard P. Reduction of ribonucleotides. Annu Rev Biochem 1979;48:133–158.
9. Hughes AL. Origin and evolution of viral interleukin-10 and other DNA virus genes with vertebrate homologues. J Mol Evol 2002;54:90–101.
10. Mineta T, Rabkin SD, Yazaki T, Hunter WD, Martuza RL. Attenuated multi-mutated herpes simplex virus-1 for the treatment of malignant gliomas. Nat Med 1995;1:938–943.
11. Todo T, Martuza RL, Rabkin SD, Johnson PA. Oncolytic herpes simplex virus vector with enhanced MHC class I presentation and tumor cell killing. Proc Natl Acad Sci U S A 2001;98:6396–6401.
12. Carew JF, Kooby DA, Halterman MW, Federoff HJ, Fong Y. Selective infection and cytolysis of human head and neck squamous cell carcinoma with sparing of normal mucosa by a cytotoxic herpes simplex virus type 1 (G207). Hum Gene Ther 1999;10:1599–1606.
13. Kooby DA, Carew JF, Halterman MW, et al. Oncolytic viral therapy for human colorectal cancer and liver metastases using a multi-mutated herpes simplex virus type-1 (G207). FASEB J 1999;13:1325–1334.
14. Bennett JJ, Delman KA, Burt BM, et al. Comparison of safety, delivery, and efficacy of two oncolytic herpes viruses (G207 and NV1020) for peritoneal cancer. Cancer Gene Ther 2002;9:935–945.
15. McAuliffe PF, Jarnagin WR, Johnson P, Delman KA, Federoff H, Fong Y. Effective treatment of pancreatic tumors with two multimutated herpes simplex oncolytic viruses. J Gastrointest Surg 2000;4:580–588.
16. Cozzi PJ, Malhotra S, McAuliffe P, et al. Intravesical oncolytic viral therapy using attenuated, replication-competent herpes simplex viruses G207 and Nv1020 is effective in the treatment of bladder cancer in an orthotopic syngeneic model. FASEB J 2001;15:1306–1308.
17. Toda M, Rabkin SD, Martuza RL. Treatment of human breast cancer in a brain metastatic model by G207, a replication-competent multimutated herpes simplex virus 1. Hum Gene Ther 1998;9: 2177–2185.
18. Sundaresan P, Hunter WD, Martuza RL, Rabkin SD. Attenuated, replication-competent herpes simplex virus type 1 mutant G207: safety evaluation in mice. J Virol 2000;74:3832–3841.
19. Todo T, Feigenbaum F, Rabkin SD, et al. Viral shedding and biodistribution of G207, a multimutated, conditionally replicating herpes simplex virus type 1, after intracerebral inoculation in aotus. Mol Ther 2000;2:588–595.
20. Bennett JJ, Delman KA, Burt BM, et al. Comparison of safety, delivery, and efficacy of two oncolytic herpes viruses (G207 and NV1020) for peritoneal cancer. Cancer Gene Ther 2002;9:935–945.
21. Papanastassiou V, Rampling R, Fraser M, et al. The potential for efficacy of the modified (ICP 34.5(-)) herpes simplex virus HSV1716 following intratumoural injection into human malignant glioma: a proof of principle study. Gene Ther 2002;9:398–406.
22. MacKie RM, Stewart B, Brown SM. Intralesional injection of herpes simplex virus 1716 in metastatic melanoma. Lancet 2001;357:525–526.
23. Stiles BM, Bhargava A, Adusumilli PS, et al. The replication-competent oncolytic herpes simplex mutant virus NV1066 is effective in the treatment of esophageal cancer. Surgery 2003;134:357–364.
24. Wong RJ, Patel SG, Kim S, et al. Cytokine gene transfer enhances herpes oncolytic therapy in murine squamous cell carcinoma. Hum Gene Ther 2001;12:253–265.
25. Hu JC, McNeish I, Shorrock C, Steiner J. A phase I clinical trial with OncoVEX$^{GM\text{-}CSF}$. Proc Am Sic Clin Oncol 2003;22:185.
26. Fraefel C, Jacoby DR, Lage C, et al. Gene transfer into hepatocytes mediated by helper virus-free HSV/AAV hybrid vectors. Mol Med 1997;3:813–825.
27. Sena-Esteves M, Saeki Y, Fraefel C, Breakefield XO. HSV-1 amplicon vectors—simplicity and versatility. Mol Ther 2000;2:9–15.
28. Fraefel C, Jacoby DR, Breakefield XO. Herpes simplex virus type 1-based amplicon vector systems. Adv Virus Res 2000;55:425–451.
29. Herrlinger U, Jacobs A, Quinones A, et al. Helper virus-free herpes simplex virus type 1 amplicon vectors for granulocyte-macrophage colony-stimulating factor-enhanced vaccination therapy for experimental glioma. Hum Gene Ther 2000;11:1429–1438.
30. Toda M, Martuza RL, Rabkin SD. Tumor growth inhibition by intratumoral inoculation of defective herpes simplex virus vectors expressing granulocyte-macrophage colony-stimulating factor. Mol Ther 2000;2:324–329.

31. Kutubuddin M, Federoff HJ, Challita-Eid PM, et al. Eradication of pre-established lymphoma using herpes simplex virus amplicon vectors. Blood 1999;93:643–654.
32. D'Angelica M, Tung C, Allen P, et al. Herpes simplex virus (HSV)-mediated ICAM-1 gene transfer abrogates tumorigenicity and induces anti-tumor immunity. Mol Med 1999;5:606–616.
33. Zager JS, Delman KA, Malhotra S, et al. Combination vascular delivery of herpes simplex oncolytic viruses and amplicon mediated cytokine gene transfer is effective therapy for experimental liver cancer. Mol Med 2001;7:561–568.
34. Bush RS, Jenkin RD, Allt WE, Beale FA, Bean H, Dembo AJ, Pringle JF. Definitive evidence for hypoxic cells influencing cure in cancer therapy. Br J Cancer Suppl 1978;37:302–306.
35. Tannock I, Guttman P. Response of Chinese hamster ovary cells to anticancer drugs under aerobic and hypoxic conditions. Br J Cancer 1981;43:245–248.
36. Shibata T, Giaccia AJ, Brown JM. Development of a hypoxia-responsive vector for tumor-specific gene therapy. Gene Ther 2000;7:493–498.
37. Reinblatt M, Pin RH, Federoff HJ, Fong Y. Utilizing tumor hypoxia to enhance oncolytic viral therapy in colorectal metastases. Ann Surg 2004;239:892–899.
38. Hauck W, Stanners CP. Transcriptional regulation of the carcinoembryonic antigen gene. Identification of regulatory elements and multiple nuclear factors. J Biol Chem 1995;270:3602–3610.
39. Chen H, Egan JO, Chiu JF. Regulation and activities of alpha-fetoprotein. Crit Rev Eukaryot Gene Expr 1997;7:11–41.
40. Cao G, Kuriyama S, Gao J, et al. Gene therapy for hepatocellular carcinoma based on tumour-selective suicide gene expression using the alpha-fetoprotein (AFP) enhancer and a housekeeping gene promoter. Eur J Cancer 2001;37:140–147.
41. Cao G, Kuriyama S, Gao J, et al. Comparison of carcinoembryonic antigen promoter regions isolated from human colorectal carcinoma and normal adjacent mucosa to induce strong tumor-selective gene expression. Int J Cancer 1998;78:242–247.
42. Schneider J, Schulze G. Comparison of tumor M2-pyruvate kinase (tumor M2-PK), carcinoembryonic antigen (CEA), carbohydrate antigens CA 19-9 and CA 72-4 in the diagnosis of gastrointestinal cancer. Anticancer Res 2003;23:5089–5093.
43. Zhou G, Ye GJ, Debinski W, Roizman B. Engineered herpes simplex virus 1 is dependent on IL13Ralpha 2 receptor for cell entry and independent of glycoprotein D receptor interaction. Proc Natl Acad Sci U S A 2002;99:15,124–15,129.

14 Cytokine Gene Therapy for Genitourinary Cancer

Terry L. Timme, PhD, *Tetsuo Fujita,* MD, *Hongyu Wang,* MD, PhD, *Koji Naruishi,* DDS, *Dov Kadmon,* MD, *Robert J. Amato,* DO, *Brian J. Miles,* MD, *Gustavo Ayala,* MD, *Thomas M. Wheeler,* MD, *Bin S. Teh,* MD, *E. Brian Butler,* MD, *and Timothy C. Thompson,* PhD

CONTENTS

Summary

This chapter will discuss the potential for delivery of cytokine molecules using neo-adjuvant/adjuvant gene therapy strategies to achieve antitumor efficacy. It focuses on two approaches for delivery of cytokine genes to achieve effective therapy; *in situ* delivery using adenoviral vectors also termed "active vaccination," and cell based approaches using specific immune cells modified with cytokine genes. These approaches have potential advantages for prostate cancer therapy and possibly other genitourinary malignancies.

Key Words: Gene therapy; adenoviral vectors; cell therapy; immunostimulatory genes; prostate cancer.

1. CHALLENGES AND OPPORTUNITIES IN PROSTATE CANCER

Prostate cancer presents specific opportunities for novel therapies such as cytokine gene therapy but also has specific challenges. Standard therapy for localized disease involves radical prostatectomy or radiation therapy which are often associated with significant morbidity (*3*). Despite a significant increase in the number of men diagnosed and treated with curative intent for localized prostate cancer, a considerable number of men develop local recurrence or distant disease following surgery or radiation performed

From: *Cancer Drug Discovery and Development: Gene Therapy for Cancer*
Edited by: K. K. Hunt, S. A. Vorburger, and S. G. Swisher © Humana Press Inc., Totowa, NJ

with curative intent. Every year tens of thousands of men experience rising serum prostate-specific antigen (PSA) levels as a result of local recurrence after presumptive definitive therapy for prostate cancer because of the limited capacity to accurately determine the virulence and stage of presumed localized disease and the limited efficacy of surgery and/or radiation therapy. Treatment options for these men are few and unproven *(5)* and the ability to predict cancer-specific mortality in this group is uncertain *(6)*. Although these patients represent a clinical challenge they also provide an opportunity to develop neo-adjuvant gene therapy protocols with cytokines to generate antimetastatic effects and perhaps develop long-term antitumor immunity. They have been the preferred treatment group for phase I trials. However, the ultimate challenge in prostate cancer research today is the development of therapies for metastatic disease. Currently, the only established therapy for metastatic prostate cancer is palliative hormone therapy *(8)*. Whereas metastatic prostate cancer is a multifocal disease, the primary metastatic site for prostate cancer is the bone, and yet, there are no therapies that specifically target prostate bone metastases.

In general, primary localized prostate cancer is slow growing and therefore offers more time for testing, evaluation, and adjustment of treatment strategies as compared with other cancers. Although the slow growth of prostate cancer limits the efficacy of conventional chemotherapy strategies, it offers a window of opportunity to temporarily delay either surgery or radiation therapy to attempt novel therapeutic interventions.

Human *(86)* and mouse *(28,44)* prostate cancer cells are generally considered to be poorly immunogenic. Cancer immunotherapy seeks, in general, to overcome deficiencies in the host immune response to malignancy that includes a significantly reduced capacity to recognize tumor cells and initiate an effective and durable systemic response *(87)*. The principal host immune response against cancer cells is the cellular type or Th1 immune response. Activation of antitumor immunity may be stimulated by Th1 promoting cytokines through enhancement of tumor cell recognition (i.e., antigenicity) as well as by the augmentation of existing cellular immune responses. Tumor antigenicity may be enhanced by initiating expression of antigenic molecules and/or by increasing the efficiency of antigen presentation. The cellular immune response against the cancer may be augmented through manipulation of any of the processes involved in its development (i.e., attraction, activation, differentiation, and amplification of specific effector cells such as $CD8^+$ T-cells). In addition to augmenting the activities of T-cell effectors, consideration must be given to abrogation of inhibitory T-reg cells which can suppress the activity of T-cell effectors *(88)*.

Intratumoral viral vector-mediated delivery of cytokines exploits the unique antigen milieu of the tumor through immune cell mediated cytotoxicity that is accompanied by release of tumor associated antigens (TAAs) (i.e., active vaccine). In addition, the availability of tumor associated immune cells (e.g., macrophage, dendritic cells [DCs], and T-cells) also provides an opportunity for straightforward initiation of a Th1 response. However, these potential advantages remain largely unrealized because of minimal understanding of the underlying molecular and cellular immunology and lack of adequate molecular tools. Systemic cancer immunotherapy also presents unique advantages and opportunities for prostate cancer. Using non-cell-based or cell-based delivery systems it is possible to specify the TAAs that are used for priming the response. There are numerous reports of potential antigens for prostate cancer including PSA *(89–92)*, prostate specific membrane antigen (PSMA) *(93,94)*, prostate associated gene (PAGE) *(95)*, and prostatic acid phosphatase (PAP) *(96,97)* as well as many additional molecules *(93,98)*.

However, it is not clear whether these antigens are sufficiently immunogenic to serve as targets for immunotherapy. Many of the purported antigens are secretory proteins that limit their usefulness in immunotherapy. In addition, these antigens are also expressed in some normal tissues such as the colon, liver, kidney, and bladder. Effective immunity elicited against these targets therefore incurs the risk of inducing autoimmunity with subsequent damage to essential organs. Certainly the identification of novel prostate cancer antigens should remain a high priority. However, it is conceivable that for optimal efficacy the development of sophisticated molecular approaches to TAA presentation will be required for this hetereogeneous and dynamic malignancy.

The expression of the desired cytokine that elicits the subsequent immune-response can be achieved through the transfection of the target cells (i.e., cancer cells) by a transgene carrying vector directly (*in situ*), or by the transfection of specialized immune-modulator cells (i.e., DCs) termed "cell mediated gene therapy." We will discuss potential opportunities of *in situ* and cell mediated cytokine gene delivery based on the results of recent preclinical studies. In addition, the results of recent clinical trials that have used cytokine gene therapy based approaches for prostate cancer are reviewed.

2. *IN SITU* CYTOKINE GENE THERAPY

The prostate and bladder are easily accessible for direct intratumoral gene therapy using routine techniques, such as transrectal ultrasound guided needle biopsy of the prostate or cystoscopy and intravesicular instillations of the bladder. Adaptation of these methods to deliver gene therapy vectors has been relatively straightforward, although there have been some difficulties overcoming the efficient gene transfer in the bladder *(11)*. Concerns related to systemic toxicity and cancer cell specificity are generally reduced in local gene therapy applications. In addition to local anti-tumor effects, cytokine genes delivered locally to prostate cancer lesions may induce systemic responses that have therapeutic impact on disseminated cancer cells. This systemic immunotherapy using local cytokine gene therapy is termed *in situ* cytokine gene therapy or "active vaccine" therapy.

2.1. Herpes Simplex Virus Thymidine Kinase Gene + Ganciclovir

One approach to the development of more effective therapies for prostate cancer is to initiate a cascade of molecular cellular events locally within the primary tumor that generate a localized and systemic antitumor immune response through the transfer of specific immunomodulatory genes. It has been considered that it might be possible to use specific genes to generate localized antitumor cytotoxicity as well as to initiate a systemic antitumor immune response. This strategy has evolved from purely cytotoxic-based gene therapies to more immunomodulatory gene therapies and various combinations to ultimately achieve the objective. Our initial gene therapy trials used the selected herpes simplex virus thymidine kinase (HSV-*tk*) gene delivered with a replication deficient adenoviral vector. HSV-*tk*+ ganciclovir (GCV) gene therapy has been shown to elicit widespread cytotoxic activities through direct and well-defined bystander activities and to elicit nonspecific and specific antitumor immunity in a variety of cancers *(20)*.

For prostate cancer, there are only limited reports of preclinical studies describing the use of nonviral vectors to deliver transgenes (e.g., liposomes) *(13–15)*. The results of some preclinical studies have demonstrated that herpes vectors *(16–18)* or canarypox vectors *(19)* can be therapeutically effective for a variety of malignancies including prostate cancer. The use of retroviral vectors for *in situ* approaches has been more limited, however they are potentially useful for ex vivo infection schemes such as those used with cell mediated therapies that will be discussed below. Thus far adenoviral vector systems have emerged as the predominant form of gene delivery for prostate cancer.

Preclinical studies were designed to assess both the efficacy and toxicity of adenoviral vector-mediated HSV-*tk* + GCV therapy using both in vivo and in vitro prostate cancer models. Mouse prostate cancer cell lines were generated from both primary and metastatic tumors initiated using the mouse prostate reconstitution model system. This model system involves the initiation of prostate cancer with the *ras* and *myc* oncogenes in wild-type C57Bl/6 mice *(21)* or mice with a targeted inactivation of one or both alleles of the p53 gene *(22,23)*.

The mouse models used are relevant to human prostate cancer because the mouse prostate cancer cell lines are inoculated orthotopically thus incorporating features unique to the prostate milieu and also incorporating the presence of the host immune system. Furthermore, the mouse cell lines used for these models resemble human prostate cancers in their expression of relevant oncogenic pathways and specific molecular markers *(24)*; possession of widespread metastatic activities *(27)*; and their low intrinsic immunogenicity *(28)*.

In our initial studies of adenoviral vector-based HSV-*tk* + GCV gene therapy, we documented cytotoxic activities in human prostate cancer cell lines in vitro and extensive cytotoxic activity through the induction of necrosis and apoptosis in subcutaneous tumors with the C57Bl/6 derived mouse prostate cancer cell line RM-1 *(29)*. A significant survival advantage was documented for the treated animals. In the clinically more relevant orthotopic models cancer cells form prostate cell lines were injected into the prostate of fully immunocompetent host mice. These inoculums develop into tumors that were still relatively small and within the confines of the host prostate. In these mice HSV-*tk*+GCV therapy led to prolonged survival *(30,31)*. To test the possibility that HSV-*tk*+GCV gene therapy could generate systemic antitumor immunity in prostate cancer, we developed a model system of pre-established lung metastasis in which mouse prostate cancer cells were simultaneously introduced into the prostate (orthotopic injection) as well as into the tail vein. Tail vein injection of these cells resulted in the establishment of lung colonies within 3 to 4 d and by the time of treatment (approx1 wk following orthotopic injection) these metastatic lesions represented pre-established metastatic targets to evaluate the systemic effects of localized *in situ* gene therapy. Interestingly, a single injection of HSV-*tk*+GCV vectors not only suppressed the growth of local orthotopic tumor through necrotic and apoptotic cell death, but also dramatically reduced the number and size of pre-established lung metastatic foci *(20)*. In nontumor bearing mice local inflammation after the administration of the HSV-*tk*+GCV vector were minimal and vector spreading outside the prostate gland was very limited and well within the limits that were perceived as being safe for human use *(32)*, thus, allowing to conduct a phase I trial in patients whose prostate cancer had recurred locally following initial radiation therapy but without any evidence of metastatic disease. The urologic gene therapy program Baylor College of Medicine thus conducted the first *in situ* gene therapy phase I clinical trial for human prostate cancer and demonstrated the safety of *in situ* HSV-*tk*+GCV gene therapy. In this clinical trial men with biochemical recurrence of localized prostate cancer following radiation therapy received a single injection of the adenoviral vector *(33)*. Although one instance of toxicity was observed at the highest dose (1×10^{11} IU), the complications ultimately resolved completely. Minimal toxicity was observed in most patients and decrease of serum PSA levels by 50% or more was noted in 3 of 18 patients *(33)*. An additional 18 patients received doses of 1–2 $\times 10^{10}$ IU, which proved to be a safe dose even when administered at multiple sites or when repeated for up to three times *(34)*. Analysis of the data from this group of patients indicated that *in situ* HSV-tk+GCV gene therapy led to an increased PSA doubling time, a significant PSA reduction, and a significantly increased mean time to return to initial PSA following vector injection, both after the initial and the repeated injections. A potential immune modulatory component in the response to HSV-*tk* gene +GCV gene therapy was demonstrated by increased levels of activated (HLA DR^+) $CD8^+$ T-cells in the peripheral blood following treatment. Interestingly, the density of $CD8^+$ T-cells in post-treatment biopsies was increased, which correlated with an increased number of apoptotic cells *(7)*.

After the safety and potential efficacy of HSV-*tk* + GCV gene therapy had been shown in men with recurrent disease, the gene therapy was tested in a neo-adjuvant setting. Men with newly diagnosed prostate cancer and clinical markers that suggested high grade disease who elected to undergo a radical prostatectomy 4 to 6 wk after vector injection entered the trial. The radical prostatectomy specimens clearly demonstrated that *in situ* gene therapy induced local inflammation within prostate cancer foci accompanied by increased infiltration of CD4 and CD8 T-cells *(35)*. In addition, necrosis within prostate cancer lesions in preference to adjacent normal prostatic tissues was noted. Additional studies confirmed that HSV-*tk*+GCV gene therapy (in this patient population) led to increased numbers of HLA DR^+ $CD8^+$ T-cells in the peripheral blood, again suggesting a systemic immune response *(36)*.

An additional phase I–II trial involved 59 patients that received two to three doses of HSV-*tk*+GCV combined with standard of care radiotherapy. Intravenous GCV was replaced with the oral bioequivalent drug valacyclovir. Men in this trial were stratified to 3 groups, 29 men with low-stage disease, 26 men with high-stage disease, and 4 men with stage D1 (regional lymph node metastases). The latter two groups also received concurrent hormonal therapy. Mild hematologic and hepatic abnormalities found in the patients were attributed to the gene therapy whereas genitourinary and gastrointestinal side effects were typical radiation related side effects. However, there was no added toxicity attributable to the combination therapeutic approach *(37)*. The combined radio-gene therapy approach appeared to provide good local control based on biopsy data, but it was not adequate for men with prostate cancer that had already spread to the pelvic lymph nodes *(38)*. Men with low-stage disease had evidence of activation of circulating CD4 and CD8 T-cells *(36)*. This translational research involving adenoviral vector mediated *in situ* gene therapy for prostate cancer set the stage for the further development of immunomodulatory active vaccines.

2.2. Interleukin-12 as Antitumor Cytokine

In our analyses we found increased in serum interleukin (IL)-12 following HSV-*tk* + GCV therapy in a significant number of patients. These led to preclinical testing of *in situ* IL-12 gene therapy. IL-12 is predominantly secreted by activated antigen presenting cells (APCs), including monocytes, macrophages, B-cells, and DCs. IL-12 interacts with specific cell receptors, which in turn can activate gene expression through the Stat4 signal transduction pathway (reviewed by Gately et al. *[39]*). The effects of IL-12 play an important role in initiating and orchestrating an immune response directed by central lymphoid effector cells, including natural killer (NK) cells, lymphokine-activated killer cells, and both $CD4^+$ and $CD8^+$ T-cells. Under the stimulation of IL-12, CD4-positive T-cells differentiate toward Th1 cells and are inhibited from differentiation into Th2 cells, a critical step in the determination of a cell vs humoral mediated immune response, respectively *(40–43)*. The clinical use of IL-12 as a recombinant protein has been limited by reports of severe toxicity after systemic application *(50–52)*. This toxicology results in part from downstream effects of interferon (IFN)-γ on the lymphohematopoietic system, intestines, liver, and lung *(53,54)*.

We evaluated effects of *in situ* IL-12 gene therapy in a orthotopical prostate cancer model. In this C57/Bl/6 derived RM-9 model, adenoviral vectors expressing IL-12 (AdIL-12) were shown to cause significant growth suppression (>50% reduction in tumor weight compared with controls). To evaluate the potential mechanisms for this response, specific immune cell populations were analyzed either biochemically or directly through quantitative immunohistochemical staining. Extensive immune cell infiltration and their activation was noted following injection of AdIL-12. The local antitumor immune effects were likely the result of:

- enhanced NK-mediated lysis during the first 7 d after vector injection,
- enhanced macrophage activities such as NOS activation, and
- increased cytokine production and possible cytolytic activity of $CD4^+$ and/or $CD8^+$ T-cells within the local tumor tissue.

In addition to local cytotoxicity preclinical studies with IL-12 encoding vectors have shown antimetastatic activities in a variety of malignancies *(55–59)*. Two different approaches were utilized to evaluate the potential for IL-12 *in situ* gene therapy to affect metastatic disease. As RM-9 cells metastasize spontaneously from the orthotopic site, we evaluated the effects of the AdmIL-12 vector on the extent of spontaneous metastasis to lymph nodes. The results indicated that localized gene therapy could significantly suppress the incidence of spontaneous lymph node metastases. In addition, IL-12 *in situ* gene therapy suppressed the formation of pre-established lung metastasis created by injection of RM-9 cells into the tail vein *(44)*. The results indicated that *in situ* IL-12 gene therapy not only led to a localized cytotoxic response through specific effector cells, but it also induced a systemic response that had an impact on metastatic disease. Antibody depletion analysis demonstrated that NK cells were predominantly responsible for the antimetastatic effects of locally administered AdIL-12 in pre-established RM-9 lung metastases. This correlated with the findings that IL-12 had been reported to induce an NK-mediated cytolytic phase followed by a T-cell phase that was characterized by CTL activity *(42,60–62)*. Although the interrelationships between the NK phase and CTL phase are poorly understood, it is well established that the generation of Th1 response is required for the CTL phase.

A phase I clinical trial was recently initiated at Baylor using *in situ* AdIL-12 in men with prostate cancer that recurred after radiotherapy. As a phase I study the objective is to assess the safety of direct intraprostatic injection of adenoviral vector expressing IL-12. The initial dose was 1×10^{10} viral particles injected directly into the prostate under ultrasound guidance. When normalized to the wet weight of the mouse prostate this dose is essentially equivalent to the effective dose and below the maximal tolerated dose for mice established in preclinical studies. Doses will be increased by $^1/_2$ log increments to a maximal dose of 5×10^{12} viral particles or until unacceptable toxicity is observed. A recently completed phase I trial of intratumoral delivery of AdIL-12 in advanced digestive tumors (e.g., liver, colorectal, and pancreatic) revealed an absence of severe adverse events even following three doses. A modest antitumor effect has been noted *(63)*.

2.3. Combination Therapy With HSV-tk + GCV + IL-12

To test whether combination gene therapy would lead to enhanced therapeutic effects when compared with either treatment alone, we used the RM-9 mouse prostate cancer cells in both orthotopic and pre-established lung metastases models of prostate cancer *(64)*. Combined treatment with a single injection of optimal doses of AdHSV-*tk*+GCV or AdIL-12 led to significantly increased suppression of local tumor growth. However, IL-12 gene therapy alone was significantly more effective in suppressing spontaneous lymph node metastases and pre-established lung metastases than AdHSV-*tk*+GCV and combination gene therapy did not result in additional antimetastatic activities. Combination gene therapy also did not achieve significantly better animal survival as compared with AdHSV-*tk*+GCV or AdmIL-12 alone. Analysis of localized antitumor activities demonstrated that AdHSV-*tk*+GCV therapy induced higher levels of necrosis compared with AdIL-12 or combination therapy. However, both treatments alone and in combination resulted in similar increase of apoptosis. To address the question of synergistic local cytotoxity we analyzed the systemic NK response and the numbers of tumor-infiltrating lymphocytes and macrophages using quantitative immunohistochemical analysis. AdHSV-*tk*+GCV therapy alone led to a slight increase of iNOS-positive cells and of $CD4^+/CD8^+$ T-cells and in a moderately increased numbers of F4/80 (macrophage selective)-positive cells within treated tumors. AdIL-12 treatment, on the other hand, elicited a robust increase of tumor infiltration by all four immune cell markers, which was similar to the response after combination therapy. Interestingly, local injection with AdHSV-*tk*+GCV induced significant cytolytic activities of splenocyte-derived NK cells reaching the maximal response 6 d after treatment, whereas AdIL-12 injection produced significantly higher NK activity with maximal response 2 d following injection. The combined treatment produced a higher systemic NK response over the 14-d treatment period. Depletion of NK cells in vivo demonstrated that this immune cell subpopulation was responsible for early locally cytotoxic activities induced by AdHSV-*tk*+GCV but not by AdIL-12 and that NK activities were largely responsible for activities against pre-established metastases demonstrated by both gene therapy protocols.

2.4. Related to Testes-Specific, Vespid, and Pathogenesis Protein (RTVP-1)

In a series of gene discovery experiments using differential display polymerase chain reaction (PCR) to identify genes relevant to prostate cancer we identified a novel mouse p53 target gene we termed *mRTVP-1 (65)*. The human homolog of this gene had also been identified in glioblastoma and was referred as glioma pathogenesis-related protein (*GliPR*) *(66)* or related to testes-specific, vespid, and pathogenesis protein (RTVP-1) *(67)*. *RTVP-1/GliPR* have also been identified as a marker of myelomonocytic differentiation in macrophages *(68)*. The RTVP-1/GliPR protein has high amino acid homology with human testis-specific protein, TPX1, and is structurally similar to group 1 of plant pathogenesis-related proteins that are implicated in plants defense response to viral, bacterial, and fungal infection *(66,67,69)*. Because the mammalian testis proteins, plant proteins, and the insect venom Ag-5 proteins are all secreted, it was speculated that RTVP-1 was a secretary protein and might play a role in human immune system *(69)*. Comparison between the deduced protein sequence of mRTVP-1 with known protein sequences revealed that this gene had 68% identity and 75% homology to the human RTVP-1 (hRTVP-1) protein *(65)*. The mRTVP-1protein contains two short in-frame deletions of two amino acids (PH) at positions 86–87 and a 9-amino acid deletion (KVSGFDALS) from amino acid 158–166 relative to hRTVP-1. Both mouse and human proteins contain extracellular protein signature motifs (sig-1 and sig-2), a transmembrane domain, a putative N-linked glycosylation site, and a hydrophobic region near the carboxyl terminus. Interestingly, both proteins also contain a putative N-terminal signal peptide which suggests that both proteins are located on the cell membrane or secreted.

In our initial studies we demonstrated that *mRTVP-1* was upregulated by p53 and was also induced by DNA damaging agents such as γ-irradiation or doxorubicin *(65)*. RTVP-1 secretion appeared to be independently regulated by specific cytokines (unpublished data). In normal prostate RTVP-1 protein was localized to epithelial cells and specific immune cells.

Multiple lines of evidence support the concept that the *RTVP-1* gene should be considered a tumor suppressor gene. Its regulation by p53, induction of apoptosis, and growth inhibition provide a functional rationale for selection for downregulation of the gene during tumor progression. Indeed *hRTVP-1* is significantly downregulated in prostate cancer compared with normal prostate tissues *(70)*. Epigenetic rather than genetic changes appear to be the prevalent mechanism of down-regulation of hRTVP-1 based on analysis of the methylation status of CpG dinucleotides in the promoter region of the *hRTVP-1* gene and increased expression in cancer cell lines following treatment with a demethylation agent *(70)*. Functional analysis of *mRTVP-1* demonstrated that overexpression induces apoptosis in multiple mouse and human cancer cell lines, like in the two widely used prostate cancer cell lines, LNCaP and TSU-Pr1, but it has minimal effects in normal cell lines *(65,70)*. To test this therapeutic potential in a preclinical model for metastatic prostate cancer mouse prostate cancer cells 178-2BMA were injected into the prostate of host 129/Sv mice leading to tumors of about 15 mm^3 after 7 d *(71)*. At this time prostate tumors were directly inject with an adenoviral vector expressing the *mRTVP-1* gene (Ad*mRTVP-1*) or a control vector (Adβgal). Fourteen days later the mice were evaluated for tumor size and metastatic spread. The mice treated with Ad*mRTVP-1* had significant suppression of tumor growth and fewer lung metastases. Quantitative immunohistochemical analysis of the tumors revealed significantly higher numbers of CD8$^+$ T-cells, as well as APCs represented by DCs and macrophage. In addition to this localized immune response, a single injection of Ad*mRTVP-1* generated a systemic antitumor immune response noted by increased NK and cytolytic T-cell activity. Hence, *mRTVP-1* appears to have great potential for antitumor therapies that are based on *in situ* transgene expression.

2.5. Other Clinical and Preclinical In Situ *Cytokine Gene Therapy Approaches*

A number of other cytokines have been proposed or used for prostate cancer gene therapy including, IL-2, IL-15, IL-18, and IL-24. In a neo-adjuvant phase I clinical trial of 24 patients with locally advanced prostate cancer, the cDNA for IL-2 was injected into the prostate as a lipid complex *(72)*. It was well tolerated with no evidence of significant toxicity and yielded some evidence of systemic immune activation in the peripheral blood and in the radical prostatectomy specimens. The IL-2 gene has also been inserted into a vaccinia virus that coexpressed the MUC-1 gene, which was then delivered as an intramuscular injection to men with advanced prostate cancer *(73)*. No toxicity was observed and one patient that received three doses had some evidence of systemic immune effects. IL-15 was shown to contribute to the development of NK and antitumor response to prostate cancer in a xenograft model with PC-3 tumors *(74)*. IL-18 may synergize with IL-12 *(75)* and although it has not been used in gene therapy strategies for prostate cancer the recombinant protein has been used in combination with IL-12 gene therapy in a bladder cancer model *(76)*. The IL-24 gene also known as a melanoma differentiation associated gene 7 (MDA-7) has been used in preclinical studies for prostate cancer gene therapy *(77)*.

Intratumoral injection of the cDNAs for interferon-γ, major histocompatability complex (MHC) class II transactivator and an antisense construct for a portion of the Ii gene has demonstrated tumor suppression in the RM-9 subcutaneous prostate cancer model *(78)*. The addition of radiation therapy led to complete tumor regression and CTL activities and the ability to reject tumor challenge in long-term survivors. The IFN-β gene has also evaluated in prostate *(79,80)*, bladder *(81)*, and renal *(82)* cancer.

Delivery of the granulocyte-macrophage colony-stimulating factor (GM-CSF) gene in either a herpesvirus vector *(83)* or a canarypox vector *(84)* has been explored in preclinical models. The GM-CSF gene was combined with IFN-α gene for liposomal delivery in a bladder cancer model *(85)*.

3. CELL MEDIATED DELIVERY OF CYTOKINE GENES

Specific protocols have been developed to allow modification of APCs via direct loading with antigen(s) or by gene modification to generate cells that have increased capacity for antigen uptake and presentation to effector immune cells including T-cells. To the extent that these modified cells are introduced systemically and depending on the cell type used there is targeting capacity associated with antigen/gene modified cell-based systemic immunotherapy. Cells that have been developed for gene-modification based immunotherapy vehicles include tumor cells, APCs (macrophages and DCs) and more recently adult stem cells. Modification of these cells with cytokine genes is particularly attractive for prostate cancer therapy.

3.1. Cytokine Modified Tumor Cell Vaccines

Antitumor vaccination with irradiated autologous cancer cells, transfected ex vivo to express cytokine genes was exemplified by the use of GM-CSF gene modified cancer cell delivery *(86,99)*. Promising initial preclinical studies with an antitumor vaccine comprised of irradiated autologous GM-CSF secreting-Dunning rat prostate carcinoma cells led to a clinical trial in which eight patients with prostate cancer were treated with autologous GM-CSF secreting, irradiated tumor cell vaccines prepared by ex vivo retroviral transduction of surgically harvested cells *(100)*. Insufficient cells were obtained from three other patients. Indeed, the major limitation of this approach was the poor prostate cancer cell recovery and growth from clinical specimens. Side effects were minimal and localized to the site of injection. The treatment resulted in DC and macrophage infiltration at the injection site. They also found activation of T- and B-cells against prostate cancer antigens, representing both Th1 and Th2 T responses, at the site of testing for a delayed type hypersensitivity response. Autologous tumor cell vaccines transduced with GM-CSF *(101,102)* have advanced to phase I studies with some evidence of immune activation.

To test the therapeutic potential of IL-12 alone or in combination with the costimulatory molecule B7-1 in a gene-modified tumor cell-based vaccine model, we transduced the mouse prostate cancer cell line RM-9 with AdIL-12 or AdIL-12/B7, irradiated the cells, and then vaccinated mice three times at weekly intervals in a conventional vaccination strategy *(103)*. Subsequent orthotopic challenge with RM-9 cells revealed a complete protection from tumor growth in 33% of the mice vaccinated with AdIL-12/B7-transduced, irradiated RM9 cells and 20% of the AdIL-12-transduced irradiated. In those animals that were not completely protected there was a significant reduction in primary tumor wet weight compared with controls that were vaccinated with nontransduced irradiated RM-9 cells *(103)*. We are currently evaluating the potential for adenoviral vector-mediated RTVP-1 gene modified tumor cell-based vaccines using the metastatic mouse prostate cancer cell line 178-2 BMA. Our preliminary results indicate that RTVP-1 gene modified cell-based vaccines may be useful in the prevention of recurrent prostate cancer and should be the focus of additional preclinical studies.

3.2. Cytokine Modified Macrophages

Tumor associated macrophages are inversely correlated with tumor progression in human prostate cancer *(104)* and they may provide important antigen presenting functions in an antitumor immune response. Studies have revealed that in radical prostatectomy specimens the macrophage marker scavenger receptor A (MSR-A) was expressed in a subset of macrophages and DCs that infiltrated prostatic tissues. The majority of MSR-A positive cells were macrophages as evidenced by coexpression of CD68 and a relatively low percentage of DC were determined by expression of S100 protein. The number of MSR-A positive cells was significantly increased in prostatic intraepithelial neoplastic lesions as compared with normal prostatic tissue. In contrast, the number of MSR-A positive cells decreased with tumor progression. This reduction in the number of MSR-A positive cells seems to demarcate tumor progression as indicated by clinical and pathological correlations. These studies may also be relevant because germ line mutations in the MSR-1 gene have been associated with increased risk of prostate cancer in some *(105,106)* but not all *(107)* studies.

To develop protocols that optimize the processing and presentation of tumor antigens we isolated peritoneal macrophages from normal adult mice and transduced them with IL-12 using an adenoviral vector. Using the 178-2 BMA mouse metastatic prostate cancer model we demonstrated that *in situ* cell therapy with AdIL-12 transduced macrophages produced significant local tumor control, decreased metastases and improved survival compared with control Adβ-gal transduced cells *(108)*. Quantitative immunohistochemical analysis demonstrated significantly increased infiltration of $CD4^+$ and $CD8^+$ T-cells in tumors injected with AdmIL-12 transduced macrophages compared with controls. Systemic immune effects were documented by enhanced splenocyte-derived NK cell activity on day 2 after AdIL-12 transduced macrophage injection and increased splenocyte-derived tumor specific cytotoxic T-lymphocyte activities on day 14. Trafficking studies with fluorescent labeled macrophages confirmed that the intratumoral injected AdIL-12 transduced macrophages migrated to draining lymph nodes more efficiently than Adβ-gal transduced macrophages. This novel approach to prostate cancer therapy demonstrates that cytokine modified macrophages should be considered for further studies as our preclinical studies revealed that they are capable of generating antitumor immune responses that provide effective antimetastatic activities in preclinical studies. Optimal isolation and transduction methods for macrophages need to be investigated further. However, our data demonstrated that AdIL-12 transduced murine peritoneal exudate macrophages secreted high levels of mIL-12 and showed increased surface expression of MHC class I and II and F4/80 antigen. It is also possible that other cytokines, such as RTVP-1, may also offer therapeutic enhancement in the *in situ* macrophage setting if they also enhance the ability of the cells to take up and process tumor antigens at the site of injection and migrate to appropriate sites such as draining lymph nodes and present antigen to downstream effector cells. As a secreted molecule, RTVP-1, like IL-12, may also have indirect benefits at the site of injection through support of effector NK and CTL cells or recruitment of additional APCs. Direct and/or indirect effects on tumor vasculature and angiogenesis may also contribute to the effectiveness of IL-12 *(108)* and RTVP-1 *(71)*.

3.3. Cytokine Modified Dendritic Cells

DCs are extremely efficient APCs that are widely dispersed in tissues and peripheral blood. Because they can be manipulated ex vivo and are perhaps the most specialized APCs they have been considered the prime candidates for cell mediated cancer therapy. A number of clinical trials using DC have been performed for prostate cancer *(109–116)* as well as other cancers (*see* ref. *117* for a review of the first 1000 trials). Although melanoma is the most commonly treated cancer using DC immunotherapy, GU cancers, notably, renal and prostate, are also being evaluated *(118)*. Most of these studies involve DC primed with specific polypeptides that will bind MHC Class I or II molecules or with tumor lysates. Tumor derived mRNA transfected into DCs is being used to circumvent the challenge of lack of identity of TAAs. In current clinical trials DCs are most often injected intradermally or subcutaneously and less commonly intravenously or into a lymph node *(118)*. A challenge with current clinical trials is proving efficacy in the patient population that is typically enrolled in phase I studies, advanced disease states typically with large tumor burdens, in whom it may be more difficult to demonstrate clinical and immunological responses *(118)*.

Cytokine modified DCs have been used less extensively but have the advantage of not requiring knowledge of specific tumor antigens. As mentioned above (*see* Section 3.1.) a significant challenge in prostate cancer immunotherapy is the lack of well-characterized tumor antigens. Because specific cytokines promote intensive antitumor cytotoxicity and can also promote a specific CTL response, potentially obviating the need to provide specific exogenous TAAs (*see* Section 2.3.), we undertook studies with IL-12 modified DCs using the 178-2 BMA metastatic mouse prostate cancer preclinical model *(119)* using tumor lysates generated either *in situ* or ex vivo. We relied on the generation of tumor lysate *in situ* by delivering adenoviral vector mediated IL-12 gene transduced DCs directly into orthotopic tumors. We compared this novel approach with DC targeting with subcutaneous delivery of adenoviral vector mediated IL-12 transduced DCs that were pulsed with tumor lysates prior to injection. Direct *in situ* delivery of IL-12 transduced DCs was moderately more effective than the subcutaneous route of administration based on enhanced local growth suppression, reductions in spontaneous metastatic activities and, importantly, a significant increase in the survival of animals. Our results also demonstrated an overlap in cellular mechanisms underlying the therapeutic responses in that both protocols had comparable increases in NK activity and CTL responses.

Clinically, cytokine modified DCs might be used in several situations. The most common delivery method for DCs in clinical trials has been intradermal or subcutaneous and it is conceivable that tumor lysates derived from radical prostatectomy specimens could be used in these protocols in men at high risk of recurrence. It has been shown that migration to lymph nodes of intradermal administered DCs is inefficient if the cells are immature *(120)*, thus cytokine modified could acquire better homing to sites where they would be more effective. It would be informative to evaluate RTVP-1 in this regard since we have shown that this secreted molecule can enhance DCs migration to tumor sites *(71)*. Our studies also suggest that cytokine modified DCs could be injected intratumorally and used in a neoadjuvant approach preradical prostatectomy or as an adjuvant to radiation therapy. Intratumoral delivery could also be used independently or potentially in combination with other systemic chemo- or immuno-therapy agents or with other *in situ* gene therapy protocols in either the neo-adjuvant or adjuvant setting. Overall, numerous studies confirm that opportunities exist for cytokine modified DCs to be used clinically in prostate cancer, however, one challenge may be the considerable financial and logistic support required for their isolation and preparation *(121)*.

3.4. Other Possible Cell Types

There are several other cell types that could be used to facilitate cytokine mediated gene therapy for GU tumors. Peripheral blood can be used not only as a source of macrophage and DC precursors but also to isolate biologically active T-cells. Over a decade ago several reports suggested that autologous T-cells could be activated in vitro with cytokines and used to treat prostate or renal cancer *(122–124)*. Tumor infiltrating T-lymphocytes isolated and treated with cytokines have also been utilized for prostate, bladder, and renal cancer *(125)*. The myriad strategies for isolation, enrichment, expansion, and possible engineering of T-cells for adoptive therapy have recently been reviewed *(126)*. In an attempt to target adoptive T-cell therapy to prostate cancer, human T-cells that were engineered to express a chimeric receptor for the tumor marker erbB2 demonstrated therapeutic potential in a xenograft models *(127)*. In another study, four of five prostate cancer patients T-cells were isolated and modified to express a receptor that recognized the PSMA lysed prostate cancer cells and expressed cytokines in response to binding to PSMA *(94)*. Attempts to isolate and propagate tumor antigen reactive T-cell clones for therapeutic use have been ongoing. Until recently, minimal success was reported but newer patient lymphodepletion conditioning protocols yielded objective clinical responses *(128)*. We are currently evaluating a model for adoptive cell therapy using *in situ* cytokine gene therapy to induce tumor reactive T-cells that can be isolated from splenocytes and subsequently transferred to naïve animals where they confer resistance to tumor challenge *(129)*. Cytokine induced killer cells isolated from the peripheral blood of patients with metastatic renal cancer and transduced with the IL-2 gene have been shown to be safe when reinjected into patients and can generate immune activities *(130)*.

Another potential cell population that holds great potential are bone marrow derived stem cells. We have developed a novel anti-bone metastasis therapy using bone marrow stem cells to transport an active IL-12 gene to the bone *(131)*. In these preliminary experiments we have used a retroviral vector, DFG-mIL12, which showed previously to efficiently transduce and mediate the expression of p35 and p40 at high levels *(132)*. DFG-eGFP, which has an identical retroviral backbone and has been shown to efficiently transduce eGFP (visualized in living and fixed tissues) served as control vector *(132)*. The distinct advantage of retroviral vectors relative to other viral vectors is their ability to stably integrate a therapeutic gene into the host cell DNA without expressing immunogenic viral proteins. Retroviral vectors may, therefore, be useful for ex vivo gene therapy applications such as production of autologous or allogeneic cancer cells as vaccines *(86,100)*. Retroviral

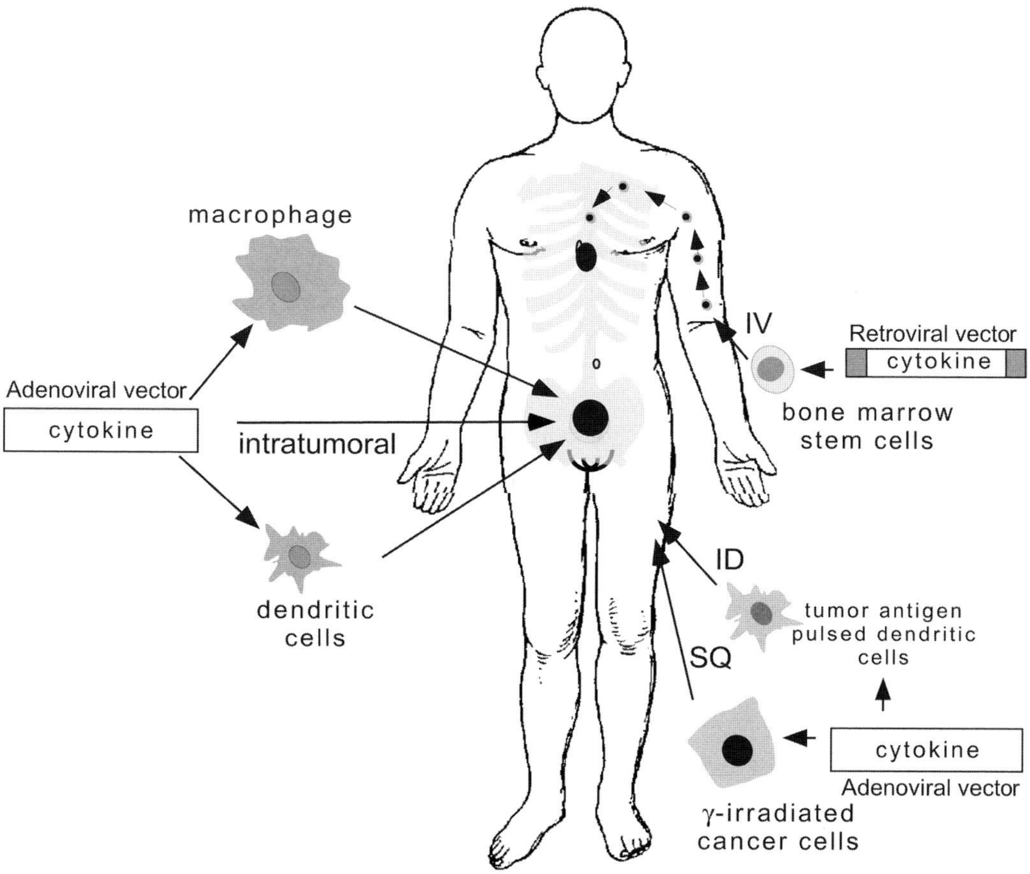

Fig. 1. *In situ* and systemic cytokine gene modified APC, cytokine gene modified vaccines, and cytokine modified bone marrow stem cell targeting for prostate cancer therapy.

vectors however, have several disadvantages with regard to clinical use. In general they only infect dividing cells, have poor cell penetration, and diffuse poorly across cells at the injection site. Retroviral vectors require specialized packaging cells which yield relatively low titers. Retroviral vectors also have a relatively small genome, limiting their carrying capacity for engineered genes. Because retroviruses randomly insert their DNA into the cell genome, they have mutagenic potential with concerns that this may cause a malignancy as in two children in gene replacement trials *(133)*.

4. CONCLUSIONS

Cytokine-mediated gene therapy holds great potential for the treatment of genitourinary cancers based on the preclinical studies described above. Cytokine gene therapy protocols have the potential to develop an "active vaccine." The active component of cytokine gene therapy involves direct (cytotoxic and apoptotic) and/or indirect (immune cell recruitment and activation) activities within the tumor following direct, *in situ* delivery of the cytokine genes by adenoviral vector-mediated transduction. These activities are capable of generating TAAs and antigen specific APCs that promote a systemic, antimetastatic immune response. Specific neoadjuvant/adjuvant approaches for cytokine gene therapy or cytokine gene-modified cell therapy together with conventional local therapies (i.e., radiation therapy or surgery), cytotoxic gene therapy, and potentially with systemic chemo-/immunotherapy may prove to be extremely beneficial for local tumor control and the induction of systemic antitumor immunity.

The ultimate success of clinical studies will rely, of course, on a number of factors. The choice of cytokine will be a key determinant. Figure 1 illustrates the various protocols for cytokine gene therapy that may have clinical utility to treat prostate cancer specifically but also have the potential to treat other genitourinary cancers. In our opinion, the cytokine IL-12 is a potent activator of the immune system whose systemic toxicity can be controlled by selective transduction with an appropriate vector and delivery method. The RTVP-1 gene is a novel gene that has cytokine-like actions as well as specific cancer cytotoxic effects that make it ideal for *in situ* gene therapy. Localized, *in situ*, cytokine or RTVP-1 gene therapy generates systemic effects mediated by factors such as a bystander effect or induction of host immunity in preclinical models. Thus, *in situ* gene therapy involving the direct injection of a viral vector into the tumor to be well suited for delivery of cytokine genes and to create an active vaccine that initiates a tumor specific immune response. Additional therapeutic interventions utilizing cytokine gene therapy approaches outlined above may build on this response to yield effective therapies for genitourinary cancers.

REFERENCES

1. Jemal A, Tiwari RC, Murray T, et al. Cancer statistics, 2004. CA Cancer J Clin 2004;54:8–29.
2. Thompson I, Leach RJ, Pollock BH, Naylor SL. Prostate cancer and prostate-specific antigen: the more we know, the less we understand. J Natl Cancer Inst 2003;95:1027–1028.
3. Wei JT, Dunn RL, Sandler HM, et al. Comprehensive comparison of health-related quality of life after contemporary therapies for localized prostate cancer. J Clin Oncol 2002;20:557–566.
4. Rioux-Leclercq NC, Chan DY, Epstein JI. Prediction of outcome after radical prostatectomy in men with organ-confined Gleason score 8 to 10 adenocarcinoma. Urology 2002;60:666–669.
5. Moul JW. Prostate specific antigen only progression of prostate cancer. J Urol 2000;163:1632–1642.
6. D'Amico AV, Moul JW, Carroll PR, Sun L, Lubeck D, Chen MH. Surrogate end point for prostate cancer-specific mortality after radical prostatectomy or radiation therapy. J Natl Cancer Inst 2003;95:1376–1383.
7. Miles BJ, Shalev M, Aguilar-Cordova E, et al. Prostate-specific antigen response and systemic T cell activation after in situ gene therapy in prostate cancer patients failing radiotherapy. Hum Gene Ther 2001;12:1955–1967.
8. Trachtenberg J. A review of hormonal treatment in advanced prostate cancer. Can J Urol 1997;4:61–64.
9. Mundy GR. Metastasis: Metastasis to bone: causes, consequences and therapeutic opportunities. Nat Rev Cancer 2002;2:584–593.
10. Teh BS, Aguilar-Cordova E, Vlachaki MT, et al. Combining radiotherapy with gene therapy (from the bench to the bedside): a novel treatment strategy for prostate cancer. Oncologist 2002;7:458–466.
11. Pagliaro LC, Keyhani A, Williams D, et al. Repeated Intravesical Instillations of an Adenoviral Vector in Patients With Locally Advanced Bladder Cancer: A Phase I Study of p53 Gene Therapy. J Clin Oncol 2003;21:2247–2253.
12. Gdor Y, Timme TL, Miles BJ, Kadmon D, Thompson TC. Gene therapy for prostate cancer. Expert Rev Anticancer Ther 2002;2:309–321.
13. Nakanishi H, Mazda O, Satoh E, et al. Nonviral genetic transfer of Fas ligand induced significant growth suppression and apoptotic tumor cell death in prostate cancer in vivo. Gene Ther 2003;10:434–442.
14. Seki M, Iwakawa J, Cheng H, Cheng PW. p53 and PTEN/MMAC1/TEP1 gene therapy of human prostate PC-3 carcinoma xenograft, using transferrin-facilitated lipofection gene delivery strategy. Hum Gene Ther 2002;13:761–773.
15. Jin RJ, Kwak C, Lee SG, et al. The application of an anti-angiogenic gene (thrombospondin-1) in the treatment of human prostate cancer xenografts. Cancer Gene Ther 2000;7:1537–1542.

16. Miyatake S, Martuza RL, Rabkin SD. Defective herpes simplex virus vectors expressing thymidine kinase for the treatment of malignant glioma. Cancer Gene Ther 1997;4:222–228.
17. Pyles RB, Warnick RE, Chalk CL, Szanti BE, Parysek LM. A novel multiply-mutated HSV-1 strain for the treatment of human brain tumors. Hum Gene Ther 1997;8:533–544.
18. Walker JR, McGeagh KG, Sundaresan P, Jorgensen TJ, Rabkin SD, Martuza RL. Local and systemic therapy of human prostate adenocarcinoma with the conditionally replicating herpes simplex virus vector G207. Hum Gene Ther 1999;10:2237–2243.
19. Kawakita M, Rao GS, Ritchey JK, et al. Effect of canarypox virus (ALVAC)-mediated cytokine expression on murine prostate tumor growth. J Natl Cancer Inst 1997;89:428–436.
20. Thompson TC. In situ gene therapy for prostate cancer. Oncol Res 1999;11:1–8.
21. Thompson TC, Southgate J, Kitchener G, Land H. Multistage carcinogenesis induced by ras and myc oncogenes in a reconstituted organ. Cell 1989;56:917–930.
22. Thompson TC, Park SH, Timme TL, et al. Loss of p53 function leads to metastasis in ras+myc-initiated mouse prostate cancer. Oncogene 1995;10:869–879.
23. Thompson TC, Timme TL, Park SH, Yang G, Ren C. Mouse prostate reconstitution model system: A series of in vivo and in vitro models for benign and malignant prostatic disease. Prostate 2000; 43:248–254.
24. Thompson TC, Timme TL, Sehgal I. Oncogenes, growth factors, and hormones in prostate cancer. In: Hormones and growth factors in development and neoplasia, Dickson RB, Salomon DS, eds. New York: Wiley-Liss, Inc. 1998;327–359.
25. Stapleton AM, Timme TL, Gousse AE, et al. Primary human prostate cancer cells harboring p53 mutations are clonally expanded in metastases. Clin Cancer Res 1997;3:1389–1397.
26. Cordon-Cardo C. Molecular alterations in bladder cancer. Cancer Surv 1998;32:115–131.
27. Timme TL, Satoh T, Tahir SA, et al. Therapeutic targets for metastatic prostate cancer. Curr Drug Targets 2003;4:251–261.
28. Lee HM, Timme TL, Thompson TC. Resistance to lysis by cytotoxic T cells: a dominant effect in metastatic mouse prostate cancer cells. Cancer Res 2000;60:1927–1933.
29. Eastham JA, Chen SH, Sehgal I, et al. Prostate cancer gene therapy: herpes simplex virus thymidine kinase gene transduction followed by ganciclovir in mouse and human prostate cancer models. Hum Gene Ther 1996;7:515–523.
30. Hall SJ, Mutchnik SE, Chen SH, Woo SL, Thompson TC. Adenovirus-mediated herpes simplex virus thymidine kinase gene and ganciclovir therapy leads to systemic activity against spontaneous and induced metastasis in an orthotopic mouse model of prostate cancer. Int J Cancer 1997;70: 183–187.
31. Hall SJ, Mutchnik SE, Yang G, et al. Cooperative therapeutic effects of androgen ablation and adenovirus- mediated herpes simplex virus thymidine kinase gene and ganciclovir therapy in experimental prostate cancer. Cancer Gene Ther 1999;6:54–63.
32. Timme TL, Hall SJ, Barrios R, Woo SL, Aguilar-Cordova E, Thompson TC. Local inflammatory response and vector spread after direct intraprostatic injection of a recombinant adenovirus containing the herpes simplex virus thymidine kinase gene and ganciclovir therapy in mice. Cancer Gene Ther 1998;5:74–82.
33. Herman JR, Adler HL, Aguilar-Cordova E, et al. In situ gene therapy for adenocarcinoma of the prostate: a phase I clinical trial. Hum Gene Ther 1999;10:1239–1249.
34. Shalev M, Kadmon D, Teh BS, et al. Suicide gene therapy toxicity after multiple and repeat injections in patients with localized prostate cancer. J Urol 2000;163:1747–1750.
35. Ayala G, Wheeler TM, Shalev M, et al. Cytopathic effect of in situ gene therapy in prostate cancer. Hum Pathol 2000;31:866–870.
36. Satoh T, Teh BS, Timme TL, et al. Enhanced systemic T-cell activation after in situ gene therapy with radiotherapy in prostate cancer patients. Int J Radiat Oncol Biol Phys 2004;59:562–571.
37. Teh BS, Aguilar-Cordova E, Kernen K, et al. Phase I/II trial evaluating combined radiotherapy and in situ gene therapy with or without hormonal therapy in the treatment of prostate cancer—a preliminary report. Int J Radiat Oncol Biol Phys 2001;51:605–613.
38. Teh BS, Ayala G, Aguilar L, et al. Phase I-II trial evaluating combined intensity-modulated radiotherapy and in situ gene therapy with or without hormonal therapy in treatment of prostate cancer-interim report on PSA response and biopsy data. Int J Radiat Oncol Biol Phys 2004;58:1520–1529.
39. Gately MK, Renzetti LM, Magram J, et al. The interleukin-12/interleukin-12-receptor system: role in normal and pathologic immune responses. Annu Rev Immunol 1998;16:495–521.

40. Stern AS, Podlaski FJ, Hulmes JD, et al. Purification to homogeneity and partial characterization of cytotoxic lymphocyte maturation factor from human B-lymphoblastoid cells. Proc Natl Acad Sci U S A 1990;87:6808–6812.
41. Gately MK. Interleukin-12: a recently discovered cytokine with potential for enhancing cell-mediated immune responses to tumors. Cancer Invest 1993;11:500–506.
42. Scott P. IL-12: initiation cytokine for cell-mediated immunity. Science 1993;260:496–497.
43. Wu CY, Demeure C, Kiniwa M, Gately M, Delespesse G. IL-12 induces the production of IFN-gamma by neonatal human CD4 T cells. J Immunol 1993;151:1938–1949.
44. Nasu Y, Bangma CH, Hull GW, et al. Adenovirus-mediated interleukin-12 gene therapy for prostate cancer: suppression of orthotopic tumor growth and pre-established lung metastases in an orthotopic model. Gene Ther 1999;6:338–349.
45. Cavallo F, Di Carlo E, Butera M, et al. Immune events associated with the cure of established tumors and spontaneous metastases by local and systemic interleukin 12. Cancer Res 1999;59:414–421.
46. Boggio K, Di Carlo E, Rovero S, et al. Ability of systemic interleukin-12 to hamper progressive stages of mammary carcinogenesis in HER2/neu transgenic mice. Cancer Res 2000;60:359–364.
47. Smyth MJ, Taniguchi M, Street SE. The anti-tumor activity of IL-12: mechanisms of innate immunity that are model and dose dependent. J Immunol 2000;165:2665–2670.
48. Robertson MJ, Cameron C, Atkins MB, et al. Immunological effects of interleukin 12 administered by bolus intravenous injection to patients with cancer. Clin Cancer Res 1999;5:9–16.
49. Kang WK, Park C, Yoon HL, et al. Interleukin 12 gene therapy of cancer by peritumoral injection of transduced autologous fibroblasts: outcome of a phase I study. Hum Gene Ther 2001;12:671–684.
50. Atkins MB, Robertson MJ, Gordon M, et al. Phase I evaluation of intravenous recombinant human interleukin 12 in patients with advanced malignancies. Clin Cancer Res 1997;3:409–417.
51. Leonard JP, Sherman ML, Fisher GL, et al. Effects of single-dose interleukin-12 exposure on interleukin-12-associated toxicity and interferon- gamma production. Blood 1997;90:2541–2548.
52. Gollob JA, Veenstra KG, Mier JW, Atkins MB. Agranulocytosis and hemolytic anemia in patients with renal cell cancer treated with interleukin-12. J Immunother 2001;24:91–98.
53. Motzer RJ, Rakhit A, Schwartz LH, et al. Phase I trial of subcutaneous recombinant human interleukin-12 in patients with advanced renal cell carcinoma. Clin Cancer Res 1998;4:1183–1191.
54. Car BD, Eng VM, Schnyder B, et al. Role of interferon-gamma in interleukin 12-induced pathology in mice. Am J Pathol 1995;147:1693–1707.
55. Siders WM, Wright PW, Hixon JA, et al. T cell- and NK cell-independent inhibition of hepatic metastases by systemic administration of an IL-12-expressing recombinant adenovirus. J Immunol 1998;160:5465–5474.
56. Hirschowitz EA, Crystal RG. Adenovirus-mediated expression of interleukin-12 induces natural killer cell activity and complements adenovirus-directed gp75 treatment of melanoma lung metastases. Am J Respir Cell Mol Biol 1999;20:935–941.
57. Mazzolini G, Qian C, Xie X, et al. Regression of colon cancer and induction of antitumor immunity by intratumoral injection of adenovirus expressing interleukin-12. Cancer Gene Ther 1999;6: 514–522.
58. Rakhmilevich AL, Janssen K, Hao Z, Sondel PM, Yang NS. Interleukin-12 gene therapy of a weakly immunogenic mouse mammary carcinoma results in reduction of spontaneous lung metastases via a T-cell-independent mechanism. Cancer Gene Ther 2000;7:826–838.
59. Worth LL, Jia SF, Zhou Z, Chen L, Kleinerman ES. Intranasal therapy with an adenoviral vector containing the murine interleukin-12 gene eradicates osteosarcoma lung metastases. Clin Cancer Res 2000;6:3713–3718.
60. Brunda MJ, Luistro L, Warrier RR, et al. Antitumor and antimetastatic activity of interleukin 12 against murine tumors. J Exp Med 1993;178:1223–1230.
61. Gately MK, Warrier RR, Honosage S, et al. Administration of recombinant IL-12 to normal mice enhances cytolytic lymphocyte activity and induces production of IFN-gamma in vivo. Int. Immunol 1994;6:157–167.
62. Banks RE, Patel PM, Selby PJ. Interleukin 12: a new clinical player in cytokine therapy. Br J Cancer 1995;71:655–659.
63. Sangro B, Mazzolini G, Ruiz J, et al. Phase I trial of intratumoral injection of an adenovirus encoding interleukin-12 for advanced digestive tumors. J Clin Oncol 2004;22:1389–1397.
64. Nasu Y, Bangma CH, Hull GW, et al. Combination gene therapy with adenoviral vector-mediated HSV-tk+GCV and IL-12 in an orthotopic mouse model for prostate cancer. Prostate Cancer Prostatic Dis 2001;4:44–55.

65. Ren C, Li L, Goltsov AA, et al. mRTVP-1, a Novel p53 Target Gene with Proapoptotic Activities. Mol Cell Biol 2002;22:3345–3357.
66. Murphy EV, Zhang Y, Zhu W, Biggs J. The human glioma pathogenesis-related protein is structurally related to plant pathogenesis-related proteins and its gene is expressed specifically in brain tumors. Gene 1995;159:131–135.
67. Rich T, Chen P, Furman F, Huynh N, Israel MA. RTVP-1, a novel human gene with sequence similarity to genes of diverse species, is expressed in tumor cell lines of glial but not neuronal origin. Gene 1996;180:125–130.
68. Gingras MC, Margolin JF. Differential expression of multiple unexpected genes during U937 cell and macrophage differentiation detected by suppressive subtractive hybridization. Exp Hematol 2000;28:65–76.
69. Szyperski T, Fernandez C, Mumenthaler C, Wuthrich K. Structure comparison of human glioma pathogenesis-related protein GliPR and the plant pathogenesis-related protein P14a indicates a functional link between the human immune system and a plant defense system. Proc Natl Acad Sci U S A 1998;95:2262–2266.
70. Ren C, Li L, Yang G, et al. RTVP-1: a tumor suppressor protein inactivated by methylation in prostate cancer. Cancer Res 2004;64:969–976.
71. Satoh T, Timme TL, Saika T, et al. Adenoviral vector-mediated mRTVP-1 gene therapy for prostate cancer. Hum Gene Ther 2003;14:91–101.
72. Belldegrun A, Tso CL, Zisman A, et al. Interleukin 2 gene therapy for prostate cancer: phase I clinical trial and basic biology. Hum Gene Ther 2001;12:883–892.
73. Pantuck AJ, van Ophoven A, Gitlitz BJ, et al. Phase I trial of antigen-specific gene therapy using a recombinant vaccinia virus encoding MUC-1 and IL-2 in MUC-1-positive patients with advanced prostate cancer. J Immunother 2004;27:240–253.
74. Suzuki K, Nakazato H, Matsui H, et al. NK cell-mediated anti-tumor immune response to human prostate cancer cell, PC-3: immunogene therapy using a highly secretable form of interleukin-15 gene transfer. J Leukoc Biol 2001;69:531–537.
75. Oshikawa K, Shi F, Rakhmilevich AL, Sondel PM, Mahvi DM, Yang NS. Synergistic inhibition of tumor growth in a murine mammary adenocarcinoma model by combinational gene therapy using IL-12, pro-IL-18, and IL-1beta converting enzyme cDNA. Proc Natl Acad Sci U S A 1999;96:13,351–13,356.
76. Yamanaka K, Hara I, Nagai H, et al. Synergistic antitumor effects of interleukin-12 gene transfer and systemic administration of interleukin-18 in a mouse bladder cancer model. Cancer Immunol Immunother 1999;48:297–302.
77. Lebedeva IV, Su ZZ, Sarkar D, et al. Melanoma differentiation associated gene-7, mda-7/interleukin-24, induces apoptosis in prostate cancer cells by promoting mitochondrial dysfunction and inducing reactive oxygen species. Cancer Res 2003;63:8138–8144.
78. Hillman GG, Xu M, Wang Y, et al. Radiation improves intratumoral gene therapy for induction of cancer vaccine in murine prostate carcinoma. Hum Gene Ther 2003;14:763–775.
79. Dong Z, Greene G, Pettaway C, et al. Suppression of angiogenesis, tumorigenicity, and metastasis by human prostate cancer cells engineered to produce interferon-beta. Cancer Res 1999;59:872–879.
80. Cao G, Su J, Lu W, et al. Adenovirus-mediated interferon-beta gene therapy suppresses growth and metastasis of human prostate cancer in nude mice. Cancer Gene Ther 2001;8:497–505.
81. Izawa JI, Sweeney P, Perrotte P, et al. Inhibition of tumorigenicity and metastasis of human bladder cancer growing in athymic mice by interferon-beta gene therapy results partially from various antiangiogenic effects including endothelial cell apoptosis. Clin Cancer Res 2002;8:1258–1270.
82. Nakanishi H, Mizutani Y, Kawauchi A, et al. Significant antitumoral activity of cationic multilamellar liposomes containing human IFN-beta gene against human renal cell carcinoma. Clin Cancer Res 2003;9:1129–1135.
83. Parkinson RJ, Mian S, Bishop MC, et al. Disabled infectious single cycle herpes simplex virus (DISC-HSV) is a candidate vector system for gene delivery/expression of GM-CSF in human prostate cancer therapy. Prostate 2003;56:65–73.
84. Griffith TS, Kawakita M, Tian J, et al. Inhibition of murine prostate tumor growth and activation of immunoregulatory cells with recombinant canarypox viruses. J Natl Cancer Inst 2001;93:998–1007.
85. Wu Q, Mahendran R, Esuvaranathan K. Nonviral cytokine gene therapy on an orthotopic bladder cancer model. Clin Cancer Res 2003;9:4522–4528.
86. Sanda MG, Ayyagari SR, Jaffee EM, et al. Demonstration of a rational strategy for human prostate cancer gene therapy. J Urol 1994;151:622–628.

87. Rini BI, Small EJ. The potential for prostate cancer immunotherapy. Crit Rev Oncol Hematol 2003;46 Suppl:S117–S125.
88. Baecher-Allan C, Viglietta V, Hafler DA. Human CD4+CD25+ regulatory T cells. Semin Immunol 2004;16:89–98.
89. Correale P, Walmsley K, Zaremba S, Zhu M, Schlom J, Tsang KY. Generation of human cytolytic T lymphocyte lines directed against prostate-specific antigen (PSA) employing a PSA oligoepitope peptide. J Immunol 1998;161:3186–3194.
90. Sanda MG, Smith DC, Charles LG, et al. Recombinant vaccinia-PSA (PROSTVAC) can induce a prostate-specific immune response in androgen-modulated human prostate cancer. Urology 1999;53:260–266.
91. Meidenbauer N, Harris DT, Spitler LE, Whiteside TL. Generation of PSA-reactive effector cells after vaccination with a PSA-based vaccine in patients with prostate cancer. Prostate 2000;43:88–100.
92. Terasawa H, Tsang KY, Gulley J, Arlen P, Schlom J. Identification and characterization of a human agonist cytotoxic T-lymphocyte epitope of human prostate-specific antigen. Clin Cancer Res 2002; 8:41–53.
93. Zhang S, Zhang HS, Reuter VE, Slovin SF, Scher HI, Livingston PO. Expression of potential target antigens for immunotherapy on primary and metastatic prostate cancers. Clin Cancer Res 1998;4:295–302.
94. Gong MC, Latouche JB, Krause A, Heston WD, Bander NH, Sadelain M. Cancer patient T cells genetically targeted to prostate-specific membrane antigen specifically lyse prostate cancer cells and release cytokines in response to prostate-specific membrane antigen. Neoplasia 1999;1:123–127.
95. Chen ME, Lin SH, Chung LW, Sikes RA. Isolation and characterization of PAGE-1 and GAGE-7. New genes expressed in the LNCaP prostate cancer progression model that share homology with melanoma-associated antigens. J Biol Chem 1998;273:17,618–17,625.
96. Fong L, Ruegg CL, Brockstedt D, Engleman EG, Laus R. Induction of tissue-specific autoimmune prostatitis with prostatic acid phosphatase immunization: implications for immunotherapy of prostate cancer. J Immunol 1997;159:3113–3117.
97. McNeel DG, Nguyen LD, Disis ML. Identification of T helper epitopes from prostatic acid phosphatase. Cancer Res 2001;61:5161–5167.
98. Dhanasekaran SM, Barrette TR, Ghosh D, et al. Delineation of prognostic biomarkers in prostate cancer. Nature 2001;412:822–826.
99. Dranoff G. GM-CSF-based cancer vaccines. Immunol Rev 2002;188:147–154.
100. Simons JW, Mikhak B, Chang JF, et al. Induction of immunity to prostate cancer antigens: results of a clinical trial of vaccination with irradiated autologous prostate tumor cells engineered to secrete granulocyte-macrophage colony-stimulating factor using ex vivo gene transfer. Cancer Res 1999;59: 5160–5168.
101. Tani K, Nakazaki Y, Hase H, et al. Progress reports on immune gene therapy for stage IV renal cell cancer using lethally irradiated granulocyte-macrophage colony-stimulating factor-transduced autologous renal cancer cells. Cancer Chemother Pharmacol 2000;46 Suppl:S73–S76.
102. Kawai K, Tani K, Yamashita N, et al. Advanced renal cell carcinoma treated with granulocyte-macrophage colony-stimulating factor gene therapy: a clinical course of the first Japanese experience. Int J Urol 2002;9:462–466.
103. Hull GW, McCurdy MA, Nasu Y, et al. Prostate cancer gene therapy: comparison of adenovirus-mediated expression of interleukin 12 with interleukin 12 plus B7-1 for in situ gene therapy and gene-modified, cell-based vaccines. Clin Cancer Res 2000;6:4101–4109.
104. Shimura S, Yang G, Ebara S, Wheeler TM, Frolov A, Thompson TC. Reduced infiltration of tumor-associated macrophages in human prostate cancer: association with cancer progression. Cancer Res 2000;60:5857–5861.
105. Xu J, Zheng SL, Komiya A, et al. Common sequence variants of the macrophage scavenger receptor 1 gene are associated with prostate cancer risk. Am J Hum Genet 2003;72:208–212.
106. Xu J, Zheng SL, Komiya A, et al. Germline mutations and sequence variants of the macrophage scavenger receptor 1 gene are associated with prostate cancer risk. Nat Genet 2002;32:321–325.
107. Wang L, McDonnell SK, Cunningham JM, et al. No association of germline alteration of MSR1 with prostate cancer risk. Nat Genet 2003;35:128–129.
108. Satoh T, Saika T, Ebara S, et al. Macrophages transduced with an adenoviral vector expressing interleukin 12 suppress tumor growth and metastasis in a preclinical metastatic prostate cancer model. Cancer Res 2003;63:7853–7860.
109. Murphy GP, Tjoa BA, Simmons SJ, et al. Infusion of dendritic cells pulsed with HLA-A2-specific prostate-specific membrane antigen peptides: a phase II prostate cancer vaccine trial involving patients with hormone-refractory metastatic disease. Prostate 1999;38:73–78.

110. Murphy GP, Tjoa BA, Simmons SJ, et al. Phase II prostate cancer vaccine trial: report of a study involving 37 patients with disease recurrence following primary treatment. Prostate 1999;39:54–59.
111. Burch PA, Breen JK, Buckner JC, et al. Priming tissue-specific cellular immunity in a phase I trial of autologous dendritic cells for prostate cancer. Clin Cancer Res 2000;6:2175–2182.
112. Small EJ, Fratesi P, Reese DM, et al. Immunotherapy of hormone-refractory prostate cancer with antigen-loaded dendritic cells. J Clin Oncol 2000;18:3894–3903.
113. Heiser A, Maurice MA, Yancey DR, et al. Induction of polyclonal prostate cancer-specific CTL using dendritic cells transfected with amplified tumor RNA. J Immunol 2001;166:2953–2960.
114. Fong L, Brockstedt D, Benike C, et al. Dendritic cell-based xenoantigen vaccination for prostate cancer immunotherapy. J Immunol 2001;167:7150–7156.
115. Correale P, Micheli L, Vecchio MT, et al. A parathyroid-hormone-related-protein (PTH-rP)-specific cytotoxic T cell response induced by in vitro stimulation of tumour-infiltrating lymphocytes derived from prostate cancer metastases, with epitope peptide-loaded autologous dendritic cells and low-dose IL-2. Br J Cancer 2001;85:1722–1730.
116. Heiser A, Coleman D, Dannull J, et al. Autologous dendritic cells transfected with prostate-specific antigen RNA stimulate CTL responses against metastatic prostate tumors. J Clin Invest 2002;109: 409–417.
117. Ridgway D. The first 1000 dendritic cell vaccinees. Cancer Invest 2003;21:873–886.
118. Figdor CG, De Vries IJ, Lesterhuis WJ, Melief CJ. Dendritic cell immunotherapy: mapping the way. Nat Med 2004;10:475–480.
119. Saika T, Satoh T, Kusaka N, et al. Route of administration influences the antitumor effects of bone marrow-derived dendritic cells engineered to produce interleukin-12 in a metastatic mouse prostate cancer model. Cancer Gene Ther 2004;11:317–324.
120. De Vries IJ, Krooshoop DJ, Scharenborg NM, et al. Effective migration of antigen-pulsed dendritic cells to lymph nodes in melanoma patients is determined by their maturation state. Cancer Res 2003;63:12–17.
121. Curiel TJ, Curiel DT. Tumor immunotherapy: inching toward the finish line. J Clin Invest 2002; 109:311–312.
122. Sawczuk IS. Autolymphocyte therapy in the treatment of metastatic renal cell carcinoma. Urol Clin North Am 1993;20:297–301.
123. Graham S, Babayan RK, Lamm DL, et al. The use of ex vivo-activated memory T cells (autolymphocyte therapy) in the treatment of metastatic renal cell carcinoma: final results from a randomized, controlled, multisite study. Semin Urol 1993;11:27–34.
124. Ross S, Liu V, Abulafia R, Hogan C, Osband M. Adoptive immunotherapy of hormone-refractory, stage D2 prostate cancer using ex vivo activated autologous T cells (autolymphocyte therapy): results from a pilot study. Biotechnol Ther 1993;4:197–211.
125. Kawakami Y, Haas GP, Lotze MT. Expansion of tumor-infiltrating lymphocytes from human tumors using the T-cell growth factors interleukin-2 and interleukin-4. J Immunother 1993;14:336–347.
126. Ho WY, Blattman JN, Dossett ML, Yee C, Greenberg PD. Adoptive immunotherapy: engineering T cell responses as biologic weapons for tumor mass destruction. Cancer Cell 2003;3:431–437.
127. Pinthus JH, Waks T, Kaufman-Francis K, et al. Immuno-Gene Therapy of Established Prostate Tumors Using Chimeric Receptor-redirected Human Lymphocytes. Cancer Res 2003;63:2470–2476.
128. Dudley ME, Wunderlich JR, Robbins PF, et al. Cancer regression and autoimmunity in patients after clonal repopulation with antitumor lymphocytes. Science 2002;298:850–854.
129. Saika T, Kusaka N, Satoh T, et al. Adoptive transfer of splenocytes from mice treated in situ with AdIL-12 results in suppression of tumor growth and metastasis and increased survival in a model for residual tumor after neo-adjuvant in situ gene therapy for prostate cancer. Mol. Ther 2002;6:S111.
130. Schmidt-Wolf IG, Finke S, Trojaneck B, et al. Phase I clinical study applying autologous immunological effector cells transfected with the interleukin-2 gene in patients with metastatic renal cancer, colorectal cancer and lymphoma. Br J Cancer 1999;81:1009–1016.
131. Wang H, Yang G, Satoh T, et al. Antimetastatic effects of IL-12 gene-modified bone marrow cells in a mouse model of metastatic prostate cancer. Mol. Ther 2003;7:S119.
132. Nishioka Y, Hirao M, Robbins PD, Lotze MT, Tahara H. Induction of systemic and therapeutic antitumor immunity using intratumoral injection of dendritic cells genetically modified to express interleukin 12. Cancer Res 1999;59:4035–4041.
133. Marshall E. Gene therapy. Second child in French trial is found to have leukemia. Science 2003;299:320.

15 Combination of Gene Therapy with Radiation

Anupama Munshi, PhD
and Raymond E. Meyn, PhD

CONTENTS

Summary

To date tremendous progress has been made in the field of cancer gene therapy. Strategies have been explored for achieving therapeutic benefit using various genes and several clinical trials for cancer gene therapy have been carried out demonstrating that gene therapy is well tolerated. However, in most cases the efficacy of gene transfer has been very limited. As an alternative, multimodality therapies are being developed with the idea of increasing the efficacy of the treatment, decreasing toxicity, and minimizing the development of resistance. Thus, simultaneous or sequential administration of gene therapy agents with conventional anticancer agents may work in a synergistic manner. Conventional radiotherapy is usually limited by a narrow therapeutic index and the combination of gene therapy with radiation is especially promising. Preclinical and clinical studies have, in fact, demonstrated significant potential for the combination of cancer gene therapy with radiotherapy that could lead to improved treatment responses. This chapter attempts to highlight some of the gene therapy approaches that have shown success both in preclinical models and in clinical trials when used in combination with conventional radiotherapy.

Key Words: Gene therapy; ionizing radiation; carcinoma; clinical trials; radiosensitization.

1. INTRODUCTION

Gene therapy has the potential to provide cancer treatments based on novel mechanisms of action that have low toxicity. Such treatments may effectively control locoregional recurrence as well as systemic micrometastases. Despite certain limitations, retroviral and adenoviral vectors can provide an effective means of delivering therapeutic genes to tumor cells. However, even if a substantial number of tumor cells are transfected,

From: *Cancer Drug Discovery and Development: Gene Therapy for Cancer*
Edited by: K. K. Hunt, S. A. Vorburger, and S. G. Swisher © Humana Press Inc., Totowa, NJ

complete eradication of the tumor is unlikely to occur. Thus, gene therapy as a single modality may not be efficacious in most cases. A multimodality approach consisting of gene therapy combined with conventional radio- or chemotherapy might, therefore, be more promising for clinical application.

Radiotherapy remains a front-line treatment for cancer. However, as is the case with other conventional therapies, radiation therapy lacks tumor specificity and the radiation dose is limited by the risk of normal tissue toxicity. Combining radiation with other anticancer agents should allow lower doses to be used, thereby minimizing side effects. Gene therapy in combination with radiation is one such promising strategy that is currently moving from laboratory studies to clinical trials. Gene therapy allows the intratumoral introduction of genetic material that may result in a radiosensitizing effect. This chapter presents an overview of the potential synergistic strategies of radiation therapy and gene transfer in the management of human malignancies.

2. GENE THERAPY APPROACHES

The basic therapeutic approaches that have been employed in cancer gene therapy combined with radiation include molecular chemotherapy, gene replacement, oncolytic viruses, and antimolecular therapy.

3. MOLECULAR CHEMOTHERAPY

3.1. Herpes Simplex Virus Thymidine Kinase

One specific molecular chemotherapy approach involves tumor cell transduction with the herpes simplex virus-thymidine kinase (HSV-*tk*) gene via a viral vector, followed by the systemic administration of the chemotherapy agent ganciclovir (GCV) *(1)*. GCV is a prodrug that must be phosphorylated initially by the HSV-*tk* gene product to a monophosphate form and, subsequently, by the mammalian kinases to the cytotoxic triphosphate form. Once activated by this process, GCV functions as a purine analog that inhibits DNA polymerase thereby preventing DNA synthesis and inducing cell death *(2,3)*. In addition, HSV-*tk* gene therapy mediates a "bystander effect," whereby nontransduced neighboring cells are also killed. This bystander effect appears to result from the transfer of active GCV metabolites through intercellular gap junctions between the transduced cells and the neighboring cells *(4,5)*. Gene therapy with HSV-*tk* coadministered with GCV has been shown to be effective in various tumor models where it delayed local tumor growth and prolonged survival *(7,8)*. Because radiation acts primarily by causing DNA strand breaks, HSV-*tk* gene therapy enhances radiation effects by interfering with DNA repair mechanisms. Other possible mechanisms may include an improved adenoviral-mediated gene transfer efficiency in irradiated cells *(6)*, and radiation-induced cellular membrane damage may facilitate the transfer of cytotoxic nucleotide analogs from HSV-*tk*-expressing cells to neighboring nontransduced cells. Chhikara et al. *(9)* demonstrated that the combination therapy has a considerably better antimetastatic effect compared with HSV-*tk* gene therapy alone. They attributed this to the induction of a potent local and systemic immune response as evidenced by the abundance of $CD4^+$ cells in the primary tumor. In a recent study Rosenberg et al. *(10)* showed that HSV-*tk* radiosensitized human glioma, U87 MG cells, after exposure to low concentrations of GCV. Importantly, this radiosensitization was most pronounced in the dose range that is used clinically (1–3 Gy). Preliminary results from an ongoing phase I/II trial evaluating the role of this combination for the treatment of prostate cancer indicate that this strategy is safe, but longer follow-up is required to demonstrate whether this therapy provides a therapeutic advantage compared with standard treatment *(11)*.

3.2. Cytosine Deaminase

Several chemotherapy agents have demonstrated activity for human cancer, including cisplatin, doxorubicin, methotrexate, vinblastine, and 5-fluorouracil (5-FU). However, the clinical utility and effectiveness of several of these drugs is generally limited by toxicity. Using the approach of gene therapy, a suicide gene encoding the bacterial and fungal enzyme cytosine deaminase (CD) can be transferred from bacteria and expressed in mammalian tumor cells. CD expressing cells can deaminate the relatively non-toxic prodrug 5-fluorocytosine (5-FC) to the highly toxic drug 5-FU. The effect of suicide gene therapy using an adenovirus vector expressing the CD gene combined with radiation therapy has been evaluated in several different tumor cell systems *(12–14)*. The interaction between CD/5-FC gene therapy and radiation was compared when radiation preceded CD/5-FC treatment vs radiation followed by CD/5-FC treatment. Enhanced cell killing was seen only when the cells were exposed to the CD/5-FC before radiation making this finding significant for the future design of treatment strategies using the combination therapy. Adenovirus-mediated delivery of the CD gene used with 5-FC has also been used to achieve increased radiation killing of tumor cells in xenograft models. In a study using a colon cancer xenograft model, a significant growth delay was observed in the irradiated, Ad-CD infected tumors treated with 5-FC compared with radiation alone or the Ad-CD infected and 5-FC-treated tumors without radiation *(15)*.

4. GENE REPLACEMENT THERAPY

Malignant cells are frequently resistant to chemotherapy and radiation-induced programmed cell death (apoptosis). Such resistance is generally the result of abnormal expression of certain oncogenes or mutations in or loss of expression of tumor suppressor genes involved in the control of apoptosis. Strategies designed to replace defective tumor suppressor genes, as well as to force expression of apoptosis-inducing genes offer promise for restoring this mode of cell death in tumor cells.

4.1. p53

The *p53* gene (also known as *TP53*) encodes a 593-amino acid phosphoprotein that plays critical roles in several cell processes including cell-cycle regulation and control of apoptosis *(16–18)*. *p53* gene mutations are frequent in tumor cells and have been associated with cancer progression and the development of resistance to both chemotherapy and radiation therapy *(19–21)*. The development of gene transfer techniques has facilitated transduction of tumor cells with wild-type *p53* (wt-p53). Preclinical studies both in vitro and in vivo have shown that restoration of wt-*p53* function can induce apoptosis in cancer cells. Intratumoral injection in animal models of retroviral or adenoviral wt-*p53* constructs results in tumor regression for a variety of different tumor histologies, including non-small-cell lung cancer (NSCLC), leukemia, glioblastoma, and breast, liver, ovarian, colon, and kidney cancers *(22–28)*. Several preclinical studies have indicated that gene therapy with Ad-p53 has useful synergistic effects when combined with certain drugs or radiation therapy. Studies from our laboratory have evaluated the ability of Ad-p53 to radiosensitize human tumor cells from cancer cells of various origins including NSCLC, prostate cancer, colorectal cancer and head and neck cancer *(19,29–32)*. In addition, we have examined the effects of Ad-p53 mediated gene transfer on normal lung fibroblast cells. These studies indicated that gene therapy using Ad-p53 in combination with radiation radiosensitized tumor cells irrespective of their *p53* status while sparing normal fibroblasts. In addition, tumor growth suppression was enhanced by this combination strategy in xenograft tumors growing in nude mice compared with Ad-p53 or radiation therapy when used alone, indicating that therapy using Ad-p53 and irradiation in combination is more effective than either treatment when used alone.

Though numerous studies have been carried out using Ad-p53 gene therapy in combination with radiation, the in vitro mechanism of radiosensitization of human tumor cells by the gene therapy vector has not been tested. In a recent study, we have demonstrated that Ad-p53 mediated radiosensitization of human tumor cells is caused by suppression of nonhomologus end joining (NHEJ), a pathway that is especially important for repairing radiation-induced DNA double strand breaks *(30)*. We found that Ad-p53 radiosensitized human tumor cells and that this effect correlated with a down-modulation of proteins involved in NHEJ. Normal human fibroblasts were not radiosensitized by Ad-p53, suggesting that Ad-p53 has a differential effect on DNA repair in tumor cells versus normal cells.

Roth et al. *(33)* were the first group to demonstrate the safety and feasibility of using a retroviral wt-*p53* construct in patients with advanced NSCLC. Currently there are several ongoing trials using adenoviral-mediated p53-based gene therapy for human cancers of the lung, brain, ovary, head and neck, and bladder *(34–38)*. Similar trials have previously shown that *p53* gene replacement therapy is feasible and safe using both retroviral and adenoviral vectors, and that it induces tumor regression in patients with advanced NSCLC and recurrent head and neck cancer *(36)*. Based on these reports, Swisher et al. *(39)* extended their previous studies of Ad-p53 as a single agent in NSCLC and initiated a clinical trial of Ad-p53 combined with external beam ionizing radiation. These investigators reported that intratumoral injection of Ad-p53 followed by radiation therapy was well tolerated, led to successful *p53* gene transfer, had low toxicity, and produced tumor regression. A high metastatic failure rate was evident in their patient population, which may have been expected because chemotherapy could not be administered to these high-risk patients. Thus, because survival in locoregionally advanced NSCLC is dependent on the control of metastatic disease, phase III randomized studies are being planned to determine whether the potential improvement in locoregional control achieved by Ad-p53 and radiation therapy can translate into improved overall survival. This group also plans to address metastatic relapse in future studies by adding chemotherapy to the combination of Ad-p53 and radiation therapy.

4.2. *mda-7*

The protein product of the *mda-7* gene, *Mda-7*/interleukin (IL)-24, is a novel cytokine that belongs to the IL-10 family of cytokines *(40)*. Gene delivery using Ad-mda-7 results in growth suppression and apoptosis in a broad-spectrum of cancer cell types including those of the lung, prostate, mesothelioma, pancreatic, breast, gliomas, renal, and human melanoma *(41–48)*. In contrast, Ad-mda-7 does not elicit deleterious effects in normal cells, including those of epithelial, fibroblast, astrocyte, melanocyte, or endothelial origin *(49)*. Based on these distinctive properties and reports of antitumor and antiangiogenic activities in human tumor xenograft animal models, a phase I/II clinical trial in patients with advanced carcinomas involving intratumoral administration of *mda-7*/IL-24 [using a replication incompetent adenovirus; ING241 (Ad-mda-7)] has been initiated. Preliminary data from this trial documents that this gene is safe and well-tolerated by patients and that a single virus injection elicits apoptosis in a majority of the tumors *(50)*.

One of the first studies demonstrating the ability of Ad-mda-7 to synergistically enhance radiosensitivity of human tumor cells was reported by the authors. We demonstrated that Ad-mda-7 can act to radiosensitize human lung carcinoma cells but has no effect on normal human fibroblasts *(51)*. We further examined the basis for this difference in the ability of Ad-mda-7 to radiosensitize tumor cells compared with normal cells. Radiation-induced apoptosis was restored in the tumor cell lines, but not in the normal cells. Ad-mda-7 enhances radiosensitivity independently of any ability to upregulate the expression of Fas or Bax in NSCLC cells and was independent of the p53 status of tumor cells. Further analysis indicated that phosphorylated c-Jun expression was increased by Ad-mda-7 in tumor cells, but not in the normal fibroblasts. To elucidate the mechanisms underlying the radiosensitizing effect of Ad-mda-7 in tumor cells, we have examined the relationship between ectopic expression of *mda-7* and the NHEJ pathway for repair of radiation-induced DNA double-strand breaks. The data indicated that the expression of proteins involved in NHEJ was downregulated in tumor cells pretreated with Ad-mda-7 compared with that in mock-treated and Ad-Luc–treated cells. Additionally, no such changes were observed in normal human fibroblasts treated with Ad-mda-7. Therefore, it appears reasonable to propose that the radiosensitizing effect of Ad-mda-7 is a result of the observed suppressed expression of NHEJ components and capacity for repair *(52)*. In addition to our previous observation related to JNK and c-Jun activation, other investigators have reported that Ad-mda7 may activate p38 *(43)*. It will therefore be important to determine which of these or other signaling pathways activated in Ad-mda-7 infected cells are responsible for the downregulation of components of NHEJ and mediating the radiosensitizing effect. There have also been studies reporting the ability of Ad-mda-7 and purified MDA-7 protein to sensitize malignant glioma cells to ionizing radiation *(41,53,54)*. Thus, the combination of Ad-mda-7 and radiation may have broad applicability to cancer treatment.

4.3. p16

The cyclin-dependent kinase inhibitor (CDK-I), p16, was identified in a yeast two-hybrid screen as a protein that inhibits the ability of cyclin-dependent kinase 4 (CDK4) and cyclin-dependent kinase 6 (CDK6) to regulate the phosphorylation status of phospho retinoblastoma (pRb), thereby controlling progression of cells into S phase. Inactivation of p16 function either through mutations or deletions has been linked to the development of many types of cancers including melanoma, esophageal, lung, pancreas, mesothelioma, bladder, head and neck, breast, brain, acute lymphocytic leukemia, osteosarcoma, ovarian, and renal cell carcinoma *(55–62)*. Restoration of p16 expression to human tumor cells using adenoviral vectors has been studied by several investigators and has been shown to arrest the cells in the G1-S phase of the cell cycle *(63)*. In addition, adenovirus-p16 (Ad-p16) was found to inhibit the growth of pre-established xenografts and prolong the survival time of the tumor-bearing mice *(64)*. Kawabe et al. *(65)* compared the ability of Ad-p16 to radiosensitize NSCLC cell lines that lack p16 but have wt-*p53*, mt-*p53*, or deleted *p53* status. Their results indicated that NSCLC cells carrying wt-*p53* were radiosensitized by Ad-p16. The NSCLC cells which did not have functional p53, were either minimally radiosensitized or not at all. These results suggested that the radiosensitization involved a restoration of apoptosis propensity that was dependent on the endogenous *p53* status of the tumor cells. They further demonstrated that NSCLC cells that lack wt-p53 could still be radiosensitized to Ad-p16 by infecting with a small quantity of Ad-p53. Because Ad-p16 has shown limited success as a single agent in preclinical models, Rhee et al. *(66)* developed a strategy to combine ionizing radiation with Ad-p16 gene transfer to radiosensitize head and neck squamous cell carcinoma. Combination of Ad-p16 and radiation showed an augmented therapeutic response in vitro. When these cell lines were grown as xenograft tumors in nude mice the antitumor response to combination therapy showed a statistically significant additive effect when compared with the response to each agent alone. They, however, did not address the significance of functional p53 in mediating this radiosensitizing effect.

4.4. Bax

Bax is a proapoptotic member of the bcl-2 family of proteins which can mediate the mitochondrial pathway of apoptosis *(67,68)*. Bax is normally sequestered in the cell and its proapoptotic effect is exerted only after a concomitant death signal, such as deprivation of a growth factor, or radiation *(69)*. Induction of apoptosis may be an important mechanism that contributes to the cytotoxicity of radiotherapy, and in many cases, its presence predicts the sensitivity to and outcome of radiation. It has been shown that adenovirus-mediated Bax expression sensitizes various human tumor cells to radiation both in vitro and in vivo. Exogenous Bax-mediated induction of apoptosis sensitizes breast and ovarian cancer cells to the effect of radiation *(70–72)*. More importantly, it has been shown that the inability of p53 to induce the activity of Bax is associated with the development of radioresistance in malignant gliomas *(73)*. Based on these observations, it can be hypothesized that Bax gene delivery into malignant gliomas would sensitize the tumor to the cytotoxic effects of radiotherapy. Investigation into the involved mechanism suggests that Bax-mediated radiosensitization occurs through both apoptosis and necrosis pathways.

4.5. Tumor Necrosis Factor-α (TNFerade™)

Tumor necrosis factor (TNF)-α is a soluble cytokine that mediates cellular immune response. It has potent antitumor properties as demonstrated using the recombinant protein in numerous preclinical models *(74–76)* and in clinical trials as a single agent. TNF-α has been shown to be directly cytotoxic to a number of cell lines through the production of hydroxyl radicals with resulting damage to DNA. As radiation therapy also produces DNA damage by free radical formation, a synergistic interaction between TNF-α and radiation might be expected and several studies have demonstrated the synergistic effect of TNF-α combined with radiation in laboratory models. However, the clinical development of TNF-α has been limited because of severe toxicity when administered systemically. If TNF-α were administered such that systemic toxicity was limited, it might be a useful anticancer agent. A gene therapy approach, using intratumoral injections of an adenovirus expressing TNF-α is one possible strategy that has been developed by Weichselbaum *(77)*. The vector, TNFerade™, is a replication deficient, second generation adenoviral vector that has the radiation-inducible immediate early growth response (Egr-1) gene promoter ligated upstream to the transcriptional start site of human TNF-α cDNA *(77)*.

The activity of TNFerade in combination with radiation has been evaluated in a number of different human xenograft models including gliomas, prostate, esophageal, and laryngeal carcinoma *(78–80)*. The effect of the combination in each of these cases was greater than the effect of either agent when used alone. Interestingly, the combination of TNFerade and radiation was found to be effective even against tumors that were resistant to radiation or TNF-α *(77)*.

Based on the promising results obtained these preclinical models, a phase-I clinical study of TNFerade was conducted in patients with various solid tumors to evaluate the safety, tolerability, and feasibility of intratumoral administration of TNFerade in combination with radiation. The results from this study demonstrated that repeated intratumoral injections of TNFerade in combination with radiation are well tolerated *(81,82)*. Thus, this novel gene therapy approach using a radiation-inducible promoter in combination with irradiation, appears to be an effective way to optimize the anticancer activity and minimize the systemic toxicity of cytotoxic agents such as TNF-α *(77)*.

4.6. EIA

Several studies have shown that Her2/neu is overexpressed in human tumors and enhances metastasis, tumorigenicity, and resistance to chemotherapeutic agents. These patients often have poor prognosis. Adenovirus type 5 carries the *EIA* gene that encodes a phosphonuclear protein which is the first viral gene product expressed in host cells after adenoviral infection *(83,84)*. *EIA* in turn activates viral gene transcription and reprograms the host's cellular gene expression to allow efficient propagation of adenovirus in the host's cells *(83,84)*. The *EIA* gene also produces proteins that inhibit Her-2/neu expression in both rodent and human cells. On the basis of this observation it was demonstrated that *E1A* gene delivered via a novel cationic liposome suppressed tumor growth and prolonged survival in orthotopic models of ovarian and breast cancer *(85,86)*. In a study by Wang et al. *(87) E1A* gene transfer was shown to slightly enhance the sensitivity of human head and neck squamous carcinoma cells to ionizing radiation. Based on the preclinical studies a phase I trial of *E1A* gene therapy using cationic liposomes as the delivery agent has been conducted for human ovarian, head and neck and breast cancer. Preliminary results demonstrated that *E1A* gene transfer was well tolerated and no dose-limiting toxicity was observed, warranting further testing *(88,89)*.

5. ONCOLYTIC VIRUSES

Successful anticancer strategies require a differential response between tumor and normal tissue (i.e., a therapeutic index). Replication-competent, E1B-attenuated adenoviruses represent a means of achieving a therapeutic index by selectively destroying tumor cells with minimal toxicity to normal cells *(90–92)*. The prototype virus, ONYX-015, is deleted for the E1B protein that binds to and inactivates cellular p53 *(90,93)*. As a result, ONYX-015 viral therapy was initially regarded as a potentially significant advancement in cancer treatment because of its ability to destroy *p53*-mutated tumors, which comprise approx 50% of all human cancers *(94)*. In addition, *p53* mutation often correlates with resistance to conventional therapies *(94,95)*. However, subsequent studies have called into question the host range specificity originally described for ONYX-015 *(91,96–101)*. Multiple groups have recently demonstrated in vitro that ONYX-015 can lyse tumor cells having a wild-type or mutant *p53* status. Because most of these studies used heterogeneous cell lines having diverse genetic backgrounds, it is possible that these conflicting observations were, in part, attributable to differences other than *p53* status.

Because ONYX-015 virus has proven to be biologically active and safe in cancer patients *(102)*, several investigators have evaluated the possible radiosensitizing effect of ONYX-015 on human tumor cells. ONYX-015 has been suggested as an effective neo-adjuvant to radiation therapy in a human colon carcinoma model and malignant glioma *(103,104)*. These studies provide evidence that ONYX-015 has an additive, even potentiating antitumor effect on irradiated human tumor xenografts supporting the use of combined treatment with this attenuated replicative adenovirus and radiation therapy.

6. ANTIMOLECULAR THERAPY

6.1. Antisense Oligonucleotides

Antisense oligonucleotides (ASONs) are a new class of molecularly targeted agents that are transitioning from the laboratory into the clinic. Clinically, these drugs are well-tolerated with favorable toxicity profiles, and laboratory studies have demonstrated that they can be feasibly combined with radiotherapy. ASONs directed against a number of important cellular targets, including the mRNA of c-myb, MDM2, bcl-2, protein kinase C-α, PKA-I, H-ras, c-raf, R1- and R2-subunit of ribonucleotide reductase, and transforming growth factor β2 *(105–108)* have been investigated in clinical trials. Laboratory studies investigating the potential value of ASONs as radiosensitizers have also been conducted. Survivin is a recently discovered member of the IAP family that plays a dual role in suppressing apoptosis and regulating cell division and interest has been generated on the use of ASONs to target survivin for downregulation *(109)*. A variety of human tumor types including lung, breast, colon, gastric, esophageal, pancreatic, liver, bladder, uterine, and ovarian cancers, large-cell non-Hodgkin's lymphomas, leukemias, neuroblastomas, gliomas, soft tissue sarcomas, melanomas and other skin cancers abnormally express survivin possibly rendering them resistant to apoptosis-inducing therapies *(110)*. A possible role for survivin in determining the radiation response of human tumor cells was revealed in a recent report indicating that survivin acts as a constitutive radioresistance factor in pancreatic cancer cells *(111)*. Specifically, using a panel of established cell lines an inverse relationship was found between survivin mRNA expression and in vitro sensitivity to radiation. ASONs against survivin attenuated survivin expression compared with the mismatch oligonucleotide, resulting in a 20% reduction of cell viability when used as a single agent. However, concurrent survivin inhibition and irradiation caused a significant shift in the survival curve of human lung cancer cells after 2 Gy and 5 Gy, suggesting that the inhibition of survivin expression produces a radiation-sensitizing effect.

Another approach to radiosensitize tumors uses ASONs designed to target DNA repair proteins that are involved in repairing radiation-induced DNA double strand breaks. One such protein complex, involved in DNA double-strand break repair and V(D)J recombination, is the DNA-dependent protein kinase (DNA-PK) complex consisting of Ku70 protein, cooperating with Ku80 and the DNA-PK catalytic subunit (DNA-PKcs). It is well established that cells deficient in any of these DNA repair proteins have increased radiosensitivity. Omori et al. *(112)* demonstrated using a human squamous cell lung carcinoma cell line that introduction of an antisense to Ku70 suppressed Ku70 protein expression as compared with controls and a small but statistically significant increase in radiosensitivity of the cells was achieved. In addition, the antisense to Ku70 increased the chemosensitivity of the cells to some DNA-damaging agents such as bleomycin.

A more recent study examined the feasibility of using adenovirus-mediated, heat-activated expression of antisense Ku70 RNA as a gene therapy approach to sensitize cells and tumors to ionizing radiation. The adenovirus vector contained antisense Ku70 under the control of hsp70 promoter. Their data showed that heat shock induces antisense Ku70 mRNA expression, reduces the endogenous Ku70 expression level, and significantly increases the radiosensitivity of cells. This approach was then extended to in vivo models where heat-shock-induced expression of antisense Ku70 mRNA using this same vector attenuated Ku70 protein expression in murine FSa-II tumors, and radiosensitized the FSa-II tumors *(113)*. Based on these results it appears that adenovirus-mediated, heat-activated antisense Ku70 expression is a novel approach to radiosensitize human tumors.

6.2. Angiogenesis Inhibitors

Over the last years, tumor-specific vasculature formation (angiogenesis) has emerged as a promising new target for inhibiting the growth of tumors *(114–118)*, using antiangiogenic agents either alone, or in combination with conventional therapies *(114,115, 117–119)*. The key advantages of this approach are that because it targets normal endothelial cells rather than tumor cells, the development of drug resistance is less likely *(114)*, and that antiangiogenic therapy can exert a powerful antitumor effect with little or no systemic toxicity to the host *(114,115,117,118)*. The combination of antiangiogenic agents with ionizing radiation has demonstrated a local synergistic antitumor interaction between the two modalities *(120–123)* for angiostatin *(120)*, antivascular endothelial growth factor antibody *(121)*, and endostatin *(122)*. Several investigators have produced adenoviral based vectors for delivering the genes that encode these or similar proteins thereby enabling future tests of antiangiogenic gene therapy in combination with radiation.

7. CONCLUSIONS

The examples presented in the above sections indicate that several novel gene therapy strategies have been discovered that may synergize with radiation to enhance therapeutic response in tumor cells. Although the examples listed above do not reflect all such available strategies, it is clear that several promising approaches targeting cell death pathways have been developed and entered into clinical trials. Ultimately, the results of these trials will help determine which if any of these strategies will become a standard of care in radiation oncology.

ACKNOWLEDGMENTS

This study was supported in part by grants R41 CA88421, PO1 CA78778, PO1 CA06294 and P30 CA16672 from the National Cancer Institute and a sponsored research agreement with Introgen Therapeutics, Inc.

REFERENCES

1. Moolten FL. Tumor chemosensitivity conferred by inserted herpes thymidine kinase genes: paradigm for a prospective cancer control strategy. Cancer Res 1986;46:5276–5281.
2. Frank KB, Chiou JF, Cheng YC. Interaction of herpes simplex virus-induced DNA polymerase with 9-(1,3-dihydroxy-2-propoxymethyl)guanine triphosphate. J Biol Chem 1984;259:1566–1569.
3. Matthews T, Boehme R. Antiviral activity and mechanism of action of ganciclovir. Rev Infect Dis 1988;10 Suppl 3:S490–S494.

4. Mesnil M, Yamasaki H. Bystander effect in herpes simplex virus-thymidine kinase/ganciclovir cancer gene therapy: role of gap-junctional intercellular communication. Cancer Res 2000;60:3989–3999.
5. Yang L, Chiang Y, Lenz HJ, et al. Intercellular communication mediates the bystander effect during herpes simplex thymidine kinase/ganciclovir-based gene therapy of human gastrointestinal tumor cells. Hum Gene Ther 1998;9:719–728.
6. Zeng M, Cerniglia GJ, Eck SL, Stevens CW. High-efficiency stable gene transfer of adenovirus into mammalian cells using ionizing radiation. Hum Gene Ther 1997;8:1025–1032.
7. Kim SH, Kim JH, Kolozsvary A, Brown SL, Freytag SO. Preferential radiosensitization of 9L glioma cells transduced with HSV-*tk* gene by acyclovir. J Neurooncol 1997;33:189–194.
8. Atkinson G, Hall SJ. Prodrug activation gene therapy and external beam irradiation in the treatment of prostate cancer. Urology 1999;54:1098–1104.
9. Chhikara M, Huang H, Vlachaki MT, et al. Enhanced therapeutic effect of HSV-tk+GCV gene therapy and ionizing radiation for prostate cancer. Mol Ther 2001;3:536–542.
10. Rosenberg E, Hawkins W, Holmes M, et al. Radiosensitization of human glioma cells in vitro and in vivo with acyclovir and mutant HSV-TK75 expressed from adenovirus. Int J Radiat Oncol Biol Phys 2002;52:831–836.
11. Teh BS, Ayala G, Aguilar L, et al. Phase I-II trial evaluating combined intensity-modulated radiotherapy and in situ gene therapy with or without hormonal therapy in treatment of prostate cancer-interim report on PSA response and biopsy data. Int J Radiat Oncol Biol Phys 2004;58:1520–1529.
12. Khil MS, Kim JH, Mullen CA, Kim SH, Freytag SO. Radiosensitization by 5-fluorocytosine of human colorectal carcinoma cells in culture transduced with cytosine deaminase gene. Clin Cancer Res 1996;2:53–57.
13. Hanna NN, Mauceri HJ, Wayne JD, Hallahan DE, Kufe DW, Weichselbaum RR. Virally directed cytosine deaminase/5-fluorocytosine gene therapy enhances radiation response in human cancer xenografts. Cancer Res 1997;57:4205–4209.
14. Pederson LC, Buchsbaum DJ, Vickers SM, et al. Molecular chemotherapy combined with radiation therapy enhances killing of cholangiocarcinoma cells in vitro and in vivo. Cancer Res 1997; 57:4325–4332.
15. Ueno M, Koyama F, Yamada Y, et al. Tumor-specific chemo-radio-gene therapy for colorectal cancer cells using adenovirus vector expressing the cytosine deaminase gene. Anticancer Res 2001; 21:2601–2608.
16. Hartwell LH, Kastan MB. Cell cycle control and cancer. Science 1994;266:1821–1828.
17. Kastan MB, Canman CE, Leonard CJ. P53, cell cycle control and apoptosis: implications for cancer. Cancer Metastasis Rev 1995;14:3–15.
18. Mukhopadhyay T, Maxwell SA, Roth JA. p53 Suppressor Gene. Austin, Texas: R. G. Landes Co., 1995.
19. Spitz FR, Nguyen D, Skibber JM, Meyn RE, Cristiano RJ, Roth JA. Adenoviral-mediated wild-type p53 gene expression sensitizes colorectal cancer cells to ionizing radiation. Clin Cancer Res 1996; 2:1665–1671.
20. Lowe SW, Schmitt EM, Smith SW, Osborne BA, Jacks T. p53 is required for radiation-induced apoptosis in mouse thymocytes. Nature 1993;362:847–849.
21. Lowe SW, Ruley HE, Jacks T, Housman DE. p53-dependent apoptosis modulates the cytotoxicity of anticancer agents. Cell 1993;74:957–967.
22. Fujiwara T, Cai DW, Georges RN, Mukhopadhyay T, Grimm EA, Roth JA. Therapeutic effect of a retroviral wild-type p53 expression vector in an orthotopic lung cancer model. J Natl Cancer Inst 1994;86:1458–1462.
23. Zhang WW, Fang X, Mazur W, French BA, Georges RN, Roth JA. High-efficiency gene transfer and high-level expression of wild-type p53 in human lung cancer cells mediated by recombinant adenovirus. Cancer Gene Ther 1994;1:5–13.
24. Kock H, Harris MP, Anderson SC, et al. Adenovirus-mediated p53 gene transfer suppresses growth of human glioblastoma cells in vitro and in vivo. Int J Cancer 1996;67:808–815.
25. Harris MP, Sutjipto S, Wills KN, et al. Adenovirus-mediated p53 gene transfer inhibits growth of human tumor cells expressing mutant p53 protein. Cancer Gene Ther 1996;3:121–130.
26. Mujoo K, Maneval DC, Anderson SC, Gutterman JU. Adenoviral-mediated p53 tumor suppressor gene therapy of human ovarian carcinoma. Oncogene 1996;12:1617–1623.
27. Nielsen LL, Dell J, Maxwell E, Armstrong L, Maneval D, Catino JJ. Efficacy of p53 adenovirus-mediated gene therapy against human breast cancer xenografts. Cancer Gene Ther 1997;4:129–138.

28. Wills KN, Maneval DC, Menzel P, et al. Development and characterization of recombinant adenoviruses encoding human p53 for gene therapy of cancer. Hum Gene Ther 1994;5:1079–1088.
29. Kawabe S, Munshi A, Zumstein LA, Wilson DR, Roth JA, Meyn RE. Adenovirus-mediated wild-type p53 gene expression radiosensitizes non-small cell lung cancer cells but not normal lung fibroblasts. Int J Radiat Biol 2001;77:185–194.
30. Sah NK, Munshi A, Nishikawa T, Mukhopadhyay T, Roth JA, Meyn RE. Adenovirus-mediated wild-type p53 radiosensitizes human tumor cells by suppressing DNA repair capacity. Mol Cancer Ther 2003;2:1223–1231.
31. Colletier PJ, Ashoori F, Cowen D, et al. Adenoviral-mediated p53 transgene expression sensitizes both wild-type and null p53 prostate cancer cells in vitro to radiation. Int J Radiat Oncol Biol Phys 2000;48:1507–1512.
32. Nishizaki M, Meyn RE, Levy LB, et al. Synergistic inhibition of human lung cancer cell growth by adenovirus-mediated wild-type p53 gene transfer in combination with docetaxel and radiation therapeutics in vitro and in vivo. Clin Cancer Res 2001;7:2887–2897.
33. Roth JA, Nguyen D, Lawrence DD, et al. Retrovirus-mediated wild-type p53 gene transfer to tumors of patients with lung cancer. Nat Med 1996;2:985–991.
34. Roth JA, Swisher SG, Merritt JA, et al. Gene therapy for non-small cell lung cancer: a preliminary report of a phase I trial of adenoviral p53 gene replacement. Semin Oncol 1998;25:33–37.
35. Lang FF, Bruner JM, Fuller GN, et al. Phase I trial of adenovirus-mediated p53 gene therapy for recurrent glioma: biological and clinical results. J Clin Oncol 2003;21:2508–2518.
36. Wen SF, Mahavni V, Quijano E, et al. Assessment of p53 gene transfer and biological activities in a clinical study of adenovirus-p53 gene therapy for recurrent ovarian cancer. Cancer Gene Ther 2003; 10:224–238.
37. Edelman J, Nemunaitis J. Adenoviral p53 gene therapy in squamous cell cancer of the head and neck region. Curr Opin Mol Ther 2003;5:611–617.
38. Pagliaro LC, Keyhani A, Williams D, et al. Repeated intravesical instillations of an adenoviral vector in patients with locally advanced bladder cancer: a phase I study of p53 gene therapy. J Clin Oncol 2003;21:2247–2253.
39. Swisher SG, Roth JA, Komaki R, et al. Induction of p53-regulated genes and tumor regression in lung cancer patients after intratumoral delivery of adenoviral p53 (INGN 201) and radiation therapy. Clin Cancer Res 2003;9:93–101.
40. Chada S, Sutton RB, Ekmekcioglu S, et al. MDA-7/IL-24 is a unique cytokine-tumor suppressor in the IL-10 Family. Int Immunopharmacol 2004;4:649–667.
41. Yacoub A, Mitchell C, Brannon J, et al. MDA-7 (interleukin-24) inhibits the proliferation of renal carcinoma cells and interacts with free radicals to promote cell death and loss of reproductive capacity. Molecular Cancer Therapeutics 2003;2:623–632.
42. Cao XX, Mohuiddin I, Chada S, et al. Adenoviral transfer of mda-7 leads to BAX up-regulation and apoptosis in mesothelioma cells, and is abrogated by over-expression of BCL-XL. Mol Med 2002;8:869–876.
43. Sarkar D, Su ZZ, Lebedeva IV, et al. mda-7 (IL-24) Mediates selective apoptosis in human melanoma cells by inducing the coordinated overexpression of the GADD family of genes by means of p38 MAPK. Proc Natl Acad Sci U S A 2002;99:10,054–10,059.
44. Saeki T, Mhashilkar A, Swanson X, et al. Inhibition of human lung cancer growth following adenovirus-mediated mda-7 gene expression in vivo. Oncogene 2002;21:4558–4566.
45. Lebedeva IV, Su ZZ, Chang Y, Kitada S, Reed JC, Fisher PB. The cancer growth suppressing gene mda-7 induces apoptosis selectively in human melanoma cells. Oncogene 2002;21:708–718.
46. Su Z, Lebedeva IV, Gopalkrishnan RV, et al. A combinatorial approach for selectively inducing programmed cell death in human pancreatic cancer cells. Proc Natl Acad Sci U S A 2001;98:10,332–10,337.
47. Su ZZ, Madireddi MT, Lin JJ, et al. The cancer growth suppressor gene mda-7 selectively induces apoptosis in human breast cancer cells and inhibits tumor growth in nude mice. Proc Natl Acad Sci U S A 1998;95:14,400–14,405.
48. Lebedeva IV, Su ZZ, Sarkar D, et al. Melanoma differentiation associated gene-7, mda-7/interleukin-24, induces apoptosis in prostate cancer cells by promoting mitochondrial dysfunction and inducing reactive oxygen species. Cancer Research 2003;63:8138–8144.
49. Mhashilkar AM, Schrock RD, Hindi M, et al. Melanoma differentiation associated gene-7 (mda-7): a novel anti-tumor gene for cancer gene therapy. Mol Med 2001;7:271–282.
50. Cunningham C. A phase I dose-escalation pharmacokinetic and phamacodynamic study of INGN 241 (Ad-mda7) in patients with advanced solid tumors. Am Soc Clin Oncol 2002; Abstract #87.

51. Kawabe S, Nishikawa T, Munshi A, Roth JA, Chada S, Meyn RE. Adenovirus-mediated mda-7 gene expression radiosensitizes non-small cell lung cancer cells via TP53-independent mechanisms. Mol Ther 2002;6:637–644.
52. Nishikawa T, Munshi A, Story MD, Chada S, Meyn RE. Adenoviral-mediated mda-7 expression suppresses DNA repair capacity and radiosensitizes non-small cell lung cancer cells. Oncogene 2004;23:7125–7131.
53. Su ZZ, Lebedeva IV, Sarkar D, et al. Melanoma differentiation associated gene-7, mda-7/IL-24, selectively induces growth suppression, apoptosis and radiosensitization in malignant gliomas in a p53-independent manner. Oncogene 2003;22:1164–1180.
54. Yacoub A, Mitchell C, Lister A, et al. Melanoma differentiation-associated 7 (interleukin 24) inhibits growth and enhances radiosensitivity of glioma cells in vitro and in vivo. Clin Cancer Res 2003; 9:3272–3281.
55. Ohta M, Nagai H, Shimizu M, et al. Rarity of somatic and germline mutations of the cyclin-dependent kinase 4 inhibitor gene, CDK4I, in melanoma. Cancer Res 1994;54:5269–5272.
56. Jen J, Harper JW, Bigner SH, et al. Deletion of p16 and p15 genes in brain tumors. Cancer Res 1994; 54:6353–6358.
57. Cairns P, Polascik TJ, Eby Y, et al. Frequency of homozygous deletion at p16/CDKN2 in primary human tumours. Nat Genet 1995;11:210–212.
58. Cheng JQ, Jhanwar SC, Klein WM, et al. p16 alterations and deletion mapping of 9p21-p22 in malignant mesothelioma. Cancer Res 1994;54:5547–5551.
59. Hebert J, Cayuela JM, Berkeley J, Sigaux F. Candidate tumor-suppressor genes MTS1 (p16INK4A) and MTS2 (p15INK4B) display frequent homozygous deletions in primary cells from T- but not from B-cell lineage acute lymphoblastic leukemias. Blood 1994;84:4038–4044.
60. Schultz DC, Vanderveer L, Buetow KH, et al. Characterization of chromosome 9 in human ovarian neoplasia identifies frequent genetic imbalance on 9q and rare alterations involving 9p, including CDKN2. Cancer Res 1995;55:2150–2157.
61. Reed AL, Califano J, Cairns P, et al. High frequency of p16 (CDKN2/MTS-1/INK4A) inactivation in head and neck squamous cell carcinoma. Cancer Res 1996;56:3630–3633.
62. Mori T, Miura K, Aoki T, Nishihira T, Mori S, Nakamura Y. Frequent somatic mutation of the MTS1/CDK4I (multiple tumor suppressor/cyclin-dependent kinase 4 inhibitor) gene in esophageal squamous cell carcinoma. Cancer Res 1994;54:3396–3397.
63. Calbo J, Marotta M, Cascallo M, et al. Adenovirus-mediated wt-p16 reintroduction induces cell cycle arrest or apoptosis in pancreatic cancer. Cancer Gene Ther 2001;8:740–750.
64. Adachi Y, Chandrasekar N, Kin Y, et al. Suppression of glioma invasion and growth by adenovirus-mediated delivery of a bicistronic construct containing antisense uPAR and sense p16 gene sequences. Oncogene 2002;21:87–95.
65. Kawabe S, Roth JA, Wilson DR, Meyn RE. Adenovirus-mediated p16INK4A gene expression radiosensitizes non-small cell lung cancer cells in a p53-dependent manner. Oncogene 2000;19:5359–5366.
66. Rhee JG, Li D, O'Malley BW, Jr, Suntharalingam M. Combination radiation and adenovirus-mediated P16(INK4A) gene therapy in a murine model for head and neck cancer. ORL J Otorhinolaryngol Relat Spec 2003;65:144–154.
67. Korsmeyer SJ, Shutter JR, Veis DJ, Merry DE, Oltvai ZN. Bcl-2/Bax: a rheostat that regulates an anti-oxidant pathway and cell death. Semin Cancer Biol 1993;4:327–332.
68. Gomez-Navarro J, Arafat W, Xiang J. Gene therapy for carcinoma of the breast: Pro-apoptotic gene therapy. Breast Cancer Res 2000;2:32–44.
69. Sakakura C, Sweeney EA, Shirahama T, et al. Overexpression of bax sensitizes human breast cancer MCF-7 cells to radiation-induced apoptosis. Int J Cancer 1996;67:101–105.
70. Sakakura C, Sweeney EA, Shirahama T, et al. Overexpression of bax enhances the radiation sensitivity in human breast cancer cells. Surg Today 1997;27:90–93.
71. Arafat WO, Gomez-Navarro J, Xiang J, et al. An adenovirus encoding proapoptotic Bax induces apoptosis and enhances the radiation effect in human ovarian cancer. Mol Ther 2000;1:545–554.
72. Arafat WO, Buchsbaum DJ, Gomez-Navarro J, et al. An adenovirus encoding proapoptotic Bax synergistically radiosensitizes malignant glioma. Int J Radiat Oncol Biol Phys 2003;55:1037–1050.
73. Shu HK, Kim MM, Chen P, Furman F, Julin CM, Israel MA. The intrinsic radioresistance of glioblastoma-derived cell lines is associated with a failure of p53 to induce p21(BAX) expression. Proc Natl Acad Sci U S A 1998;95:14,453–14,458.

74. Asher A, Mule JJ, Reichert CM, Shiloni E, Rosenberg SA. Studies on the anti-tumor efficacy of systemically administered recombinant tumor necrosis factor against several murine tumors in vivo. J Immunol 1987;138:963–974.
75. Fukumura D, Salehi HA, Witwer B, Tuma RF, Melder RJ, Jain RK. Tumor necrosis factor alpha-induced leukocyte adhesion in normal and tumor vessels: effect of tumor type, transplantation site, and host strain. Cancer Res 1995;55:4824–4829.
76. Balkwill FR, Lee A, Aldam G, et al. Human tumor xenografts treated with recombinant human tumor necrosis factor alone or in combination with interferons. Cancer Res 1986;46:3990–3993.
77. Rasmussen H, Rasmussen C, Lempicki M, et al. TNFerade Biologic: preclinical toxicology of a novel adenovector with a radiation-inducible promoter, carrying the human tumor necrosis factor alpha gene. Cancer Gene Ther 2002;9:951–957.
78. Chung TD, Mauceri HJ, Hallahan DE, et al. Tumor necrosis factor-alpha-based gene therapy enhances radiation cytotoxicity in human prostate cancer. Cancer Gene Ther 1998;5:344–349.
79. Staba MJ, Mauceri HJ, Kufe DW, Hallahan DE, Weichselbaum RR. Adenoviral TNF-alpha gene therapy and radiation damage tumor vasculature in a human malignant glioma xenograft. Gene Ther 1998;5:293–300.
80. Gupta VK, Park JO, Jaskowiak NT, et al. Combined gene therapy and ionizing radiation is a novel approach to treat human esophageal adenocarcinoma. Ann Surg Oncol 2002;9:500–504.
81. Senzer N, Mani S, Rosemurgy A, et al. TNFerade biologic, an adenovector with a radiation-inducible promoter, carrying the human tumor necrosis factor alpha gene: a phase I study in patients with solid tumors. J Clin Oncol 2004;22:592–601.
82. Sharma A, Mani S, Hanna N, et al. Clinical protocol. An open-label, phase I, dose-escalation study of tumor necrosis factor-alpha (TNFerade Biologic) gene transfer with radiation therapy for locally advanced, recurrent, or metastatic solid tumors. Hum Gene Ther 2001;12:1109–1131.
83. Nevins JR, Raychaudhuri P, Yee AS, Rooney RJ, Kovesdi I, Reichel R. Transactivation by the adenovirus E1A gene. Biochem Cell Biol 1988;66:578–583.
84. Nevins JR. Adenovirus E1A-dependent trans-activation of transcription. Semin Cancer Biol 1990; 1:59–68.
85. Yu D, Matin A, Xia W, Sorgi F, Huang L, Hung MC. Liposome-mediated in vivo E1A gene transfer suppressed dissemination of ovarian cancer cells that overexpress HER-2/neu. Oncogene 1995; 11:1383–1388.
86. Chang JY, Xia W, Shao R, et al. The tumor suppression activity of E1A in HER-2/neu-overexpressing breast cancer. Oncogene 1997;14:561–568.
87. Wang XL, Qian XL, Zhao QZ, Xu ZG, Tang PZ. [Effect of E1A gene on in vitro growth inhibition and radiochemosensitivity of lymph node metastasis cells of human head and neck squamous cell carcinoma]. Ai Zheng 2003;22:1140–1146.
88. Hortobagyi GN, Ueno NT, Xia W, et al. Cationic liposome-mediated E1A gene transfer to human breast and ovarian cancer cells and its biologic effects: a phase I clinical trial. J Clin Oncol 2001; 19:3422–3433.
89. Yoo GH, Hung MC, Lopez-Berestein G, et al. Phase I trial of intratumoral liposome E1A gene therapy in patients with recurrent breast and head and neck cancer. Clin Cancer Res 2001;7:1237–1245.
90. Bischoff JR, Kirn DH, Williams A, et al. An adenovirus mutant that replicates selectively in p53-deficient human tumor cells. Science 1996;274:373–376.
91. Heise C, Sampson-Johannes A, Williams A, McCormick F, Von Hoff DD, Kirn DH. ONYX-015, an E1B gene-attenuated adenovirus, causes tumor-specific cytolysis and antitumoral efficacy that can be augmented by standard chemotherapeutic agents. Nat Med 1997;3:639–645.
92. Freytag SO, Rogulski KR, Paielli DL, Gilbert JD, Kim JH. A novel three-pronged approach to kill cancer cells selectively: concomitant viral, double suicide gene, and radiotherapy. Hum Gene Ther 1998;9:1323–1333.
93. Yew PR, Berk AJ. Inhibition of p53 transactivation required for transformation by adenovirus early 1B protein. Nature 1992;357:82–85.
94. Hollstein M, Sidransky D, Vogelstein B, Harris CC. p53 mutations in human cancers. Science 1991; 253:49–53.
95. Bergh J, Norberg T, Sjogren S, Lindgren A, Holmberg L. Complete sequencing of the p53 gene provides prognostic information in breast cancer patients, particularly in relation to adjuvant systemic therapy and radiotherapy. Nat Med 1995;1:1029–1034.

96. Goodrum FD, Ornelles DA. The early region 1B 55-kilodalton oncoprotein of adenovirus relieves growth restrictions imposed on viral replication by the cell cycle. J Virol 1997;71:548–561.
97. Rothmann T, Hengstermann A, Whitaker NJ, Scheffner M, zur Hausen H. Replication of ONYX-015, a potential anticancer adenovirus, is independent of p53 status in tumor cells. J Virol 1998; 72:9470–9478.
98. Hall SJ, Sanford MA, Atkinson G, Chen SH. Induction of potent antitumor natural killer cell activity by herpes simplex virus-thymidine kinase and ganciclovir therapy in an orthotopic mouse model of prostate cancer. Cancer Res 1998;58:3221–3225.
99. Turnell AS, Grand RJ, Gallimore PH. The replicative capacities of large E1B-null group A and group C adenoviruses are independent of host cell p53 status. J Virol 1999;73:2074–2083.
100. Harada JN, Berk AJ. p53-Independent and -dependent requirements for E1B-55K in adenovirus type 5 replication. J Virol 1999;73:5333–5344.
101. Goodrum FD, Ornelles DA. p53 status does not determine outcome of E1B 55-kilodalton mutant adenovirus lytic infection. J Virol 1998;72:9479–9490.
102. Nemunaitis J, Cunningham C, Buchanan A, et al. Intravenous infusion of a replication-selective adenovirus (ONYX-015) in cancer patients: safety, feasibility and biological activity. Gene Ther 2001;8:746–759.
103. Rogulski KR, Freytag SO, Zhang K, et al. In vivo antitumor activity of ONYX-015 is influenced by p53 status and is augmented by radiotherapy. Cancer Res 2000;60:1193–1196.
104. Geoerger B, Grill J, Opolon P, et al. Potentiation of radiation therapy by the oncolytic adenovirus dl1520 (ONYX-015) in human malignant glioma xenografts. Br J Cancer 2003;89:577–584.
105. Jen KY, Gewirtz AM. Suppression of gene expression by targeted disruption of messenger RNA: available options and current strategies. Stem Cells 2000;18:307–319.
106. Crooke ST. Vitravene—another piece in the mosaic. Antisense Nucleic Acid Drug Dev 1998; 8:vii–viii.
107. Wang H, Prasad G, Buolamwini JK, Zhang R. Antisense anticancer oligonucleotide therapeutics. Curr Cancer Drug Targets 2001;1:177–196.
108. Agrawal S, Kandimalla ER. Antisense and/or immunostimulatory oligonucleotide therapeutics. Curr Cancer Drug Targets 2001;1:197–209.
109. Altieri DC, Marchisio PC, Marchisio C. Survivin apoptosis: an interloper between cell death and cell proliferation in cancer. Lab Invest 1999;79:1327–1333.
110. Altieri DC. The molecular basis and potential role of survivin in cancer diagnosis and therapy. Trends Mol Med 2001;7:542–547.
111. Asanuma K, Moriai R, Yajima T, et al. Survivin as a radioresistance factor in pancreatic cancer. Jpn J Cancer Res 2000;91:1204–1209.
112. Omori S, Takiguchi Y, Suda A, et al. Suppression of a DNA double-strand break repair gene, Ku70, increases radio- and chemosensitivity in a human lung carcinoma cell line. DNA Repair (Amst) 2002;1:299–310.
113. Li GC, He F, Shao X, et al. Adenovirus-mediated heat-activated antisense Ku70 expression radiosensitizes tumor cells in vitro and in vivo. Cancer Res 2003;63:3268–3274.
114. Folkman J. Angiogenesis in cancer, vascular, rheumatoid and other disease. Nat Med 1995;1:27–31.
115. Mauceri HJ, Seetharam S, Beckett MA, et al. Angiostatin potentiates cyclophosphamide treatment of metastatic disease. Cancer Chemother Pharmacol 2002;50:412–418.
116. O'Reilly MS, Holmgren L, Shing Y, et al. Angiostatin: a novel angiogenesis inhibitor that mediates the suppression of metastases by a Lewis lung carcinoma. Cell 1994;79:315–328.
117. O'Reilly MS, Boehm T, Shing Y, et al. Endostatin: an endogenous inhibitor of angiogenesis and tumor growth. Cell 1997;88:277–285.
118. Teicher BA, Holden SA, Ara G, et al. Potentiation of cytotoxic cancer therapies by TNP-470 alone and with other anti-angiogenic agents. Int J Cancer 1994;57:920–925.
119. Teicher BA, Sotomayor EA, Huang ZD. Antiangiogenic agents potentiate cytotoxic cancer therapies against primary and metastatic disease. Cancer Res 1992;52:6702–6704.
120. Gorski DH, Beckett MA, Jaskowiak NT, et al. Blockage of the vascular endothelial growth factor stress response increases the antitumor effects of ionizing radiation. Cancer Res 1999;59:3374–3378.
121. Hanna NN, Seetharam S, Mauceri HJ, et al. Antitumor interaction of short-course endostatin and ionizing radiation. Cancer J 2000;6:287–293.
122. Gridley DS, Loredo LN, Slater JD, et al. Pilot evaluation of cytokine levels in patients undergoing radiotherapy for brain tumor. Cancer Detect Prev 1998;22:20–29.
123. Maniwa Y, Okada M, Ishii N, Kiyooka K. Vascular endothelial growth factor increased by pulmonary surgery accelerates the growth of micrometastases in metastatic lung cancer. Chest 1998;114:1668–1675.

16 Gene Transfer for Chemoprotection and Enrichment of Hematopoietic Stem Cells

Justin C. Roth, PhD *and Stanton L. Gerson,* MD

CONTENTS

Summary

Hematopoietic stem cells (HSCs) have been the archetypal target for therapeutic gene transfer strategies, due to the ease with which these cells are obtained and cultured ex vivo, as well as their capacity for reconstituting an entire tissue type. The myelosuppressive consequence of neoplastic disease treatment has provided additional thrust for the development of HSC drug-resistance and gene transfer strategies. In this regard, significant advances in vector design have been achieved by careful evaluation of different promoter and enhancer sequences, as well as exogenous elements, that contribute to high gene expression levels and resist positional effect variegation. Gene transfer efficiencies have also been improved by the identification of envelope pseudotypes that recognize receptors expressed in the more primitive hematopoietic populations. In addition, several natural and synthetic gene products have been evaluated as tools for amplifying or enriching gene-modified HSCs in vivo. These include the homeobox transcription factors, selective amplifier genes, and drug resistance genes. The ability to enrich and repopulate the hematopoietic compartment with therapeutic gene-corrected cells requires strategies that act on primitive progenitor populations, and vectors that efficiently express multiple gene products. The realization of insertional mutagenesis has demonstrated the importance of therapy-related risk assessment and the need for vectors with inherent cell-type specificities. These advances have culminated in enhanced HSC gene transfer and enrichment, while highlighting areas requiring further development.

Key Words: Drug resistance genes; hematopoietic stem cell; in vivo selection; stem cell amplification; insertional mutagenesis.

From: *Cancer Drug Discovery and Development: Gene Therapy for Cancer*
Edited by: K. K. Hunt, S. A. Vorburger, and S. G. Swisher © Humana Press Inc., Totowa, NJ

1. INTRODUCTION

Once achieved, efficient and stable gene transfer into hematopoietic stem cells (HSCs) has the potential for curing hematologic disease, or alleviating the myelosuppressive consequences of antineoplastic chemotherapy. Regardless of the therapeutic endpoint, HSC gene transfer efficiency is limited, and the proportion of gene-modified cells is further diluted by the vast excess of unmanipulated cells upon transplant. These limitations have spurred efforts aimed at improving the specificity of HSC gene therapy vectors and the development of methods for enriching gene-modified stem cells in vivo. This chapter describes the common viral vector systems used for stable gene transfer into HSCs, and the main strategies used for protecting and enriching these cells in vivo.

1.1. Stable Gene Transfer Vectors

The requirement for high gene transfer and expression levels in HSC gene therapy has been a driving force in the development of viral vector delivery systems. Viruses that integrate into the host genome, such as adeno-associated viruses (AAV), retroviruses (RV), and lentiviruses (LV), are of particular interest due to their stable transmission and expression of the transgene. Significant progress has been made in identifying cis- and *trans*-acting elements, from endogenous and exogenous sources, that influence the efficiency of vector packaging, integration, and expression.

Vectors derived from murine leukemia virus (MuLV), myeloproliferative sarcoma virus (MPSV), spleen focus-forming virus (SFFV), and other oncoretroviruses have been generated *(1–4)*. Extensive characterization of these vectors has revealed both positive and negative regulatory elements that affect transgene expression in primitive hematopoietic cells *(4–7)*. Exogenous sequences have also been inserted into these vectors to improve transgene expression levels. In this regard, scaffold attachment regions *(8,9)* and insulator elements *(10–12)* reduce silencing and positional effects, whereas post-transcriptional regulatory elements (PREs), such as that from the Woodchuck hepatitis virus, improve expression levels by increasing transcript export and stability *(13)*. The cell division requirement for retroviral integration and the quiescent nature of HSCs has limited retrovirus-based transduction efficiencies. However, insight into the roles specific cytokines play in hematopoiesis has led to the identification of cytokine cocktails that promote stem-cell cycling and transduction, while limiting commitment towards differentiation *(14,15)*.

Many of the recent HSC gene transfer models have utilized lentivirus vectors, such as those based on the human immunodeficiency virus (HIV-1). Lentiviruses actively transport the reverse-transcribed transgene across the nuclear envelope and therefore do not require cell division for access to the host genome *(16)*. This active transport process enables lentiviruses to transduce nondividing HSCs. However, lentiviral transduction efficiencies are dramatically improved after cytokine stimulation, indicating that at least partial entry into the cell cycle may be necessary for key steps in viral entry *(17–19)*. As with retroviral vectors, key *cis*-acting elements in the lentiviral backbone have been identified as essential components for efficient transduction and expression. The central DNA flap, composed of the central polypurine tract and the central termination sequence (cPPT/CTS), has been proposed to play an important role in nuclear translocation of the reverse-transcribed genome *(20)*. Reinsertion of this sequence into lentiviral vectors was shown to dramatically improve transduction of HSCs *(21,22)*. Self-inactivating (SIN) vectors, originally described for retroviral vectors and duplicated in lentiviral vectors, have been generated by deleting promoter and enhancer sequences from the U3 region of the 3′LTR *(23–25)*. Following reverse transcription, this modification is duplicated to form the 5′U3 region. Thus, promoter and enhancer functions are effectively removed from both proviral LTRs. SIN vectors are a major improvement in safety, as they reduce the capacity for recombination or rescue from exogenous virus, and deletion of the 3′U3 sequences may reduce the frequency of insertional activation. Transgene expression in SIN vectors is achieved by the insertion of an internal promoter, a range of which have been evaluated for HSC gene therapy, including the ubiquitous cytomegalovirus (CMV), elongation factor 1α (EF-1α), and phosphoglycerate kinase (PGK) promoters *(17,26)*. Vector comparisons utilizing the green fluoorescent protein (GFP) reporter indicate that the EF-1α promoter provides the most robust multilineage hematopoietic expression levels *(26)*. Additional studies have utilized cellular promoter and enhancer sequences to restrict expression to specific hematopoietic lineages *(27,28)*. Many of the enhancer sequences developed in oncoretroviral vectors for strong hematopoietic expression have also been functionally transferred into the lentivector systems *(29,30)*. The first clinical trial using lentiviral vectors was recently approved for anti-HIV therapy *(31)*. This particular study should also determine whether or not SIN lentivectors are truly innocuous in the presence of high wild-type virus loads.

1.2. Envelope Pseudotypes

Viral envelope proteins are responsible for cell type specificity and viral membrane stability. In addition to combining sequence elements for improved vector expression, vast efforts have gone into evaluating envelope proteins from other viral species for functional substitution of retro- and lentivirus envelope proteins to improve virion stability and transduction efficiency. This type of substitution is known as pseudotyping. Overexpression of a foreign envelope protein is often sufficient to generate a pseudotyped a virus. The amphotropic murine and gibbon ape leukemia virus envelope proteins were favored in early hematopoietic gene transfer applications, but subsequent studies have shown that the receptors for these envelopes are limiting in the more primitive stem cell populations *(32)*. The reduced stability of these envelope proteins also limits production of concentrated viral stocks.

The vesicular stomatitis virus G glycoprotein (VSVG) is the most widely used pseudotype for lentivirus gene transfer. This protein enables the transduction of a wide range of species and cell types, as it utilizes a ubiquitous phospholipid for membrane fusion, rather than a protein receptor, for entry *(33)*. In addition, VSVG-pseudotyped viruses are much more stable, allowing virus-enriched media to be concentrated to levels over 10^8 transducing units/ml. The main drawback of VSVG is its cytotoxicity. This toxicity has prompted the development of inducible VSVG packaging cell lines *(34,35)*. Despite the reduced expression of the amphotropic receptor in early stem cells, von Laer et al. reported that retroviral particles pseudotyped with VSVG or the amphotropic envelope appear to transduce human hematopoietic progenitors with similar efficiency *(36)*.

Vectors pseudotyped with the feline endogenous virus envelope protein, RD114, have also been described *(37)*. RD114-pseudoyped virions can be concentrated and the lack of toxicity has permitted the generation of stable packaging cell lines *(38)*. Hanawa et al. compared lentivectors pseudotyped with VSVG, RD114, or amphotropic envelopes for their ability to be concentrated and transduce primitive human hematopoietic $CD34^+$ cells *(39)*. The amphotropic and RD114 particles excelled over VSVG at transducing cord blood-derived CD34$^+$ progenitors, and the amphotropic particles were more efficient at transducing SCID repopulating cells derived from G-CSF-mobilized peripheral blood CD34$^+$ cells. Relander et al. recently compared lentivectors pseudotyped with modified gibbon ape leukemia virus, RD114, or amphotropic envelopes for transduction efficiency of NOD/SCID-repopulating human CD34$^+$ cells *(40)*. In the presence of cytokine stimulation, the modified RD114-pseudotyped vectors generated the highest percentage of transduced cells. Many other pseudotypes are being evaluated for use in a variety of applications. The best pseudotype for any particular situation will ultimately depend on several factors, including the type of vector, the transduction protocol, and the type and source of the target cells.

2. HSC EXPANSION: INDUCERS OF PROLIFERATION AND SELF-RENEWAL

Limited gene transfer efficiency into HSCs and the myelotoxicity associated with neoplastic drug treatments have led to efforts aimed at enriching gene-modified cells in vivo. Genes that are utilized to specifically enrich transduced stem cells in vivo can be divided into two main classes: those that induce HSC proliferation and expansion, and those that protect cells from cytotoxic drug treatments (*see* Fig. 1). The particular strategy employed will likely be determined by the type and severity of the disorder for which gene transfer is needed. Disorders such as chronic granulomatous disease that can be alleviated by low levels of gene-corrected cells may favor stem cell expansion strategies. Other diseases, such as sickle cell anemia in which uncorrected cells negatively impact on survival, may favor drug selection strategies. Multigene vectors offer the additional potential for linking the advantages of each strategy and will be discussed later in the chapter.

2.1. Endogenous Genes for HSC Expansion

Gene products that contribute to stem cell self renewal and proliferation are highly sought after as tools for overcoming the limited cell numbers associated with stem cell therapies. Considerable progress has been made in identifying growth factors that can maintain or expand the stem cell pool ex vivo *(41)*. However, growth factors act on natural receptors, and thus cannot be used to specifically enrich transduced stem cell population in vivo. Therefore, genes that provide an intrinsic proliferative advantage to stem cells are being evaluated as tools for enriching transduced populations. Endogenous genes, which have a natural role in stem cell self renewal, as well as recombinant genes engineered for this activity, have been assessed as candidates for this approach.

Although gene products that have a natural role in stem cell self renewal and proliferation will likely have the most potential for this type of application, many have also been implicated in leukemogenesis. The homeobox transcription factors are a good example of this. This gene family was initially discovered for its role in embryogenesis, but many of the hox genes have an ongoing role in hematopoiesis. Several members from the *hoxA, B,* and *C* gene clusters have distinct expression patterns that are restricted to different lineages or stages of hematopoietic differentiation *(42–44)*. Ectopic expression of these genes, either with retroviral vectors, or by naturally occurring translocation events, has also been linked to major perturbations in hematopoiesis *(45)*. The HoxB4 transcription factor appears to be an exception. Transduction of murine or human HSCs with HoxB4 has been shown to induce expansion in vitro and

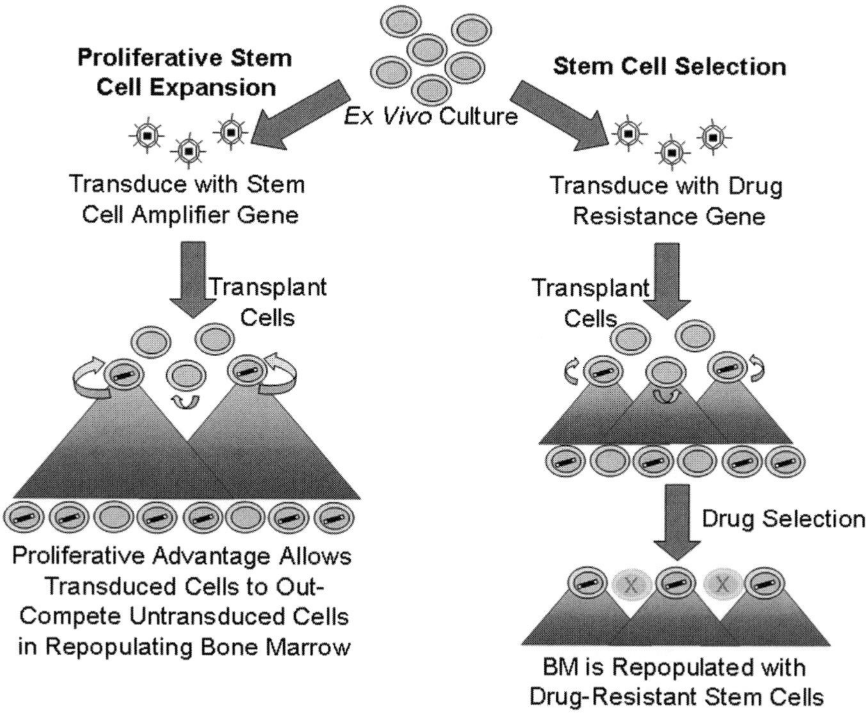

Fig. 1. Enrichment of transduced HSCs in vivo. Transduced HSCs can be enriched in vivo using genes that provide a proliferative advantage *(left)* or a survival advantage *(right)* over untransduced cells.

in vivo *(46–51)*. Murine HSCs that overexpress HoxB4 have up to a 50-fold competitive repopulation advantage over untransduced cells. In these HoxB4 studies stem cell expansion did not progress beyond normal stem cell levels, which suggests the existence of an environmental sensor of stem cell density *(47)*. The level of HoxB4 expression also seems to determine its biological activity. Beslu et al. demonstrated that increased HoxB4 expression levels correlated with increased repopulating potential *(52)*. HoxB4 applied to cells in protein form has also been shown to allow ex vivo stem cell expansion *(49,50)*. This strategy offers the potential for preloading stem cells prior to transplant, allowing transient expansion without a requirement for stable expression. Delivery of other hox members with this strategy may allow for transient expansion of specific lineages without the associated risk of leukemogenesis. HoxB4 expression in human $CD34^+$ cord blood cells has been reported to impair lymphomyeloid differentiation *(51)*. Thus, the necessary feedback signals that appear to be present in the all-murine model may not be recognized by human cells when expanded ex vivo or transplanted into NOD/SCID mice.

2.2. Recombinant Genes for HSC Expansion

Another strategy for stem cell expansion utilizes chimeric gene products, called selective amplifier genes (SAGs). SAGs are composed of a dimerization and a signaling domain, which become activated by specific molecules called chemical inducers of dimerization (CID). Dimerization activates the SAG signaling domains to induce cell proliferation (*see* Fig. 2). Several variations of this theme have been evaluated for both in vitro and in vivo expansion in response to CID administration.

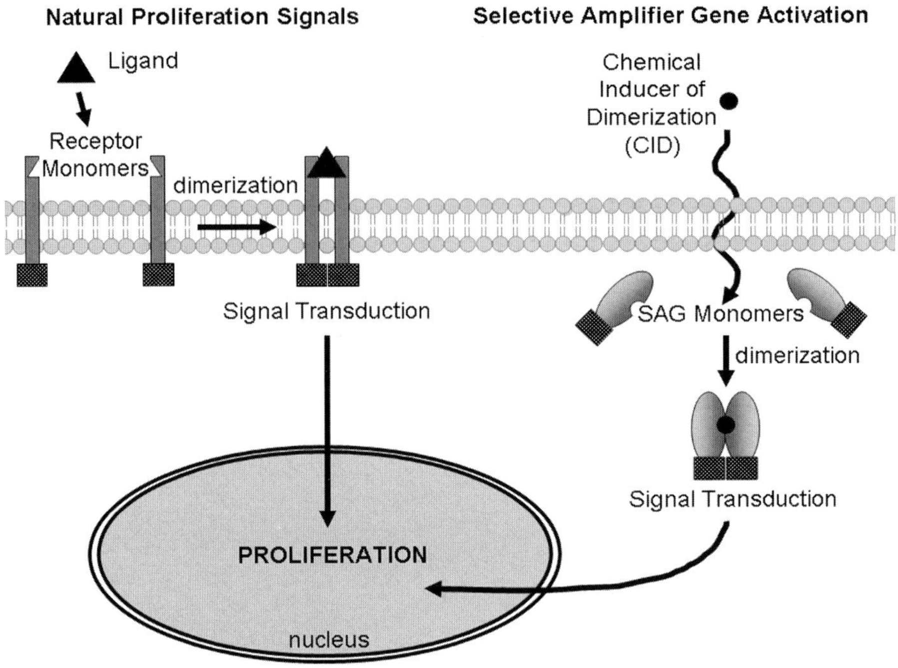

Fig. 2. Selective amplifier genes (SAGs). SAGs are chimeric gene products consisting of dimerization and signaling domains. Chemical inducers of dimerization (CIDs) bring two SAG monomers together, which activates the signaling domains to induce cell proliferation.

Initial studies utilized the FK506-binding domain of the immunophilin FKBP12 linked to the intracellular signaling domain of either the erythropoietin or c-kit receptors *(53,54)*. The feasibility of this strategy was demonstrated using an interleukin (IL)-3-dependent cell line; addition of the CID (FK1012) to the media rescued transduced cells from IL-3 deprivation *(53,54)*. The intracellular signaling domain of the thrombopoietin receptor was evaluated in subsequent studies *(55)*. Murine bone marrow cells transduced with this construct could be expanded ex vivo only in the presence of FK1012. Although multilineage expansion was demonstrated at early time points, megakaryocytic cells dominated the cultures at later time points. CID-mediated expansion of $CD34^+$ cord blood progenitors was achieved in later experiments using a similar construct *(56)*. Whereas the expanded murine cultures favored megakaryocytic differentiation, erythroid cells dominated the CID-expanded human cell cultures.

SAG-mediated HSC expansion has also been evaluated in vivo. Zhao et al. recently demonstrated that SAGs derived from Jak family members may be the key to amplifying specific hematopoietic lineages *(57)*. Experiments carried out with a SAG construct containing the JH1 domain of murine Jak2 linked to a tandem binding site for the CID, AP20187, were evaluated in a murine transplant model. Administration of the CID resulted in a rapid expansion of transduced erythrocytes. However, the effect was short-lived, and the transduced erythrocyte population declined to pretreatment levels after CID withdrawal. Another SAG, consisting of the erythropoietin (EPO) receptor dimerization domain fused to the thrombopoietin receptor signaling domain, was recently evaluated in cynomogus macaques *(58)*. Transduced $CD34^+$ cells were transplanted directly into irrigated femurs and humeri in unconditioned animals. In the absence of

CID administration (in this case EPO), 2–30% of colony-forming units (CFU) and less than 0.1% of peripheral mononucleocytes were transgene positive after 1 yr. Peripheral blood marking levels in animals treated with daily injections of EPO peaked at 8–9% over the same time period, with polyclonal marking detected in multiple lineages. However, as seen in previous studies, marked cell percentages returned to baseline levels shortly after each CID treatment *(58)*.

Selective amplification strategies reported to date have demonstrated promising results. However, the marking levels obtained in animal models remain low, and depend on continuous CID administration. It remains unclear whether the chimeric gene products are only effective at expanding less primitive cell populations, or decline as a result of an immune response. However, rather than returning to baseline levels, an immune response would likely clear even the more primitive SAG-expressing cells upon CID withdrawal. One advantage SAG-mediated stem cell expansion has over drug selection schemes is the limited toxicities associated with selection. No obvious adverse events were detected from transgene expression or CID treatment in the animal models. Nevertheless, it will be essential to determine whether cells transduced with these constructs exhibit normal checkpoint controls in response to DNA damage when faced with such strong proliferative signals. This issue needs to be addressed, especially if attempts will be made to link SAG and drug selection strategies. Additional candidates for SAG-mediated HSC expansion should come from transcriptional profiling studies underway.

3. SELECTIVE ENRICHMENT OF HSCs: DRUG-RESISTANCE GENE TRANSFER

Drug resistance genes offer another approach to enriching transduced stem cell populations in vivo. Whereas selective amplifier genes confer a proliferative advantage, allowing transduced stem cells to outgrow untransduced cells, drug resistance genes provide a survival advantage to transduced stem cells in response to cytotoxic drug treatment. The most common restriction to neoplastic drug treatment is the associated myelotoxicity. Chemotherapy resistant genes transferred to HSCs should reduce treatment-related morbidity and permit dose escalation to levels needed for neoplastic cell toxicity. In addition, drug resistance genes offer the potential to specifically select transduced cells at the expense of unmodified cells in vivo. Several drug resistance genes have been evaluated as tools for either increasing the therapeutic index of cancer therapies, or for selective enrichment of gene corrected stem cells.

3.1. Multidrug-Resistance Proteins

P-glycoprotein (P-gp) is encoded by the multidrug-resistance-1 gene (*mdr1*) and is the prototypic member of the ATP-binding cassette family of drug resistance proteins. P-gp was identified as the cellular protein responsible for the pleiotropic cross-resistance certain cell lines acquired to unrelated chemotherapy drugs, such as anthracyclins, epipodophyllotoxins, taxanes, and vinca-alkaloids *(59,60)*. Drug resistance is established by the ATP-dependent efflux of these compounds from the cell, preventing intracellular concentrations from becoming cytotoxic (*see* Fig. 3).

The potential for using P-gp to protect bone marrow from myelosuppression was first demonstrated in transgenic mice *(61,62)*. High level P-gp expression in transgenic bone marrow protected animals from daunomycin and taxol treatments that caused myelosuppression in normal mice. Transplantation of *mdr1*-transgenic bone marrow

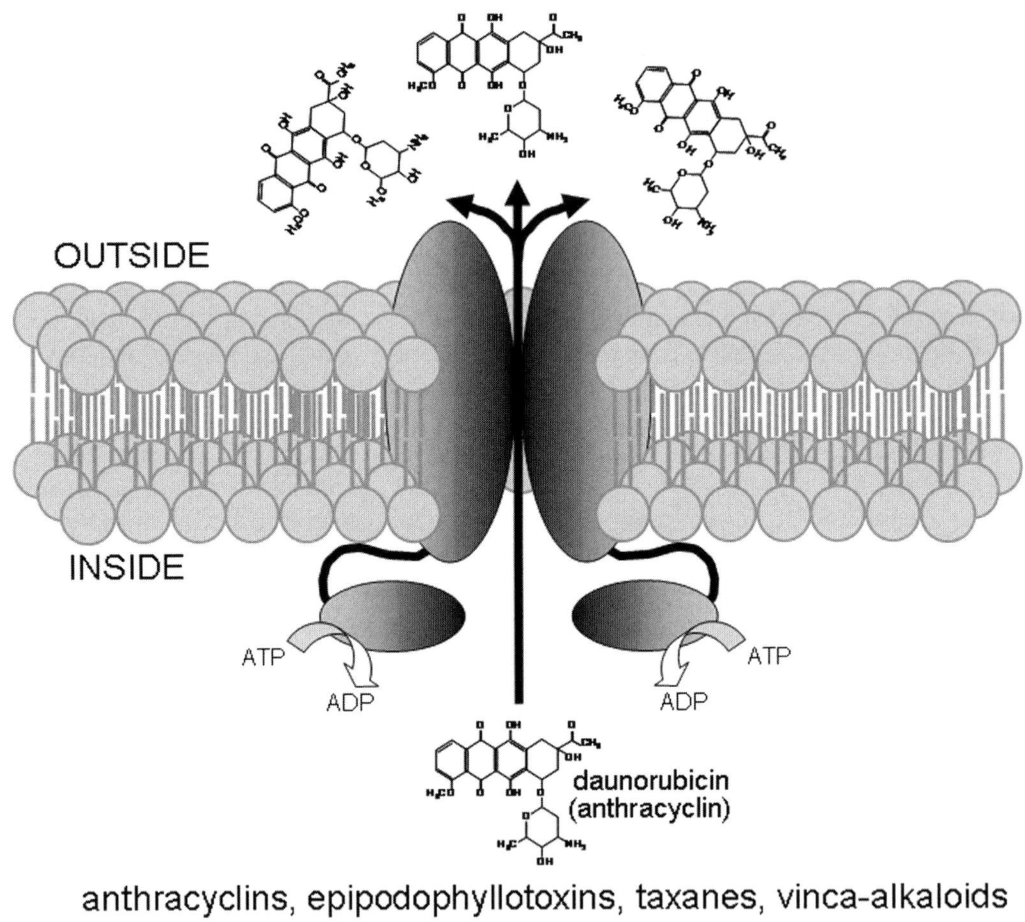

Fig. 3. Drug efflux pumps. The ABC-family of drug efflux proteins are localized in the plasma membrane where they actively export cytotoxic drugs from the cytosol to the extracellular space. Cells that overexpress these proteins are protected from higher drug concentrations.

into lethally-irradiated control animals was sufficient to transfer long-term drug resistance to recipient animals *(63)*. These results set the framework for retroviral gene transfer experiments. In 1992 two groups demonstrated that retroviral delivery of *mdr1* to bone marrow progenitor cells resulted in increased drug tolerance that correlated with enrichment for the transduced population *(64,65)*. Transduction of long-term repopulating cells with *mdr1* was subsequently shown to protect murine transplant recipients from repetitive administration of normally myelotoxic chemotherapy treatments *(66,67)*, while simultaneously sensitizing tumor cells *(68)*. More recent in vivo selection studies using *mdr1* have been carried out in other animal models. Schiedlmeier et al. demonstrated the first significant evidence of *mdr1*-mediated selection of human hematopoietic progenitors *in vivo*, using NOD/SCID recipients treated with paclitaxel *(69)*.

Clinical trials have also been carried out to evaluate the use of *mdr1* gene transfer for cancer patients receiving autologous transplants to reduce treatment-induced myelosuppression *(70–75)*. Early trials were limited by poor transduction efficiencies and resulted in transient marking levels indicative of short-term repopulating cell contributions. Higher marking rates (up to 52%) have been obtained using plates coated with

agents in vivo. Increased resistance to multiple doses of BCNU correlated with increased percentages of MGMT-transduced murine progenitors in the bone morrow *(104)*. Human CD34$^+$ hematopoietic progenitor cells transduced with MGMT were also shown to tolerate higher doses of BCNU *(105)*.

Just as high BM AGT expression reduces alkylating agent-induced myelosuppression, tumor cells with upregulated AGT are also tolerant to these treatments *(106–108)*. Therefore, the modest levels of protection achieved by MGMT gene transfer experiments are unlikely to have a dramatic therapeutic impact. However, two major advancements brought MGMT-mediated chemoprotection to the forefront. First was the discovery of the potent MGMT inactivator, O^6-benzylguanine (BG). BG provided a mechanism for depleting AGT activity, sensitizing tumors to drug treatment *(109–111)*. However, BG-mediated inactivation of AGT is not specific, and thus sensitizes both tumor and bone marrow cells to alkylating agents *(112)*. The second major advancement came from the identification of specific point mutations in MGMT that conferred significant resistance to BG inactivation without altering the O^6-alkyltransferase activity *(113)*. Additional BG-resistant MGMT mutants were identified from randomized MGMT libraries using BG and O^6-alkylating agent selection schemes *(114,115)*. Specific MGMT mutants were then shown to efficiently protect transduced human bone marrow progenitors from BG-mediated sensitization to chloroethylating *(116)* and methylating *(117)* agent toxicity (*see* Fig. 4). Davis et al. demonstrated that murine bone marrow progenitors transduced with the BG-resistant MGMT-G156A point mutant could be enriched in vivo with combined doses of BG and BCNU, and this enrichment protected transplant recipients from doses that were lethal to animals transplanted with control bone marrow cells *(118)*. Other MGMT point mutants were also shown to protect mice from combined BG and temozolomide *(119)*, or BG and BCNU treatments *(120)*. These studies also demonstrated that selective enrichment occurred at the stem cell level.

The true potential for using MGMT mutants for stem cell selection was demonstrated by Davis et al. using nonmyeloablated transplant recipients *(121)*. Transduced bone marrow CFU were enriched up to 47% in mice infused with as few as 5×10^4 transduced cells and selected with three rounds of BG and BCNU treatments. Enrichment to 97% was obtained when 1×10^5 cells were infused prior to drug treatments. In vivo enrichment for MGMT-transduced human CD34$^+$ cord blood progenitors has also been achieved in NOD/SCID recipients preconditioned with irradiation *(122)* or a mild dose of BG and BCNU *(123)*. The potency of MGMT-mediated stem cell selection has recently been demonstrated in a large animal canine model *(124,125)*. Transgene-expressing granulocytes were enriched to over 98% in both animals studied (from 3 and 16% initial cell expression percentages), following incremental dosing with BG and temozolomide. Remarkably, polyclonal marking and long-term expression was achieved with an average of only one integration event per cell.

The use of MGMT point mutants to differentially protect the hematopoietic compartment while sensitizing tumors has also been reported in animal xenograft models *(126–128)*. Clinical trials using gene transfer of MGMT have been proposed by several investigators, and one phase I trial in patients with advanced malignancies such as melanoma, sarcoma and other solid tumors is in progress *(129)*. The objective of this trial is to protect bone marrow stem cells from the toxic effects of chemotherapy and select for MGMT-G156A transduced cells during treatment. This strategy is expected to result in less toxicity to bone marrow and blood cells while enriching for the number of genetically altered drug resistant stem cells over time, perhaps even from undetectable levels. The hypothesis of this study is based on preclinical data that shows this gene can provide HSCs with more than 500-fold survival advantage compared with HSCs not carrying the gene. In this clinical protocol, peripheral blood stem cells are collected from patients, exposed to a MMLRV containing the G156A MGMT gene in the laboratory and immediately reinfused into the patient. Starting 2 d prior to cell infusion and every 6 wk thereafter, patients are treated with BG and BCNU to inhibit tumor growth and provide selective resistance to the stem cells carrying the gene. To date, 5 patients have been enrolled and the level of gene transfer into the stem cells before infusion ranged from 11 to 36%. No complications related to cell infusion or chemotherapy administration have been observed. In one patient, evidence of genetically altered cells was observed by molecular analysis in the bone marrow 5 wk after the infusion and prior to the chemotherapy treatment. Although preliminary, these results indicate that infusion of HSCs transduced with retroviral mutant MGMT is feasible and safe. This is an important trial because stem cell selection with MGMT may be useful in other planned clinical applications including the use of MGMT in combination with therapeutic genes to correct for genetic disorders and the use of MGMT stem cell protection during allogeneic transplantation as a selection strategy to encourage donor engraftment. Because the theoretical risks of oncogenesis associated with oncoretroviral vector integration has now been observed in a successful human gene therapy trial for SCID XI *(130)*, the next generation of gene therapy trials will likely incorporate lentiviral vectors. These vectors are thought to have a decreased risk of insertional oncogenesis, and their increased stem cell transduction efficiencies indicate that lower multiplicities of infection (MOIs) may be used to achieve the same endpoint.

3.3. Nucleoside and Folate Analog Resistance

Several other drug resistance genes have been evaluated for in vivo selection or chemoprotection, including cytidine deaminase (CDA), and dihydrofolate reductase (DHFR). CDA belongs to a class of enzymes involved in pyrimidine metabolism and salvage pathways. CDA can also inactivate cytosine nucleoside analogs, (e.g., cytarabine), which are used as antineoplastic agents. Transduction of murine bone marrow cells with CDA was shown to increase hematopoietic CDA expression levels in recipient animals, but showed little evidence of drug protection *(131)*. The selection stringency for CDA-transduced bone marrow cells ex vivo is also dependent on cell density, indicating that release of CDA into the media may inactivate these drugs, reucing the toxicity of untransduced cells *(132)*.

DHFR converts folate into tetrahydrofolate, a cofactor required for thymidylate and purine biosynthesis. Folate analogs such as methotrexate (MTX) and trimetrexate (TMTX) bind to DHFR with greater affinity, thereby inhibiting DNA synthesis (*see* Fig. 5). Specific DHFR mutations have been identified that are resistant to these antifolates *(133,134)*. Early experiments showed that murine bone marrow transduced with DHFR mutants efficiently protected irradiated recipients from methotrexate-induced marrow toxicity *(133,135)*. Allay et al. demonstrated that nucleoside transport inhibitors, such as nitrobenzylmercaptopurineriboside phosphate (NBMPR-P), increased the sensitivity of primitive hematopoietic cells to folate analogs *(136)*. Subsequent murine transplant experiments, using both TMTX and NBMPR-P for in vivo selection, resulted in a significant expansion of DHFR-transduced progenitors *(137)*. However, only transient and limiting levels of DHFR-mediated enrichment was observed in nonhuman primate

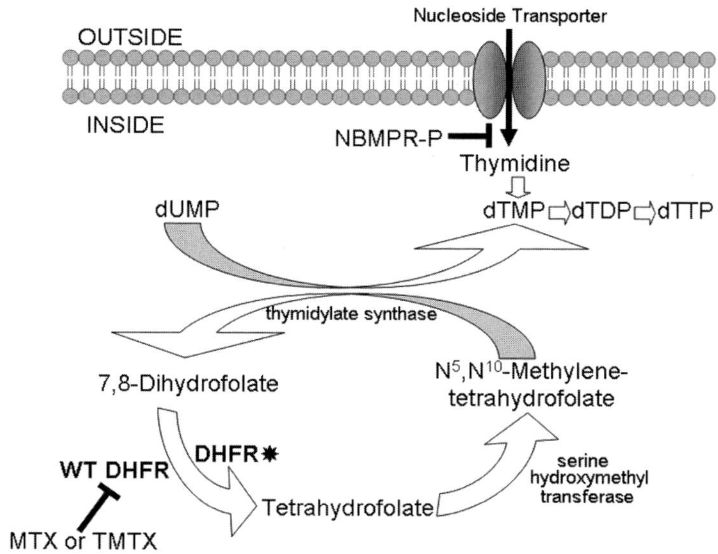

Fig. 5. The role of DHFR in pyrimidine biosynthesis. Antifolates (e.g., MTX) competitively bind to DHFR, blocking tetrahydrofolate synthesis. DHFR mutants (DHFR*) are resistant to antifolate inhibition. Nucleoside transporters allow cells to salvage nucleosides. NBMPR-P inhibits nucleoside transporters, further sensitizing untransduced cells to antifolate drugs.

models in vivo, following combined TMTX and NBMPR-P treatment *(138)*. Increased toxicity was also evident in this model. Further, pretreatment with cytokines failed to significantly increase the selection stringency for long-term repopulating cells transduced with DHFR. Thus, DHFR and CDA may reduce treatment-related toxicities, but may not provide additional protection to transduced HSCs.

4. DUAL-GENE TRANSFER STRATEGIES

Although a major focus for in vivo HSC enrichment methods has been to reduce myelosuppression, another emphasis has been to use this strategy to repopulate a diseased hematopoietic compartment with gene-corrected cells. This application requires vectors that are capable of efficiently expressing both the selectable marker and the therapeutic gene. The selectable marker gene allows the transduced cells to be enriched, and the therapeutic gene restores function to the diseased cells. Several vector designs have been generated for this endpoint.

Bicistronic vectors are constructed using internal ribosome entry site (IRES) sequences. If two genes are positioned in the vector in tandem they will be transcribed as a bicistronic message. However, in this configuration the first gene will be translated by the normal cap-dependent mechanism, but the second gene will only extend the 3′-untranslated region. An IRES element positioned between the two genes will reinitiate translation to generate the second gene product. IRES elements were initially discovered in viral genomes, but have now been identified in many other organisms. The majority of the IRES sequences used for dual-gene vectors are derived from the polio virus or encephalomyocarditis virus genomes. IRES-initiated translation is typically less efficient than cap-mediated translation *(139,140)*. Thus, the orientation of the two genes in a bicistronic vector must be taken into account for each application. For instance, selection of cells transduced with a *therapeutic*-IRES-*drug-resistance* gene configuration might lead to an oligoclonal population with high-therapeutic gene expression, because high levels of the bicistronic transcript will compensate for low-IRES translation rates. The same genes configured in the opposite orientation (with respect to the IRES) might result in a polyclonal population with low-therapeutic gene expression. IRES elements with tissue-specific or inducible expression patterns have also been identified, some of which are being developed for gene therapy applications *(141,142)*. Several gene therapy models have used IRES elements to couple drug resistance genes to therapeutic or reporter gene expression. Bicistronic vectors containing two separate drug resistance genes have also been used to expand HSC resistance to additional classes of chemotherapy drugs *(143)*.

The foot and mouth disease virus (FMDV) 2a element has also been utilized in many dual-gene vectors *(144,145)*. The 54-bp sequence encoding FMDV-2a is positioned between two genes, the first of which has the stop codon removed. Thus, both genes and the 2a element are joined as one open reading frame. After the first gene and 2a sequence are translated, *cis*-acting hydrolase activity within the 2a residues cause ribosomes to "skip" the last peptide bond in 2a. Thus, the first gene product is released with 17 residues from the 2a element fused to its C-terminus. The ribosome then continues translating the second gene product, which contains an N-terminal proline from the 2a sequence *(146)*. Like IRES elements, the efficiency of ribosome slippage sequences appears to be sensitive to the specific gene combinations used *(145)*. Further, the activity of the first gene product can be perturbed by the 2a residues that remain fused to its C-terminus *(147)*.

Alternative splicing mechanisms have also been utilized to create dual gene vectors *(148,149)*. These vectors are constructed by adding an extra splice acceptor site in front of the second gene. If the first splice acceptor is recognized, the first gene is translated and the second gene becomes an extended 3′-untranslated region. If the second splice acceptor is recognized the first gene becomes part of the excised intron and the second gene is translated. However, stringent selection can result in the amplification of cells that preferentially splice out the therapeutic gene in favor of drug resistance gene expression. Additional transcription cassettes can also be inserted into vectors to coexpress two genes. This strategy can be complicated by transcriptional interference, resulting in the silencing of one gene in favor of the other *(150)*. Recently Amendola et al. created lentivectors containing synthetic promoters that are bidirectional. These synthetic promoters allow two genes in opposite orientations to be expressed from the same promoter *(151)*.

Another strategy utilizes a mixture of separate single-gene lentiviral vectors to cotransduce cells. This strategy allows the rapid evaluation of two genes without a need for dual-gene vector construction. Cotransduction with lentiviral vectors has only been described in vitro *(152,153)*. In these studies separate VSV-G pseudotyped LV were shown to cotransduce cell lines or primary human neurons at a frequency proportional to the transduction efficiency of each virus. Frimpong et al. also reported efficient cotransduction of cells with two bicistronic vectors, each with a unique drug resistance gene, for in vitro selection of only dual positive cells *(153)*. Cotransduction of hematopoietic cells has not been evaluated. In the context of ex vivo gene therapy, the vast excess of unmodified endogenous cells in vivo would limit the efficacy of selection prior to transplant. The prolonged ex vivo culturing periods required for preselection have also been shown to correlate with reduced cell pluripotency and engraftment *(154,155)*. Therefore, brief transduction schemes followed by in vivo enrichment has been a focus of most hematopoietic drug resistance gene transfer strategies.

5. TARGETED TRANSDUCTION

Because there is an apparent tradeoff between specificity and transduction efficiency with natural viral proteins, many attempts to engineer viruses with specificity towards clinically relevant target cells have been made. Previous strategies have focused on localizing the MuLV-based vectors to target cells through the use of antibody bridges *(156–158)* or envelopes that display ligands such as erythropoietin, heregulin, and hepatocyte growth factor *(159–161)*. However these experiments required co-expression of the wild-type envelope, or only moderately improved the transduction efficiency.

Other strategies have utilized the insertion of sequences within the surface domain (SU) of viral envelopes that force transduction through new receptors. These insertions are usually ligands *(161,162)* or single-chain antibodies with binding specificity for specific proteins expressed in the target cell *(163–169)*. Although many insertions have been shown to fold correctly and are presented on the virion surface, the transduction efficiency is often limited by perturbations in the transmembrane domain's (TM) fusion activity. Flexible linkers inserted between the ligand-SU junction have only moderately improved transduction efficiencies *(170)*. The process of infection involves SU trimerization, receptor binding, and conformational changes that expose TM for fusion. Thus, the insert must be presented in a way that redirects binding without perturbing SU trimerization or fusion. Recently, Chandrashekran et al. demonstrated that expression of a membrane-bound form of stem cell factor in an ecotropic packaging cell line resulted in virions containing the ecotropic envelope and stem cell factor on their surface, which were able to specifically transduce human cells expressing the SCF receptor *(171)*. Thus, the ecotropic envelope may be able to utilize the human receptor or induce receptor-independent fusion upon gaining entry into endosomes. Regardless, this study demonstrates that envelope modifications may be unnecessary when other targeting molecules are present.

Additional strategies have involved the use of retroviral display by randomizing the receptor binding domains and using entry-based screens to identify targeted virions *(172,173)*. However, the titers obtained with retroviral vectors restrict the size of the libraries that can be screened. Because structural information for many envelope proteins remains elusive, strategies utilizing inserted targeting motifs may benefit from the combined use of randomization strategies. Randomization of the residues flanking the targeting motif might aid in the identification of a display configuration that allows both targeted binding and functional envelope fusion activities. Alternatively, other viral envelope proteins that are much more tolerant of insertions, may permit more efficient targeted delivery vehicles.

6. BALANCING SAFETY WITH EFFICACY

Great strides have been made in vector development with much of the focus aimed at increasing viral titers and tropism. While this improves the range of applications for a given system, it has also led to the trend of maximizing expression without regard for the cumulative number of integrations. Theoretical concerns over insertional mutations arising from gene therapy vectors have now been realized in three patients enrolled in X-linked severe combined immunodeficiency (X-SCID) gene therapy trials *(174)*. These adverse events have encouraged investigators to reevaluate copy number and weigh the risks of insertional mutagenesis for gene therapy models used for preclinical relevance. Woods et al. have demonstrated that even early hematopoietic progenitors are susceptible to multiple lentiviral integration events when transduced with high MOIs *(175)*. The finding that transcriptionally active regions of the genome are hotspots for integration further emphasizes the need for caution *(176)*. These issues point to the need for standards, beyond expression level, for evaluating the potency of a given vector and delivery system. An index based on expression level per insertion may be one such standard, but would require further standardization of the techniques used for copy number analysis. Kustikova et al. have pointed to the importance for such a standard by demonstrating the nonlinear relationship between insertion and expression levels *(177)*. They concluded that expression-based gene transfer efficiencies should be targeted to 30% or less to attain the highest expression level with the fewest insertions. Standardized cell lines and protocols for determining viral titer are also nonexistent, as each group tends to have a different method for defining MOI. The use of virus-loaded fibronectin plates and spinoculation protocols for transduction further complicates the use of MOI as an informative index. Ultimately, the number of insertions per cell and total cell dose required for therapeutic efficacy will have to be established for clinical trial risk assessment. The statistical risk of insertional mutagenesis and the need for elevated titers could be reduced by minimizing the number of nontarget cell transductions. For this reason, continued emphasis should be placed on the development of vectors with integration site or target cell specificity.

7. CONCLUSION

In summary, many advances have been, and continue to be made in HSC gene transfer and selection technologies. However, multiple factors must be taken into account for each unique application. The efficacy of *cis*- and *trans*-acting vector determinants, such as promoters, dual-gene linkage elements, and envelope pseudotypes, often vary based on the genes used, the cell source, the intended cell targets, and the methods used for transduction. The risks associated with each disease should obviously outweigh those associated with therapy. Defining the general risk of insertional mutagenesis and in vivo selection will provide essential insight, but these risks should also be evaluated for each application.

REFERENCES

1. Artelt P, et al. Vectors for efficient expression in mammalian fibroblastoid, myeloid and lymphoid cells via transfection or infection. Gene 1988;68(2):213–219.
2. Hawley G, et al. Transplantable myeloproliferative disease induced in mice by an interleukin 6 retrovirus. J Exp Med 1992;176(4):1149–1163.
3. Tumas B, et al. High-frequency cell surface expression of a foreign protein in murine hematopoietic stem cells using a new retroviral vector. Blood 1996;87(2):509–517.
4. Halene S, et al. Improved expression in hematopoietic and lymphoid cells in mice after transplantation of bone marrow transduced with a modified retroviral vector. Blood 1999;94(10):3349–3357.
5. Baum C, Richters A, Ostertag W. Retroviral vector-mediated gene expression in hematopoietic cells. Curr Opin Mol Ther 1999;1(5):605–612.
6. Cherry R, et al. Retroviral expression in embryonic stem cells and hematopoietic stem cells. Mol Cell Biol 2000;20(20):7419–7426.
7. Ketteler R, et al. Enhanced transgene expression in primitive hematopoietic progenitor cells and embryonic stem cells efficiently transduced by optimized retroviral hybrid vectors. Gene Ther 2002;9(8):477–487.
8. Agarwal M, et al. Scaffold attachment region-mediated enhancement of retroviral vector expression in primary T cells. J Virol 1998;72(5):3720–3728.

9. Murray L, et al. Addition of the human interferon beta scaffold attachment region to retroviral vector backbones increases the level of in vivo transgene expression among progeny of engrafted human hematopoietic stem cells. Hum Gene Ther 2000;11(14):2039–2050.
10. Inoue T, et al. Position-independent human beta-globin gene expression mediated by a recombinant adeno-associated virus vector carrying the chicken beta- globin insulator. J Hum Genet 1999;44(3):152–162.
11. Emery W, et al. A chromatin insulator protects retrovirus vectors from chromosomal position effects. Proc Natl Acad Sci U S A 2000;97(16):9150–9155.
12. Rivella S, et al. The cHS4 insulator increases the probability of retroviral expression at random chromosomal integration sites. J Virol 2000;74(10):4679–4687.
13. Popa I, et al. CRM1-dependent function of a *cis*-acting RNA export element. Mol Cell Biol 2002;22(7):2057–2067.
14. Luens KM, et al. Thrombopoietin, kit ligand, and flk2/flt3 ligand together induce increased numbers of primitive hematopoietic progenitors from human CD34+Thy-1+Lin- cells with preserved ability to engraft SCID-hu bone. Blood 1998;91(4):1206–1215.
15. Dao A, et al. FLT3 ligand preserves the ability of human CD34+ progenitors to sustain long-term hematopoiesis in immune-deficient mice after ex vivo retroviral-mediated transduction. Blood 1997;89(2):446–456.
16. Naldini L, et al. In vivo gene delivery and stable transduction of nondividing cells by a lentiviral vector. Science 1996;272(5259):263–267.
17. Sutton E, et al. Transduction of human progenitor hematopoietic stem cells by human immunodeficiency virus type 1-based vectors is cell cycle dependent. J Virol 1999;73(5):3649–3660.
18. Douglas L, et al. Efficient human immunodeficiency virus-based vector transduction of unstimulated human mobilized peripheral blood CD34+ cells in the SCID-hu Thy/Liv model of human T cell lymphopoiesis. Hum Gene Ther 2001;12(4):401–413.
19. Zielske P, Gerson SL. Cytokines, including stem cell factor alone, enhance lentiviral transduction in nondividing human LTCIC and NOD/SCID repopulating cells. Mol Ther 2003;7(3):325–333.
20. Zennou V, et al. HIV-1 genome nuclear import is mediated by a central DNA flap. Cell 2000;101(2):173–185.
21. Sirven A, et al. The human immunodeficiency virus type-1 central DNA flap is a crucial determinant for lentiviral vector nuclear import and gene transduction of human hematopoietic stem cells. Blood 2000;96(13):4103–4110.
22. Follenzi A, et al. Gene transfer by lentiviral vectors is limited by nuclear translocation and rescued by HIV-1 pol sequences. Nat Genet 2000;25(2):217–222.
23. Yu SF, et al. Self-inactivating retroviral vectors designed for transfer of whole genes into mammalian cells. Proc Natl Acad Sci U S A 1986;83(10):3194–3198.
24. Miyoshi H, et al. Development of a self-inactivating lentivirus vector. J Virol 1998;72(10): 8150–8157.
25. Zufferey R, et al. Self-inactivating lentivirus vector for safe and efficient in vivo gene delivery. J Virol 1998;72(12):9873–9880.
26. Salmon P, et al. High-level transgene expression in human hematopoietic progenitors and differentiated blood lineages after transduction with improved lentiviral vectors. Blood 2000;96(10): 3392–3398.
27. Moreau-Gaudry F, et al. High-level erythroid-specific gene expression in primary human and murine hematopoietic cells with self-inactivating lentiviral vectors. Blood 2001;98(9):2664–2672.
28. Lotti F, et al. Transcriptional targeting of lentiviral vectors by long terminal repeat enhancer replacement. J Virol 2002;76(8):3996–4007.
29. Choi K, et al. Hybrid HIV/MSCV LTR enhances transgene expression of lentiviral vectors in human CD34(+) hematopoietic cells. Stem Cells 2001;19(3):236–246.
30. Demaison C, et al. High-level transduction and gene expression in hematopoietic repopulating cells using a human immunodeficiency [correction of imunodeficiency] virus type 1-based lentiviral vector containing an internal spleen focus forming virus promoter. Hum Gene Ther 2002;13(7):803–813.
31. Manilla P, et al. Regulatory considerations for novel gene therapy products: a review of the process leading to the first clinical lentiviral vector. Hum Gene Ther 2005;16(1):17–25.
32. Thomsen S, et al. Lack of functional Pit-1 and Pit-2 expression on hematopoietic stem cell lines. Acta Haematol 1998;99(3):148–155.
33. Carneiro A, et al. Membrane recognition by vesicular stomatitis virus involves enthalpy-driven protein-lipid interactions. J Virol 2002;76(8):3756–3764.

34. Farson D, et al. A new-generation stable inducible packaging cell line for lentiviral vectors. Hum Gene Ther 2001;12(8):981–997.
35. Pacchia AL, et al. An inducible packaging cell system for safe, efficient lentiviral vector production in the absence of HIV-1 accessory proteins. Virology 2001;282(1):77–86.
36. von Laer D, et al. Amphotropic and VSV-G-pseudotyped retroviral vectors transduce human hematopoietic progenitor cells with similar efficiency. Bone Marrow Transplant 2000;25 Suppl 2:S75–S79.
37. Kelly F, et al. RD114-pseudotyped oncoretroviral vectors. Biological and physical properties. Ann N Y Acad Sci 2001;938:262–276; discussion 276–277.
38. Ward M, et al. A stable murine-based RD114 retroviral packaging line efficiently transduces human hematopoietic cells. Mol Ther 2003;8(5):804–812.
39. Hanawa H, et al. Comparison of various envelope proteins for their ability to pseudotype lentiviral vectors and transduce primitive hematopoietic cells from human blood. Mol Ther 2002;5(3):242–251.
40. Relander T, et al. Gene Transfer to Repopulating Human CD34(+) Cells Using Amphotropic-, GALV-, or RD114-Pseudotyped HIV-1-Based Vectors from Stable Producer Cells. Mol Ther 2005;11(3):452–459.
41. Sauvageau G, Iscove NN, Humphries RK. In vitro and in vivo expansion of hematopoietic stem cells. Oncogene 2004;23(43):7223–7232.
42. Giampaolo A, et al. Key functional role and lineage-specific expression of selected HOXB genes in purified hematopoietic progenitor differentiation. Blood 1994;84(11):3637–3647.
43. Moretti P, et al. Identification of homeobox genes expressed in human haemopoietic progenitor cells. Gene 1994;144(2):213–219.
44. Sauvageau G, et al. Differential expression of homeobox genes in functionally distinct CD34+ subpopulations of human bone marrow cells. Proc Natl Acad Sci U S A 1994;91(25):12,223–12,227.
45. Grier DG, et al. The pathophysiology of HOX genes and their role in cancer. J Pathol 2005;205(2): 154–171.
46. Sauvageau G, et al. Overexpression of HOXB4 in hematopoietic cells causes the selective expansion of more primitive populations in vitro and in vivo. Genes Dev 1995;9(14):1753–1765.
47. Thorsteinsdottir U, Sauvageau G, Humphries RK. Enhanced in vivo regenerative potential of HOXB4-transduced hematopoietic stem cells with regulation of their pool size. Blood 1999;94(8):2605–2612.
48. Antonchuk J, Sauvageau G, Humphries RK. HOXB4-induced expansion of adult hematopoietic stem cells ex vivo. Cell 2002;109(1):39–45.
49. Amsellem S, et al. Ex vivo expansion of human hematopoietic stem cells by direct delivery of the HOXB4 homeoprotein. Nat Med 2003;9(11):1423–1427 Epub 2003 Oct 26.
50. Krosl J, et al. In vitro expansion of hematopoietic stem cells by recombinant TAT-HOXB4 protein. Nat Med 2003;9(11):1428–1432 Epub 2003 Oct 26.
51. Schiedlmeier B, et al. High-level ectopic HOXB4 expression confers a profound in vivo competitive growth advantage on human cord blood CD34+ cells, but impairs lymphomyeloid differentiation. Blood 2003;101(5):1759–1768 Epub 2002 Oct 24.
52. Beslu N, et al. Molecular interactions involved in HOXB4-induced activation of HSC self-renewal. Blood 2004;104(8):2307–2314 Epub 2004 Jun 29.
53. Blau A, et al. A proliferation switch for genetically modified cells. Proc Natl Acad Sci U S A 1997;94(7):3076–3081.
54. Jin L, Asano H, Blau CA, Stimulating cell proliferation through the pharmacologic activation of c-kit. Blood 1998;91(3):890–897.
55. Jin L, et al. Targeted expansion of genetically modified bone marrow cells. Proc Natl Acad Sci U S A 1998;95(14):8093–8097.
56. Richard E, et al. Expansion of genetically modified primary human hemopoietic cells using chemical inducers of dimerization. Blood 2000;95(2):430–436.
57. Zhao S, et al. In vivo selection of genetically modified erythroid cells using a jak2-based cell growth switch. Mol Ther 2004;10(3):456–468.
58. Ueda K, et al. High-level in vivo gene marking after gene-modified autologous hematopoietic stem cell transplantation without marrow conditioning in nonhuman primates. Mol Ther 2004;10(3):469–477.
59. Juliano RL, Ling V. A surface glycoprotein modulating drug permeability in Chinese hamster ovary cell mutants. Biochim Biophys Acta 1976;455(1):152–162.
60. Kartner N, et al. Detection of P-glycoprotein in multidrug-resistant cell lines by monoclonal antibodies. Nature 1985;316(6031):820–823.
61. Galski H, et al. Expression of a human multidrug resistance cDNA (MDR1) in the bone marrow of transgenic mice: resistance to daunomycin-induced leukopenia. Mol Cell Biol 1989;9(10):4357–4363.

62. Mickisch GH, et al. Chemotherapy and chemosensitization of transgenic mice which express the human multidrug resistance gene in bone marrow: efficacy, potency, and toxicity. Cancer Res 1991;51(19):5417–5424.
63. Mickisch GH, et al. Transplantation of bone marrow cells from transgenic mice expressing the human MDR1 gene results in long-term protection against the myelosuppressive effect of chemotherapy in mice. Blood 1992;79(4):1087–1093.
64. Podda S, et al. Transfer and expression of the human multiple drug resistance gene into live mice. Proc Natl Acad Sci U S A 1992;89(20):9676–9680.
65. Sorrentino BP, et al. Selection of drug-resistant bone marrow cells in vivo after retroviral transfer of human MDR1. Science 1992;257(5066):99–103.
66. Hanania EG, Deisseroth AB. Serial transplantation shows that early hematopoietic precursor cells are transduced by MDR-1 retroviral vector in a mouse gene therapy model. Cancer Gene Ther 1994;1(1):21–25.
67. Carpinteiro A, et al. Genetic protection of repopulating hematopoietic cells with an improved MDR1-retrovirus allows administration of intensified chemotherapy following stem cell transplantation in mice. Int J Cancer 2002;98(5):785–792.
68. Hanania EG, Deisseroth AB. Simultaneous genetic chemoprotection of normal marrow cells and genetic chemosensitization of breast cancer cells in a mouse cancer gene therapy model. Clin Cancer Res 1997;3(2):281–286.
69. Schiedlmeier B, et al. Multidrug resistance 1 gene transfer can confer chemoprotection to human peripheral blood progenitor cells engrafted in immunodeficient mice. Hum Gene Ther 2002;13(2):233–242.
70. Hanania EG, et al. Results of MDR-1 vector modification trial indicate that granulocyte/macrophage colony-forming unit cells do not contribute to posttransplant hematopoietic recovery following intensive systemic therapy. Proc Natl Acad Sci U S A 1996;93(26):15,346–15,351.
71. Hesdorffer C, et al. Phase I trial of retroviral-mediated transfer of the human MDR1 gene as marrow chemoprotection in patients undergoing high-dose chemotherapy and autologous stem-cell transplantation. J Clin Oncol 1998;16(1):165–172.
72. Vahdat LT, et al. Phase I trial of sequential high-dose chemotherapy with escalating dose paclitaxel, melphalan, and cyclophosphamide, thiotepa, and carboplatin with peripheral blood progenitor support in women with responding metastatic breast cancer. Clin Cancer Res 1998;4(7):1689–1695.
73. Moscow JA, et al. Engraftment of MDR1 and NeoR gene-transduced hematopoietic cells after breast cancer chemotherapy. Blood 1999;94(1):52–61.
74. Cowan KH, et al. Paclitaxel chemotherapy after autologous stem-cell transplantation and engraftment of hematopoietic cells transduced with a retrovirus containing the multidrug resistance complementary DNA (MDR1) in metastatic breast cancer patients. Clin Cancer Res 1999;5(7):1619–1628.
75. Abonour R, et al. Efficient retrovirus-mediated transfer of the multidrug resistance 1 gene into autologous human long-term repopulating hematopoietic stem cells. Nat Med 2000;6(6):652–658.
76. Abbott BL. ABCG2 (BCRP) expression in normal and malignant hematopoietic cells. Hematol Oncol 2003;21(3):115–130.
77. Goodell MA, et al. Isolation and functional properties of murine hematopoietic stem cells that are replicating in vivo. J Exp Med 1996;183(4):1797–1806.
78. Zhou S, et al. The ABC transporter Bcrp1/ABCG2 is expressed in a wide variety of stem cells and is a molecular determinant of the side-population phenotype. Nat Med 2001;7(9):1028–1034.
79. Zhou S, et al. Bcrp1 gene expression is required for normal numbers of side population stem cells in mice, and confers relative protection to mitoxantrone in hematopoietic cells in vivo. Proc Natl Acad Sci U S A 2002;99(19):12,339–12,344 Epub 2002 Sep 06.
80. Bunting KD, et al. Enforced P-glycoprotein pump function in murine bone marrow cells results in expansion of side population stem cells in vitro and repopulating cells in vivo. Blood 2000;96(3):902–909.
81. Modlich U, et al. Leukemias following retroviral transfer of multidrug resistance 1 (MDR1) are driven by combinatorial insertional mutagenesis. Blood 2005;15:15.
82. Kim M, et al. The multidrug resistance transporter ABCG2 (breast cancer resistance protein 1) effluxes Hoechst 33342 and is overexpressed in hematopoietic stem cells. Clin Cancer Res 2002;8(1):22–28.
83. Scharenberg CW, Harkey MA, Torok-Storb B. The ABCG2 transporter is an efficient Hoechst 33342 efflux pump and is preferentially expressed by immature human hematopoietic progenitors. Blood 2002;99(2):507–512.
84. Uchida N, Leung FY, Eaves CJ. Liver and marrow of adult mdr-1a/1b(-/-) mice show normal generation, function, and multi-tissue trafficking of primitive hematopoietic cells. Exp Hematol 2002;30(8):862–869.

85. Sellers SE, et al. The effect of multidrug-resistance 1 gene versus neo transduction on ex vivo and in vivo expansion of rhesus macaque hematopoietic repopulating cells. Blood 2001;97(6):1888–1891.
86. Hafkemeyer P, et al. Chemoprotection of hematopoietic cells by a mutant P-glycoprotein resistant to a potent chemosensitizer of multidrug-resistant cancers. Hum Gene Ther 2000;11(4):555–565.
87. Ujhelly O, et al. Application of a human multidrug transporter (ABCG2) variant as selectable marker in gene transfer to progenitor cells. Hum Gene Ther 2003;14(4):403–412.
88. Pegg AE, et al. Purification and properties of *O*6-methylguanine-DNA transmethylase from rat liver. J Biol Chem 1983;258(4):2327–2333.
89. Srivenugopal KS, et al. Ubiquitination-dependent proteolysis of *O*6-methylguanine-DNA methyltransferase in human and murine tumor cells following inactivation with *O*6-benzylguanine or 1,3-bis(2-chloroethyl)-1-nitrosourea. Biochemistry 1996;35(4):1328–1334.
90. Gerson SL, Miller K, Berger NA. O6 alkylguanine-DNA alkyltransferase activity in human myeloid cells. J Clin Invest 1985;76(6):2106–2114.
91. Gerson SL, et al. Repair of O6-alkylguanine during DNA synthesis in murine bone marrow hematopoietic precursors. Cancer Res 1987;47(1):89–95.
92. Moriwaki S, et al. Analysis of *N*-methyl-*N*-nitrosourea-induced mutations in a shuttle vector plasmid propagated in mouse *O*6-methylguanine-DNA methyltransferase-deficient cells in comparison with proficient cells. Cancer Res 1991;51(23 Pt 1):6219–6223.
93. Karran P, Bignami M. DNA damage tolerance, mismatch repair and genome instability. Bioessays 1994;16(11):833–839.
94. Dolan ME, et al. Effect of O6-methylguanine on DNA interstrand cross-link formation by chloroethylnitrosoureas and 2-chloroethyl(methylsulfonyl)methanesulfonate. Cancer Res 1988;48(13):3603–3606.
95. Gonzaga PE, Brent TP. Affinity purification and characterization of human *O*6-alkylguanine-DNA alkyltransferase complexed with BCNU-treated, synthetic oligonucleotide. Nucleic Acids Res 1989;17(16):6581–6590.
96. Margison GP, Cooper DP, Brennand J. Cloning of the *E. coli* O6-methylguanine and methylphosphotriester methyltransferase gene using a functional DNA repair assay. Nucleic Acids Res 1985;13(6): 1939–1952.
97. Brennand J, Margison GP. Reduction of the toxicity and mutagenicity of alkylating agents in mammalian cells harboring the *Escherichia coli* alkyltransferase gene. Proc Natl Acad Sci U S A 1986;83 (17):6292–6296.
98. Samson L, Derfler B, Waldstein EA. Suppression of human DNA alkylation-repair defects by *Escherichia coli* DNA-repair genes. Proc Natl Acad Sci U S A 1986;83(15):5607–5610.
99. Ishizaki K, et al. Transfer of the *E. coli O*6-methylguanine methyltransferase gene into repair-deficient human cells and restoration of cellular resistance to *N*-methyl-*N′*-nitro-*N*-nitrosoguanidine. Mutat Res 1986;166(2):135–141.
100. Jelinek J, et al. Transfection of murine multi-potent haemopoietic stem cells with an E. coli DNA alkyltransferase gene confers resistance to the toxic effects of alkylating agents. Carcinogenesis 1988;9(1):81–87.
101. Harris LC, et al. Retroviral transfer of a bacterial alkyltransferase gene into murine bone marrow protects against chloroethylnitrosourea cytotoxicity. Clin Cancer Res 1995;1(11):1359–1368.
102. Allay JA, et al. Retroviral transduction and expression of the human alkyltransferase cDNA provides nitrosourea resistance to hematopoietic cells. Blood 1995;85(11):3342–3351.
103. Moritz T, et al. Retrovirus-mediated expression of a DNA repair protein in bone marrow protects hematopoietic cells from nitrosourea-induced toxicity in vitro and in vivo. Cancer Res 1995;55(12): 2608–2614.
104. Allay JA, Davis BM, Gerson SL. Human alkyltransferase-transduced murine myeloid progenitors are enriched in vivo by BCNU treatment of transplanted mice. Exp Hematol 1997;25(10):1069–1076.
105. Allay JA, et al. Retroviral-mediated gene transduction of human alkyltransferase complementary DNA confers nitrosourea resistance to human hematopoietic progenitors. Clin Cancer Res 1996;2(8): 1353–1359.
106. Citron M, et al. *O*6-methylguanine-DNA methyltransferase in human normal and tumor tissue from brain, lung, and ovary. Cancer Res 1991;51(16):4131–4134.
107. Schold SC, Jr, et al. *O*6-alkylguanine-DNA alkyltransferase and sensitivity to procarbazine in human brain-tumor xenografts. J Neurosurg 1989;70(4):573–577.
108. Brent TP, Houghton PJ, Houghton JA. *O*6-Alkylguanine-DNA alkyltransferase activity correlates with the therapeutic response of human rhabdomyosarcoma xenografts to 1-(2-chloroethyl)-3-(*trans*-4-methylcyclohexyl)-1-nitrosourea. Proc Natl Acad Sci U S A 1985;82(9):2985–2989.

109. Dolan ME, Moschel RC, Pegg AE. Depletion of mammalian O6-alkylguanine-DNA alkyltransferase activity by *O*6-benzylguanine provides a means to evaluate the role of this protein in protection against carcinogenic and therapeutic alkylating agents. Proc Natl Acad Sci U S A 1990;87(14):5368–5372.
110. Dolan ME, et al. Effect of *O*6-benzylguanine on the sensitivity of human colon tumor xenografts to 1,3-*bis*(2-chloroethyl)-1-nitrosourea (BCNU). Biochem Pharmacol 1993;46(2):285–290.
111. Pegg AE, et al. Increased killing of prostate, breast, colon, and lung tumor cells by the combination of inactivators of *O*6-alkylguanine-DNA alkyltransferase and *N,N′-bis*(2-chloroethyl)-*N*-nitrosourea. Biochem Pharmacol 1995;50(8):1141–1148.
112. Fairbairn LJ, et al. *O*6-benzylguanine increases the sensitivity of human primary bone marrow cells to the cytotoxic effects of temozolomide. Exp Hematol 1995;23(2):112–116.
113. Crone TM, et al. Mutations in human *O*6-alkylguanine-DNA alkyltransferase imparting resistance to *O*6-benzylguanine. Cancer Res 1994;54(23):6221–6227.
114. Christians FC, et al. Creation of human alkyltransferases resistant to *O*6-benzylguanine. Cancer Res 1997;57(10):2007–2012.
115. Xu-Welliver M, Kanugula S, Pegg AE. Isolation of human *O*6-alkylguanine-DNA alkyltransferase mutants highly resistant to inactivation by *O*6-benzylguanine. Cancer Res 1998;58(9):1936–1945.
116. Reese JS, et al. Retroviral transduction of a mutant methylguanine DNA methyltransferase gene into human CD34 cells confers resistance to *O*6-benzylguanine plus 1,3-*bis*(2-chloroethyl)-1-nitrosourea. Proc Natl Acad Sci U S A 1996. 93(24):14,088–14,093.
117. Hickson I, et al. Chemoprotective gene transfer I: transduction of human haemopoietic progenitors with *O*6-benzylguanine-resistant *O*6-alkylguanine-DNA alkyltransferase attenuates the toxic effects of *O*6-alkylating agents in vitro. Gene Ther 1998;5(6):835–841.
118. Davis BM, et al. Selection for G156A *O*6-methylguanine DNA methyltransferase gene-transduced hematopoietic progenitors and protection from lethality in mice treated with *O*6-benzylguanine and 1,3-*bis*(2-chloroethyl)-1-nitrosourea. Cancer Res 1997;57(22):5093–5099.
119. Chinnasamy N, et al. Chemoprotective gene transfer II: multilineage in vivo protection of haemopoiesis against the effects of an antitumour agent by expression of a mutant human *O*6-alkylguanine-DNA alkyltransferase. Gene Ther 1998;5(6):842–847.
120. Ragg S, et al. Direct reversal of DNA damage by mutant methyltransferase protein protects mice against dose-intensified chemotherapy and leads to in vivo selection of hematopoietic stem cells. Cancer Res 2000;60(18):5187–5195.
121. Davis BM, Koc ON, Gerson SL. Limiting numbers of G156A O(6)-methylguanine-DNA methyltransferase-transduced marrow progenitors repopulate nonmyeloablated mice after drug selection. Blood 2000;95(10):3078–3084.
122. Pollok KE, et al. In vivo selection of human hematopoietic cells in a xenograft model using combined pharmacologic and genetic manipulations. Hum Gene Ther 2003;14(18):1703–1714.
123. Zielske SP, et al. In vivo selection of MGMT(P140K) lentivirus-transduced human NOD/SCID repopulating cells without pretransplant irradiation conditioning. J Clin Invest 2003;112(10):1561–1570.
124. Neff T, et al. Methylguanine methyltransferase-mediated in vivo selection and chemoprotection of allogeneic stem cells in a large-animal model. J Clin Invest 2003;112(10):1581–1588.
125. Neff T, et al. Polyclonal chemoprotection against temozolomide in a large-animal model of drug resistance gene therapy. Blood 2005;105(3):997–1002 Epub 2004 Oct 19.
126. Koc ON, et al. DeltaMGMT-transduced bone marrow infusion increases tolerance to *O*6-benzylguanine and 1,3-*bis*(2-chloroethyl)-1-nitrosourea and allows intensive therapy of 1,3-*bis*(2-chloroethyl)-1-nitrosourea-resistant human colon cancer xenografts. Hum Gene Ther 1999;10(6):1021–1030.
127. Reese JS, et al. Simultaneous protection of G156A methylguanine DNA methyltransferase gene-transduced hematopoietic progenitors and sensitization of tumor cells using *O*6-benzylguanine and temozolomide. Clin Cancer Res 1999;5(1):163–169.
128. Kreklau EL, et al. Hematopoietic expression of O(6)-methylguanine DNA methyltransferase-P140K allows intensive treatment of human glioma xenografts with combination *O*(6)-benzylguanine and 1,3-*bis*-(2-chloroethyl)-1-nitrosourea. Mol Cancer Ther 2003;2(12):1321–1329.
129. Reese JS, et al. Preliminary results of a phase I trial using retroviral gene transfer of G156A MGMT to protect hematopoiesis during BG and BCNU therapy of advanced malignancies. Mol Ther 2004; 9:S385.
130. Kaiser J. Gene therapy. Seeking the cause of induced leukemias in X-SCID trial. Science 2003;299 (5606):495.
131. Eliopoulos N, et al. Retroviral transfer and long-term expression of human cytidine deaminase cDNA in hematopoietic cells following transplantation in mice. Gene Ther 1998;5(11):1545–1551.

132. Beausejour CM, et al. Selection of drug-resistant transduced cells with cytosine nucleoside analogs using the human cytidine deaminase gene. Cancer Gene Ther 2001;8(9):669–676.
133. Zhao SC, et al. Long-term protection of recipient mice from lethal doses of methotrexate by marrow infected with a double-copy vector retrovirus containing a mutant dihydrofolate reductase. Cancer Gene Ther 1994;1(1):27–33.
134. Lewis WS, et al. Methotrexate-resistant variants of human dihydrofolate reductase with substitutions of leucine 22. Kinetics, crystallography, and potential as selectable markers. J Biol Chem 1995;270 (10):5057–5064.
135. Corey CA, et al. Serial transplantation of methotrexate-resistant bone marrow: protection of murine recipients from drug toxicity by progeny of transduced stem cells. Blood 1990;75(2):337–343.
136. Allay JA, et al. Sensitization of hematopoietic stem and progenitor cells to trimetrexate using nucleoside transport inhibitors. Blood 1997;90(9):3546–3554.
137. Allay JA, et al. In vivo selection of retrovirally transduced hematopoietic stem cells. Nat Med 1998;4(10):1136–1143.
138. Persons DA, et al. Transient in vivo selection of transduced peripheral blood cells using antifolate drug selection in rhesus macaques that received transplants with hematopoietic stem cells expressing dihydrofolate reductase vectors. Blood 2004;103(3):796–803 Epub 2003 Aug 14.
139. Zhou Y, et al. Co-expression of human adenosine deaminase and multidrug resistance using a bicistronic retroviral vector. Hum Gene Ther 1998;9(3):287–293.
140. Yu X, et al. Lentiviral vectors with two independent internal promoters transfer high-level expression of multiple transgenes to human hematopoietic stem-progenitor cells. Mol Ther 2003;7(6): 827–838.
141. Creancier L, et al. Fibroblast growth factor 2 internal ribosome entry site (IRES) activity ex vivo and in transgenic mice reveals a stringent tissue-specific regulation. J Cell Biol 2000;150(1):275–281.
142. Warnakulasuriyarachchi D, et al. Translational induction of the inhibitor of apoptosis protein HIAP2 during endoplasmic reticulum stress attenuates cell death and is mediated via an inducible internal ribosome entry site element. J Biol Chem 2004;279(17):17,148–17,157 Epub 2004 Feb 11.
143. Jelinek J, et al. A novel dual function retrovirus expressing multidrug resistance 1 and *O*6-alkylguanine-DNA-alkyltransferase for engineering resistance of haemopoietic progenitor cells to multiple chemotherapeutic agents. Gene Ther 1999;6(8):1489–1493.
144. de Felipe P, et al. Use of the 2A sequence from foot-and-mouth disease virus in the generation of retroviral vectors for gene therapy. Gene Ther 1999;6(2):198–208.
145. Milsom MD, et al. Enhanced in vivo selection of bone marrow cells by retroviral-mediated coexpression of mutant *O*6-methylguanine-DNA-methyltransferase and HOXB4. Mol Ther 2004;10(5):862–873.
146. de Felipe P. Skipping the co-expression problem: the new 2A "CHYSEL" technology. Genet Vaccines Ther 2004;2(1):13.
147. Lengler J, et al. FMDV-2A sequence and protein arrangement contribute to functionality of CYP2B1-reporter fusion protein. Anal Biochem 2005;12:12.
148. Bowtell DD, et al. Comparison of expression in hemopoietic cells by retroviral vectors carrying two genes. J Virol 1988;62(7):2464–2473.
149. Zhu Y, et al. Multigene lentiviral vectors based on differential splicing and translational control. Mol Ther 2001;4(4):375–382.
150. Emerman M, Temin HM. Genes with promoters in retrovirus vectors can be independently suppressed by an epigenetic mechanism. Cell 1984;39(3 Pt 2):449–467.
151. Amendola M, et al. Coordinate dual-gene transgenesis by lentiviral vectors carrying synthetic bidirectional promoters. Nat Biotechnol 2005;23(1):108–116 Epub 2004 Dec 26.
152. Reiser J, et al. Development of multigene and regulated lentivirus vectors. J Virol 2000;74(22): 10,589–10,599.
153. Frimpong K, Spector SA. Cotransduction of nondividing cells using lentiviral vectors. Gene Ther 2000;7(18):1562–1569.
154. Kittler EL, et al. Cytokine-facilitated transduction leads to low-level engraftment in nonablated hosts. Blood 1997;90(2):865–872.
155. Gothot A, et al. Cell cycle-related changes in repopulating capacity of human mobilized peripheral blood CD34(+) cells in non-obese diabetic/severe combined immune-deficient mice. Blood 1998;92(8):2641–2649.
156. Etienne-Julan M, et al. The efficiency of cell targeting by recombinant retroviruses depends on the nature of the receptor and the composition of the artificial cell-virus linker. J Gen Virol 1992; 73(Pt 12):3251–3255.

157. Etienne-Julan M, et al. Cell targeting by murine recombinant retroviruses. Bone Marrow Trans 1992;9:139–142.
158. Roux P, Jeanteur P, Piechaczyk M. A versatile and potentially general approach to the targeting of specific cell types by retroviruses: application to the infection of human cells by means of major histocompatibility complex class I and class II antigens by mouse ecotropic murine leukemia virus-derived viruses. Proc Natl Acad Sci U S A 1989;86(23):9079–9083.
159. Han X, Kasahara N, Kan YW. Ligand-directed retroviral targeting of human breast cancer cells. Proc Natl Acad Sci U S A 1995;92(21):9747–9751.
160. Kasahara N. Tissue-Specific Targeting of Retroviral Vectors Through Ligand-Receptor Interactions. Science 1994;266:1373–1376.
161. Nguyen TH, et al. Amphotropic retroviral vectors displaying hepatocyte growth factor- envelope fusion proteins improve transduction efficiency of primary hepatocytes. Hum Gene Ther 1998;9(17):2469–2479.
162. Cosset F-L. Retroviral Retargeting by Envelopes Expressing an N-Terminal Binding Domain. J Virol 1995;69(10):6314–6322.
163. Chu TH, Dornburg R. Retroviral vector particles displaying the antigen-binding site of an antibody enable cell-type-specific gene transfer. J Virol 1995;69(4):2659–2663.
164. Somia NV, Zoppe M, Verma IM. Generation of targeted retroviral vectors by using single-chain variable fragment: an approach to in vivo gene delivery. Proc Natl Acad Sci U S A 1995;92(16):7570–7574.
165. Russell SJ. Retroviral vectors displaying functional antibody fragments. Nucl Acids Res1993;21(5): 1081–1085.
166. Marin M. Targeted Infection of Human Cells via Major Histocompatibility Complex Class I Molecules by Moloney Murine Leukemia Virus-Derived Viruses Displaying Single-Chain Antibody Fragment-Envelope Fusion Proteins. J Virol 1996;70(5):2957–2962.
167. Ager S, et al. Retroviral display of antibody fragments: interdomain spacing strongly influences vector infectivity. Hum Gene Ther 1996;7(17):2157–2164.
168. Konishi H. Targeting Strategy for Gene Delivery to Carcinoembryonic Antigen-Producing Cancer Cells by Retrovirus Displaying a Sigle-Chain Fragment Antibody. Hum Gene Ther 1998;9:235–248.
169. Jiang A, et al. Cell-type-specific gene transfer into human cells with retroviral vectors that display single-chain antibodies. J Virol 1998;72(12):10,148–10,156.
170. Valsesia-Wittmann S, et al. Improvement of retroviral retargeting by using amino acid spacers between an additional binding domain and the N terminus of Moloney murine leukemia virus SU. J Virol 1996;70(3):2059–2064.
171. Chandrashekran A, Gordon MY, Casimir C. Targeted retroviral transduction of c-kit+ hematopoietic cells using novel ligand display technology. Blood 2004;104(9):2697–2703 Epub 2004 Jul 15.
172. Bupp K, Roth MJ. Altering retroviral tropism using a random-display envelope library. Mol Ther 2002;5(3):329–335.
173. Roth J, Gerson S. Screening mutant ecotropic MuLV envelope libraries for altered host range. Mol Ther 2002;5(5):S177.
174. Hacein-Bey-Abina S, et al. A serious adverse event after successful gene therapy for X-linked severe combined immunodeficiency. N Engl J Med 2003;348(3):255–256.
175. Woods NB, et al. Lentiviral vector transduction of NOD/SCID repopulating cells results in multiple vector integrations per transduced cell: risk of insertional mutagenesis. Blood 2003;101(4):1284–1289.
176. Laufs S, et al. Retroviral vector integration occurs in preferred genomic targets of human bone marrow-repopulating cells. Blood 2003;101(6):2191–2198.
177. Kustikova OS, et al. Dose finding with retroviral vectors: correlation of retroviral vector copy numbers in single cells with gene transfer efficiency in a cell population. Blood 2003;102(12):3934–3937 Epub 2003 Jul 24.

17 Nonviral Genetic Vaccines for Cancer

Steven R. Little, PhD, *Daniel G. Anderson,* PhD,
and Robert Langer, ScD

CONTENTS

Summary

Genetic vaccination has tremendous potential for the treatment and prevention of cancer. This chapter briefly discusses the advances in research aimed at increasing the effectiveness of genetic vaccine formulations. Particular emphasis is placed on in vivo nonviral delivery technologies and modifications to safely achieve optimal antigen expression. We will also discuss implications for the future of genetic vaccines.

Key Words: DNA vaccines; genetic vaccines; nonviral; cancer; delivery; electroporation; liposomes; microparticles; nanoparticles; adjuvants.

1. INTRODUCTION

In the early 1990s, it was demonstrated that the simple injection of plasmid DNA in saline into the muscle of mice led to the expression of the encoded gene *(1)*. Shortly thereafter it was shown that DNA vaccination could produce antibodies against an encoded antigen *(2)*, cytotoxic T-cell responses, and protection from lethal doses of influenza *(3,4)*. The elicitation of an immune response using plasmid DNA encoding an antigen, rather than the antigen itself was thereafter defined as genetic vaccination.

Genetic vaccination has tremendous therapeutic potential for the prevention and treatment of diseases, the screening of pathogenic genome libraries for the determination of protective antigens *(5)*, and the high-throughput generation of high specificity monoclonal antibodies *(6)*. The immunobiology of antigen presentation along with the potential mechanisms involved with the induction of immune response in genetic vaccines are beyond the scope of this chapter, and in depth examination of these mechanisms can be found in several excellent reviews *(7,8)*. Instead, this review will examine advances in non-viral delivery technologies for genetic vaccines.

From: *Cancer Drug Discovery and Development: Gene Therapy for Cancer*
Edited by: K. K. Hunt, S. A. Vorburger, and S. G. Swisher © Humana Press Inc., Totowa, NJ

2. GENETIC VACCINES FOR CANCER THERAPY

2.1. The Elusive Cancer Cell

The processes of malignancy, such as invasion and rapid growth of tumor cells, naturally cause inflammation. Dendritic cells (DCs), the most powerful antigen presenting cell (APC), should become activated to the presence of cancer cells and present sampled antigen in association with surface major histocompatibility complexes (MHC). The presentation of these tumor associated antigens (TAA), along with the appropriate costimulatory signals, leads to activation of antigen specific $CD8^+$ T-cells. These T-cells recognize and bind that TAA on the MHC class I of tumor cells. Subsequent secretion of perforin and granzymes can induce caspase-dependent apoptosis. However, in the many reported cases of human cancer, this process obviously does not seem to occur efficiently enough to destroy the tumor cells.

Cancer cells may evade recognition by the immune system through several mechanisms *(9)*: (1) down-regulation of antigen processing and presentation, (2) loss of some TAA which may alert the immune system, and (3) secretion of soluble signals which can modify the ability of DCs to effectively present antigens to naïve T-cells. Examples of such secreted factors include interleukin (IL)-10, which inhibits DC maturation, and transforming growth factor (TGF)-β, which is secreted by cells in the eye to prohibit destructive inflammation *(9,10)*. Although it is unclear to what extent these mechanisms are involved in tumor persistence, it is clear that tumor cells have developed ways to avoid immune rejection.

2.2. Genetic Vaccines for Cancer Therapy

A primary focus of current research on genetic vaccination is the development of strategies to activate nonresponsive antigen specific T-cells. The first consideration of any tumor therapy is the choice of cancer antigen in a genetic construct. Much effort has been devoted to the optimization of TAAs, and this work is described in detail elsewhere *(11,12)*. Despite this optimization and the large number of genetic vaccine clinical trials for cancer[a], DNA vaccination in humans has not elicited as potent immune responses as observed in smaller animal models. For example, eliciting an immune response with intramuscular (im) naked DNA vaccination (plasmid DNA with no delivery vehicle) requires as much as 5mg of plasmid DNA in nonhuman primates *(13)*, but only 50 to 300 μg in mice *(4)*. Although high doses of plasmid are generally well tolerated in humans *(14)*, the need for additional technologies to boost the effectiveness of genetic vaccines is apparent.

One of the earliest advances in DNA delivery was the gene gun. This device delivers DNA coated onto the surface of tiny gold beads which are then accelerated to a high speed into the skin by a high pressure helium source *(15)*. Immune responses elicited by vaccination using gene gun delivery to the skin requires much less plasmid DNA, on the order of several hundred to several thousand times less than naked DNA *(4,16)*. This may partially result from the large amount of dendritic cells present in the skin, called Langerhan's cells *(17)*. However, immune responses to gene gun vaccines are usually Th2 polarized, and there are questions as to the viability of this technology commercially.

Viral vectors are inherently efficient at gene delivery and are powerfully immunogenic. However, the potential toxicity of viral vectors is well known, and is particularly relevant

[a]There are currently 114 clinical trials worldwide for the treatment of cancer, representing 89% of all genetic vaccine clinical trials. (Journal of Gene Medicine trial online database.)

in patients with compromised immunity resulting from the progression of cancer and chemotherapy. Furthermore, the common requirement of multiple vaccinations can be problematic using viral vectors. Recently, it was shown that restimulation with adenovirally transduced DCs actually decreased the antigen-specific immune response in favor of strong antiadenovirus specific immune reactions in melanoma patients *(18)*. Pre-existing immunity can also inhibit delivery using viral vectors. Attenuated bacteria has also shown promise for vaccine delivery, but are associated with safety concerns as well *(19)*.

Synthetic nonviral delivery of plasmid DNA vaccines, although potentially safer, has proven much less effective at eliciting strong immune responses. However, recent advances have significantly increased their efficacy and therapeutic potential. It is these current advances which this chapter focuses on.

3. METHODS OF DNA VACCINE DELIVERY

3.1. Electroporation

Elecroporation is a common in vitro transfection method. Through the application of electric pulses, the cellular membrane is temporarily disrupted. This, combined with physical translocation of ionic plasmid DNA (ionophoresis), can result in efficient gene transfection. In vivo, the application of electroporation involves the use of probes or clamp electrodes to the site of plasmid administration. This method has been shown to induce long-term expression of reporter gene in vivo. Adapting the process parameters from low voltage, long pulses to high voltage, short pulses resulted in a 500× increase in expression in muscle *(20)*.

Studies on the delivery of TAA antigens using electroporation have yielded promising results. Mendiratta et al. reported vaccination using electroporation with both plasmid encoded human GP100 and mouse TPR2 antigen elicited complete protection from melanoma challenge *(21)*. Lohr et al. demonstrated that introduction of plasmid encoding IL-2 and IL-12 (inflammatory cytokine signals) by electroporation at tumor sites caused transduction and inhibition of murine melanoma without the systemic cytokine levels experienced after adenoviral gene transfer *(22)*. Further investigations have shown that electroporation can be used to facilitate the discovery of novel antigen encoded plasmid constructs. For example, Kalat et al. used electroporation methods to optimize tyrosinase related protein-2 antigens to elicit $CD8^+$ responses and inhibition of melanoma growth in two challenge models *(23)*. This same group later demonstrated that electroporation was capable of inducing immune responses comparable to that of viral infection *(24)*.

It has been suggested that increase in gene transfection is responsible for the amplification of immune responses observed, but it is also possible that tissue damage which occurs at the immunization site may recruit APCs, effectively increasing immunogenicity *(25)*. Unfortunately, electroporation can be destructive to tissues, and some have reported pain in patients during clinical trials *(26)*.

3.2. Cationic Liposomes/Lipoplexes

Cationic lipids (*see* Fig. 1) are one of the most widely used transfection reagents in vitro and in vivo. Through the formation of lipid bi-layers, and association with anionically charged DNA, cationic liposomes can spontaneously condense DNA by charge neutralization. These particles are commonly called lipoplexes. These formulations can

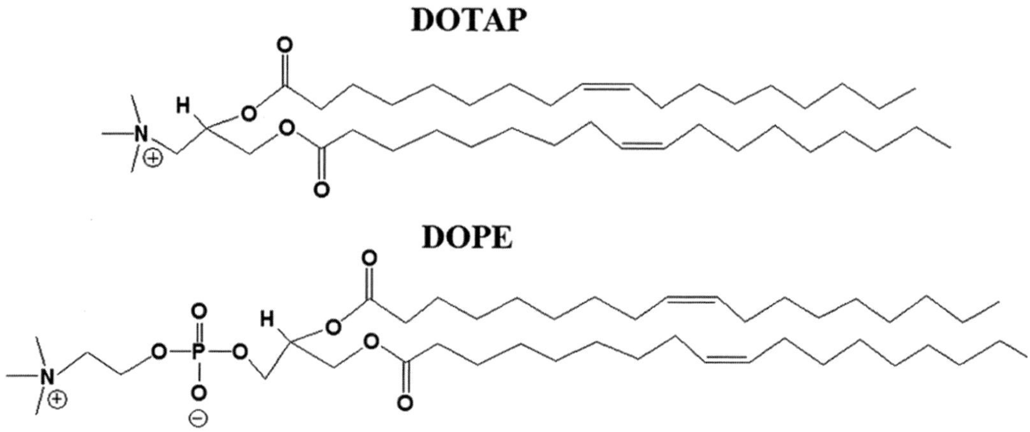

Fig. 1. Chemical structures of DOTAP and DOPE, two commonly used lipids in liposomal formulations.

include neutral components such as DOPE or cholesterol that can introduce endosomal disruption properties *(27)*. It was originally believed that fusion with cell membranes was the primary mechanism to gain cytoplasmic access. It is now widely accepted that this process occurs through an endocytic or phagocytic event, and access to the cytoplasm is mediated through a destabilization of the endosomal membrane *(28)*.

Alternatively, it has been shown that plasmid DNA can be encapsulated within a lipid vesicle called a dehydrated-rehydrated vesicle (DRV) *(29)*. DRVs are formed by freeze drying lipoplexes to increase the association of plasmid DNA with the flattened liposomal vesicles. Subsequent rehydration of these dried complexes results in the apparent entrapment of plasmid inside the lipid bilayer. Although early studies demonstrated that cationic liposomes seem to inhibit expression of plasmid DNA when delivered instrmuscularly, DRVs have shown the ability to generate improved cellular immunity and secretion of 100× greater IgG1 levels than that obtainable by cationic lipoplexes or naked DNA *(29)*. Various lipids can be included in these formulations to increased immune response *(30)* and enhance oral delivery of DRVs *(31)*. Finally, the incorporation of viral fusogenic peptides from hemaglutinating virus Japan (HVJ) or influenza into liposomes can enhance responses against tumor-associated antigens (Table 1).

Cationic lipid formulations are relatively easy to prepare, and protect the plasmid DNA from nucleases in the extracellular environment. However, the polycationic nature of the lipoplex/liposomal formulations impart a degree of cellular promiscuity in the transfection of cells, along with an inherent ability to bind to serum proteins. This can severely limit the stability and targetability of plasmid/lipid formulations. Creating targeted liposome vectors with improved serum stability could significantly enhance the potency of liposomal delivery vectors.

3.3. Polymeric Microparticles and Nanoparticles

The delivery of DNA vaccines through polymeric plasmid encapsulation or electrostatic binding has proven to be an extremely promising method of genetic vaccine delivery. First, these particles offer substantial protection of payload from extracellular degradation *(32)*. Second, these formulations are generally able to carry large payloads, making codelivery of many plasmids, or other immunostimulatory agents possible. Third, these particles, depending on their size, offer a passive targeting mechanism, since

Table 1
Examples of Cancer Models Using Liposomal Delivery of DNA Vaccines

TAA	*Liposome type*	*Delivery route*	*Ab*	*CTL*	*Protection*	*Ref.*
MAGE 1 & 3	HVJ fusogenic	im	+	ND	ND	*(135)*
gp100 melanoma	HVJ fusogenic	im	+	+	+	*(136)*
Hsp65 (for mesothelioma)	Cationic lipoplex	ip	ND	+	*90% (AC29) [a]40% (AB12)	*(137)*
gp100 + TRP2 melanoma	HVJ fusogenic	im[b], in	+Th1	+Th2	+	*(138)*
PTH-rP Prostate carcinoma	Influenza fusogenic	in	ND	+	ND	*(139,140)*

Notes: + = positive response, ND= experiment not performed.
[a]% of long term survivors post-tumor challenge (approx 150 d) AB12 more aggressive than AB12.
[b]Im route demonstrated better CTL response than in.

phagocytic APCs are capable of phagocytosing microparticles in the range of 1 to 10 μm. Fourth, surface modifications are possible to further enhance targeting and uptake *(33)*. Finally, these particles have been shown to be associated with an adjuvant effect.

Several mechanisms have been proposed to explain the microparticulate adjuvant effect. First, it may result in part from their physical size being characteristic of pathogens *(34)*. Uptake of 1 μm latex microparticles by monocytes results in differentiation into DCs and migration to the lymph nodes *(35)*. DC phagocytosis of latex beads also induces phenotypic maturation of the DCs, as shown by CD83 up-regulation *(36)*. Alternatively, the delivery system's ability to serve as a controlled release depot of antigen or plasmid DNA (which contains immunostimulatory CpG motifs recognized by toll-like receptors on DCs *[37]*) may be responsible.

3.3.1. Plasmid Encapsulated in PLGA Microparticles

By far, the most commonly used polymer to encapsulate drugs including protein antigen and plasmid DNA is polylactic–coglycolic acid (PLGA) (*see* Fig. 2). This Food and Drug Administration (FDA) approved, biodegradable and biocompatible polymer was originally used for sutures *(38)*. It decomposes by acid and base hydrolysis (and possibly through enzyme catalyzed degradation *[39]*) to lactic and glycolic acid, which are metabolized to CO_2.

It has been used for numerous early applications ranging from delivery of narcotic agonists *(40)*, contraceptives *(41)*, pesticides *(42)*, and the healing of bone fractures *(43)* and ligaments *(44)*. Applications of PLGA for delivery of protein or peptide antigen in the context of vaccines have been frequent, and have been previously reviewed *(34,45)*.

There are several ways to encapsulate plasmid in PLGA microparticles (*see* Fig. 3, *left*), but the most commonly used is the double emulsion, solvent evaporation technique (reviewed in *[47]*). Spray drying is used less frequently for encapsulation of DNA *(47)*, but in either system, the aqueous plasmid solution is first emulsified with an organic solvent containing PLGA. Release of plasmid from PLGA microparticles tends to occur in burst phases as a result of the "bulk eroding" property of PLGA *(48,49)*. The release rate of plasmid is completely adjustable by choice of molecular weight and ratio of hydrophobic lactide to hydrophilic glycolide in the copolymer's repeating unit.

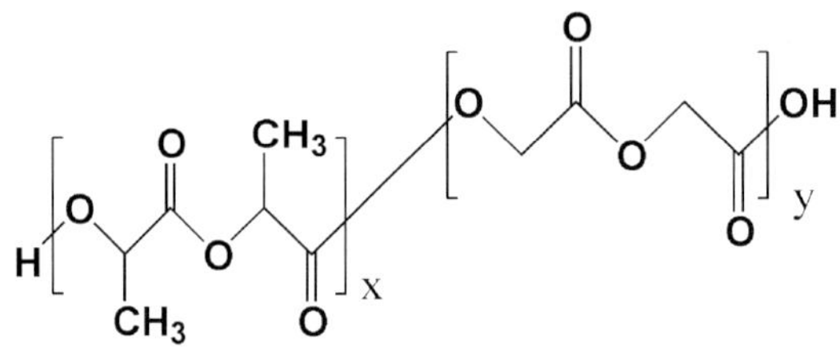

Fig. 2. Structure of PLGA. Ratio of lactide to glycolide is x:y.

Stronger CTL responses could be elicited by delivery of plasmid encoding VSV antigen in PLGA microparticles subcutaneous and intraperitoneal (ip) when compared with naked DNA vaccinations *(50)*. Phase 1 clinical trials using this delivery system for treatment of anal dysplasia showed 83% of patients demonstrated immune response to the antigen encoded in plasmid (HPV-16 E7) and continued to demonstrate a response 6 mo later *(51)*. Furthermore, a phase 1 clinical trial for cervical intraepithelial neoplasia demonstrated no adverse side effects, with 73% of patients exhibiting with specific immune responses along with 33% of patients exhibiting complete histologic responses *(52)*. In addition, Chen et al. demonstrated that oral immunization with plasmid DNA could elicit protective immunity using a rotavirus challenge model when encapsulated into PLGA microparticles *(53)*.

Although these studies show the potential of PLGA for genetic vaccine delivery, acidic degradation products can build up internally in the microparticle structure. The low pH environment has been shown to stabilize some drugs *(54)*, but it can seriously damage the integrity of supercoiled plasmid. Plasmid released from the initial burst phase remains relatively intact, but it was demonstrated plasmid released at a later time was transcriptionally inactive *(49)*. Further analysis has revealed that particles undergo a drop in pH to less than 3.5 after only 3 d of incubation in saline *(55)*.

Addition of agents to increase immunogenicity of PLGA microparticles, such as lypophilic additives (taurocholic acid [TA] and polyethylene glycol-distearoylphosphatidylethanolamine [PEG-DSPE]) substantially increases antibody response and CTL induction. More importantly for this review, these formulations were able to demonstrate protective immune responses against intravenous (iv) tumor challenge as measured by the number of pulmonary metastases *(56)*. The mechanism behind the immunogenicity of the lipophilic additive used in these formulations is unknown, but it may have been involved in membrane disruption, or protecting the plasmid DNA from the acidic microclimate of PLGA microparticles.

The microparticle formulation process itself can cause substantial damage to encapsulated material through sheer stress associated with sonication and homogenization, organic/aqueous interfaces which can denature proteins, and freeze drying. Ando et al. demonstrated a "cryo" technique for fabrication of plasmid microparticles which virtually eliminated these effects by freezing the internal aqueous phase, thereby eliminating sheer stress *(57)*. Also stabilization agents, such as sugars can be added to the plasmid to eliminate most degradation observed in freeze drying.

3.3.2. Cationic Microparticles and Nanoparticles

To completely avoid processing of plasmid DNA during the encapsulation process, Singh et al. devised a method to fabricate cationic microparticles that could be used to bind polyanionic plasmid DNA. Addition of the cationic surfactant cetyltrimethylammonium bromide (CTAB) (*see* Fig. 4) produced a positively charged surface in

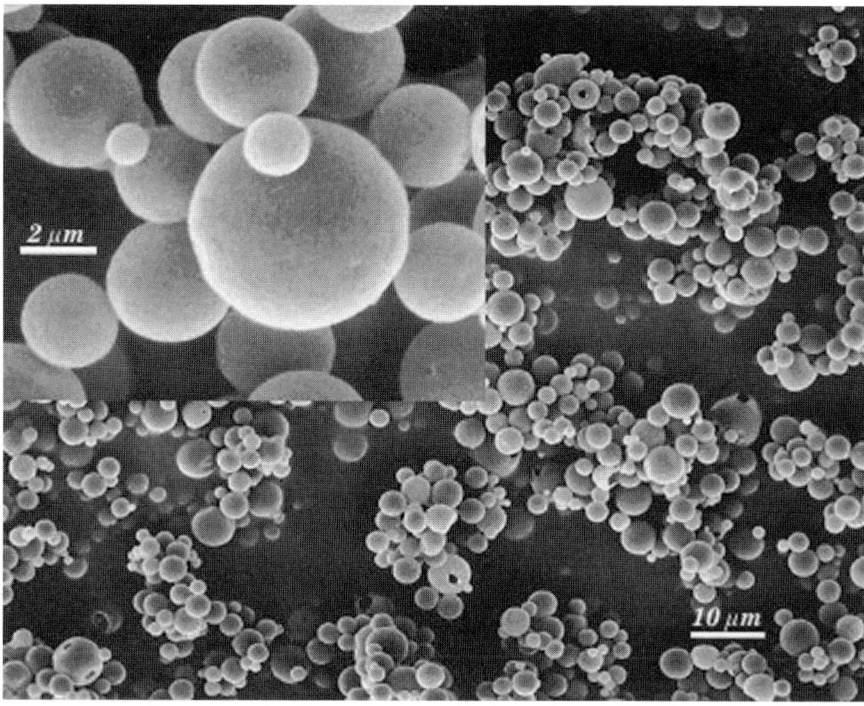

Fig. 3. PLGA microparticles prepared by the double emulsion/solvent evaporation technique. Body is ×1000 and inset is ×5000 magnification.

contrast to conventional negatively charged particles from the use of surfactants such as polyvinyl alcohol (PVA). Through an unknown mechanism (which may involve direct uptake of plasmid coated microparticles by DCs or disruption of the phagosomal membrane by CTAB) these cationic microparticles were capable of eliciting humoral responses 250× greater than naked DNA and substantially higher CTL response in a HIV p55 gag model using a relatively small dose of DNA (1 μg intramuscular) *(58)*. More recently, these microparticles have been shown to transfect primary DCs, albeit to a low extent *(59)*, and these particles could be found in draining lymph nodes 3 h after intramuscular injection *(60)*. O'Hagan et al. demonstrated use of these particles for delivery of a polyvalent p55 gag/gp120/gp140 env genetic vaccine *(61)*. Although naked DNA worked best in this study at the higher dosages, the effect was almost completely diminished upon injection of lower doses DNA. Conversely, the particles with surface adsorbed plasmid maintained high levels of Ab and CTL response with 1000× less plasmid DNA *(61)*.

Application of this efficient genetic vaccine delivery system to a TAA was first directed toward carcinoembryonic antigen (CEA) by Luo et al. *(62)*.Vaccination with this formulation inhibited the growth of injected colon adenocarcinoma expressing the CEA antigen in a population of vaccinated mice *(62)*. Addition of boosting regimens with naked DNA im encoding granulocyte-macrophage colony-stimulating factor (GM-CSF) (as will be discussed later in this review), resulted in an increased number of responders and further inhibition of growth in the non responding mice *(62)*.

One extremely simple method for creating cationic nanoparticles using a hot cetyl alcohol-polysorbate 80 wax/aqueous emulsion formed by adding cationic surfactant was

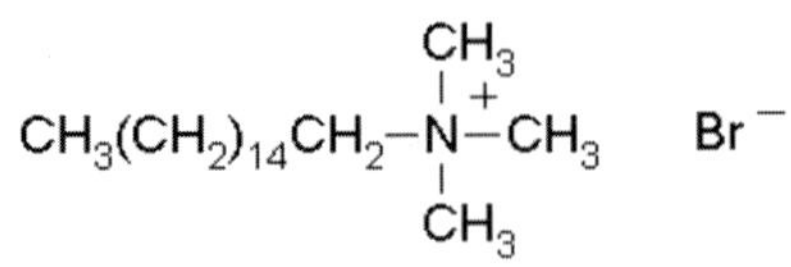

Fig. 4. The structure of the cationic surfactant, CTAB.

recently described *(63)*. Subsequent cooling produces cationic microparticles approximately 100 nm in diameter. This method has several advantages including simplicity, uniformity of size, cationic surfaces capable of binding plasmid DNA, and elimination of toxic organic solvents. These plasmid coated nanoparticles elicit immune induction by a variety of routes, all resulting in high antibody and Th1 cell mediated responses *(64–67)*.

3.3.3. DNA Encapsulated in pH Sensitive Polymer Microparticles

Recently, Wang et al. demonstrated the use of biodegradable and biocompatible, polyortho esters (POE) (*see* Fig. 5) for microparticulate genetic vaccines. Unlike bulk degradation of PLGA, POE degrades by erosion of the surface, allowing acidic byproducts to diffuse away rather than building up inside the polymer matrix. Particularly interesting is the ability of these polymers to degrade more rapidly at endosomal (acidic) pH than at physiologic pH. One of these polymers led to higher levels of secreted antibody and greater $CD8^+$ T-cell responses than PLGA microparticle delivery. In addition, mice vaccinated with the POE formulations demonstrated inhibited growth of tumor cells expressing a class I restricted epitope. The difference in immunogenicity of the formulations was attributed to the ability of the microparticles to release plasmid in a time frame that corresponds to the induction of immune response by processing and presentation of peptide on the surface of activated DCs *(68)*.

We have recently demonstrated the use of a pH sensitive, degradable poly β- amino ester (PBAE) (*see* Fig. 6) along with low molecular weight PLGA in a hybrid microparticle DNA vaccine delivery system *(148,149)*. This PBAE has been previously described as capable of binding plasmid DNA and is amenable to microsphere fabrication *(69,70)*. It has a pH sensitive solubility in the range of phagosomal acidification, making it particularly suitable for delivery to DCs. Also, the tertiary amines in the PBAE acts as a weak base, which can partially neutralize the acidic microclimate of PLGA and possibly mediate phagosomal disruption through a proton-sponge mechanism *(71)*. Formulations resulting from the mixture of PBAE and PLGA have exhibited enhanced delivery of plasmid DNA for expression by APCs when compared with PLGA alone and have an interesting ability to mediate the strong costimulatory up-regulation of primary DCs in vitro. In a model weak antigen system, we demonstrated that mice vaccinated with these PBAE microparticle formulations were able to demonstrate antigen specific rejection of subcutaneous (sc) lethal tumor challenge *(148)*. Initial evidence suggests that the response observed was most likely a polyclonal $CD8^+$ response, but the possibility of $CD4^+$ T-cell help cannot be ruled out. The mechanism behind the particles' inherent ability to activate primary DCs is unknown and currently under investigation.

4. ENHANCING THE IMMUNOGENICITY OF GENETIC VACCINES

4.1. Adjuvants and Costimulation

Numerous attempts have been made to increase the potency of nonviral genetic vaccines through genetic modifications, targeting strategies, and boosting regimens, to

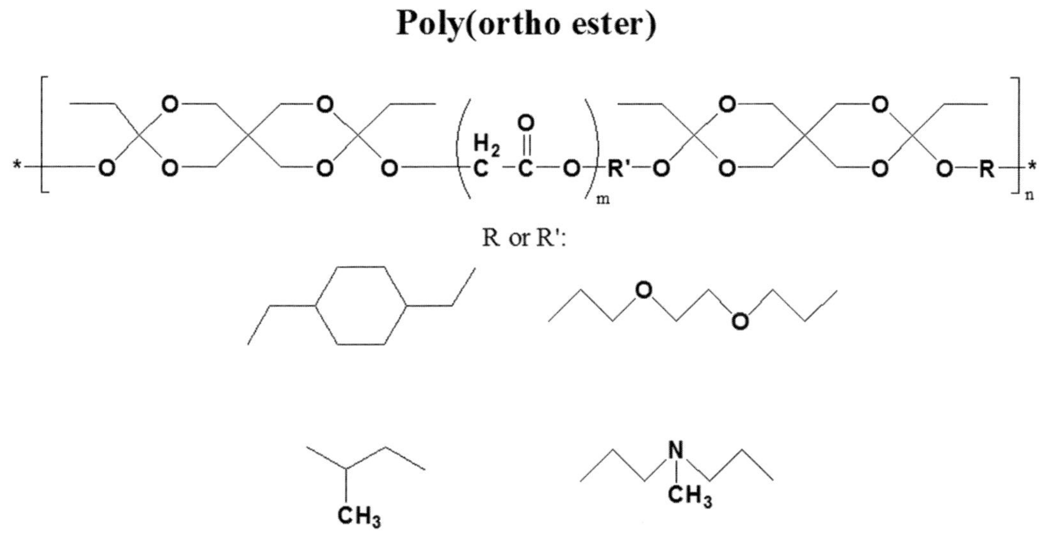

Fig. 5. The structure of the poly (ortho ester) used by Wang et al. *(147)*. R or R′ is shown below the polymer chain.

name just a few. Adjuvants are defined as anything added to a vaccine that increases the immune response in terms of magnitude, duration, or time of onset *(72)*. By this definition even micro-injury during inoculation with vaccine formulations *(73–75)* or the haplotype of an individual *(76)* can be conceivably called an adjuvant. As it relates to DCs, adjuvancy can be more tightly defined as anything that induces progression toward an optimal level of signal 1 (antigen presentation enhancements such as in delivery systems) and signal 2 (such as costimulatory molecule and cytokine up-regulations by using "immunostimulatory adjuvants"). Enhancing the presentation to signal 1 seems fairly straightforward by increasing expression of the antigen in the proper cell type. However, methods for enhancing the optimal presentation of signal 2 remain unclear, in part because of the complex dialogue between lymphocytes.

It is clear, however, that signal 2 requires the up-regulation of costimulatory molecules and the secretion of Th1 and Th2 cytokines. What causes this reaction to a stimulus is not fully understood. One theory states that the immune system is finely tuned to react to "danger signals" *(77)*. These signals distinguish between when to mount an attack, in the case of an invading pathogen, and when to suppress immune rejection, in the case of regularly surveyed "self/nondangerous" antigens. The current dogma is that the immune system induces tolerance to some antigens in certain circumstances (e.g., without signal 2 or in the presence of some other signal), and that tumor cells may have the ability to down-regulate this signal *(9)*. Attempts to modulate the immunostimulatory properties of genetic vaccines have resulted in incremental increases in vaccine potency and understanding of the immune system.

4.2. Traditional and Genetic "Adjuvants"

Perhaps the most straightforward way to facilitate T-cell stimulation during DNA vaccination is to deliver genes encoding for the known costimulatory and secreted cytokine signals. The numerous types and variations of these signals are too many to discuss here, but are reviewed thoroughly elsewhere *(78)*. Examples of secreted

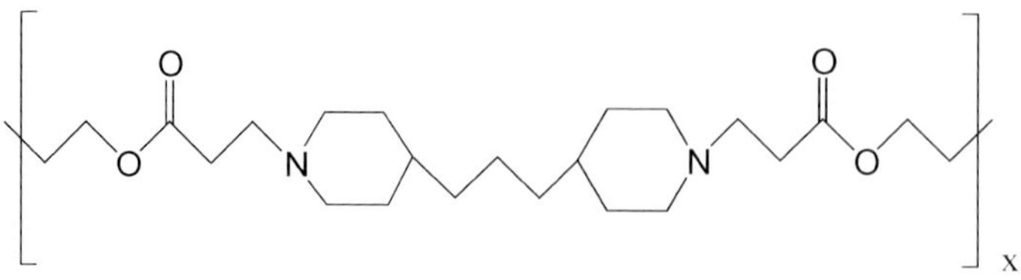

Fig. 6. The structure of the PBAE used in hybrid microparticles described above.

cytokines signals are the Th1 cytokines such as IL-2, and IL-12, Th2 cytokines such as IL-4 and IL-10, and the seemingly nonpolarized GM-CSF, the most commonly used genetic adjuvant. The timing and administration with respect to antigen plasmid administration can significantly affect the outcome of a genetic cytokine vaccination. Also, combinations of two or more of these cytokine signals can have a more pronounced effect than either of the two alone. There are indications that modifications can be made to certain known immunostimulatory cytokines which can alter their systemic toxicity profile while still retaining their antitumor effects *(79)*. Genes encoding for the T-cell activating costimulatory molecules such as B7.1 and B7.2 are promising candidates for increasing potency, but results have been conflicting *(78,80)*.

Some fusion partners have an inherent immunogenicity to which they can impart upon an antigen. Examples of this are tetanus toxoid *(81)*, plant viral proteins *(82)*, and HSP70 *(83)*. Addition of these fusion constructs is associated with large increases in potency. Mechanisms of this increased immunogenicity are thought to involve induction of helper T-cell responses through processing of the fusion proteins by the MHC class II pathway.

A range of traditional adjuvants have also been explored by coadministration with the genetic vaccine formulation. As previously discussed, the delivery systems themselves can have adjuvant properties. Even the gold beads used in gene gun immunization have adjuvant properties. A recent study has shown gold beads in tandem with in vivo electroporation led to an increase in observed immune responses *(84)*. Importantly, this did not enhance gene expression, but may have acted as a recruiting factor for DCs *(84)*. Other examples include alum (aluminum salts) and Freund's oil-in-water adjuvant (a powerful, yet toxic adjuvant containing mycobacterial materials). It is doubtful that the latter will ever be used in humans despite the fact that modifications have been made to decrease toxicity of this system. A cationic emulsion, called MF59, has been used to adsorb and increase the persistence of plasmid DNA encoding HIV p55 gag at the injection site, which resulted in increased serum IgG titers when compared with naked plasmid in mice and rabbits *(85)*.

4.3. Targeting Genetic Vaccines

There are three primary ways to target an antigen to a particular cell or organ: (1) targeting the delivery system for uptake by a specific cell, (2) linking the antigen to a targeting ligand, or (3) using DNA that is transcriptionally regulated to only become active in the target cell. For a specific cell type, modifications can be made to the antigen to direct it to different pathways of antigen processing and presentation.

4.3.1. Targeting Uptake

There are a variety of surface receptors that are potential targets for APC specific DNA or post-transcriptional antigen delivery. Fc receptors are thought to bind immune complexes and facilitate the opsonization of particulates. This binding activates DCs by up-regulation of costimulatory molecules *(86)*. CTLA-4 is another ligand that has been used to target DCs, and is thought to bind B7.1/B7.2 at a high affinity. Some chemokines act through binding to DC cell surface receptors and can be employed as well. Certain proteins such as CD36 and αβ5 integrins are involved with receptor mediated phagocytosis *(87)* and others such as DEC205 (or the human homolog LY75) and DC-SIGN, which are DC markers mediate receptor mediated endocytosis *(88)*. All of these are potential targets for use in directing DNA or antigen specifically to APCs (Table 2). A good example is the addition of mannose or mannan to a delivery system to target the mannose receptor on the DC surface. Targeting this receptor has led to 2-fold increase in phagocytosis of particle formulations by APC in vitro *(89)* and has also been used to increase transfection of cultured DCs *(90)*. The addition of mannan to the surface has also been associated with an increase in antibody and cell mediated immune responses in vivo *(65)*.

4.3.2. Intracellular Targeting

Targeting of antigen to different cellular compartments may influence the way that antigen is processed and presented. Conceivably, an antigen normally processed by the MHC class II pathway that is instead presented on the MHC class I pathway could lead to immune responses that primarily elicit CTL activity instead of antibody secretion (isotype switching), and possibly a more relevant therapy for cancer.

One of the most common cellular localization sequences used for targeting an antigen fusion partner to the MHC class I pathway is ubiquitin. Ubiquitin marks proteins for degradation by the proteosome into small peptides which are then transported to the endoplasmic reticulum for loading onto MHC class I molecules. Addition of ubiquitin to plasmid fusion constructs usually increases CTL responses at the cost of humoral responses *(91–95)*. However, in one study, a ubiquitin fusion construct demonstrated a decrease in humoral response whereas CTL response remained unchanged *(96)*. Further examination of ubiquitin fusion constructs will be required for generalization of this strategy. Calreticulin (CRT) is a particularly interesting candidate for cancer vaccines because it has both MHC class I targeting capacity and antiangiogenesis properties (the ability to inhibit blood vessel growth to the site of a tumor) *(97–100)*. Addition of CRT to fusion constructs has shown to exhibit notable antitumor activity when given as a DNA vaccine for HPV-16 E7 antigen. It is believed that the antiangiogenesis properties of CRT are involved in this observed response *(101)*.

Targeting the MHC class II pathway may also be a logical strategy if a humoral response is desired. This pathway can be targeted through fusion with lysosomal associated proteins such as LAMP-1 *(102–104)* or LIMP II *(91)*. An antigen can also be targeted to the cell surface *(105)*. Another apparent mechanism for increasing MHC class II processing is targeting antigen for secretion. This antigen could then be taken up by a DC and associated with class II molecules in the lysosome. Interestingly, both humoral and/or cell mediated immunity are increased by using this strategy *(106,107)*. This phenomenon may involve a cross-priming mechanism to allow antigen to enter the cytoplasm.

4.3.3. Transcriptional Targeting

One of the most commonly used mammalian promoters in genetic vaccines is the cytomegalovirus promoter (pCMV). This is an extremely strong viral promoter that is capable of mediating high levels of antigen expression in many cell types. However, some of the expression products in a genetic vaccine, such as the immunomodulating

Table 2
Some Examples of the Genetic Vaccine Targeting Strategies[a]

Ligand	*Target*	*Ref.*
IgG F_C Fragment	DC F_C receptor	*(141)*
CTLA-4	DC B7.1 & B7.2	*(142–144)*
L-selectin	Endothelial CD34 (lymph node)	*(142,143)*
RANTES chemokine	DC chemokine receptor	*(145)*
IP-10 chemokine	DC chemokine receptor	*(146)*
MCP-3 chemokine	DC chemokine receptor	*(146)*
Mannose/Mannan	DC MR	*(65,90)*
DEC205 mAb	DC receptor mediated endocytosis	*(150)*
CD36/αβ5 integrin Ligands	DC receptor mediated phagocytosis	ND

[a]ND=These targets, to our knowledge, have not been investigated in genetic vaccine formulations.

cytokines discussed earlier, may generate toxicity if expression is not controlled. Also, persisting expression of low levels of antigen after vaccination may induce tolerance to the expressed antigen *(108)*. Alternatively, one strategy is to use transient promoters capable of transfecting a targeted subset of cells, such as DCs. One such DC specific promoter is the lectin promoter, which was used with GFP plasmid to demonstrate transfection of DCs in vivo and anti-green fluorescent protein (GFP) CTL response *(109)*. Another example is the mature DC specific fascin promoter, which demonstrated a distinct Th1 response as compared with Th2 responses observed when using pCMV *(110,111)*. The isotype switching of responses by transcriptional targeting may prove to be a powerful method to alter the way the immune system reacts to an antigen.

4.4. Increasing Gene Expression

DCs have proven to be a notoriously difficult cell to transfect *(59,90,112–115)*. Increasing transfection of these cells seems to be a logical way to increase vaccine potency. Although some evidence suggests that greater antigen expression does not always lead to greater immune responses *(116)*, others have shown that increasing the magnitude and duration of antigen expression is a viable way to increase the immunogenicity of genetic vaccines. Some examples of these strategies are: (1) optimization of the plasmid construct, (2) avoiding degradation in the lysosomes, (3) increased DC lifespan, and (4) self-replicating antigen constructs.

4.4.1. Plasmid Modifications

One of the most straightforward ways to increase gene expression is through the addition of multiple gene expression cassettes in the same plasmid vector. Sasaki et al. used these dual-antigen expression vectors to generate significantly higher expression than that obtained by using 2× the amount of single expression vector cassettes. Vaccinations with these plasmids correspondingly led to increased IL-4 and IFN-γ secretion by isolated splenocytes *(117)*. Haas et al. demonstrated that optimizing codon usage, which can be significantly different in mammals relative to bacteria, led to increases in antibody and CTL responses in mice using a HIV gp120 antigen construct *(118)*. Another example is codon optimized plasmid encoding for a MHC class I restricted listeria antigen, which showed increases in CTL responses and partial protection from listerial challenge while unoptimized plasmid remained ineffective *(119)*.

4.4.2. Avoiding Lysosomal Degradation of Plasmid

Other attempts to increase gene expression are aimed at avoiding lysosomal degradation of the plasmid DNA. Trehalose 6,6′-dimycolate (TDM) has been shown to cause inhibition of fusion between the lysosome and phagosome *(120)* and this inhibition may allow more time for the transfer of DNA from phagosomal compartments to cytoplasm of APCs before lysosomal degradation. Inclusion of TDM in PLGA microparticle vaccine formulations induces stronger resistance to mycobacterium tuberculosis in mice *(121)*. Other strategies attempt to avoid the lysosomal pathway altogether by adding mechanisms for traversing the plasma membrane *(122)*. Using a plasmid encoding either the protein transduction domains for HSV-1 (VP-22) *(123)*, or *Pseudomonas aeruginosa* exotoxin A (ETA(dII)) *(124)*, fused with HPV type 16 E7 antigen, Hung et al. observed a 50× increase in the amount of responding $CD8^+$ T-cells along with the increased ability of vaccinated mice to react to E7 expressing tumors.

4.4.3. Dendritic Cell Life Span

Increasing the lifetime of an antigen expressing DCs in vivo is yet another strategy to increase the immune presentation. Kim et al. investigated the effect of including a plasmid encoding antiapoptotic proteins such as Bcl-x_L *(125)* and serine protease inhibitor 6 (SPI-6) *(126)* to antigen fusion constructs with MHC class II targeting signals. These antiapoptotic proteins increased avidity of T-cells and elicited stronger tumor protection. Interestingly, covaccination with genes such as Fas *(127)* and caspases 2 or 3 *(128)* (apoptotic proteins) can also increase the potency of genetic vaccine formulations. While the exact mechanism of immune stimulation is unclear, it is possible that cross presentation of antigen from the apoptotic cells to a DCs may serve as an appropriate "danger" signal.

4.4.4. Replicons

Self-replicating RNA antigen constructs, or replicons, are based on alpha viruses such as the Venezuelan equine encephalitis virus, Sindbis Virus, and Semliki Forest Virus. Plasmid replicons contain the information for the transcription of a positive strand of RNA, which in turn encodes for both a 5′ replicase complex, and a negative strand of antigen encoding RNA (*see* Fig. 7). These vectors do not produce viral structural proteins, leaving no possibility for recombinant events. This is accomplished by replacing the viral gene for the structural proteins with a heterologous gene. Replicons have also been called "suicide vectors" because the presence of large quantities of dsRNA is thought to induce apoptosis shortly after transfection. Because of the infection process occurring in the cytoplasm, there is little possibility of chromosomal integration.

It should be noted that by using a defective helper gene encoding structural proteins, an infection competent, but replication incompetent, viral particle can be produced. These particles can target DCs *(129,130)* and have higher gene transfection efficiency than replicon plasmids alone. However, there is a small probability that recombination events could occur, leading to infectious particles. The reader is directed to a recent review on alphaviral vectors for more detail on this topic *(131)*.

Replicons have proven to be powerful enhancements to DNA vaccination, and are capable of eliciting antibody and tumor protective responses at up to 1000 times lower titers than conventional naked DNA vaccines in a β-gal expressing tumor model *(132)*. Vaccination with replicons has also induced protective immunity to melanoma challenge in a TRP-1 expression system, unlike conventional DNA vaccines *(133)*. Although it is

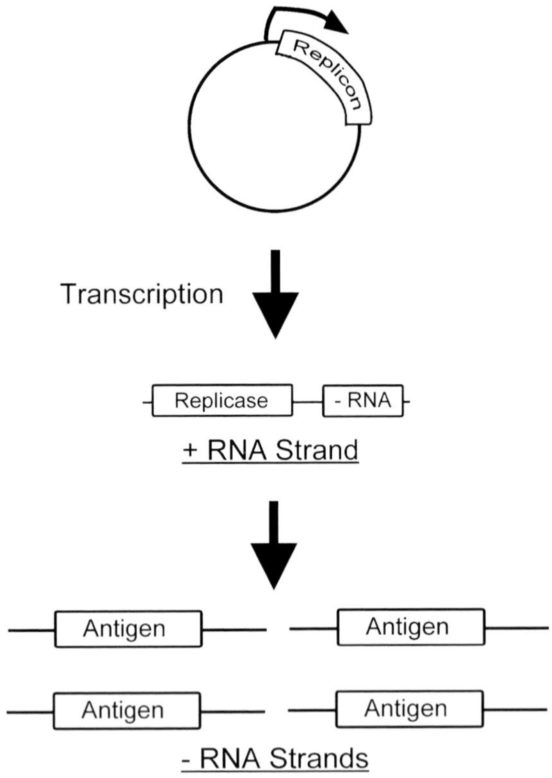

Fig. 7. Self-replicating plasmid replicons.

logical to infer that increased antigen expression is the reason for this enhancement, it is widely accepted that is rather results from the presence of dsRNA. The formation of dsRNA can activate antiviral apoptosis pathways, which subsequently lead to cross-priming of antigen in the presence of a danger signal *(133)*.

5. TOMORROW'S GENETIC VACCINES

The efficiency of nonviral gene delivery is still far below that of viral vectors. However, research in the field has come a long way toward identifying key mechanisms responsible for optimizing immune response. For example, the use of protein transduction domains and alphaviral replicons has allowed fundamental viral mechanisms to be incorporated into completely synthetic delivery systems. There is no reason to doubt that further understanding of viral gene delivery mechanisms will inspire synthetic versions of these functionalities which will serve the same purpose, and someday allow for completely synthetic, yet fully potent, gene delivery with minimal safety concerns.

This "ideal" genetic vaccine formulation has already been described as having the following properties: (1) low dose/frequency, (2) low cost, (3) effective immune response, (4) high reproducibility, (5) pharmaceutical acceptability, and (6) a high safety profile *(134)*. However, "effective immune response," by definition, requires a strong elicitation of the immune system, a process which is currently believed to be intimately tied to "danger signals" *(77)*. It is reasonable then to question whether effective genetic vaccines will have this "high safety profile" until our limited understanding of adjuvancy is substantially increased. One indication of this challenge is apparent in FDA clinical trials for conventional adjuvants. With approx 80 yr having passed since the first usage of alum in humans, there are still no additional FDA approved adjuvants. This could be the result of crude "adjuvancy" and low toxicity being mutually exclusive traits. In the short term, mastering the intricate balance between these two properties is the key to the first FDA approved genetic vaccine formulation. Until we are able to reconcile the apparent incompatibility between toxicity and immunogenicity, the most potent vaccines may be reserved only for extreme circumstances, such as terminally malignant cancer or severe pathogenic outbreaks.

REFERENCES

1. Wolff JA, Malone RW, Williams P, et al. Direct Gene-Transfer into Mouse Muscle In vivo. Science 1990;247:1465–1468.
2. Tang DC, De Vit M, Johnston SA. Genetic immunization is a simple method for eliciting an immune response. Nature 1992;356:152–154.
3. Ulmer JB, Donnelly JJ, Parker SE, et al. Heterologous protection against influenza by injection of DNA encoding a viral protein. Science 1993;259:1745–1749.
4. Fynan EF, Webster RG, Fuller DH, Haynes JR, Santoro JC, Robinson HL. DNA vaccines: protective immunizations by parenteral, mucosal, and gene-gun inoculations. Proc Natl Acad Sci U S A 1993; 90:11,478–11,482.
5. Johnston SA, Barry MA. Genetic to genomic vaccination. Vaccine 1997;15:808–809.
6. Chambers RS, Johnston SA. High-level generation of polyclonal antibodies by genetic immunization. Nat Biotechnol 2003;21:1088–1092.
7. Coombes BK, Mahony JB. Dendritic cell discoveries provide new insight into the cellular immunobiology of DNA vaccines. Immunol Lett 2001;78:103–111.
8. Banchereau J, Steinman RM. Dendritic cells and the control of immunity. Nature 1998;392:245–252.
9. Pardoll D. Does the immune system see tumors as foreign or self? Ann Rev Immunol 2003;21:807–839.
10. Marincola FM, Jaffee EM, Hicklin DJ, Ferrone S. Escape of human solid tumors from T-cell recognition: molecular mechanisms and functional significance. Adv Immunol 2000;74:181–273.
11. Houghton AN. Cancer antigens: immune recognition of self and altered self. J Exp Med 1994; 180:1–4.
12. Pardoll DM. Spinning molecular immunology into successful immunotherapy. Nat Rev Immunol 2002;2:227–238.
13. Barouch DH, Santra S, Schmitz JE, et al. Control of viremia and prevention of clinical AIDS in rhesus monkeys by cytokine-augmented DNA vaccination. Science 2000;290:486–492.
14. Le TP, Coonan KM, Hedstrom RC, et al. Safety, tolerability and humoral immune responses after intramuscular administration of a malaria DNA vaccine to healthy adult volunteers. Vaccine 2000; 18:1893–1901.
15. Williams RS, Johnston SA, Riedy M, DeVit MJ, McElligott SG, Sanford JC. Introduction of foreign genes into tissues of living mice by DNA-coated microprojectiles. Proc Natl Acad Sci U S A 1991; 88:2726–2730.
16. Pertmer TM, Eisenbraun MD, McCabe D, Prayaga SK, Fuller DH, Haynes JR. Gene gun-based nucleic acid immunization: elicitation of humoral and cytotoxic T lymphocyte responses following epidermal delivery of nanogram quantities of DNA. Vaccine 1995;13:1427–1430.
17. Bergstresser PR, Fletcher CR, Streilein JW. Surface densities of Langerhans cells in relation to rodent epidermal sites with special immunologic properties. J Invest Dermatol 1980;74:77–80.
18. Tuettenberg A, Jonuleit H, Tuting T, Bruck J, Knop J, Enk AH. Priming of T-cells with ad-transduced DC followed by expansion with peptide-pulsed DC significantly enhances the induction, of tumor-specific CD8(+) T-cells: implications for an efficient vaccination strategy. Gene Ther 2003; 10:243–250.
19. Dietrich G, Spreng S, Favre D, Viret JF, Guzman CA. Live attenuated bacteria as vectors to deliver plasmid DNA vaccines. Curr Opin Mol Ther 2003;5:10–19.
20. Vicat JM, Boisseau S, Jourdes P, et al. Muscle transfection by electroporation with high-voltage and short-pulse currents provides high-level and long-lasting gene expression. Hum Gene Ther 2000; 11:909–916.

21. Mendiratta SK, Thai G, Eslahi NK, et al. Therapeutic tumor immunity induced by polyimmunization with melanoma antigens gp100 and TRP-2. Cancer Res 2001;61:859–863.
22. Lohr F, Lo DY, Zaharoff DA, et al. Effective tumor therapy with plasmid-encoded cytokines combined with in vivo electroporation. Cancer Res 2001;61:3281–3284.
23. Kalat M, Kupcu Z, Schuller S, et al. In vivo plasmid electroporation induces tumor antigen-specific CD8+ T-cell responses and delays tumor growth in a syngeneic mouse melanoma model. Cancer Res 2002;62:5489–5494.
24. Paster W, Zehetner M, Kalat M, Schuller S, Schweighoffer T. In vivo plasmid DNA electroporation generates exceptionally high levels of epitope-specific CD8+ T-cell responses. Gene Ther 2003; 10:717–724.
25. Babiuk S, Baca-Estrada ME, Foldvari M, et al. Electroporation improves the efficacy of DNA vaccines in large animals. Vaccine 2002;20:3399–3408.
26. Rodriguez-Cuevas S, Barroso-Bravo S, Almanza-Estrada J, Cristobal-Martinez L, Gonzalez-Rodriguez E. Electrochemotherapy in primary and metastatic skin tumors: phase II trial using intralesional bleomycin. Arch Med Res 2001;32:273–276.
27. Zabner J. Cationic lipids used in gene transfer. Adv Drug Deliv Rev 1997;27:17–28.
28. Xu Y, Szoka FC, Jr. Mechanism of DNA release from cationic liposome/DNA complexes used in cell transfection. Biochemistry 1996;35:5616–5623.
29. Gregoriadis G, Saffie R, de Souza JB. Liposome-mediated DNA vaccination. FEBS Lett 1997; 402:107–110.
30. Perrie Y, Frederik PM, Gregoriadis G. Liposome-mediated DNA vaccination: the effect of vesicle composition. Vaccine 2001;19:3301–3310.
31. Perrie Y, Obrenovic M, McCarthy D, Gregoriadis G. Liposome (Lipodine (TM))-mediated DNA vaccination by the oral route. J Lipo Res 2002;12:185–197.
32. Jones DH, Corris S, McDonald S, Clegg JC, Farrar GH. Poly(DL-lactide-co-glycolide)-encapsulated plasmid DNA elicits systemic and mucosal antibody responses to encoded protein after oral administration. Vaccine 1997;15:814–817.
33. Kempf M, Mandal B, Jilek S, et al. Improved stimulation of human dendritic cells by receptor engagement with surface-modified microparticles. J Drug Target 2003;11:11–18.
34. O'Hagan DT, Singh M, Gupta RK. Poly(lactide-co-glycolide) microparticles for the development of single-dose controlled-release vaccines. Adv Drug Deliv Rev 1998;32:225–246.
35. Randolph GJ, Inaba K, Robbiani DF, Steinman RM, Muller WA. Differentiation of phagocytic monocytes into lymph node dendritic cells in vivo. Immunity 1999;11:753–761.
36. Thiele L, Rothen-Rutishauser B, Jilek S, Wunderli-Allenspach H, Merkle HP, Walter E. Evaluation of particle uptake in human blood monocyte-derived cells in vitro. Does phagocytosis activity of dendritic cells measure up with macrophages? J Control Release 2001;76:59–71.
37. Hemmi H, Takeuchi O, Kawai T, et al. A Toll-like receptor recognizes bacterial DNA. Nature 2000; 408:740–745.
38. Frazza EJ, Schmitt EE. A new absorbable suture. J Biomed Mater Res 1971;5:43–58.
39. Williams DF, Mort E. Enzyme-Accelerated Hydrolysis of Polyglycolic Acid. J Bioeng 1977; 1:231–238.
40. Woodland JH, Yolles S. Long-Acting Delivery Systems for Narcotic Antagonists. 1. J Med Chem 1973;16:897–901.
41. Beck LR, Cowsar DR, Lewis DH, Gibson JW, Flowers CE. New Long-Acting Injectable Microcapsule Contraceptive System. Am J Obstet Gynecol 1979;135:419–426.
42. Sinclair RG. Slow-Release Pesticide System - Polymers of Lactic and Glycolic Acids as Ecologically Beneficial, Cost-Effective Encapsulating Materials. Environ Sci Technol 1973;7:955–956.
43. Rokkanen P, Bostman O, Vainionpaa S, et al. Biodegradable implants in fracture fixation: early results of treatment of fractures of the ankle. Lancet 1985;1:1422–1424.
44. Bercovy M, Goutallier D, Voisin MC, et al. Carbon-PGLA prostheses for ligament reconstruction. Experimental basis and short-term results in man. Clin Orthop 1985:159–168.
45. Langer R, Cleland JL, Hanes J. New advances in microsphere-based single-dose vaccines. Adv Drug Deliv Rev 1997;28:97–119.
46. Odonnell PB, McGinity JW. Preparation of microspheres by the solvent evaporation technique. Adv Drug Deliv Rev 1997;28:25–42.
47. Gander B, Wehrli E, Alder R, Merkle HP. Quality improvement of spray-dried, protein-loaded D,L-PLA microspheres by appropriate polymer solvent selection. J Microencapsul 1995;12:83–97.

48. Wang D, Robinson DR, Kwon GS, Samuel J. Encapsulation of plasmid DNA in biodegradable poly(D, L-lactic-co-glycolic acid) microspheres as a novel approach for immunogene delivery. J Control Release 1999;57:9–18.
49. Walter E, Moelling K, Pavlovic J, Merkle HP. Microencapsulation of DNA using poly(DL-lactide-co-glycolide): stability issues and release characteristics. J Control Release 1999;61:361–374.
50. Hedley ML, Curley J, Urban R. Microspheres containing plasmid-encoded antigens elicit cytotoxic T-cell responses. Nat Med 1998;4:365–368.
51. Klencke B, Matijevic M, Urban RG, et al. Encapsulated plasmid DNA treatment for human papillomavirus 16-associated anal dysplasia: a Phase I study of ZYC101. Clin Cancer Res 2002;8:1028–1037.
52. Sheets EE, Urban RG, Crum CP, et al. Immunotherapy of human cervical high-grade cervical intraepithelial neoplasia with microparticle-delivered human papillomavirus 16 E7 plasmid DNA. Am J Obstet Gynecol 2003;188:916–926.
53. Chen SC, Jones DH, Fynan EF, et al. Protective immunity induced by oral immunization with a rotavirus DNA vaccine encapsulated in microparticles. J Virol 1998;72:5757–5761.
54. Shenderova A, Burke TG, Schwendeman SP. The acidic microclimate in poly(lactide-co-glycolide) microspheres stabilizes camptothecins. Pharm Res 1999;16:241–248.
55. Fu K, Pack DW, Klibanov AM, Langer R. Visual evidence of acidic environment within degrading poly(lactic-co-glycolic acid) (PLGA) microspheres. Pharm Res 2000;17:100–106.
56. McKeever U, Barman S, Hao T, et al. Protective immune responses elicited in mice by immunization with formulations of poly(lactide-co-glycolide) microparticles. Vaccine 2002;20:1524–1531.
57. Ando S, Putnam D, Pack DW, Langer R. PLGA microspheres containing plasmid DNA: Preservation of supercoiled DNA via cryopreparation and carbohydrate stabilization. J Pharm Sci 1999; 88:126–130.
58. Singh M, Briones M, Ott G, O'Hagan D. Cationic microparticles: A potent delivery system for DNA vaccines. Proc Natl Acad Sci U S A 2000;97:811–8116.
59. Denis-Mize KS, Dupuis M, MacKichan ML, et al. Plasmid DNA adsorbed onto cationic microparticles mediates target gene expression and antigen presentation by dendritic cells. Gene Ther 2000; 7:2105–2112.
60. Denis-Mize KS, Dupuis M, Singh M, et al. Mechanisms of increased immunogenicity for DNA-based vaccines adsorbed onto cationic microparticles. Cell Immunol 2003;225:12–20.
61. O'Hagan D, Singh M, Ugozzoli M, et al. Induction of potent immune responses by cationic microparticles with adsorbed human immunodeficiency virus DNA vaccines. J Virol 2001;75:9037–9043.
62. Luo YP, O'Hagan D, Zhou H, et al. Plasmid DNA encoding human carcinoembryonic antigen (CEA) adsorbed onto cationic microparticles induces protective immunity against colon cancer in CEA-transgenic mice. Vaccine 2003;21:1938–1947.
63. Cui Z, Mumper RJ. Plasmid DNA-entrapped nanoparticles engineered from microemulsion precursors: in vitro and in vivo evaluation. Bioconjug Chem 2002;13:1319–1327.
64. Cui Z, Mumper RJ. Topical immunization using nanoengineered genetic vaccines. J Control Release 2002;81:173–184.
65. Cui Z, Mumper RJ. Genetic immunization using nanoparticles engineered from microemulsion precursors. Pharm Res 2002;19:939–946.
66. Cui Z, Mumper RJ. Intranasal administration of plasmid DNA-coated nanoparticles results in enhanced immune responses. J Pharm Pharmacol 2002;54:1195–1203.
67. Cui Z, Baizer L, Mumper RJ. Intradermal immunization with novel plasmid DNA-coated nanoparticles via a needle-free injection device. J Biotechnol 2003;102:105–115.
68. Wang C, Ge Q, Ting D, et al. Molecularly engineered poly(ortho ester) microspheres for enhanced delivery of DNA vaccines. Nat Mater 2004;3:190–196.
69. Lynn DM, Langer R. Degradable poly(beta-amino esters): Synthesis, characterization, and self-assembly with plasmid DNA. J Am Chem Soc 2000;122:10,761–10,768.
70. Lynn DM, Amiji MM, Langer R. pH-responsive polymer microspheres: Rapid release of encapsulated material within the range of intracellular pH. Ang Chem-IntEd 2001;40:1707–1710.
71. Boussif O, Lezoualch F, Zanta MA, et al. A Versatile Vector for Gene and Oligonucleotide Transfer into Cells in Culture and in-Vivo - Polyethylenimine. Proc Natl Acad Sci U S A 1995;92:7297–7301.
72. Schijns VE. Immunological concepts of vaccine adjuvant activity. Curr Opin Immunol 2000; 12:456–463.
73. Pardoll DM, Beckerleg AM. Exposing the immunology of naked DNA vaccines. Immunity 1995; 3:165–169.

74. Hohlfeld R, Engel AG. The immunobiology of muscle. Immunol Today 1994;15:269–274.
75. Porgador A, Irvine KR, Iwasaki A, Barber BH, Restifo NP, Germain RN. Predominant role for directly transfected dendritic cells in antigen presentation to CD8(+)T-cells after gene gun immunization. J Exp Med 1998;188:1075–1082.
76. Hoon DS, Okamoto T, Wang HJ, et al. Is the survival of melanoma patients receiving polyvalent melanoma cell vaccine linked to the human leukocyte antigen phenotype of patients? J Clin Oncol 1998;16:1430–1437.
77. Matzinger P. The danger model: a renewed sense of self. Science 2002;296:301–305.
78. Scheerlinck JY. Genetic adjuvants for DNA vaccines. Vaccine 2001;19:2647–2656.
79. Hakim I, Levy S, Levy R. A nine-amino acid peptide from IL-1beta augments antitumor immune responses induced by protein and DNA vaccines. J Immunol 1996;157:5503–5511.
80. Agadjanyan MG, Kim JJ, Trivedi N, et al. CD86 (B7-2) can function to drive MHC-restricted antigen-specific CTL responses in vivo. J Immunol 1999;162:3417–3427.
81. Stevenson FK. DNA vaccines against cancer: From genes to therapy. Ann Oncol 1999;10:1413–1418.
82. Savelyeva N, Munday R, Spellerberg MB, Lomonossoff GP, Stevenson FK. Plant viral genes in DNA idiotypic vaccines activate linked CD4(+) T-cell mediated immunity against B-cell malignancies. Nat Biotechnol 2001;19:760–764.
83. Chen CH, Wang TL, Hung CF, et al. Enhancement of DNA vaccine potency by linkage of antigen gene to an HSP70 gene. Cancer Res 2000;60:1035–1042.
84. Zhang L, Widera G, Bleecher S, Zaharoff DA, Mossop B, Rabussay D. Accelerated immune response to DNA vaccines. DNA Cell Biol 2003;22:815–822.
85. Ott G, Singh M, Kazzaz J, et al. A cationic sub-micron emulsion (MF59/DOTAP) is an effective delivery system for DNA vaccines. J Control Release 2002;79:1–5.
86. Regnault A, Lankar D, Lacabanne V, et al. Fcgamma receptor-mediated induction of dendritic cell maturation and major histocompatibility complex class I-restricted antigen presentation after immune complex internalization. J Exp Med 1999;189:371–380.
87. Albert ML, Pearce SF, Francisco LM, et al. Immature dendritic cells phagocytose apoptotic cells via alphavbeta5 and CD36, and cross-present antigens to cytotoxic T lymphocytes. J Exp Med 1998; 188:1359–1368.
88. Jiang W, Swiggard WJ, Heufler C, et al. The receptor DEC-205 expressed by dendritic cells and thymic epithelial cells is involved in antigen processing. Nature 1995;375:151–155.
89. Cui Z, Hsu CH, Mumper RJ. Physical characterization and macrophage cell uptake of mannan-coated nanoparticles. Drug Dev Ind Pharm 2003;29:689–700.
90. Diebold SS, Lehrmann H, Kursa M, Wagner E, Cotten M, Zenke M. Efficient gene delivery into human dendritic cells by adenovirus polyethylenimine and mannose polyethylenimine transfection. Hum Gene Ther 1999;10:775–786.
91. Rodriguez F, Harkins S, Redwine JM, de Pereda JM, Whitton JL. CD4(+) T-cells induced by a DNA vaccine: immunological consequences of epitope-specific lysosomal targeting. J Virol 2001; 75:10,421–10,430.
92. Rodriguez F, An LL, Harkins S, et al. DNA immunization with minigenes: low frequency of memory cytotoxic T lymphocytes and inefficient antiviral protection are rectified by ubiquitination. J Virol 1998;72:5174–5181.
93. Rodriguez F, Zhang J, Whitton JL. DNA immunization: ubiquitination of a viral protein enhances cytotoxic T-lymphocyte induction and antiviral protection but abrogates antibody induction. J Virol 1997;71:8497–8503.
94. Delogu G, Howard A, Collins FM, Morris SL. DNA vaccination against tuberculosis: expression of a ubiquitin-conjugated tuberculosis protein enhances antimycobacterial immunity. Infect Immun 2000;68:3097–3102.
95. Tobery T, Siliciano RF. Cutting edge: induction of enhanced CTL-dependent protective immunity in vivo by N-end rule targeting of a model tumor antigen. J Immunol 1999;162:639–642.
96. Fu TM, Guan L, Friedman A, Ulmer JB, Liu MA, Donnelly JJ. Induction of MHC class I-restricted CTL response by DNA immunization with ubiquitin-influenza virus nucleoprotein fusion antigens. Vaccine 1998;16:p1711–p1717.
97. Sadasivan B, Lehner PJ, Ortmann B, Spies T, Cresswell P. Roles for calreticulin and a novel glycoprotein, tapasin, in the interaction of MHC class I molecules with TAP. Immunity 1996;5:103–114.
98. Spee P, Neefjes J. TAP-translocated peptides specifically bind proteins in the endoplasmic reticulum, including gp96, protein disulfide isomerase and calreticulin. Eur J Immunol 1997;27:2441–2449.
99. Pike SE, Yao L, Jones KD, et al. Vasostatin, a calreticulin fragment, inhibits angiogenesis and suppresses tumor growth. J Exp Med 1998;188:2349–2356.

100. Pike SE, Yao L, Setsuda J, et al. Calreticulin and calreticulin fragments are endothelial cell inhibitors that suppress tumor growth. Blood 1999;94:2461–2468.
101. Cheng WF, Hung CF, Chai CY, et al. Tumor-specific immunity and antiangiogenesis generated by a DNA vaccine encoding calreticulin linked to a tumor antigen. J Clin Invest 2001;108:669–678.
102. Rowell JF, Ruff AL, Guarnieri FG, et al. Lysosome-associated membrane protein-1-mediated targeting of the HIV-1 envelope protein to an endosomal/lysosomal compartment enhances its presentation to MHC class II-restricted T-cells. J Immunol 1995;155:1818–1828.
103. Ji H, Wang TL, Chen CH, et al. Targeting human papillomavirus type 16 E7 to the endosomal/lysosomal compartment enhances the antitumor immunity of DNA vaccines against murine human papillomavirus type 16 E7-expressing tumors. Hum Gene Ther 1999;10:2727–2740.
104. Wu TC, Guarnieri FG, Staveley-O'Carroll KF, et al. Engineering an intracellular pathway for major histocompatibility complex class II presentation of antigens. Proc Natl Acad Sci U S A 1995; 92:11,671–11,675.
105. Forns X, Emerson SU, Tobin GJ, Mushahwar IK, Purcell RH, Bukh J. DNA immunization of mice and macaques with plasmids encoding hepatitis C virus envelope E2 protein expressed intracellularly and on the cell surface. Vaccine 1999;17:1992–2002.
106. Geissler M, Bruss V, Michalak S, et al. Intracellular retention of hepatitis B virus surface proteins reduces interleukin-2 augmentation after genetic immunizations. J Virol 1999;73:4284–4292.
107. Rice J, King CA, Spellerberg MB, Fairweather N, Stevenson FK. Manipulation of pathogen-derived genes to influence antigen presentation via DNA vaccines. Vaccine 1999;17:3030–3038.
108. Steinman RM, Hawiger D, Nussenzweig MC. Tolerogenic dendritic cells. Ann Rev Immunol 2003; 21:685-711.
109. Morita A, Ariizumi K, Ritter R, 3rd, et al. Development of a Langerhans cell-targeted gene therapy format using a dendritic cell-specific promoter. Gene Ther 2001;8:1729–1737.
110. Ross R, Sudowe S, Beisner J, et al. Transcriptional targeting of dendritic cells for gene therapy using the promoter of the cytoskeletal protein fascin. Gene Ther 2003;10:1035–1040.
111. Sudowe S, Ludwig-Portugall I, Montermann E, Ross R, Reske-Kunz AB. Transcriptional targeting of dendritic cells in gene gun-mediated DNA immunization favors the induction of type 1 immune responses. Mol Ther 2003;8:567–575.
112. Irvine AS, Trinder PK, Laughton DL, et al. Efficient nonviral transfection of dendritic cells and their use for in vivo immunization. Nat Biotechnol 2000;18:1273–1278.
113. Walter E, Merkle HP. Microparticle-mediated transfection of non-phagocytic cells in vitro. J Drug Target 2002;10:11–21.
114. Walter E, Thiele L, Merkle HP. Gene delivery systems to phagocytic antigen-presenting cells. Stp Pharma Sciences 2001;11:45–56.
115. Arthur JF, Butterfield LH, Roth MD, et al. A comparison of gene transfer methods in human dendritic cells. Cancer Gene Ther 1997;4:17–25.
116. Haensler J, Verdelet C, Sanchez V, et al. Intradermal DNA immunization by using jet-injectors in mice and monkeys. Vaccine 1999;17:628–638.
117. Sasaki S, Takeshita F, Oikawa T, et al. Improvement of DNA vaccine immunogenicity by a dual antigen expression system. Biochem Biophys Res Commun 2004;315:38–43.
118. Andre S, Seed B, Eberle J, Schraut W, Bultmann A, Haas J. Increased immune response elicited by DNA vaccination with a synthetic gp120 sequence with optimized codon usage. J Virol 1998; 72:1497–1503.
119. Uchijima M, Yoshida A, Nagata T, Koide Y. Optimization of codon usage of plasmid DNA vaccine is required for the effective MHC class I-restricted T cell responses against an intracellular bacterium. J Immunol 1998;161:5594–5599.
120. Crowe LM, Spargo BJ, Ioneda T, Beaman BL, Crowe JH. Interaction of cord factor (alpha, alpha'-trehalose-6,6'-dimycolate) with phospholipids. Biochim Biophys Acta 1994;1194:53–60.
121. Lima KM, Santos SA, Lima VMF, Coelho-Castelo AAM, Rodrigues JM, Silva CL. Single dose of a vaccine based on DNA encoding mycobacterial hsp65 protein plus TDM-loaded PLGA microspheres protects mice against a virulent strain of Mycobacterium tuberculosis. Gene Ther 2003; 10:678–685.
122. Ford KG, Souberbielle BE, Darling D, Farzaneh F. Protein transduction: an alternative to genetic intervention? Gene Ther 2001;8:1–4.
123. Hung CF, Cheng WF, Chai CY, et al. Improving vaccine potency through intercellular spreading and enhanced MHC class I presentation of antigen. J Immunol 2001;166:5733–5740.
124. Hung CF, Cheng WF, Hsu KF, et al. Cancer immunotherapy using a DNA vaccine encoding the translocation domain of a bacterial toxin linked to a tumor antigen. Cancer Res 2001;61:3698–3703.

125. Kim TW, Hung CF, Boyd D, et al. Enhancing DNA vaccine potency by combining a strategy to prolong dendritic cell life with intracellular targeting strategies. J Immunol 2003;171:2970–2976.
126. Kim TW, Hung CF, Boyd DA, et al. Enhancement of DNA vaccine potency by coadministration of a tumor antigen gene and DNA encoding serine protease inhibitor-6. Cancer Res 2004;64:400–405.
127. Chattergoon MA, Kim JJ, Yang JS, et al. Targeted antigen delivery to antigen-presenting cells including dendritic cells by engineered Fas-mediated apoptosis. Nat Biotechnol 2000;18:974–979.
128. Sasaki S, Amara RR, Oran AE, Smith JM, Robinson HL. Apoptosis-mediated enhancement of DNA-raised immune responses by mutant caspases. Nat Biotechnol 2001; 19:543–547.
129. Davis NL, Brown KW, Johnston RE. A viral vaccine vector that expresses foreign genes in lymph nodes and protects against mucosal challenge. J Virol 1996;70:3781–787.
130. Ohno K, Sawai K, Iijima Y, Levin B, Meruelo D. Cell-specific targeting of Sindbis virus vectors displaying IgG-binding domains of protein A. Nat Biotechnol 1997;15:763–767.
131. Schlesinger S, Dubensky TW. Alphavirus vectors for gene expression and vaccines. Curr Opin Biotechnol 1999;10:434–439.
132. Leitner WW, Ying H, Driver DA, Dubensky TW, Restifo NP. Enhancement of Tumor-specific Immune Response with Plasmid DNA Replicon Vectors. Cancer Res 2000;60:51–55.
133. Leitner WW, Hwang LN, deVeer MJ, et al. Alphavirus-based DNA vaccine breaks immunological tolerance by activating innate antiviral pathways. Nat Med 2003;9:33–39.
134. Mumper RJ, Ledebur HC. Dendritic cell delivery of plasmid DNA - Applications for controlled genetic immunization. Mol Biotechnol 2001;19:79–95.
135. Okamoto T, Kaneda Y, Yuzuki D, Huang SK, Chi DD, Hoon DS. Induction of antibody response to human tumor antigens by gene therapy using a fusigenic viral liposome vaccine. Gene Ther 1997; 4:969–976.
136. Zhou WZ, Kaneda Y, Huang S, Morishita R, Hoon D. Protective immunization against melanoma by gp100 DNA-HVJ-liposome vaccine. Gene Ther 1999;6:1768–1773.
137. Lanuti M, Rudginsky S, Force SD, et al. Cationic lipid: bacterial DNA complexes elicit adaptive cellular immunity in murine intraperitoneal tumor models. Cancer Res 2000;60:2955–2963.
138. Tanaka M, Kaneda Y, Fujii S, et al. Induction of a systemic immune response by a polyvalent melanoma-associated antigen DNA vaccine for prevention and treatment of malignant melanoma. Mol Ther 2002;5:291–299.
139. Correale P, Cusi MG, Sabatino M, et al. Tumour-associated antigen (TAA)-specific cytotoxic T-cell (CTL) response in vitro and in a mouse model, induced by TAA-plasmids delivered by influenza virosomes. Eur J Cancer 2001;37:2097–2103.
140. Scardino A, Correale P, Firat H, et al. In vivo study of the GC90/IRIV vaccine for immune response and autoimmunity into a novel humanised transgenic mouse. Br J Cancer 2003;89:199–205.
141. You ZY, Huang X, Hester J, Toh HC, Chen SY. Targeting dendritic cells to enhance DNA vaccine potency. Cancer Research 2001;61:3704–3711.
142. Boyle JS, Brady JL, Lew AM. Enhanced responses to a DNA vaccine encoding a fusion antigen that is directed to sites of immune induction. Nature 1998;392:408–411.
143. Lew AM, Brady BJ, Boyle BJ. Site-directed immune responses in DNA vaccines encoding ligand-antigen fusions. Vaccine 2000;18:1681–1685.
144. Chaplin PJ, De Rose R, Boyle JS, et al. Targeting improves the efficacy of a DNA vaccine against Corynebacterium pseudotuberculosis in sheep. Infect Immun 1999;67:6434–6438.
145. Kim SJ, Suh D, Park SE, et al. Enhanced immunogenicity of DNA fusion vaccine encoding secreted hepatitis B surface antigen and chemokine RANTES. Virology 2003;314:84–91.
146. Biragyn A, Tani K, Grimm MC, Weeks S, Kwak LW. Genetic fusion of chemokines to a self tumor antigen induces protective, T-cell dependent antitumor immunity. Nat Biotechnol 1999;17:253–258.
147. Wang B, Merva M, Dang K, et al. DNA inoculation induces protective in vivo immune responses against cellular challenge with HIV-1 antigen-expressing cells. AIDS Res Hum Retroviruses 1994; 10:S35–S41.
148. Little SR, Lynn DM, Ge Q, et al. Poly-beta amino ester-containing microparticles enhance the activity of nonviral genetic vaccines. Proc Natl Acad Sci USA 2004;101:9534–9539.
149. Little SR, Lynn DM, Puram SV, Langer R. Formulation and characterization of poly (beta amino ester) microparticles for genetic vaccine delivery. J Control Release 2005;107:449–462.
150. Demangel C, Zhou J, Choo AB, Shoebridge G, Halliday GM, Britton WJ. Single chain antibody fragments for the selective targeting of antigens to dendritic cells. Mol Immunol 2005;42:979–985.

18 Gene Therapy Targeted at Angiogenesis and Lymphangiogenesis for Cancer Treatment

Anita T. Tandle, PhD *and Steven K. Libutti,* MD

CONTENTS

Summary

Angiogenesis and lymphangiogenesis play an important role in several normal and pathological conditions such as wound healing, reproduction, inflammation, and cancer growth and metastasis. A tight regulation between angiogenic/lymphangiogenic growth factors and inhibitors determines the balance between a progrowth or inhibitory phenotype. Hence, inhibition of angiogenesis/lymphangiogenesis using gene therapy is a potentially important strategy to inhibit the growth of primary tumors and to inhibit their metastatic spread.

This chapter reviews the more recent data available in the field of angiogenesis/lymphangiogenesis. The focus of the chapter is on using gene therapy to achieve sustained physiological levels of antiangiogenic inhibitors with minimal systemic toxicity as well as ways to achieve tumor targeted antiangiogenic gene therapy.

Key Words: Angiogenesis; lymphangiogenesis; tumor targeting; targeted gene therapy; antiangiogenic inhibitors; VEGF; nanoparticles.

1. INTRODUCTION

Angiogenesis is a fundamental biological process involved in reproduction and wound healing. Under these conditions, neovascularization is tightly regulated. However, unregulated angiogenesis is thought to be indispensable for cancer growth and metastasis *(1)*. The process is composed of two main phases, an activation phase and a resolution phase *(2)*. The phase of activation encompasses increased vascular permeability, extravascular fibrin deposition, vessel wall disassembly, basement membrane degradation, cell migration, extracellular matrix invasion, endothelial cell (EC) proliferation, and capillary lumen formation. The phase of resolution includes inhibition of EC proliferation, cessation of cell migration, basement membrane reconstitution,

From: *Cancer Drug Discovery and Development: Gene Therapy for Cancer*
Edited by: K. K. Hunt, S. A. Vorburger, and S. G. Swisher © Humana Press Inc., Totowa, NJ

junctional complex maturation, and vessel wall assembly, including recruitment and differentiation of smooth muscle cells and pericytes. Implicit in the definition of the resolution phase is the establishment of blood flow within the newly formed vessel.

Within a given microenvironment, the angiogenic response is determined by a net balance between pro- and antiangiogenic regulators released from activated ECs, monocytes, smooth muscle cells, and platelets *(3)*. The principal growth factors driving angiogenesis are vascular endothelial growth factor (VEGF), basic fibroblast growth factor (bFGF), angiopoietin-1 (Ang-1), platelet-derived growth factor (PDGF), angiotropin, angiogenin, epidermal growth factor (EGF), and interleukins (ILs) (-1, -6, and -8), matrix proteins such as collagen, and the integrins *(4)*. The proteolytic enzymes critical to angiogenesis and tumor spread include cathepsin, urokinase-type plasminogen activator (uPAR), gelatinases A/B, and stromelysin *(5)*. The angiogenic inhibitors include naturally occurring inhibitors such as endostatin, thrombospondin (TSP), angiostatin, inhibitors of EC growth (TNP-470, thalidomide, IL-12 etc), inhibitors of proangiogenic molecules (antibodies, antisense RNA and soluble receptors for FGF, VEGF), agents that interfere with basement membrane and extracellular matrix, tissue inhibitors of metalloproteinases, antibodies to adhesion molecules ($\alpha V\beta 3$), and small inhibitors of receptor tyrosine kinases. Tumor necrosis factor-α (TNF-α), transforming growth factor-β (TGF-β), and IL-4 are bifunctional modulators. These molecules are either stimulators or inhibitors depending on the amount, the site, the microenvironment, and the presence of other cytokines.

The growth of lymphatic vessels is called lymphangiogenesis and also plays an important role in several normal and pathological conditions such as wound healing, inflammation, and cancer metastasis *(6)*. The development of lymphatic system may consist of two mechanisms—venous origin of the lymphatic vessels and *de novo* formation of primary lymph sacs in the mesenchyme *(7)*. Insufficient lymphangiogenesis causes incapacitating lymphedema, whereas lymphatic growth around tumors may facilitate metastatic spread of malignant cells that ultimately kill the patient *(8)*. Although, the lymphatic vessels are composed of ECs, they lack supporting pericytes which are present in blood vessels *(9,10)*. The key lymphatic growth factors are VEGF-C, VEGF-D, and their receptor VEGFR3 *(7)*. Although the two processes share some common similarities there are major differences as shown in Fig. 1.

The present chapter reviews the recent literature on antiangiogenesis and lymphangiogenesis. The inhibition of molecular targets specific for these two processes has been discussed. The chapter focuses on preclinical tumor targeted gene therapy to inhibit angiogenesis and lymphangiogenesis. Finally, it addresses the need for in depth research required to take especially antiangiogenic gene therapy to clinic.

2. ANGIOGENESIS/LYMPHANGIOGENESIS

2.1. Requirement for Tumor Growth and Metastasis

It is a well accepted fact that a tumor growth is angiogenesis dependent, with more than 2500 scientific reports showing angiogenesis linked to tumor growth *(11,12)*. Angiogenic switch occurs during the precancerous stage, thus angiogenesis might be important in tumor initiation *(13,14)*. The degree of vascularization of the primary tumor correlates directly with presence of bone marrow micrometastases at diagnosis in breast cancer patients *(15)*. Intratumoral vascularization has a prognostic value for

	Angiogenesis	Lymphangiogenesis
Vessles	Tight lining of endothelial cells	Discontinuous lining of endothelial cells
	Tight interendothelial junctions	Lack tight interendothelial junctions, more permeable
	A continuous basement membrane	A discontinuous basement membrane
	Presence of Pericytes, platelets	No pericytes and platelets
	High pressure	Low pressure
Tumor spread	Penetration through basement membrane, not so easy	Easy penetration by tumor cells
Role	Supply of oxygen and nutrients to tumor cells, and indirectly in metastasis	Lymphatic spread of malignant tumor
Major molecular players	VEGF, VEGFR-1, -2, FGF, MMP's	VEGF-C, -D, VEGFR-2, -3
Molecular markers	CD31, CD34, vWF, P1H12, CEC's	VEGFR-3, LYVE-1, Podoplanin, Prox-1, Nrp-2

Fig. 1. Angiogenesis and Lymphangiogenesis. The flowchart depicts the major differences between angiogenesis and lymphangiogenesis *(8)*.

cancers of the breast, colon, cervix, lung, and melanoma, as well as others *(13)*. The recent data has shown that not only solid tumors but hematopoietic malignancies as well are also dependent on angiogenesis *(16,17)*. Bone marrow angiogenesis has been seen in acute lymphoblastic leukemia and multiple myeloma and hence antiangiogenic therapy can prove beneficial in treating these malignancies *(18–20)*.

The first systematic description of the lymphatic system was carried out in 1627 and metastatic spread of breast cancer through lymphatic vessels in 1977 *(21,22)*. Although the physiological importance of the lymphatic system has been recognized for a long time, the knowledge about its involvement in the metastatic cascade has been hampered by major interests surrounding the formation of tumor-associated blood vessels. Clinical and pathological evidence now confirms that the metastatic spread of tumors via lymphatic vessels to local/regional lymph nodes is an early event in metastatic disease for many human solid tumors. The recent understanding about lymphangiogenesis has come from our knowledge of VEGF-C, VEGF-D, and their receptor VEGFR3. The lymphatic growth factors play a central role in generating new lymphatic vessels in and around the primary tumor and is responsible for lymphatic metastasis *(23)*. Several reports have shown expression of VEGF-C and -D in multiple human malignancies such as gastric, colon, breast, lung, and malignant melanoma *(7,24–28)*. Metastasis of breast cancer occurs primarily through the lymphatic system, and the extent of lymph node involvement is a key prognostic factor for the disease, determining further therapy *(29)*. The recent studies have extended the similar findings to many other tumor types *(7)*.

2.2. Molecular Regulators

Several published reports have reviewed molecules involved mainly in angiogenesis and to a lesser extent in lymphangiogenesis *(30–33)*. The following section describes important regulators in both the processes.

2.2.1. The VEGF Family and VEGF Receptors

The VEGF family currently consist of six known factors: VEGF-A, VEGF-B, VEGF-C, VEGF-D, VEGF-E, and placenta growth factor, with homology to platelet derived growth factor *(34)*. The most important single angiogenic growth factor, VEGF (VEGF-A) induces angiogenesis through binding to its relevant receptors, VEGFR1 and VEGFR2 that are mainly expressed in ECs. It is the most extensively studied growth factor, with a variety of EC specific effects, such as induction of EC proliferation, extracellular matrix degradation, migration, and tube formation *(35)*. VEGF seems to modulate 46 different signaling molecules *(34,36)*. VEGF-C and VEGF-D are predominantly lymphangiogenic factors; however, they have been shown to promote angiogenesis *(8,37)*. The biological effects of VEGF-C and -D are mediated mainly through VEGFR3 *(38–40)*.

VEGF-D can induce both tumor angiogenesis and lymphangiogenesis, whereas VEGF induces tumor angiogenesis but not lymphangiogenesis. Importantly, VEGF-D promotes lymphatic spread of tumors whereas VEGF does not *(41)*. In VEGF-C$^{-/-}$ mice, endothelial ECs commit to the lymphatic lineage but do not sprout to form lymph vessels and results into prenatal death *(42)*. Recent work in animal models showed that the incidence of metastasis is increased in tumors expressing VEGF-C and VEGF-D *(25,41)*. Furthermore, tumor derived expression of VEGF-C and VEGF-D may indicate, lymphatic invasion, lymph node metastasis, poor survival and is a predictor of poor outcome *(7,25)*. Expression of VEGF-C, VEGF-D, and VEGFR3 show differences in expression pattern at different stages of cervical cancer *(43)*. VEGFR3 is related to the VEGF receptors, but does not bind VEGF and its expression becomes restricted mainly to lymphatic endothelia during development.

2.2.2. Basic Fibroblast Growth Factor

Basic fibroblast growth factor (bFGF) was one of the first angiogenic factors to be characterized and since then has been studied extensively. It induces tube formation in collagen gels, modulates integrin expression and gap junction intercellular communication, and it upregulates VEGF, VEGFR2, and uPAR in vitro *(44)*. bFGF stimulates both lymphangiogenesis and angiogenesis in a mouse corneal lymphangiogenesis model and up-regulats VEGF-C expression in vascular endothelial and perivascular cells *(45)*. It is one of the most potent angiogenic factors and high serum levels upon diagnosis are associated with poor outcomes for cases of lung cancer *(46)*.

2.2.3. Tie/Angiopoietin (Ang) System

Together with VEGF and bFGF, the Angs constitute an important regulatory system for the development and maintenance of functional blood and lymphatic vessels. The important members of this family include Ang-1 and Ang-2, which both bind solely to the Tie-2 receptor and control blood vessel stabilization signals *(47,48)*. VEGF and Ang-1 appear to work in complementary fashion during early vascular development, with VEGF initiating vascular formation and Ang-1 promoting subsequent vascular remodeling, maturation, and stabilization, perhaps in part by supporting interactions between ECs and surrounding support cells and matrix *(49–51)*. Ang-2 seems to be required for the proper development of the lymphatic vessels. Mice lacking Ang-2 exhibit profound defects in the patterning and function of the lymphatic vasculature *(52)*.

2.2.4. Matrix Metalloproteinases

Matrix metalloproteinases (MMPs) are a family of extracellular and membrane-associated endopeptidases, collectively digest almost all extracellular matrix and

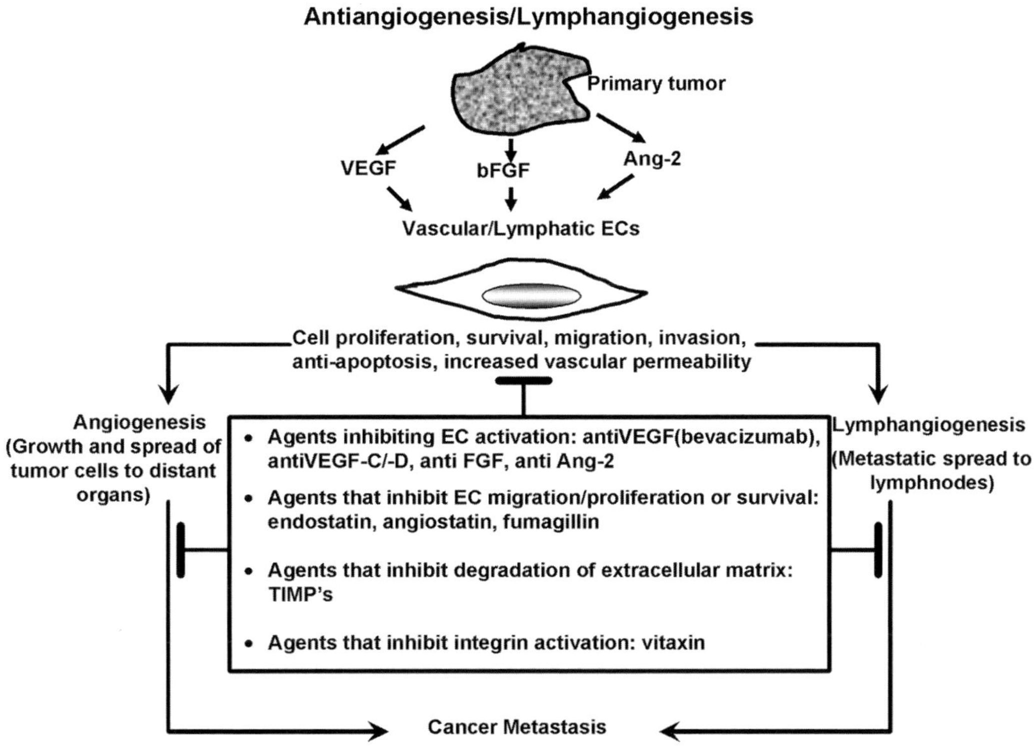

Fig. 2. Therapeutic Approaches: Antiangiogenesis/Antilymphangiogenesis. The flowchart shows some of the therapeutic approaches to inhibit angiogenesis and lymphangiogenesis.

basement membrane components, and thus play an important role in tumor progression *(44,53)*. MMPs promote tumor angiogenesis by mobilizing or activating proangiogenic factors, such as bFGF, VEGF, and TGF-β *(54)*. Indeed, recent studies have revealed that MMPs are important during the early stages of tumor development, before metastasis occurs *(54)*. The most important proteases are MMP -2 and -9, considered as a marker for tumor invasion and metastasis and recurrence of the disease *(55,56)*. By cleavage of the proapoptotic FAS ligand, MMP-7 allows tumor cells to become resistant to apoptosis signals *(57)*.

2.2.5. Integrins

The important category of cell surface receptors which shows regulated expression on vasculature in the normal tissues but enhanced expression on the tumor endothelium are integrins *(58,59)*. Endothelial cells have been shown to express at least 13 different integrins—depending on their state of development, differentiation, and function—and are required for embryonic vascular development and postnatal angiogenesis *(60)*. Integrin expression on the surface of activated ECs regulate distinct biologic events such as cell migration, proliferation, and differentiation during angiogenesis *(61)*. One widely studied integrin, αVβ3, is a receptor for extracellular matrix harboring a tripeptide (RGD) sequence, including vitronectin, fibronectin, and fibrinogen *(62)*. Vascular expression of integrin αVβ3 in tumor vascular "hot spots" was found to be the most significant prognostic factor predictive of relapse-free survival in both node-negative and node-positive breast cancer patients *(63)*. However, the most recent reports shows that αVβ3 may have both positive and negative functions *(60,64)*.

2.2.6. Hypoxia

The hypoxic environment in solid tumors results from oxygen consumption by rapid proliferation of tumor cells. Hypoxia has been shown to facilitate the survival of tumor cells and to be a cause of malignant transformation thus playing a critical role in tumor biology *(65)*. It inhibits TNF-related apoptosis-inducing ligand (TRAIL) -induced apoptosis by blocking Bax translocation to the mitochondria *(65)*. Intratumoral hypoxia has been shown to be a prognostic parameter in variety of human cancers *(66)*. In hypoxic tissue the hypoxia inducible factor-1 (HIF-1) has been proven to play a central role in inducing the transcription of genes that are involved in angiogenesis, including VEGF *(67)*. Activation of HIF-1 in combination with activated signaling pathways is implicated in tumor progression and prognosis *(68)*. Increased levels of HIF-1 α are potentially associated with more aggressive breast cancer and treatment failure and/or patient mortality in oropharyngeal squamous cell cancer *(69–71)*.

2.2.7. Other Players

Other factors that seem to be involved in lymphangiogenesis include the, Prox1, T1α/podoplanin, neuropilin-2, and integrin α9β1 *(7)*. Prox1 a homeobox gene is a specific and required regulator of the development of the lymphatic system and lymphatic programming *(72,73)*. Prox1-deficient mice are devoid of lymphatic vasculature, and in these animals ECs fail to acquire the lymphatic phenotype; instead, they remain as blood vascular endothelium *(72)*.

Podoplanin/T1 α, a membrane mucoprotein, is predominantly expressed by lymphatic endothelium, and recent studies have shown that it is regulated by Prox1 gene *(73)*. Podoplanin(–/–) mice have defects in lymphatic system, but not blood vessel pattern formation. Inhibition of podoplanin expression can decrease lymphatic endothelial cell (LEC) adhesion in cell culture *(74)*. Neuropilin-2 (NRP-2) acts as a coreceptor for VEGF-C with VEGFR-3 *(75)*. It is particularly required for the formation of small lymphatics *(76)*. The α9β1 integrin is required for the normal development of the lymphatic system *(77)*.

2.3. A Crosstalk Between Different Modulators

There are certain molecules seem to play multiple roles. A crosstalk between the various modulators of angiogenesis and lymphangiogenesis has been described recently *(78)*. VEGF a key player in the induction of angiogenesis, also induces a strong lymphangiogenic response *(79)*. The lymphatics generated by VEGF are giant and structurally and functionally abnormal. VEGF-C may cooperate with VEGF in regulating embryonic vascular development and can activate VEGFR-2. VEGF-C signaling through VEGFR-2 works synergistically with VEGF, the binding of VEGF-C to VEGFR-3 consequently regulates VEGFR-2 signaling *(80)*. Also, it may compensate for the loss of VEGF in VEGF deficient mice. Under certain experimental conditions, VEGF-C promotes angiogenesis *(37)*. Targeted inactivation of VEGFR-3 results in defective blood vessel development in early mouse embryos *(81)*. Further, the inactivation of VEGFR-3 by a MAb suppresses tumor growth by inhibiting the neoangiogenesis through the disruption of endothelial lining *(82)*. The biologic effects of VEGF-D are tissue-specific and dependent on the abundance of blood vessels and lymphatics expressing the receptors for VEGF-D in a given tissue; however, it is capable of inducing EC proliferation, angiogenesis, and lymphangiogenesis *(83)*.

3. GENE THERAPY: ANTIANGIOGENESIS/ANTILYMPHANGIOGENESIS

Considering the importance of angiogenesis/lymphangiogenesis in various human malignancies, therapeutic approaches targeting the tumor endothelium may provide long-term effective control of the disease. Antiangiogenic therapy has potential advantages over traditional modes of cancer treatment: (1) it is less toxic than conventional chemotherapy, (2) there is less development of resistance, and (3) it controls tumor growth independently of growth fraction or tumor cell type *(84)*. The following section summarizes antiangiogenic/lymphangiogenic inhibitors for gene therapy. The later section focuses on targeted gene therapy to tumor vasculature to combat any systemic toxicity.

3.1. Why Gene Therapy?

Gene therapy using nonviral/viral vectors offers an approach to the long-term delivery of therapeutic proteins to maintain physiological circulating levels of antiangiogenic inhibitors. The different nonviral vectors available are naked DNA/peptides, antibodies, antisense RNA, siRNA, liposomes, and nanoparticles. The major viruses used in the field are selected depending on requirements such as transduction efficiency, level of transgene expression, level of integration, and target cell type. Examples of these viral vectors include adenoviruses (Ad), retroviruses, adeno-associated viruses (AAV), lentiviruses, herpes simplex-1 viruses (HSV) and a new category of bacteriophages *(85,86)*. Viral vectors can be produced in high titer and they can efficiently infect a variety of replicating or nonreplicating cells to yield high-level expression of exogenous proteins. However, viral vectors can be associated with serious and sometimes life threatening health risks including potentially severe immune responses to the virus and the unintended activation of nontarget genes predisposing the target cell to cancer or other abnormalities *(87)*. The following section describes the uses of different vectors and target genes for anti-angiogenic/antilymphangiogenic gene therapy and are listed in table (Table 1).

3.2. Targets for Antiangiogenic/Antilymphangiogenic Gene Therapy

3.2.1. Inhibition of Proangiogenic/Lymphangiogenic Growth Factors

3.2.1.1. VEGF and VEGFR-1/-2. It is well-known that vascular endothelial growth factor with its receptor plays an important role in tumor-induced angiogenesis and has emerged as a critical target for antiangiogenic therapy *(88)*. Inhibition of VEGF or its signaling pathway has been shown to suppress tumor angiogenesis and tumor growth. An adenovirus containing antisense VEGF cDNA was shown to down-regulate VEGF expression and significantly inhibit the growth of established experimental breast tumors *(89)*. Recently, the Food and Drug Administration (FDA) approved Avastin (bevacizumab), a humanized MAb, as a first-line treatment for patients with metastatic colorectal cancer.

Simultaneously targeting VEGF production with antisense oligonucleotide and VEGF receptor signaling with receptor tyrosine kinase inhibitors enhances the anticancer efficacy of either therapy alone *(90)*. Some focus has been given to the preclinical gene therapy with soluble truncated forms of VEGFR-2 (sVEGFR-2). This molecule functions in two ways: by sequestering VEGF and, in a dominant-negative fashion, by forming inactive heterodimers with membrane-spanning VEGFRs *(91,92)*. Recently, murine fibrosarcoma and melanoma cells transduced with a retrovirus expressing sVEGFR-2, showed tumor growth reduction by inhibition of angiogenesis; however, it did not show

Table 1
Gene Therapy for Angiogenesis/Lymphangiogenesis

Inhibitor	*Vector (Nonviral/viral)*	*Findings*	*Ref.*
Inhibition of growth factors and receptors			
Antisense VEGF	Adenovirus	Tumor growth inhibition	*(89)*
Anti VEGF-D antibody	–	Reduction in vessels, inhibition of tumor growth	*(41)*
Antisense VEGF+VEGFR tyrosine kinase	–	EC growth inhibition and tumor delay	*(90)*
sVEGFR-2 and VEGFR-1	Adenovirus/Retrovirus	Reduction in MVD, delay in tumor growth, tumor reduction, inhibition of lymph node metastasis, increase in survival	*(93–95)*
sVEGFR-3	Adenovirus	Inhibits fetal lymphangiogenesis, induces regression of already formed lymphatic vessels with no effect on blood vasculature, suppression of tumor lymphangiogenesis	*(97,98)*
sTie2 receptor	Adenovirus	Inhibited both the growth of well established primary tumors and vascularization and growth of established and spontaneous lung metastases	*(103)*
Increase in endogenous angiogenic inhibitors			
Endostatin plasmid DNA/	Naked plasmid/cationic lipid	Tumor reduction, suppression of lung metastasis, increase in survival, decrease in tumor vessels, markedly narrowed or collapsed lumens	**(248–250)*
Endostatin	Adenovirus/Retrovirus/ AAV	Inhibition of tumor growth, antiproliferative activity towards endothelial cells and direct anticancer action against certain colon cancer cells	*(114,115, 113,251, 252)*
Angiostatin	Adenovirus	Inhibition of tumor growth and intratumoral angiogenesis with marked increase in apoptotic cells	*(138)*
Angiostatin	AAV	Sustained levels of circulating angiostatin, tumor suppression and long term survival, diminished vessel densities and increased apoptosis of tumor cells surrounding the neovessel	*(139,140, 253)*
Endostatin+ Angiostatin	AAV	Complete protection from tumor development in combination treatment	*(232)*

(*Continued*)

Table 1 (*Continued*)

Inhibitor	*Vector (Nonviral/viral)*	*Findings*	*Ref.*
TSP-1	Liposome	Inhibition of growth of tumor xenograft, induction of necrosis and decrease in MVD in tumors overexpressing TSP-1	*(254)*
TSP-1	Adenovirus	Inhibition of growth of human leukemia xenografts caused by inhibition of tumor angiogenesis	*(130)*
TIMP-2	Adenovirus	Inhibition of tumor growth, metastasis, angiogenesis index and increased survival	*(137)*
TIMP-2	Retrovirus	Increase the accumulation of connective tissue proteins in tumor tissue, to inhibit growth, and to prevent local invasion	*(135)*
PF-4	Adenovirus/ Retrovirus	Downregulation of ascites formation, tumor growth, vascularity, and prolongation of animal survival, decrease in secreted VEGF by tumor cells	*(116, 144)*
Canstatin	Recombinant purified protein	Suppression of tumor growth in xenograft model	*(255)*
Tumstatin	Recombinant purified protein	Decreased tumor growth, decreased numbers of CD31-positive blood vessels and VEGFR2-positive circulating endothelial cells	*(146)*

The table summarizes the preclinical gene therapy data available for antiangiogenesis/lymphangiogenesis with major finding.

AAV: adeno-associated virus; TSP-1: thrombospondin-1; TIMP-2: tissue inhibitor of metalloproteinases-2, MVD: microvessel density; VEGF: vascular endothelial growth factor, VEGFR: VEGF receptor.

reduction in VEGF levels compared with control *(93)*. A recombinant adenovirus expressing sVEGFR-2 is also effective in reducing lymphatic metastases and a decrease in the frequency of regional metastases in transgenic mice with spontaneous prostate tumors *(94)*. The sVEGFR-1 could inhibit the growth of follicular thyroid carcinoma by 70% by suppressing intratumoral angiogenesis *(95)*. These results lend support to the use of human sVEGFR-1 in anticancer therapy. Thus, gene therapy with soluble VEGFR-1 and -2 seems to be a reasonable approach to inhibit angiogenesis.

3.2.1.2. VEGF-C/-D and VEGFR-3. As these are the important molecules in the generation of lymphangiogenesis, they also represent the best targets to inhibit lymphangiogenesis. Recently a MAb VD1 was shown to compete with VEGF-D in binding to both VEGFR2 and VEGFR3, indicating that the binding epitopes on VEGF-D for these two receptors may be in close proximity *(96)*. Subcutaneous tumors grown in severe combined immunodeficiency (SCID) mice by injecting VEGF-D overexpressing 293EBNA cells were inhibited by VD1 antibody *(41)*. Also, treatment with the VD1 antibody reduced the abundance of vessels in the tumors as assessed by immunohistochemistry. Thus, it is possible that a single agent could inhibit both the receptors. There are few reports showing inhibition of VEGFR-3 by either a soluble receptor or using a specific antibody. A soluble form of VEGFR-3 is a potent inhibitor of VEGF-C/VEGF-D signaling, and when expressed in the skin of transgenic mice, it inhibits fetal lymphangiogenesis and induces a regression of already formed lymphatic vessels, though the blood vasculature remains normal *(97)*. Expression of the VEGFR-3-Ig fusion protein induces apoptosis in LECs *(97)*. A highly metastatic human lung cancer cell line, LNM35 expressing VEGFR-3-Ig was generated *(98)*. Mice bearing LNM35 expressing VEGFR-3-Ig, tumors, showed inhibition of lymphatic vessels compared with non-expresser. Histologic analysis demonstrated that most axillary lymph nodes of mice bearing the control LNM35 tumors were almost completely occupied by the tumor cells, but only one lymph node had macroscopic evidence of metastasis in mice bearing VEGFR-3-Ig-expressing tumors, indicating suppression of lymph node metastasis from a primary tumor. Similar inhibition of lymph node metastasis has been seen in a syngeneic mammary tumor model *(99)*. Moreover, it is not clear whether lymphangiogenesis alone is sufficient for lymph node metastasis, as overexpression of VEGF-C can induce growth of lymphatic vessels, but not increase the incidence of lymph node metastasis in poorly metastatic tumor cells *(98)*. Karpanen et al. used adenovirus expressing a soluble fusion protein VEGFR-3, to inhibit growth of lymphatic vessels, in MCF7 tumors *(100)*. Systemic administration of anti-VEGFR-3 blocking antibodies resulted in the inhibition of regional lymph node metastasis and reduction of lymphatic vessel density in the primary tumors *(101)*. Administration of blocking anti-VEGFR-3 antibodies could also inhibit the bFGF induced lymphangiogenesis. These findings show that VEGFR-3 can be effective in inhibiting lymphangiogenesis induced by other growth factors also *(45)*.

3.2.1.3. Tie2. As shown by Lin et al., a single application of a soluble form of the extracellular domain of murine Tie2 inhibited the growth of a mammary tumor by >75% and tumor vascular density by 40% *(102)*. The same group also demonstrated that administration of adenovirus expressing Tie2 significantly inhibited the growth rate of mammary adenocarcinoma and melanoma tumors *(103)*. A single intravenous administration of virus produced >1 mg/mL of circulating levels of Tie2. The coadministration of tumor cells with virus expressing Tie2 could suppress the growth of tumor metastases. Only small, avascular metastases could be seen in the lungs of treated mice. Administration of Ad-Tie2 also inhibited tumor metastasis when delivered at the time of surgical excision of primary tumors. The same construct could inhibit experimental retinal and choroidal neovascularization *(104)*.

3.2.2. Augmentation of Antiangiogenic/Antilymphangiogenic Inhibitors

Increasing levels of endogenous inhibitors can have mixed results. The increase can have a direct action on EC function, such as inhibition of cell proliferation, tube formation, cell migration, and induction of apoptosis but may also have indirect effects on inhibiting the secretion of proangiogenic growth factors from tumor cells.

3.2.2.1. Endostatin. Endostatin, a 20-kDa fragment of collagen XVIII, is a member of a group of endogenous antiangiogenic proteins *(105)*. It is a multifunctional molecule; which activates a number of signaling molecules, blocks VEGF/VEGFR signaling, inhibits MMPs, and downregulates c-*myc*, and cyclin-D1 *(106–111)*. Endostatin inhibits endothelial cell proliferation, migration/invasion, and tube formation. The inhibitory effect by endostatin has been proposed to involve binding to the receptor $\alpha_5\beta_1$ and also glycopican on ECs *(112)*. In addition to its antiangiogenic activity, endostatin exerts a direct anticancer action that appears to be restricted to some tumor cell lines *(113)*. Earlier work from our laboratory has reported very high plasma levels of endostatin after administration of a recombinant adenovirus expressing endostatin. This construct inhibited growth of MC38 adenocarcinoma by 40%, which is relatively resistant to adenoviral infection *(114)*. A retroviral construct expressing endostatin showed dramatic reduction in tumor volume and increased overall survival in treated mice *(115)*. Adenovirus expressing endostatin, angiostatin, and/or platelet factor 4 (PF4) significantly inhibited ascites formation, tumor growth, vascularity, and caused prolongation of animal survival after intraperitoneal treatment in three different ascites tumor models *(116)*. Combined treatment proved to be more effective than treatment with one vector alone. Recently, a lentivirus expressing endostatin/angiostatin was developed, which inhibited EC proliferation in a coculture experiment *(117)*.

3.2.2.2. Fumagillin. Fumagillin, a natural product isolated from *Aspergillus fumigatus*, was found to strongly inhibit endothelial cell proliferation by selective inhibition of methionine aminopeptidase type 2 *(118,119)*. TNP-470 (a fumagilin analogue) was found to have greater potency and lower toxicity than fumagillin, and it was one of the first inhibitors of angiogenesis to reach clinical trials *(120)*. Most of the reports have used TNP-470 as an inhibitor. TNP-470, inhibits tumor growth and tumor angiogenesis in number of animal models tested so far, including rhabdomyosarcoma and head and neck cancers *(121–123)*. However, detailed studies are needed to study the effect of fumagillin in the gene therapy set up.

3.2.2.3. Thrombospondin 1 (TSP-1). TSP-1 is a heparin-binding glycoprotein constitutively secreted by many cell types including ECs *(124)*. It is a multimodular, 420-kDa homotrimeric glycoprotein that participates in cellular response to growth factors, cytokines, and injury. It regulates cell proliferation, migration, and apoptosis in a variety of physiological and pathological settings, including wound healing, inflammation, angiogenesis and neoplasia and it inhibits EC proliferation and angiogenesis *(125–127)*. Expression of TSP-1 has been inversely correlated with vascularization and malignant progression of breast-, lung cancers and melanomas *(128)*. TSP-1 is a potent inhibitor of angiogenesis and tumor growth *(129)*. In a human leukemia xenograft model, adenovirus-mediated TSP-1 gene transfer greatly inhibited K562-derived tumor growth and angiogenesis in animals *(130)*. Human glioma cell line U-251 MG (with mutated p53) transduced with wild-type p53, led to the enhanced expression of thrombospondin-1 mRNA and protein in these cells *(131)*. It has been shown that, p53 can stimulate the endogenous TSP-1 gene and positively regulate TSP-1 promoter sequences *(132)*. Thus, these studies suggest that mutation of the p53 gene endows gliomas with an angiogenic phenotype by reducing TSP-1 production as well as enhancing the angiogenesis inducers in the early phase of malignant progression.

3.2.2.4. TIMP-2. It is a natural MMP inhibitor that prevents the degradation of extracellular matrix proteins. It abolishes the hydrolytic activity of all activated members of the metalloproteinase family and in particular that of MT1-MMP, MMP-2, and MMP-9, which are selective for type IV collagenolysis *(133)*. Overexpression of TIMP-2 in the stroma of colorectal carcinomas correlates with a longer survival time *(134)*. Overexpression of TIMP-2 by a retrovirus inhibits tumor growth and invasion *(135)*. TIMP-2 overexpression mediated by a retrovirus significantly inhibited migration as well as invasion and metastatic progression of H-ras transformed MCF10A human breast cancer cells in a dose-dependent manner *(136)*. A single local injection of AdTIMP-2 into pre-established lung, colon, and breast tumors significantly reduced tumor growth rates by 60 to 80% and tumor-associated angiogenesis index by 25 to 75% *(137)*. Lung metastasis of LLC tumor were inhibited by more than 90%. In addition, AdTIMP-2-treated mice showed a significantly prolonged survival in all the cancer models tested.

3.2.2.5. Angiostatin. Angiostatin is a cleavage product of plasminogen. It acts especially on ECs without affecting tumor cells. Angiostatin delivery by a defective adenovirus expressing a secretable angiostatin K3 molecule could selectively inhibit EC proliferation and disrupt the G2/M transition *(138)*. A single intratumoral injection of the virus into pre-established rat C6 glioma or human MDA-MB-231 breast carcinoma resulted in a significant inhibition of tumor growth, which was associated with a suppression of neovascularization and induction of apoptosis. The intratumoral injection of a high-titer AAV-angiostatin expressing virus resulted in tumor suppression of malignant brain tumors and long-term survival in 40% of the treated rats *(139)*. Combined gene therapy of an adenoviral vector carrying the suicidal thymidine kinase gene along with the AAV-angiostatin vector offered the best tumor-suppressive effect and increased long-term survival of up to 55% in the treated rats *(139)*. AAV-mediated stable expression of angiostatin inhibited tumor burden in the highly aggressive B16F10 melanoma and Lewis lung carcinoma models of experimental metastasis resulting in prolonged survival of treated mice *(140)*.

3.2.2.6. Platelet Factor-4 (PF-4). PF-4 is a heparin binding protein normally stored within the α-granules of platelets. It is a potent inhibitor of EC proliferation and migration, and it is able to interact directly with bFGF and VEGF and inhibit their interaction with cell surface receptors *(141)*. A phase I clinical trial in metastatic colorectal cancer with recombinant PF-4 protein was well tolerated (although no clinical responses were observed) *(142)*. Adenovirus/retrovirus mediated soluble PF-4 therapy selectively inhibited EC proliferation and angiogenesis resulting in prolonged animal survival *(143,144)*. A recombinant adenovirus expressing PDF-4 reduced VEGF production by tumor cells and led to increased survival rates in an animal model *(116)*.

3.2.2.7. Canstatin and Tumstatin. These proteins are degradation products of type IV collagen. Both are antiangiogenic and are involved in the inhibition of EC tube formation, and proliferation, induction of apoptosis, and both show antitumor activity *(145,146)*. Tumstatin exerts its biological activity by binding to αVβ3 integrin *(112)*. Canstatin inhibits Akt activation and induces Fas-dependent apoptosis in ECs *(147)*. Our laboratory is currently in the process of producing adenoviral and retroviral vectors expressing canstatin.

3.2.2.8. TNF-α. Numerous preclinical models and clinical trials have shown potent antivascular properties of TNF-α *(148)*. It has been shown to have vasculotoxic effects at high concentrations, whereas at low concentrations it promotes angiogenesis *(149)*. It has been shown to induce tumor vessel destruction and improve vascular permeability to drugs in clinical settings and it, furthermore, induces significant bystander effects *(150)*. The antiangiogenic properties of TNF-α can be augmented by endothelial monocyte activating polypeptide-II *(151)*. The severe systemic toxicity of TNF-α has limited its use to isolated organ- and limb perfusions *(152,153)*. However, if the systemic toxicity can be controlled, it is a useful anticancer agent leading to objective tumor responses *(154)*. The local expression of TNF-α from adenovirus vector infected tumor cells induced intratumoral necrosis; with considerable toxicity *(155)*. In mice bearing small tumors, intratumoral injection of Ad-TNF-α virus with a repeated booster treatment results in complete regression *(156)*.

3.2.3. Pericytes and Vascular Smooth Muscle Cells as Targets

The blood vessels develop through the assembly of the two principal cell types—ECs and pericytes (PCs). ECs first form tubes, which are subsequently surrounded by a layer of PCs. They form a basal lamina beneath the endothelial layer, thus contributing to the stability of the capillary wall *(157)*. Disruption of endothelial-pericyte associations results in excessive regression of vascular loops and abnormal remodeling *(158)*. Platelet derived growth factor-β (PDGF-β) and its receptor (PDGFR-β) are critically involved in the recruitment of pericytes to blood capillaries and communication between the ECs and PCs appears to be essential for normal blood vessel development *(159)*.

In comparison with normal vessels, tumor blood vessels are different structurally as well as at the molecular level *(160,161)*. PCs show clear differences in their association with ECs between normal and tumor vessels *(162)*. A receptor tyrosine kinase (RTK) inhibitor incorporating selectivity for PDGFRs (SU6668) has been shown to block further growth of end-stage tumors *(163)*.

Bergers et al. used a RIPtag2 transgenic model to combine the SU5416 and SU6668 RTK inhibitors *(163)*. RIPTag2 mice have been particularly instructive about parameters of angiogenesis. By virtue of expressing the SV40 virus oncoprotiens in the pancreatic islet β cells, RIPTag2 mice develop islet carcinomas in multiple stages of hyperplastic/dysplastic islet, angiogenic displastic islet, solid tumors, and invasive carcinomas. The two kinase inhibitors (SU5416 and SU6668) were more efficacious against all stages of islet carcinogenesis than either single agent alone. It can be expected that the combination of different RTKs will be more efficient in treating multiple stages of tumorigenesis. Gene therapy approaches combining inhibition of pericytes and ECs will further increase the therapeutic efficacy.

3.2.4. Integrins

Another antiangiogenic approach is to target the upregulated cell surface receptors on tumor neovasculature. The αVβ3 integrin expressed on a variety of tumor cells is more consistently expressed at higher levels on neovascular ECs. VEGF induced EC migration requires interaction between VEGFR-2 and αVβ3 to drive the activation of downstream mitogenic pathways. Various studies suggest a role for αVβ3 in selective tumor cell intracellular signaling, generation of growth and survival signals, migration and generation of MMPs *(62)*. Thus, selective targeting of upregulated αVβ3 and VEGFR-2 on the neovasculature of tumors is a novel antiangiogenesis strategy for treating a wide variety of solid tumors. It has been shown that inhibition of αVβ3 or αVβ5 integrins by either monoclonal antibodies (MAbs) or cyclic peptides could suppress tumor angiogenesis in mice *(60)*. However, a recent report showed that knock-out mice that lack β3- or β3/β5-integrins demonstrated increased primary tumor growth and angiogenesis *(164)*. This can be explained by the inactivation of the antiangiogenic effect of endostatin and tumstatin who act via α5β1 and αVβ3 receptors *(112)*.

4. TARGETED GENE THERAPY

The development of strategies to achieve effective targeted gene expression and to enable appropriate regulation of gene expression may help to maximize therapeutic efficacy and minimize systemic toxicity. As important players in angiogenesis/lymphangiogenesis, VEGF helps to maintain normal bone marrow microvascular endothelial function and bFGF serves to modulate the proliferation of mesenchymal cells *(124)*. Systemic administration of a synthetic analogue of fumagillin (a strong inhibitor of endothelial cell proliferation) to nonpregnant female mice inhibited endometrial maturation and corpora luteum formation whereas in pregnant mice it resulted in complete failure of embryonic growth *(165)*. To avoid these unwanted effect of antiangiogenic agents on normal functions a targeted approach (i.e., by gene therapy) is necessary *(166)*.

Targeted gene therapy offers the possibility of systemic application, which is advantageous because it can prevent recurrence of distant metastases after surgery or radiotherapy, and it can be used in combination with conventional chemotherapy, vaccine therapy, immunotherapy or in combination with other types of gene therapy, for example, delivery of tumor suppressor genes *(84)*. However, efforts to influence antiangiogenic therapy by gene delivery have been hampered by a lack of targeting vectors specific for ECs in diseased tissues. The next section reviews the different modes of tissue targeting, vector availability and specific targets on tumor endothelium. Some of the tumor targeted gene therapy reports are listed in table (Table 2).

4.1. Tumor Targeting

4.1.1. Transcriptional Targeting

Transcriptional targeting can be achieved by the use of an expression cassette which is activated by tissue specific promoters (TSPs) *(167)*. The options are to use either a promoter with a high activity in tumor cells/tumor ECs or to use inducible promoters to achieve therapeutic transgene expression. Examples of promoters with high tumor-selective activity (minimal expression in normal cells) are, CXCR4, cyclooxygenase-2 (COX-2), survivin (a member of the inhibitor of apoptosis protein family) and pre-proendothelin-1 (PPE-1) a precursor protein for endothelin-1. The human CXCR4 gene is expressed at high levels in many types of cancers, but is repressed in the liver. Thus, the CXCR4 promoter has a "tumor-on" and "liver-off" status in vitro and in vivo, which make it a good candidate TSP for targeted cancer gene therapy approaches, (i.e., for melanoma and breast cancers) *(168)*. COX-2, a key enzyme in the synthesis of prostaglandins and thromboxanes, is highly up-regulated in tumor cells, stromal cells and angiogenic ECs during tumor progression *(60)*. COX-2 of EC promotes integrin $\alpha V\beta 3$-mediated EC adhesion, spreading, migration and angiogenesis *(169)*. The COX-2 promoter has been used to direct expression of caspases to COX-2-overexpressing cancer cells, inducing apoptosis while normal cells showed no caspase activation *(170)*. Similarly, systemic application of an adenovirus containing a reporter gene expressed from the survivin promoter resulted in high levels of reporter gene expression in tumor cells only *(171)*. PPE-1 is the precursor protein for endothelin-1 (a potent vasoconstrictor and smooth muscle cell mitogen) and is synthesized by ECs. The murine PPE-1 promoter contains a hypoxia-responsive element that increases the promoter activity in hypoxic tissue, like in marginally vascularized tumors *(172,173)*. Greenberger et al. used a chimeric death receptor transgene, coding for Fas and TNF receptor 1 under the control of the PPE-1 promoter, to sensitize cancer cells to the proapoptotic effect of TNF-α and to induce specific apoptosis of ECs in vitro *(174)*.

Table 2
Tumor Targeted Antiangiogenic Gene Therapy

Vector	*Targeting motif*	*Target*	*Ref.*
Polycation polyethylenimine	COX-2 promoter	Tumor cells	*(170)*
RGD peptide conjugated to PEG-liposomes	αVβ3 integrin	ECs	*(215)*
Cationic liposome	Chemotheraputic drug paclitaxel	ECs	*(210)*
Peptides	Receptor binding domain of VEGF	VEGF	*(186)*
Peptides	Peptide binding to VEGFR-2	VEGFR-2	*(187,188)*
Peptides	Aminopeptidase N (CD13) and RGD ligands carrying TNF-α	CD13 and αv integrins on ECs	*(190,191)*
Endothelium homing peptide	TNF-α	ECs	*(190)*
Nanoparticles	Integrin antagonist and radionucleotide	ECs	*(222)*
Nanoparticles	αVβ3 integrin	ECs	*(221)*
Quantum dots	Endothelium homing peptide	ECs/lymphatic vessels	*(226)*
Antibody	E-selectinAb-dexamethasone conjugate	ECs	*(182,198)*
Adenovirus	Pre-proendothelin-1 promoter	ECs	*(174)*
Adenovirus	VEGFR-2 and endoglin promoter	ECs	*(175)*
Adenovirus	Angiotensin-converting enzyme and flt-1 promoter	Lung	*(183)*
Adenovirus	RGD ligand	αvβ3 on ECs	*(179,228)*
Adenovirus	Radiosensitive EGR-1 promoter expressing TNF-α	Tumor	*(176)*
AAV	Hypoxia responsive element	Retina	*(239)*

The table list the possible vectors and targeting motif available for tumor targeted antiangiogenic gene therapy.

EC's Endothelial cells; AAV: Adeno-associated virus; VEGF: vascular endothelial growth factor; VEGFR: VEGF receptor; TCF-α: Tumor necrosis factor-α.

Recently, another tumor targeted approach with a conditionally replicating adenovirus capable of targeting dividing ECs was described *(175)*. The adenovirus has two promoters with the regulatory elements of VEGFR-2 and endoglin genes, which have been shown to be highly overexpressed in angiogenic ECs, to drive the adenoviral replication sequence. Hallahan and colleagues used another adenovirus vector expressing TNF-α under the control of radiation-inducible Egr-1 promoter (Ad5.Egr-TNF) *(176)*. Combined treatment with Ad5.Egr-TNF and 5000 cGy (rad) resulted in increased intratumoral TNF-α production and improved tumor control, without associated damage to normal tissue.

4.1.2. Transductional Targeting or Receptor Targeting

Transductional targeting involves the chemical or genetic modification of a vector, redirecting its tropism to a new target expressed preferentially on the target cell. This can be achieved either by direct targeting or indirect targeting. In direct targeting, the cell-specific targeting of the vector is mediated by a ligand that is directly inserted into the viral capsid *(177)*. However, this direct, ligand-mediated targeting, has its prerequisites that have to be considered, as there should be a good internalization site, the ligand should be structure independent, not too large to avoid the destabilization of the entire capsid, the ligand should be cell-type specific, the ligand-receptor complex should be internalized in a way that allows an efficient transport of the virus and the release of the viral DNA in the cell nucleus *(178)*. Recently, the arginine-glycine-aspartic acid (RGD) containing peptide ligands targeted to integrin receptors expressed on activated ECs have been studied *(179)*.

In indirect targeting the interaction between the viral vector and the target cell is mediated by an associated molecule (e.g., a glycoside molecule or a bispecific antibody), which is bound to the viral surface and interacts with a specific cell surface molecule *(178,180)*. A bispecific antibody containing Fab arms of $\alpha IIb\beta 3$ integrin and AAV capsid antibodies, could target AAV to cells, which are not normally permissive for AAV infection *(181)*. Everts et al. used this targeting strategy to the selective delivery of dexamethasone to activated ECs, using an E-selectin-directed drug-Ab conjugate *(182)*. Because E-selectin is not expressed in inactive EC the dexamethasone-Ab conjugate did not bind to resting ECs.

To achieve cell-specific transgene expression in pulmonary endothelium, Reynolds et al. used an adenoviral vector system that combined transductional and transcriptional targeting *(183)*. The combination of transductional targeting to a pulmonary endothelial marker (angiotensin-converting enzyme [ACE]) and to an endothelial-specific promoter (VEGFR-1) resulted in a synergistic, 300,000-fold increased selectivity of transgene expression to lung tissue compared with non-targeted vectors, that, after systemic application usually sequestrate in the liver.

4.2. Vectors for Targeted Gene Therapy

The biggest problem of any gene therapy is the availability of suitable vectors. The success of gene therapy is mainly dependent on the delivery of a therapeutic gene and, hence, on the development of an adequate gene delivery vector. The vector systems can be broadly divided in non-viral vectors and viral vectors.

4.2.1. Non-Viral Vectors

Several physical and chemical criteria have been put together to generate better vectors *(184)*. The important barriers to gene delivery are chemicals including particulates, lipids, and polymer complexes that optimize DNA complexation/condensation, membrane fusion, endosomal release, and nuclear targeting. Although viral vectors are more advantageous by most criteria than nonviral vectors, they bear the problems of systemic cytotoxicity and immunogenicity. Ideally, a vector could mimic the beneficial aspects of viral vectors without their disadvantages. A variety of nonviral gene delivery systems have been developed, including cationic liposomes, nanoparticles, and quantum dots. The endothelial cell specific peptides, MAbs, antisense RNA, small interfering RNA, and plasmid DNA, can all be complexed with either lipids, polymers or nanoparticles to avoid undesired interaction with nontarget sites and to enhance uptake into the target cells *(167)*.

4.2.1.1. Endothelial Specific Peptides and Antibodies. A number of endothelial specific peptides have been identified using in vivo biopanning of peptide phage-display libraries, which can be used as tumor-specific vascular targeting agents *(185)*. Phage based peptide libraries have identified peptides that bind to VEGF and prevent its binding to VEGFR *(186,187)*. The ATWLPPR peptide specifically inhibited VEGF-mediated proliferation of human vascular ECs and totally abolished VEGF-induced angiogenesis in a rabbit corneal model *(188)*. Another peptide identified by Hetian et al. could functionally disrupt the interaction between VEGF and the VEGFR2 and significantly inhibited tumor growth and metastasis *(189)*. The dose-limiting systemic toxicity of TNF-α has been minimized by conjugating it to endothelium targeting peptide (CNGRC) an aminopeptidase N (CD13) ligand that targets activated blood vessels in tumors *(190)*. It was 12 to 15× more efficient than murine TNF in decreasing tumor burden. Similarly, the peptide conjugated human TNF induced stronger antitumor effects than human TNF alone, even at 30× lower doses *(190)*. Further, fusion of TNF with the ACDCRGDCFCG peptide, a ligand of αV integrins, demonstrated that subnanogram doses of this conjugate were sufficient to induce antitumor effects in tumor-bearing mice when combined with melphalan, a chemotherapeutic drug *(191)*.

Human antibodies can be used to target anticancer agents to cancer cells with improved therapeutic efficacy because of reduced immunogenicity *(193,194)*. Endoglin/CD105 is a membrane protein involved in the TGF-β receptor signaling pathway. Its expression is strongly elevated in the angiogenic endothelium in tumors *(195)*. Antiendoglin antibody have been shown to preferentially bind to tumor endothelium, which resulted in tumor growth inhibition without significant systemic toxicity *(196,197)*. Similarly, antibodies against E-selectin have been used to target transgenes to activated endothelium *(198)*.

4.2.1.2. Antisense RNA and siRNA. Antisense oligodeoxynucleotides (ODNs) are synthetic molecules that block mRNA translation. Use of ODNs against VEGF, its receptors and Ang-1, suppressed tumor growth and angiogenesis and induced tumor cell apoptosis *(199–201)*. Equally, downregulation of the integrin subunit β3 expression by antisense RNA inhibited microvascular endothelial cell capillary tube formation *(202)*. RNAi is a conserved surveillance system that responds to double-stranded RNA by silencing mRNAs with homology to the double-stranded RNA trigger. siRNA targeted to either subunit of the α6β4 integrin (a laminin adhesion receptor) led to reduced cell surface expression of this integrin and resulted in decreased invasion of MDA-MB-231 breast carcinoma cells in a mouse model *(203)*. In another approach, increased expression of the antiangiogenic factor TSP-1 and decreased expression of VEGF in human breast or ovarian cancer has been provoked by siRNA-knockdown of Her-2/neu. This may be an effective antitumor strategy for Her-2/neu-overexpressing cancers as antibody therapy against Her-2/neu showed good efficacy in breast carcinoma in the clinical setting *(204)*.

DNA-vector based RNAi, in which RNAi sequences targeting VEGF isoforms, has potential applications in isoform-specific knock-down of VEGF *(205)*. Rubinson et al. and Hemann et al. have demonstrated that RNAi delivered by retroviral and lentiviral vectors can silence genes in mice *(206,207)*. With these reports and creation of transgenic mice expressing siRNA, it will now be possible to knockdown diseased genes in vivo and test these concepts *(208)*.

4.2.1.3. Cationic Liposomes. Cationic liposomes have a natural "tropism" to tumor ECs, as they are taken up 15- to 33-fold more than into corresponding normal ECs *(209)*. Thus, the encapsulation of antineoplastic drugs into cationic liposomes is a promising approach to improve selective drug delivery by targeting tumor vasculature. Strieth et al. selectively targeted paclitaxel to tumor ECs by cationic liposomes to achieve vascular targeted chemotherapy *(210)*. It resulted in significantly delayed metastasis to regional lymph nodes *(211)*. The intravenous administration of a plasmid expressing endostatin, complexed with a cationic lipid system, led to significant levels of endostatin in the lung and in the serum, which blocked systemic angiogenesis resulting in reduced tumor proliferation in murine models *(212)*.

Yet another way to home liposomes to tumor cells or tumor EC is by conjugating them to specific molecules like, antibodies, proteins, and small peptides *(213)*. Liposomes with antitumor agents modified with an angiogenic homing peptide for EC showed strong tumor suppression compared with unmodified liposomes *(214)*. Janssen et al. showed, that the coupling of cyclic RGD-peptides to the surface of PEG-liposomes could, indeed, target tumor endothelium *(215,216)*.

4.2.1.4. Nanoparticles and Quantum Dots (qdots). Nanoparticles (NPs) are submicron-sized polymeric colloidal particles with a therapeutic agent of interest encapsulated within their polymeric matrix or adsorbed or conjugated onto the surface *(217)*. The NPs are mostly composed of lipids that crosslink to form liquid crystal structures that self-assemble through polymerization. They have received considerable attention because of their smaller size, which led to improved cellular uptake over microparticles. NPs are used to improve oral bioavailability, to sustain drug/gene effect in target tissue, to solubilize drugs for intravascular delivery, and to increase the stability of therapeutic agents against enzymatic degradation *(218)*. They are less immunogenic than viral vectors, which offers the possibility to deliver therapeutic genes repeatedly to angiogenic blood vessels for long-term treatment of diseases. NPs can also be conjugated to a biospecific ligand, which then direct them to a specific tissue or organ. Recently, it was discovered that dense inorganic silica NPs, which by themselves do not deliver DNA, were able to enhance DNA transfection mediated by other commonly used transfection reagents *(219)*. A three component system, consisting of silica NPs, transfection agent SuperFect™ and DNA has been developed *(220)*. The silica NPs serve as an uptake-enhancing component by physical concentration at the cell surface; enhanced transfection resulting from the particles is seen with almost every transfection reagent tested with little toxicity *(220)*. The synthetic polyester based NPs, PLGA, escapes rapidly from the degradative endo-lysosomal compartment to the cytoplasmic compartment, thus protecting the therapeutic agent from degradation resulting from lysosomal enzymes *(217)*.

A cationic NP coupled to an integrin αVβ3-targeting ligand can deliver genes selectively to angiogenic blood vessels in tumor-bearing mice *(221)*. Systemic injection of the NP attached to mutant Raf gene (*ATP^{μ}-Raf*), which blocks endothelial signaling and angiogenesis in response to multiple growth factors into mice, resulted in apoptosis of the tumor-associated endothelium, ultimately leading to tumor cell apoptosis and sustained regression of established primary and metastatic tumors. Li et al. used radiolabeled NP with ^{90}Y to target murine melanoma and colon adenocarcinoma using the small molecule integrin antagonist (IA) and a MAb against murine VEGFR-2 *(222)*. The combination of radiolabeled NP either with IA or Anti-VEGFR-2 caused a significant tumor growth delay compared with single agents alone.

Recent advances in nanomaterials have produced a new class of fluorescent labels by conjugating semiconductor quantum dots (Qdots) with biorecognition molecules *(223)*. Qdots are small (<10 nm) inorganic nanocrystals that possess unique luminescent properties; their fluorescence emission is stable and tuned by varying the particle size or composition. Earlier, Erkki Ruoslahti and colleagues, identified peptides homing specifically to tumor blood vessels and tumor lymphatic vessels *(224,225)*. In a recent report, the group has demonstrated that, these peptides specifically direct qdots to blood vessels or lymphatic vessels in tumors *(226)*. The other tested organs such as, brain, heart, kidney, or skin did not contain detectable qdots, however, accumulation was seen in both the liver and spleen, in addition to the targeted tissues. Adding polyethylene glycol to the qdot coating reduced the accumulation in the liver and spleen by about 95%, without noticeably altering qdot accumulation in tumor tissue.

4.2.2. Viral Vectors

Several studies utilize viral vectors to target gene therapy to tumor endothelium (Table 2). In one approach adenovirus has been created that selectively replicates in and lyses dividing ECs *(175)*. Jin and colleagues used cytotoxic T-lymphocytes to deliver a retroviral VEGF-toxin fusion protein to its specific leukemia cell target in vivo to inhibit tumor growth *(227)*. Melanoma cells with low levels of adenoviral receptor (CAR) can be transduced successfully by a recombinant adenoviral containing RGD motif in their fiber knob *(228,229)*. The same vector revealed dramatic antitumor efficacy through hemolytic necrosis in an established melanoma model at a much lower dose *(228)*. Nakamura et al. used RGD targeted adenovirus to deliver human IL-2 to CAR deficient melanomas *(179)*. TNFerade™, a new class of vector consisting of an adenovirus expressing the human TNF-α cDNA under the control of a radiation-inducible promoter combining the therapeutic synergy between radiation and TNF-α has been generated *(230)*. Recently, TNFerade was tested in a phase I safety and toxicity trial *(231)*. The results of the study demonstrated that the treatment was well tolerated in patients with predominantly prior treatment-refractory solid tumors.

In another approach, it was shown that intraperitoneal injection of a bicistronic recombinant AAV coding for both endostatin and angiostatin resulted in a complete protection from development of human ovarian cancer in nude mice *(232)*. Furthermore, retroviruses have been engineered so that they can be coated with an VEGFR-2 antibody for the selective delivery of genes to tumor endothelium *(233)*.

Within recent years, bacteriophage vectors have become an alternative vector system, which combine desirable properties of both viral and nonviral systems minimizing the typical drawbacks of both the systems *(86)*. Phage vectors engineered to express specific ligands can be targeted to tumor cells. Bacteriophage containing fibroblast growth factor (FGF) as a ligand can be used to express a reporter gene in FGF receptor positive cells but not to the receptor negative cells *(234)*. Long-term transgene expression was established, indicating that with the appropriate targeted tropism, phage vectors could be used target gene therapeutic effects to mammalian cells. Multivalent phage vectors have been shown to increase the transduction efficiency compared with monovalent phage systems *(235)*. These observations have been confirmed with phages displaying single chain antibody against the HER2 receptor *(236)*. The main concern about phage vectors is the low-transduction efficiency which can be improved by certain genotoxic treatment *(237)*. However, the efficacy of this novel vector system using different preclinical models has yet to prove its applicability in more clinical models.

Phage display can also be used to alter the tropism of AAV to the vasculature *(192)*. The vector uptake is principally independent of native AAV tropism and mediated via the peptide.

4.3. Newer Concepts

4.3.1. Use of Tumor Microenvironment

An interesting, newly emerging approach tries to couple transgene expression to changes in the tumor microenvironment. The classical change of peritumoral tissue is the occurrence of hypoxia resulting from limited oxygen supply caused by the exponential cellular proliferation compared with the linear increase in the vascular supply. This universal property of human cancer can be used to achieve hypoxia-regulated expression of antiangiogenic molecules. The synthetic hypoxia-responsive element (HRE) OBHRE combines low-basal expression in normoxic conditions with high-level activated expression when the oxygen concentration is low *(238)*. The recombinant AAV containing HRE targets reporter gene expression to sites of neovascularization and results in expression that is not sustained beyond the period of active angiogenesis *(239)*. Thus, HRE-driven gene expression offers an attractive strategy for the targeted and regulated delivery of angiostatic proteins in the management of neovascular disorders including cancer.

5. CONCLUSIONS AND FUTURE CHALLENGES

Recent results from clinical studies strongly support antiangiogenic/antilymphangiogenic gene therapy in treating human malignancies. The advantage of tumor targeted gene therapy is, that it can be used across all tumor types with tolerable systemic toxicity. However, the field needs to concentrate on developing better vectors, vector delivery systems and appropriate targets for gene therapy. Extending our knowledge of ECs of blood and lymphatic origin and tumor cell interactions might help to achieve this goal.

Combining traditional treatment modalities such as radiation/chemotherapy with antiangiogenic inhibitors as well as using combinations of different antiangiogenic inhibitors may have therapeutic benefits in stopping the progression of cancer and preventing metastasis *(243,244)*. The antiangiogenic therapy can normalize tumor vasculature, improving drug delivery by pruning the immature and inefficient vessels *(245)*. This leads to the new concept to treat cancer as a chronic manageable disease with angiogenesis inhibitors. Since tumor progression depends crucially on the balance between the *in situ* tumor's total angiogenic output and an individual's total angiogenic defense, a beneficial long-term balance may be achieved *(246)*. However, in order to have long-term tumor-free survival by using antiangiogenic therapy, the factors controlling tumor neovasculature need to be systemically maintained at stable therapeutic levels.

The field of lymphangiogenesis has long been scrutinized and overshadowed by antiangiogenesis research. Increasing the understanding of lymphatic system development, lymphatic markers, and how to target vectors to lymphatic vessels could help future therapies to selectively target lymphatic vessel invasion by tumor cells without affecting the immune response nurtured from the lymphatic flow. In the future, the identification of molecules involved in the development of lymphatic system will support this task to selectively inhibit lymphangiogenesis.

In spite of these remaining challenges, the field of targeted antiangiogenesis and antilymphangiogenesis therapy is moving exceedingly fast towards its clinical application in biological tumor therapy.

REFERENCES

1. Hanahan D. A flanking attack on cancer, Nat Med 1998;4:13–14.
2. Pepper MS. Role of the matrix metalloproteinase and plasminogen activator-plasmin systems in angiogenesis, Arterioscler Thromb Vasc Biol 2001;21:1104–1117.
3. Carmeliet P, Jain RK. Angiogenesis in cancer and other diseases, Nature 2000;407:249–257.
4. Folkman J, Klagsbrun M. Angiogenic factors, Science 1987;235:442–447.
5. Ribatti D, Vacca A, Presta M. The discovery of angiogenic factors: a historical review, Gen Pharmacol 2000;35:227–231.
6. Junghans BM, Collin HB. Limbal lymphangiogenesis after corneal injury: an autoradiographic study, Curr Eye Res 1989;8:91–100.
7. He Y, Karpanen T, Alitalo K. Role of lymphangiogenic factors in tumor metastasis, Biochim Biophys Acta 2004;1654:3–12.
8. Alitalo K, Carmeliet P. Molecular mechanisms of lymphangiogenesis in health and disease, Cancer Cell 2002;1:219–227.
9. Leak LV. Electron microscopic observations on lymphatic capillaries and the structural components of the connective tissue-lymph interface, Microvasc Res 1970;2:361–391.
10. Casley-Smith JR, Florey HW. The structure of normal small lymphatics, Q J Exp Physiol Cogn Med Sci 1961;46:101–106.
11. Folkman J. Tumor angiogenesis: therapeutic implications, N Engl J Med 1971;285:1182–1186.
12. Brem S. Angiogenesis and Cancer Control: From Concept to Therapeutic Trial, Cancer Control 1999;6:436–458.
13. Kitadai Y, et al.Angiogenic switch occurs during the precancerous stage of human esophageal squamous cell carcinoma, Oncol Rep 2004;11:315–319.
14. Ravazoula P. et al. Assessment of angiogenesis in human cervical lesions, Anticancer Res 1996;16:3861–3864.
15. Fox SB, et al. Association of tumor angiogenesis with bone marrow micrometastases in breast cancer patients, J Natl Cancer Inst 1997;89:1044–1049.
16. Bikfalvi A, Han ZC. Angiogenic factors are hematopoietic growth factors and vice versa, Leukemia 1994;8:523–529.
17. Vacca A, et al. A paracrine loop in the vascular endothelial growth factor pathway triggers tumor angiogenesis and growth in multiple myeloma, Haematologica 2003;88:176–185.
18. Perez-Atayde AR, et al. Spectrum of tumor angiogenesis in the bone marrow of children with acute lymphoblastic leukemia, Am J Pathol 1997;150:815–821.
19. Rajkumar SV, Fonseca R, Witzig TE, Gertz MA, Greipp PR. Bone marrow angiogenesis in patients achieving complete response after stem cell transplantation for multiple myeloma, Leukemia 1999;13:469–472.
20. Scappaticci FA, et al. Combination angiostatin and endostatin gene transfer induces synergistic antiangiogenic activity in vitro and antitumor efficacy in leukemia and solid tumors in mice, Mol Ther 2001;3:186–196.
21. Fontaine R. [Lymphology from the early 17th century to the beginning of the 20th century. First part: Aseli to Pecquet (author's transl)], Ann Chir 1977;31:91–99.
22. Reis-Filho JS, Schmitt FC. Lymphangiogenesis in tumors: what do we know?, Microsc Res Tech 2003;60:171–180.
23. Stacker SA, Baldwin ME, Achen MG. The role of tumor lymphangiogenesis in metastatic spread, FASEB J 2002;16:922–934.
24. Yanai Y, et al. Vascular endothelial growth factor C promotes human gastric carcinoma lymph node metastasis in mice, J Exp Clin Cancer Res 2001;20:419–428.
25. Skobe M, et al. Induction of tumor lymphangiogenesis by VEGF-C promotes breast cancer metastasis, Nat Med 2001;7:192–198.
26. Skobe M, et al. Concurrent induction of lymphangiogenesis, angiogenesis, and macrophage recruitment by vascular endothelial growth factor-C in melanoma, Am J Pathol 2001; 159:893–903.
27. Kajita T, et al. The expression of vascular endothelial growth factor C and its receptors in non-small cell lung cancer, Br J Cancer 2001;85:255–260.
28. Akagi K, et al. Vascular endothelial growth factor-C (VEGF-C) expression in human colorectal cancer tissues, Br J Cancer 2000;83:887–891.

29. Schoppmann SF, Horvat R, Birner P. Lymphatic vessels and lymphangiogenesis in female cancer: mechanisms, clinical impact and possible implications for anti-lymphangiogenic therapies (Review), Oncol Rep 2002;9:455–460.
30. Tonini T, Rossi F, Claudio PP. Molecular basis of angiogenesis and cancer, Oncogene 2003;22:6549–6556.
31. Folkman J. Fundamental concepts of the angiogenic process, Curr Mol Med 2003;3:643–651.
32. Korpelainen EI, Alitalo K. Signaling angiogenesis and lymphangiogenesis, Curr Opin Cell Biol 1998;10:159–164.
33. Karkkainen MJ, Alitalo K. Lymphatic endothelial regulation, lymphoedema, and lymph node metastasis, Semin Cell Dev Biol 2002;13:9–18.
34. Ton NC, Jayson GC. Resistance to anti-VEGF agents, Curr Pharm Des 2004;10:51–64.
35. Pepper MS, Montesano R, Mandriota SJ, Orci L, Vassalli JD. Angiogenesis: a paradigm for balanced extracellular proteolysis during cell migration and morphogenesis, Enzyme Protein 1996;49:138–162.
36. Zachary I, Gliki G. Signaling transduction mechanisms mediating biological actions of the vascular endothelial growth factor family, Cardiovasc Res 2001;49:568–581.
37. Witzenbichler B, et al. Vascular endothelial growth factor-C (VEGF-C/VEGF-2) promotes angiogenesis in the setting of tissue ischemia, Am J Pathol 1998;153:381–394.
38. de Vries C, et al. The fms-like tyrosine kinase, a receptor for vascular endothelial growth factor, Science 1992;255:989–991.
39. Terman BI, et al. Identification of the KDR tyrosine kinase as a receptor for vascular endothelial cell growth factor, Biochem Biophys Res Commun 1992;187:1579–1586.
40. Pajusola K, et al. FLT4 receptor tyrosine kinase contains seven immunoglobulin-like loops and is expressed in multiple human tissues and cell lines, Cancer Res 1992;52:5738–5743.
41. Stacker SA, et al. VEGF-D promotes the metastatic spread of tumor cells via the lymphatics, Nat Med 2001;7:186–191.
42. Karkkainen MJ, et al. Vascular endothelial growth factor C is required for sprouting of the first lymphatic vessels from embryonic veins, Nat Immunol 2004;5:74–80.
43. Van Trappen PO, et al. Expression of vascular endothelial growth factor (VEGF)-C and VEGF-D, and their receptor VEGFR-3, during different stages of cervical carcinogenesis, J Pathol 2003;201:544–554.
44. Mignatti P, Rifkin DB. Plasminogen activators and matrix metalloproteinases in angiogenesis, Enzyme Protein 1996;49:117–137.
45. Kubo H, et al. Blockade of vascular endothelial growth factor receptor-3 signaling inhibits fibroblast growth factor-2-induced lymphangiogenesis in mouse cornea, Proc Natl Acad Sci U S A 2002;99: 8868–8873.
46. Joensuu H, et al. Soluble syndecan-1 and serum basic fibroblast growth factor are new prognostic factors in lung cancer, Cancer Res 2002;62:5210–5217.
47. Liekens S, De Clercq E, Neyts J. Angiogenesis: regulators and clinical applications, Biochem Pharmacol 2001;61:253–270.
48. Yancopoulos GD, et al. Vascular-specific growth factors and blood vessel formation, Nature 2000;407:242–248.
49. Carmeliet P, et al. Abnormal blood vessel development and lethality in embryos lacking a single VEGF allele, Nature 1996;380:435–439.
50. Sato TN, et al. Distinct roles of the receptor tyrosine kinases Tie-1 and Tie-2 in blood vessel formation, Nature 1995;376:70–74.
51. Suri C, et al. Requisite role of angiopoietin-1, a ligand for the TIE2 receptor, during embryonic angiogenesis, Cell 1996;87:1171–1180.
52. Gale NW, et al. Angiopoietin-2 is required for postnatal angiogenesis and lymphatic patterning, and only the latter role is rescued by Angiopoietin-1, Dev Cell 2002;3:411–423.
53. Lode HN, Wenkel J, Gaedicke G. Angiogenesis, views and news. The 93rd Annual Meeting of the American Association for Cancer Research, Expert Opin Biol Ther 2002;2:671–676.
54. Egeblad M, Werb A. New functions for the matrix metalloproteinases in cancer progression, Nat Rev Cancer 2002;2:161–174.
55. Nagakawa Y, Aoki T, Kasuya K, Tsuchida A, Koyanagi Y. Histologic features of venous invasion, expression of vascular endothelial growth factor and matrix metalloproteinase-2 and matrix metalloproteinase-9, and the relation with liver metastasis in pancreatic cancer, Pancreas 2002;24:169–178.
56. Okada M, et al. Matrix metalloproteinase-2 and matrix metalloproteinase-9 expressions correlate with the recurrence of intracranial meningiomas, J Neurooncol 2003;66:29–37.

57. Fingleton B, Vargo-Gogola T, Crawford HC, Matrisian LM. Matrilysin [MMP-7] expression selects for cells with reduced sensitivity to apoptosis, Neoplasia 2001;3:459–468.
58. Bello L, et al. Alpha(v)beta3 and alpha(v)beta5 integrin expression in meningiomas, Neurosurgery 2000;47:1185–1195.
59. Max R, et al. Immunohistochemical analysis of integrin alpha vbeta3 expression on tumor-associated vessels of human carcinomas, Int J Cancer 1997;71:320–324.
60. Ruegg C, Dormond O, Mariotti A. Endothelial cell integrins and COX-2: mediators and therapeutic targets of tumor angiogenesis, Biochim Biophys Acta 2004;1654:51–67.
61. Brooks PC, Clark RA, Cheresh DA. Requirement of vascular integrin alpha v beta 3 for angiogenesis, Science 1994;264:569–571.
62. Marshall JF, Hart IR. The role of alpha v-integrins in tumour progression and metastasis, Semin Cancer Biol 1996;7:129–138.
63. Gasparini G, et al. Vascular integrin alpha(v)beta3: a new prognostic indicator in breast cancer, Clin Cancer Res 1998;4:2625–2634.
64. Hynes RO. A reevaluation of integrins as regulators of angiogenesis, Nat Med 2002;8:918–921.
65. Kim M, et al. Hypoxia Inhibits Tumor Necrosis Factor-Related Apoptosis-Inducing Ligand-Induced Apoptosis by Blocking Bax Translocation, Cancer Res 2004;64:4078–4081.
66. Stone HB, Brown JM, Phillips TL, Sutherland RM. Oxygen in human tumors: correlations between methods of measurement and response to therapy. Summary of a workshop held November 19–20, 1992, at the National Cancer Institute, Bethesda, Maryland, Radiat Res 1993;136:422–434.
67. Ryan HE, Lo J, Johnson RS. HIF-1 alpha is required for solid tumor formation and embryonic vascularization, EMBO J 1998;17:3005–3015.
68. Shi YH, Fang WG. Hypoxia-inducible factor-1 in tumour angiogenesis, World J Gastroenterol 2004;10:1082–1087.
69. Bos R, et al. Levels of hypoxia-inducible factor-1 alpha during breast carcinogenesis, J Natl Cancer Inst 2001;93:309–314.
70. Aebersold DM, et al. Expression of hypoxia-inducible factor-1alpha: a novel predictive and prognostic parameter in the radiotherapy of oropharyngeal cancer, Cancer Res 2001;61:2911–2916.
71. Semenza G. Signal transduction to hypoxia-inducible factor 1, Biochem Pharmacol 2002;64:993–998.
72. Wigle JT, Oliver G. Prox1 function is required for the development of the murine lymphatic system, Cell 1999;98:769–778.
73. Hong YK, et al. Prox1 is a master control gene in the program specifying lymphatic endothelial cell fate, Dev Dyn 2002;225:351–357.
74. Schacht V, et al. T1alpha/podoplanin deficiency disrupts normal lymphatic vasculature formation and causes lymphedema, EMBO J 2003;22:3546–3556.
75. Stacker SA, Hughes RA, Achen MG. Molecular targeting of lymphatics for therapy, Curr Pharm Des 2004;10:65–74.
76. Yuan L, et al. Abnormal lymphatic vessel development in neuropilin 2 mutant mice, Development 2002;129:4797–4806.
77. Huang XZ, et al. Fatal bilateral chylothorax in mice lacking the integrin alpha9beta1, Mol Cell Biol 2000;20:5208–5215.
78. Scavelli X, Vacca A, Di Pietro G, Dammacco FRibatti D. Crosstalk between angiogenesis and lymphangiogenesis in tumor progression, Leukemia 2004;18:1054–1058.
79. Nagy JA, et al. Vascular permeability factor/vascular endothelial growth factor induces lymphangiogenesis as well as angiogenesis, J Exp Med 2002;196:1497–1506.
80. Hamada K, et al. VEGF-C signaling pathways through VEGFR-2 and VEGFR-3 in vasculoangiogenesis and hematopoiesis, Blood 2000;96:3793–3800.
81. Dumont DJ, et al. Cardiovascular failure in mouse embryos deficient in VEGF receptor-3, Science 1998;282:946–949.
82. Kubo H, et al. Involvement of vascular endothelial growth factor receptor-3 in maintenance of integrity of endothelial cell lining during tumor angiogenesis, Blood 2000;96:546–553.
83. Byzova TV, et al. Adenovirus encoding vascular endothelial growth factor-D induces tissue-specific vascular patterns in vivo, Blood 2002;99:4434–4442.
84. 84 Folkman J. Antiangiogenic gene therapy, Proc Natl Acad Sci U S A 1998;95:9064–9066.
85. Thomas CE, Ehrhardt A, Kay MA. Progress and problems with the use of viral vectors for gene therapy, Nat Rev Genet 2003;4:346–358.
86. Larocca D, et al. Evolving phage vectors for cell targeted gene delivery, Curr Pharm Biotechnol 2002;3:45–57.

87. Cavazzana-Calvo M, Thrasher A, Mavilio F. The future of gene therapy, Nature 2004;427:779–781.
88. Jain RK. Tumor angiogenesis and accessibility: role of vascular endothelial growth factor, Semin Oncol 2002;29:3–9.
89. Im SA, et al. Inhibition of breast cancer growth in vivo by antiangiogenesis gene therapy with adenovirus-mediated antisense-VEGF, Br J Cancer 2001;84:1252–1257.
90. Shi W, Siemann DW. Simultaneous targeting of VEGF message and VEGF receptor signaling as a therapeutic anticancer approach, Anticancer Res 2004;24:213–218.
91. Lin P, et al. Inhibition of tumor growth by targeting tumor endothelium using a soluble vascular endothelial growth factor receptor, Cell Growth Differ 1998;9:49–58.
92. Goldman CK, et al. Paracrine expression of a native soluble vascular endothelial growth factor receptor inhibits tumor growth, metastasis, and mortality rate, Proc Natl Acad Sci U S A 1998;95: 8795–8800.
93. Kou B, et al. In vivo inhibition of tumor angiogenesis by a soluble VEGFR-2 fragment, Exp Mol Pathol 2004;76:129–137.
94. Becker CM, et al. Gene therapy of prostate cancer with the soluble vascular endothelial growth factor receptor Flk1, Cancer Biol Ther 2002;1:548–553.
95. Ye C, et al. sFlt-1 gene therapy of follicular thyroid carcinoma, Endocrinology 2004;145:817–822.
96. Achen MG, et al. Monoclonal antibodies to vascular endothelial growth factor-D block its interactions with both VEGF receptor-2 and VEGF receptor-3, Eur J Biochem 2000;267:2505–2515.
97. Makinen T, et al. Inhibition of lymphangiogenesis with resulting lymphedema in transgenic mice expressing soluble VEGF receptor-3, Nat Med 2001;7:199–205.
98. He Y, et al. Suppression of tumor lymphangiogenesis and lymph node metastasis by blocking vascular endothelial growth factor receptor 3 signaling, J Natl Cancer Inst 2002;94:819–825.
99. Krishnan J, et al. Differential in vivo and in vitro expression of vascular endothelial growth factor (VEGF)-C and VEGF-D in tumors and its relationship to lymphatic metastasis in immunocompetent rats, Cancer Res 2003;63:713–722.
100. Karpanen T, et al. Vascular endothelial growth factor C promotes tumor lymphangiogenesis and intralymphatic tumor growth, Cancer Res 2001;61:1786–1790.
101. Shimizu K, et al. Suppression of VEGFR-3 signaling inhibits lymph node metastasis in gastric cancer, Cancer Sci 2004;95:328–333.
102. Lin P, et al. Inhibition of tumor angiogenesis using a soluble receptor establishes a role for Tie2 in pathologic vascular growth, J Clin Invest 1997;100:2072–2078.
103. Lin P, et al. Antiangiogenic gene therapy targeting the endothelium-specific receptor tyrosine kinase Tie2, Proc Natl Acad Sci U S A 1998;95:8829–8834.
104. Hangai M, et al. Systemically expressed soluble Tie2 inhibits intraocular neovascularization, Hum Gene Ther 2001;12:1311–1321.
105. O'Reilly MS, et al. Endostatin: an endogenous inhibitor of angiogenesis and tumor growth, Cell 1997;88:277–285.
106. Hajitou A, et al. The antitumoral effect of endostatin and angiostatin is associated with a down-regulation of vascular endothelial growth factor expression in tumor cells, FASEB J 2002;16: 1802–1804.
107. Kim YM, et al. Endostatin blocks vascular endothelial growth factor-mediated signaling via direct interaction with KDR/Flk-1, J Biol Chem 2002;277:27,872–27,879.
108. Kim YM, et al. Endostatin inhibits endothelial and tumor cellular invasion by blocking the activation and catalytic activity of matrix metalloproteinase, Cancer Res 2000;60:5410–5413.
109. Hanai J, et al. Endostatin causes G1 arrest of endothelial cells through inhibition of cyclin D1, J Biol Chem 2002;277:16,464–16,469.
110. Shichiri M, Hirata Y. Antiangiogenesis signals by endostatin, FASEB J 2001;15:1044–1053.
111. Abdollahi A, et al. Endostatin's antiangiogenic signaling network, Mol Cell 2004;13:649–663.
112. Sudhakar A, et al. Human tumstatin and human endostatin exhibit distinct antiangiogenic activities mediated by alpha v beta 3 and alpha 5 beta 1 integrins, Proc Natl Acad Sci U S A 2003;100: 4766–4771.
113. Dkhissi F, et al. Endostatin exhibits a direct antitumor effect in addition to its antiangiogenic activity in colon cancer cells, Hum Gene Ther 2003;14:997–1008.
114. Feldman AL, et al. Antiangiogenic gene therapy of cancer utilizing a recombinant adenovirus to elevate systemic endostatin levels in mice, Cancer Res 2000;60:1503–1506.
115. Feldman AL, et al. Effect of retroviral endostatin gene transfer on subcutaneous and intraperitoneal growth of murine tumors, J Natl Cancer Inst 2001;93:1014–1020.

116. Hampl M, et al. Therapeutic effects of viral vector-mediated antiangiogenic gene transfer in malignant ascites, Hum Gene Ther 2001;12:1713–1729.
117. Shichinohe T, et al. Development of lentiviral vectors for antiangiogenic gene delivery, Cancer Gene Ther 2001;8:879–889.
118. Ingber D, et al. Synthetic analogues of fumagillin that inhibit angiogenesis and suppress tumour growth, Nature 1990;348:555–557.
119. Sin N, et al. The anti-angiogenic agent fumagillin covalently binds and inhibits the methionine aminopeptidase, MetAP-2, Proc Natl Acad Sci U S A 1997;94:6099–6103.
120. Pyun HJ, et al. Investigation of novel fumagillin analogues as angiogenesis inhibitors, Bioorg Med Chem Lett 2004;14:91–94.
121. Landuyt W, et al. Effect of TNP-470 (AGM-1470) on the growth of rat rhabdomyosarcoma tumors of different sizes, Cancer Invest 2001;19:35–40.
122. Kawano T, Yanoma S, Nishimura G, Tsukuda M. The inhibitory effects of TNP470 on tumour growth of head and neck carcinoma cell producing interleukin-8, J Laryngol Otol 2001;115:802–807.
123. Emoto M, Ishiguro M. Iwasaki H, Kikuchi M, Kawarabayashi T. Effect of angiogenesis inhibitor TNP-470 on the growth, blood flow, and microvessel density in xenografts of human uterine carcinosarcoma in nude mice, Gynecol Oncol 2003;89:88–94.
124. Kong HL, Crystal RG. Gene therapy strategies for tumor antiangiogenesis, J Natl Cancer Inst 1998;90:273–286.
125. Sengupta K, Banerjee S, Saxena NK, Banerjee SK. Thombospondin-1 disrupts estrogen-induced endothelial cell proliferation and migration and its expression is suppressed by estradiol, Mol Cancer Res 2004;2:150–158.
126. Lawler J. The structural and functional properties of thrombospondin, Blood 1986;67:1197–1209.
127. Chen H, Herndon ME, Lawler J. The cell biology of thrombospondin-1, Matrix Biol 2000;19: 597–614.
128. Zabrenetzky V, Harris CC, Steeg PS, Roberts DD. Expression of the extracellular matrix molecule thrombospondin inversely correlates with malignant progression in melanoma, lung and breast carcinoma cell lines, Int J Cancer 1994;59:191–195.
129. Streit M, et al. Overexpression of thrombospondin-1 decreases angiogenesis and inhibits the growth of human cutaneous squamous cell carcinomas, Am J Pathol 1999;155:441–452.
130. Liu P, et al. Adenovirus-mediated gene therapy with an antiangiogenic fragment of thrombospondin-1 inhibits human leukemia xenograft growth in nude mice, Leuk Res 2003;27:701–708.
131. Harada H, et al. Introduction of wild-type p53 enhances thrombospondin-1 expression in human glioma cells, Cancer Lett 2003;191:109–119.
132. Dameron KM, Volpert OV, Tainsky MA, Bouck N. Control of angiogenesis in fibroblasts by p53 regulation of thrombospondin-1, Science 1994;265:1582–1584.
133. Gomez DE, Alonso DF, Yoshiji H, Thorgeirsson UP. Tissue inhibitors of metalloproteinases: structure, regulation and biological functions, Eur J Cell Biol 1997;74:111–122.
134. Ring P, Johansson K, Hoyhtya M, Rubin K, Lindmark G. Expression of tissue inhibitor of metalloproteinases TIMP-2 in human colorectal cancer—a predictor of tumour stage, Br J Cancer 1997;76:805–811.
135. Imren S, Kohn DB, Shimada H, Blavier L, DeClerck YA. Overexpression of tissue inhibitor of metalloproteinases-2 retroviral-mediated gene transfer in vivo inhibits tumor growth and invasion, Cancer Res 1996;56:2891–2895.
136. Ahn SM, Jeong SJ, Kim YS, Sohn Y, Moon A. Retroviral delivery of TIMP-2 inhibits H-ras-induced migration and invasion in MCF10A human breast epithelial cells, Cancer Lett 2004;207:49–57.
137. Li H, et al. AdTIMP-2 inhibits tumor growth, angiogenesis, and metastasis, and prolongs survival in mice, Hum Gene Ther 2001;12:515–526.
138. Griscelli F, et al. Angiostatin gene transfer: inhibition of tumor growth in vivo by blockage of endothelial cell proliferation associated with a mitosis arrest, Proc Natl Acad Sci U S A 1998;95:6367–6372.
139. Ma HI, et al. Intratumoral gene therapy of malignant brain tumor in a rat model with angiostatin delivered by adeno-associated viral (AAV) vector, Gene Ther 2002;9:2–11.
140. Lalani AS, et al. Anti-tumor efficacy of human angiostatin using liver-mediated adeno-associated virus gene therapy, Mol Ther 2004;9:56–66.
141. Bikfalvi A, Gimenez-Gallego G. The control of angiogenesis and tumor invasion by platelet factor-4 and platelet factor-4-derived molecules, Semin Thromb Hemost 2004;30:137–144.
142. Belman N, Bonnem EM, Harvey HA, Lipton A. Phase I trial of recombinant platelet factor 4 (rPF4) in patients with advanced colorectal carcinoma, Invest New Drugs 1996;14:387–389.

143. Tanaka T, Manome Y, Wen P, Kufe DW, Fin HA. Viral vector-mediated transduction of a modified platelet factor 4 cDNA inhibits angiogenesis and tumor growth, Nat Med 1997;3:437–442.
144. Li Y, et al. Suppression of tumor growth by viral vector-mediated gene transfer of N-terminal truncated platelet factor 4, Cancer Biother Radiopharm 2003;18:829–840.
145. Kamphaus GD, et al. Canstatin, a novel matrix-derived inhibitor of angiogenesis and tumor growth, J Biol Chem 2000;275:1209–1215.
146. Hamano Y, et al. Physiological levels of tumstatin, a fragment of collagen IV alpha3 chain, are generated by MMP-9 proteolysis and suppress angiogenesis via alphaV beta3 integrin, Cancer Cell 2003;3:589–601.
147. Panka DJ, Mier JW. Canstatin inhibits Akt activation and induces Fas-dependent apoptosis in endothelial cells, J Biol Chem 2003;278:37,632–37,636.
148. Friedl J, et al. Induction of permeability across endothelial cell monolayers by tumor necrosis factor (TNF) occurs via a tissue factor-dependent mechanism: relationship between the procoagulant and permeability effects of TNF, Blood 2002;100:1334–1339.
149. Fajardo LF, Kwan HH, Kowalski J, Prionas SD, Allison AC. Dual role of tumor necrosis factor-alpha in angiogenesis, Am J Pathol 1992;140:539–544.
150. Lejeune FJ, Ruegg C, Lienard D. Clinical applications of TNF-alpha in cancer, Curr Opin Immunol 1998;10:573–580.
151. Kayton ML, Libutti SK. Endothelial monocyte activating polypeptide II (EMAP II) enhances the effect of TNF on tumor-associated vasculature, Curr Opin Investig Drugs 2001;2:136–138.
152. Feldman ED, et al. Treatment of patients with unresectable primary hepatic malignancies using hyperthermic isolated hepatic perfusion, J Gastrointest Surg 2004;8:200–207.
153. Lans TE, et al. Improved antitumor response to isolated limb perfusion with tumor necrosis factor after upregulation of endothelial monocyte-activating polypeptide II in soft tissue sarcoma, Ann Surg Oncol 2002;9:812–819.
154. Thom AK, et al. Cytokine levels and systemic toxicity in patients undergoing isolated limb perfusion with high-dose tumor necrosis factor, interferon gamma, and melphalan, J Clin Oncol 1995;13:264–273.
155. Marr RA, Hitt M, Muller WJ, Gauldie J, Graham FL. Tumour therapy in mice using adenovirus vectors expressing human TNFa, Int J Oncol 1998;12:509–515.
156. Wright P, et al. Adenovirus-mediated TNF-alpha gene transfer induces significant tumor regression in mice, Cancer Biother Radiopharm 1999;14:49–57.
157. Saharinen P, Alitalo K. Double target for tumor mass destruction, J Clin Invest 2003;111:1277–1280.
158. Benjamin LE, Hemo I, Keshet E. A plasticity window for blood vessel remodelling is defined by pericyte coverage of the preformed endothelial network and is regulated by PDGF-B and VEGF, Development 1998;125:1591–1598.
159. Hellstrom M, Kalen M, Lindahl P, Abramsson A, Betsholtz C. Role of PDGF-B and PDGFR-beta in recruitment of vascular smooth muscle cells and pericytes during embryonic blood vessel formation in the mouse, Development 1999;126:3047–3055.
160. Jain RK, Munn LL, Fukumura D. Dissecting tumour pathophysiology using intravital microscopy, Nat Rev Cancer 2002;2:266–276.
161. St Croix B, et al. Genes expressed in human tumor endothelium, Science 2000;289:1197–1202.
162. Morikawa S, et al. Abnormalities in pericytes on blood vessels and endothelial sprouts in tumors, Am J Pathol 2002;160:985–1000.
163. Bergers G, Song S, Meyer-Morse N, Bergsland E, Hanahan D. Benefits of targeting both pericytes and endothelial cells in the tumor vasculature with kinase inhibitors, J Clin Invest 2003;111:1287–1295.
164. Taverna D, et al. Increased primary tumor growth in mice null for beta3- or beta3/beta5-integrins or selectins, Proc Natl Acad Sci U S A 2004;101:763–768.
165. Klauber N, Rohan RM, Flynn E, D'Amato RJ. Critical components of the female reproductive pathway are suppressed by the angiogenesis inhibitor AGM-1470, Nat Med 1997;3:443–446.
166. Sedlacek HH. Pharmacological aspects of targeting cancer gene therapy to endothelial cells, Crit Rev Oncol Hematol 2001;37:169–215.
167. Wagner E, Kircheis R, Walker GF. Targeted nucleic acid delivery into tumors: new avenues for cancer therapy, Biomed Pharmacother 2004;58:152–161.
168. Zhu ZB, et al. Transcriptional targeting of adenoviral vector through the CXCR4 tumor-specific promoter, Gene Ther 2004;11:645–648.
169. Dormond O, Bezzi M, Mariotti A, Ruegg C. Prostaglandin E2 promotes integrin alpha Vbeta 3-dependent endothelial cell adhesion, rac-activation, and spreading through cAMP/PKA-dependent signaling, J Biol Chem 2002;277:45,838–45,846.

170. Godbey WT, Atala A. Directed apoptosis in Cox-2-overexpressing cancer cells through expression-targeted gene delivery, Gene Ther 2003;10:1519-1527.
171. Zhu ZB, et al. Transcriptional targeting of tumors with a novel tumor-specific survivin promoter, Cancer Gene Ther 2004;11:256–262.
172. Yanagisawa M, Kurihara H, Kimura S, Goto K, Masaki, T. A novel peptide vasoconstrictor, endothelin, is produced by vascular endothelium and modulates smooth muscle Ca2+ channels, J Hypertens 1988;6:S188–S191.
173. Hu J, Discher DJ, Bishopric NH, Webster KA. Hypoxia regulates expression of the endothelin-1 gene through a proximal hypoxia-inducible factor-1 binding site on the antisense strand, Biochem Biophys Res Commun 1998;245:894–899.
174. Greenberger S, et al. Transcription-controlled gene therapy against tumor angiogenesis, J Clin Invest 2004;113:1017–1024.
175. Savontaus MJ, Sauter BV, Huang TG, Woo SL. Transcriptional targeting of conditionally replicating adenovirus to dividing endothelial cells, Gene Ther 2002;9:972–979.
176. Hallahan DE, et al. Spatial and temporal control of gene therapy using ionizing radiation, Nat Med 1995;1:786–791.
177. Walther W, Stein U. Cell type specific and inducible promoters for vectors in gene therapy as an approach for cell targeting, J Mol Med 1996;74:379–392.
178. Buning H, et al. Receptor targeting of adeno-associated virus vectors, Gene Ther 2003;10: 1142–1151.
179. Nakamura T, Sato K, Hamada H. Effective gene transfer to human melanomas via integrin-targeted adenoviral vectors, Hum Gene Ther 2002;13:613–626.
180. Miller AD. Cell-surface receptors for retroviruses and implications for gene transfer, Proc Natl Acad Sci U S A 1996;93:11,407–11,413.
181. Bartlett JS, Kleinschmidt J, Boucher RC, Samulski RJ. Targeted adeno-associated virus vector transduction of nonpermissive cells mediated by a bispecific F(ab'gamma)2 antibody, Nat Biotechnol 1999;17:181–186.
182. Everts M, et al. Selective intracellular delivery of dexamethasone into activated endothelial cells using an E-selectin-directed immunoconjugate, J Immunol 2002;168:883–889.
183. Reynolds PN, et al. Combined transductional and transcriptional targeting improves the specificity of transgene expression in vivo, Nat Biotechnol 2001;19:838–842.
184. Niidome T, Huang L. Gene therapy progress and prospects: nonviral vectors, Gene Ther 2002;9: 1647–1652.
185. Pasqualini R, Koivunen E, Ruoslahti E. A peptide isolated from phage display libraries is a structural and functional mimic of an RGD-binding site on integrins, J Cell Biol 1995;130:1189–1196.
186. Fairbrother WJ, et al. Novel peptides selected to bind vascular endothelial growth factor target the receptor-binding site, Biochemistry 1998;37:17,754–17,764.
187. Wu J, et al. [Development of toxin targeting to VEGF-KDR], Zhonghua Zhong Liu Za Zhi 2004;26: 78–81.
188. Binetruy-Tournaire R, et al. Identification of a peptide blocking vascular endothelial growth factor (VEGF)-mediated angiogenesis, EMBO J 2000;19:1525-1533.
189. Hetian L, et al. A novel peptide isolated from a phage display library inhibits tumor growth and metastasis by blocking the binding of vascular endothelial growth factor to its kinase domain receptor, J Biol Chem 2002;277:43,137–43,142.
190. Curnis F, et al. Enhancement of tumor necrosis factor alpha antitumor immunotherapeutic properties by targeted delivery to aminopeptidase N (CD13), Nat Biotechnol 2000;18:1185–1190.
191. Curnis F, Gasparri A, Sacchi A, Longhi R, Corti A. Coupling tumor necrosis factor-alpha with alphaV integrin ligands improves its antineoplastic activity, Cancer Res 2004;64:565–571.
192. White SJ, et al. Targeted gene delivery to vascular tissue in vivo by tropism-modified adeno-associated virus vectors, Circulation 2004;109:513–519.
193. Clark M. Antibody humanization: a case of the 'Emperor's new clothes'?, Immunol Today 2000;21: 397–402.
194. Volkel T, Muller R, Kontermann RE. Isolation of endothelial cell-specific human antibodies from a novel fully synthetic scFv library, Biochem Biophys Res Commun 2004;317:515–521.
195. Miller DW, et al. Elevated expression of endoglin, a component of the TGF-beta-receptor complex, correlates with proliferation of tumor endothelial cells, Int J Cancer 1999;81:568–572.
196. Seon BK, Matsuno F, Haruta Y, Kondo M, Barcos M. Long-lasting complete inhibition of human solid tumors in SCID mice by targeting endothelial cells of tumor vasculature with antihuman endoglin immunotoxin, Clin Cancer Res 1997;3:1031–1044.

197. Tabata M, Kondo M, Haruta Y, Seon BK. Antiangiogenic radioimmunotherapy of human solid tumors in SCID mice using (125)I-labeled anti-endoglin monoclonal antibodies, Int J Cancer 1999;82:737–742.
198. Tan PH, et al. Antibody targeted gene transfer to endothelium, J Gene Med 2003;5:311–323.
199. Im SA, et al. Antiangiogenesis treatment for gliomas: transfer of antisense-vascular endothelial growth factor inhibits tumor growth in vivo, Cancer Res 1999;59:895–900.
200. Marchand GS, Noiseux N, Tanguay JF, Sirois MG. Blockade of in vivo VEGF-mediated angiogenesis by antisense gene therapy: role of Flk-1 and Flt-1 receptors, Am J Physiol Heart Circ Physiol 2002;282:H194–H204.
201. Shim WS, Teh M, Mack PO, Ge R. Inhibition of angiopoietin-1 expression in tumor cells by an antisense RNA approach inhibited xenograft tumor growth in immunodeficient mice, Int J Cancer 2001;94:6–15.
202. Dallabrida SM, De Sousa MA, Farrell DH. Expression of antisense to integrin subunit beta 3 inhibits microvascular endothelial cell capillary tube formation in fibrin, J Biol Chem 2000;275:32,281–32,288.
203. Lipscomb EA, Dugan AS, Rabinovitz I, Mercurio AM. Use of RNA interference to inhibit integrin (alpha6beta4)-mediated invasion and migration of breast carcinoma cells, Clin Exp Metastasis 2003;20:569–576.
204. Yang G, Cai KQ, Thompson-Lanza JA, Bast RC, Jr, Liu J. Inhibition of breast and ovarian tumor growth through multiple signaling pathways by using retrovirus-mediated small interfering RNA against Her-2/neu gene expression, J Biol Chem 2004;279:4339–4345.
205. Zhang L, Yang N, Mohamed-Hadley A, Rubin SC, Coukos G. Vector-based RNAi, a novel tool for isoform-specific knock-down of VEGF and anti-angiogenesis gene therapy of cancer, Biochem Biophys Res Commun 2003;303:1169–1178.
206. Rubinson DA, et al. A lentivirus-based system to functionally silence genes in primary mammalian cells, stem cells and transgenic mice by RNA interference, Nat Genet 2003;33:401–406.
207. Hemann MT, et al. An epi-allelic series of p53 hypomorphs created by stable RNAi produces distinct tumor phenotypes in vivo, Nat Genet 2003;33:396–400.
208. Hasuwa H, Kaseda K, Einarsdottir T, Okabe M. Small interfering RNA and gene silencing in transgenic mice and rats, FEBS Lett 2002;532:227–230.
209. Thurston G, et al. Cationic liposomes target angiogenic endothelial cells in tumors and chronic inflammation in mice, J Clin Invest 1998;101:1401–1413.
210. Strieth S, et al. Neovascular targeting chemotherapy: Encapsulation of paclitaxel in cationic liposomes impairs functional tumor microvasculature, Int J Cancer 2004;110:117–124.
211. Schmitt-Sody M, et al. Neovascular targeting therapy: paclitaxel encapsulated in cationic liposomes improves antitumoral efficacy, Clin Cancer Res 2003;9:2335–2341.
212. Blezinger P, et al. Intravenous delivery of an endostatin gene complexed in cationic lipid inhibits systemic angiogenesis and tumor growth in murine models, Angiogenesis 1999;3:205–210.
213. Marty C, et al. Cytotoxic targeting of F9 teratocarcinoma tumours with anti-ED-B fibronectin scFv antibody modified liposomes, Br J Cancer 2002;87:106–112.
214. Kondo M, et al. Anti-neovascular therapy by liposomal drug targeted to membrane type-1 matrix metalloproteinase, Int J Cancer 108 (2004) 301–306.
215. Janssen AP, et al. Peptide-targeted PEG-liposomes in anti-angiogenic therapy, Int J Pharm 2003;254:55–58.
216. Pastorino F, et al. Vascular damage and anti-angiogenic effects of tumor vessel-targeted liposomal chemotherapy, Cancer Res 2003;63:7400–7409.
217. Panyam J, Labhasetwar V. Biodegradable nanoparticles for drug and gene delivery to cells and tissue, Adv Drug Deliv Rev 2003;55:329–347.
218. Moghimi SM, Hunter AC, Murray JC. Long-circulating and target-specific nanoparticles: theory to practice, Pharmacol Rev 2001;53:283–318.
219. Luo D, Saltzman WM. Enhancement of transfection by physical concentration of DNA at the cell surface, Nat Biotechnol 2000;18:893–895.
220. Luo S, Han E, Belcheva N, Saltzman WM. A self-assembled, modular DNA delivery system mediated by silica nanoparticles, J Control Release 2004;95:333–341.
221. Hood JD, et al. Tumor regression by targeted gene delivery to the neovasculature, Science 2002;296:2404–2407.
222. Li L, et al. A novel antiangiogenesis therapy using an integrin antagonist or anti-Flk-1 antibody coated 90Y-labeled nanoparticles, Int J Radiat Oncol Biol Phys 2004;58:1215–1227.
223. Chan WC, et al. Luminescent quantum dots for multiplexed biological detection and imaging, Curr Opin Biotechnol 2002;13:40–46.

224. Porkka K, Laakkonen P, Hoffman JA, Bernasconi M, Ruoslahti E. A fragment of the HMGN2 protein homes to the nuclei of tumor cells and tumor endothelial cells in vivo, Proc Natl Acad Sci U S A 2002;99:7444–7449.
225. Laakkonen P, Porkka K, Hoffman JA, Ruoslahti, E. A tumor-homing peptide with a targeting specificity related to lymphatic vessels, Nat Med 2002;8:751–755.
226. Akerman ME, Chan WC, Laakkonen P, Bhatia SN, Ruoslahti E. Nanocrystal targeting in vivo, Proc Natl Acad Sci U S A 2002;99:12,617–12,621.
227. Jin N, Chen W, Blazar BR, Ramakrishnan S, Vallera DA. Gene therapy of murine solid tumors with T cells transduced with a retroviral vascular endothelial growth factor—immunotoxin target gene, Hum Gene Ther 2002;13:497–508.
228. Okada Y, et al. Tumor Necrosis Factor alpha-Gene Therapy for an Established Murine Melanoma Using RGD (Arg-Gly-Asp) Fiber-mutant Adenovirus Vectors, Jpn J Cancer Res 2002;93: 436–444.
229. Bilbao G, et al. Genetically modified adenovirus vector containing an RGD peptide in the HI loop of the fiber knob improves gene transfer to nonhuman primate isolated pancreatic islets, Am J Transplant 2002;2:237–243.
230. Rasmussen H, et al. TNFerade Biologic: preclinical toxicology of a novel adenovector with a radiation-inducible promoter, carrying the human tumor necrosis factor alpha gene, Cancer Gene Ther 2002;9:951–957.
231. Senzer N, et al. TNFerade biologic, an adenovector with a radiation-inducible promoter, carrying the human tumor necrosis factor alpha gene: a phase I study in patients with solid tumors, J Clin Oncol 2004;22:592–601.
232. Ponnazhagan S, et al. Adeno-associated virus 2-mediated antiangiogenic cancer gene therapy: long-term efficacy of a vector encoding angiostatin and endostatin over vectors encoding a single factor, Cancer Res 2004;64:1781–1787.
233. Masood R, et al. Retroviral vectors bearing IgG-binding motifs for antibody-mediated targeting of vascular endothelial growth factor receptors, Int J Mol Med 2001;8:335–343.
234. Larocca S, Witte A, Johnson W, Pierce GF, Baird A. Targeting bacteriophage to mammalian cell surface receptors for gene delivery, Hum Gene Ther 1998;9:2393–2399.
235. Larocca D, Jensen-Pergakes K, Burg MA, Baird A. Receptor-targeted gene delivery using multivalent phagemid particles, Mol Ther 2001;3:476–484.
236. Poul MA, Marks JD. Targeted gene delivery to mammalian cells by filamentous bacteriophage, J Mol Biol 1999;288:203–211.
237. Burg MA, et al. Enhanced phagemid particle gene transfer in camptothecin-treated carcinoma cells, Cancer Res 2002;62:977–981.
238. Boast K, et al. Characterization of physiologically regulated vectors for the treatment of ischemic disease, Hum Gene Ther 1999;10:2197–2208.
239. Bainbridge JW, et al. Hypoxia-regulated transgene expression in experimental retinal and choroidal neovascularization, Gene Ther 2003;10:1049–1054.
240. Kerbel RS, Kamen BA. The anti-angiogenic basis of metronomic chemotherapy, Nat Rev Cancer 2004;4:423–436.
241. Vacca A, et al. Docetaxel versus paclitaxel for antiangiogenesis, J Hematother Stem Cell Res 2002;11:103–118.
242. Kruczynski A, Hill BT. Vinflunine, the latest Vinca alkaloid in clinical development. A review of its preclinical anticancer properties, Crit Rev Oncol Hematol 2001;40:159–173.
243. Emanuel S, et al. A VEGF-R2 kinase inhibitor potentiates the activity of the conventional chemotherapeutic agents paclitaxel and doxorubicin in tumor xenograft models, Mol Pharmacol 2004; 66:635–647.
244. Emmenegger U, et al. A comparative analysis of low-dose metronomic cyclophosphamide reveals absent or low-grade toxicity on tissues highly sensitive to the toxic effects of maximum tolerated dose regimens, Cancer Res 2004;64:3994–4000.
245. Jain RK. Normalizing tumor vasculature with anti-angiogenic therapy: a new paradigm for combination therapy, Nat Med 2001;7:987–989.
246. Folkman J, Kalluri R. Cancer without disease, Nature 2004;427:787.
247. Mousa SA, Mousa AS. Angiogenesis inhibitors: current & future directions, Curr Pharm Des 2004;10:1–9.
248. Barnett FH, et al. Intra-arterial delivery of endostatin gene to brain tumors prolongs survival and alters tumor vessel ultrastructure, Gene Ther 2004;11:1283–1289.

249. Nakashima Y, et al. Endostatin gene therapy on murine lung metastases model utilizing cationic vector-mediated intravenous gene delivery, Gene Ther 2003;10:123–130.
250. Jia S, Zhu F, Li H, He F, Xiu R. Anticancer treatment of endostatin gene therapy by targeting tumor neovasculature in C57/BL mice, Clin Hemorheol Microcirc 23 2000;23:251-257.
251. Wang X, Liu F, Li X, Li J, Xu G. Anti-tumor effect of human endostatin mediated by retroviral gene transfer in nude mice, Chin Med J (Engl) 2002;115:1664–1669.
252. Shi W, Teschendorf C, Muzyczka N, Siemann DW. Adeno-associated virus-mediated gene transfer of endostatin inhibits angiogenesis and tumor growth in vivo, Cancer Gene Ther 2002;9:513–521.
253. Ma HI, et al. Suppression of intracranial human glioma growth after intramuscular administration of an adeno-associated viral vector expressing angiostatin, Cancer Res 2002;62:756–763.
254. Jin RJ, et al. The application of an anti-angiogenic gene (thrombospondin-1) in the treatment of human prostate cancer xenografts, Cancer Gene Ther 2000;7:1537–1542.
255. He GA, Luo JX, Zhang TY, Wang FY, Li RF. Canstatin-N fragment inhibits in vitro endothelial cell proliferation and suppresses in vivo tumor growth, Biochem Biophys Res Commun 2003; 312:801–805.

19 Tumor-Specific Replicating Adenoviruses

Δ 24 for Human Gliomas

Giacomo G. Vecil, MD, *Juan Fueyo*, MD, *and Frederick F. Lang*, MD

CONTENTS

Summary

Recent advances in the fundamental understanding of brain tumor biology have suggested that exploiting the molecular pathways underlying gliomagenesis may provide novel molecularly based approaches to brain tumor treatment. One such molecular approach is the application of replication-competent viruses as therapeutic agents for gliomas. With this approach, the capacity of viruses to infect, replicate within, and lyse cells is exploited to therapeutic advantage (oncolysis). In this context, by deleting 24 base pairs from the E1A gene, our group developed a conditionally replication-competent adenovirus, Δ24. Because the mutant E1A protein is unable to bind Rb (the critical protein involved in regulating entry into the cell cycle), Δ 24 selectively replicates in tumor cells, but not in normal cells with intact Rb. This chapter reviews the biology and therapeutic effects of Δ 24, and outlines modifications to this virus that have resulted in second-generation Δ 24 constructs that display increased tumor cell selectivity (Δ 24-RGD), reduced normal cell toxicity (CB1), and augmented tumoricidal capacity (Δ 24-CD and Δ 24-p53).

Key Words: Adenovirus; Δ 24; E1A; E1B; gene therapy; oncolysis; replication-competent; vector.

1. INTRODUCTION

Brain tumors are a significant therapeutic challenge. Despite advances in neurosurgical techniques, improvements in radiation therapy, and the addition of new chemotherapeutic agents, there has been little change over the last forty years in the outcome of patients with malignant glioma, particularly glioblastoma multiforme (GBM), the most common adult primary tumor. Indeed, the median survival time of

From: *Cancer Drug Discovery and Development: Gene Therapy for Cancer*
Edited by: K. K. Hunt, S. A. Vorburger, and S. G. Swisher © Humana Press Inc., Totowa, NJ

patients with GBM remains at less than 2 years *(1,2)*. However, recent advances in the fundamental understanding of brain tumor biology have suggested that exploiting the molecular pathways underlying gliomagenesis may provide alternative molecularly based approaches to brain tumor treatment.

One such molecular approach is the application of replication-competent viruses as therapeutic agents for gliomas. With this approach, the capacity of viruses to infect, replicate within, and lyse cells is exploited to therapeutic advantage (oncolysis) *(3–5)*. Although oncolytic viruses have been developed for a variety of viral types, including herpes simplex virus (HSV) *(6)*, influenza virus *(7)*, Newcastle disease virus *(8)*, poliovirus *(9)*, reovirus *(10)*, vaccinia virus *(11)*, and vesicular stomatitis virus *(12)*, adenoviruses have been particularly applicable to viral-based tumor therapy because they are minimally pathogenic in humans, can be manufactured in high titers, can infect a wide range of cells, and because much is known about their molecular biology. This last feature has allowed for the engineering of adenoviruses that are cytotoxic to gliomas but safe in normal brain cells *(5,13–16)*.

In an effort to improve therapy for gliomas, our group developed a conditionally replication-competent adenovirus (Δ 24) that, because of a deletion in the viral E1A protein, selectively replicates in tumor cells whose retinoblastoma (Rb) protein is functionally inactive *(17)*. The purpose of this chapter is to review the features of Δ 24. We first describe the biology and therapeutic effects of Δ 24, and then we outline modifications to this virus that have resulted in second-generation Δ 24 viruses that display increased tumor cell selectivity (Δ 24-RGD; *[18]*), reduced normal cell toxicity (CB1; *[19]*), and augmented tumoricidal capacity (Δ 24-CD; *[20,21]*). We emphasize the use of Δ 24 against brain tumors, recognizing that Δ 24 has also been shown to be effective in other cancer types *(14,21–24)*.

2. ONCOLTYIC VIRUSES: THE CHALLENGE OF BRAIN TUMORS

Brain tumors are generally considered to be amenable to local therapies, such as gene therapy, because in contrast with many other cancers, gliomas rarely metastasize, and their recurrence typically results from the failure of local control. Nevertheless, the promise of many local therapies, including gene therapy, has not been achieved for brain tumors because local therapies have proved incapable of delivering therapeutic agents to the majority of the tumor *(25,26)*. Although malignant gliomas do not metastasize outside the central nervous system, they are capable of widespread infiltration throughout the brain, and it is not uncommon for tumor cells to invade the hemisphere opposite the main tumor mass (*see* Fig. 1) *(27)*. Consequently, for local therapies to be effective they must have the capacity to reach cells distant from the site of initial delivery. In contrast with many other therapies, replication competent adenoviruses have the potential for spreading throughout a brain tumor and for reaching the infiltrating tumor cells because each round of infection-replication-lysis not only kills the infected tumor cells but also produces larger numbers of viral particles that can infect and lyse surrounding contiguous cells. This feature makes replication-competent adenoviruses especially attractive in the treatment of human gliomas (*see* Fig. 2).

The capacity of viruses to potentially spread throughout the target organ requires them to be selective for tumor cells rather than normal cells. Selective killing is especially critical for brain tumors because the tumor cells that infiltrate far from the solid tumor mass are typically intermingled with normal supportive cells (astrocytes) and

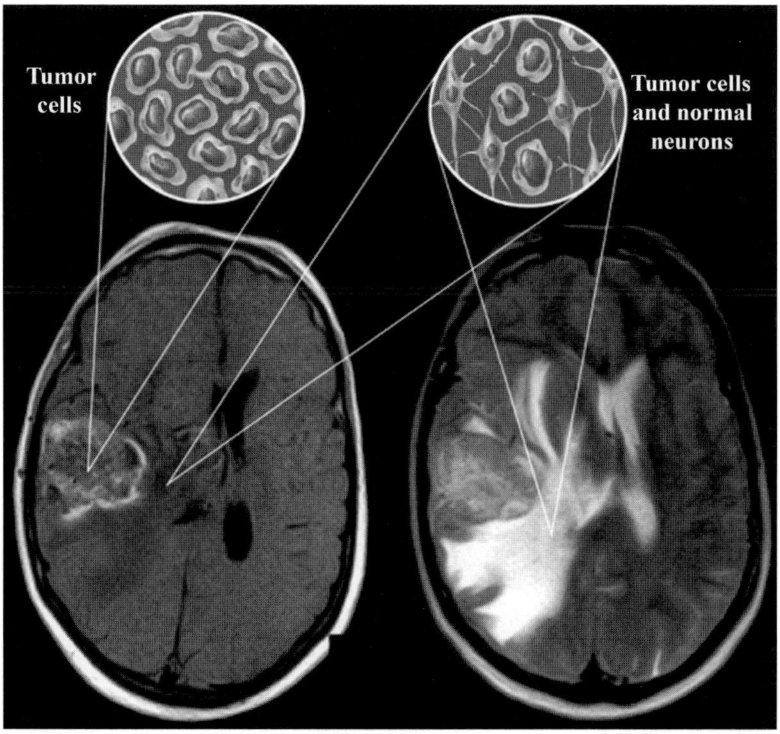

Fig. 1. The histological composition of a GBM. T1-weighted magnetic resonance (MR) image *(left)* demonstrates a contrast-enhancing tumor mass (white) that when viewed under the microscope *(left inset)* is composed of abutting tumor cells. T2-weighted MR image *(right)* shows areas of hyperintensity (white zone) surrounding the mass; as viewed microscopically *(right inset)*, this zone is composed of infiltrating tumor cells. (Reproduced with permission from ref. *27*.)

functioning neurons, the loss of which results in neurological deficit. Indeed, most therapies for brain tumors fail because of the inability to selectively kill the invading tumor cells without damaging the normal infiltrated brain. Although wild-type adenoviruses were used clinically as early as the 1950s *(28,29)*, concerns about normal tissue injury forestalled this approach, and it was never applied to brain tumors. In the modern era, however, these concerns have been addressed by genetically manipulating viruses to replicate selectively in malignant cells rather than normal cells, while at the same time maintaining their oncolytic potential (virulence). This ability to create tumor-selective viruses has allowed the treatment of brain tumors with adenoviruses.

3. Δ 24: BIOLOGY AND THERAPY

3.1. Molecular Biology of Δ 24

In order to avoid toxicity to normal cells, replication-competent adenoviruses have been designed to be tumor selective. Although targeting (selectivity) can be achieved by a variety of approaches *(30)*, in the context of adenoviruses, tumor selectivity has been most successfully accomplished by altering the viral genes that are required for viral replication in normal cells but are dispensable in cancer cells *(31,32)*. This approach was first pursued by Bischoff et al., who developed a conditionally replicative adenovirus, ONYX-015, that contains a deletion in the viral p53-binding protein E1B-55kDa and

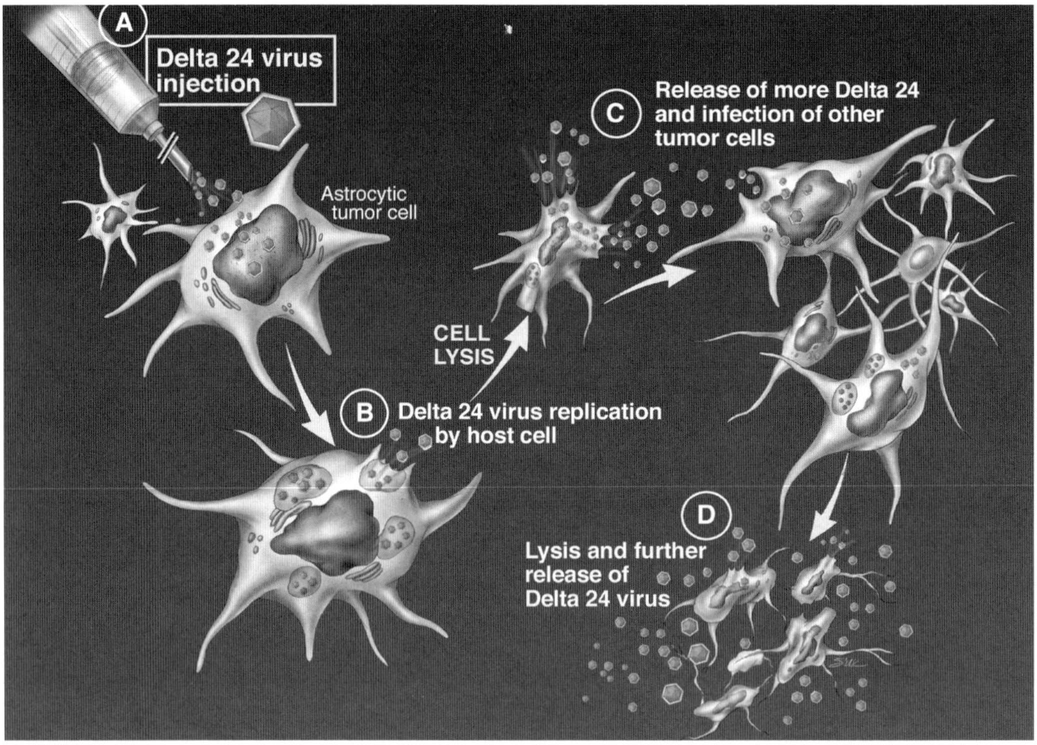

Fig. 2. Adenoviruses as oncolytic agents. Infection of a few cells by replication-competent adenoviruses, such as Δ 24, results in amplification of the virus with subsequent release and infection of surrounding cells. Each round of infection and lysis not only kills the infected cells but also increases the number of viral particles. Selectivity for tumor cells is determined by genetically engineering the virus. (Reproduced with permission from ref. *64.*)

that was intended to selectively replicate in tumor cells containing an inactivated p53 protein *(31)*. Fueyo et al. also used this approach to develop Δ 24, whose selectivity is based on a deletion in the E1A viral protein and which, therefore, selectively replicates in tumor cells containing inactivated retinoblastoma (Rb) protein *(17)*. To understand the basis of the selectivity of Δ 24 for tumor cells vs normal cells, the roles of cellular Rb protein and viral E1A protein in cell cycle regulation and viral replication must be understood (*see* Fig. 3).

3.1.1. Regulation of the Cell Cycle: The Rb Protein

The control of cell division is a complex process (for review *see 33,34*), but to a first approximation, the critical regulator of entry from G1 to S-phase is the retinoblastoma (Rb) protein *(35)*, a 110-kDa phosphoprotein whose phosphorylation status regulates the activity of E2F, a transcription factor that is important in activating genes involved in DNA replication (S-phase) and other components of cell proliferation *(35–39)*. Hypophosphorylated Rb binds E2F, and the resulting E2F/Rb complex represses the expression of E2F-target genes, thereby arresting cells in G1. Phosphorylation of Rb diminishes the repression of E2F by Rb, resulting in transcriptional activation of E2F-target genes and progression into S-phase (*see* Fig. 3). Phosphorylation of Rb is accomplished through cyclin-dependent kinases (in particular, cdks 4 and 6), a group of serine/threonine kinases whose activity requires association with regulatory subunits or

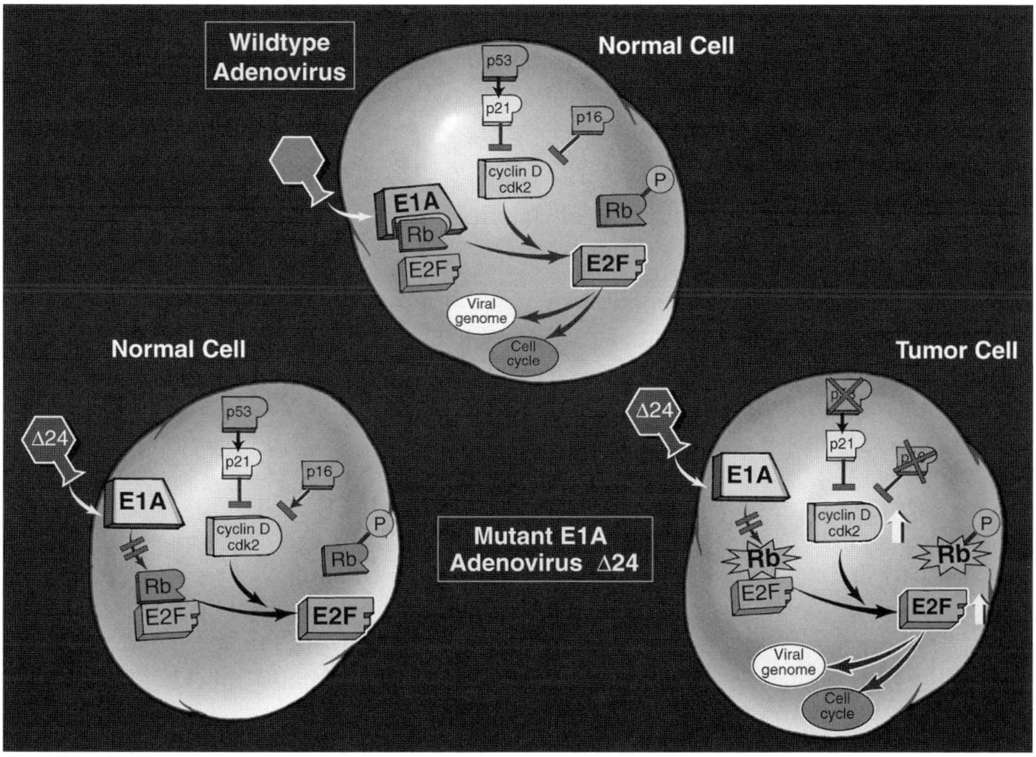

Fig. 3. The basis of tumor selectivity for Δ 24. Wild-type adenovirus commandeers the cellular replication machinery by inactivating Rb protein by binding the E1A protein *(top)*. This interaction frees up E2F, thereby driving the cell into S-phase and promoting viral replication. Because it harbors a mutant E1A protein, Δ 24 is unable to inactivate Rb *(bottom left)* and thus cannot replicate in normal cells. Nevertheless, tumor cells typically contain an inactivated Rb pathway, rendering the mutant E1A of Delta 24 unnecessary for promoting cell cycle progression, and viral replication proceeds unhindered.

cyclins (cyclin D1 is most critical in the Rb pathway). Cdks and their inhibitors (CDKIs, particularly p16/INK4a and p21) are important checkpoint proteins in regulating Rb and thus cell-cycle progression *(40)*.

3.1.2. Inactivation of Rb in Tumor Cells

Evidence is accumulating that nearly all tumors, including gliomas, harbor some defect in Rb or its regulatory pathway *(40,41)*. Although mutational inactivation of Rb is less common in gliomas than in other cancers, loss of p16INK4a (CDK-inhibitor upstream of Rb) or overexpression of cdks 4 and 6 or cyclin D are common defects in gliomas *(42)*. This loss of Rb function in tumor cells results in high levels of E2F, causing unregulated entry into the cell cycle and unfettered cellular proliferation, a cardinal feature of cancer *(43)* (*see* Fig. 3).

3.1.3. Forced Entry by Adenoviruses into the Cell Cycle: E1A Inactivation of Rb

Inactivation of Rb is also fundamental to the replication of most viruses, including adenoviruses *(44,45)*. After entry into cells, viruses replicate their DNA and produce the proteins of the structural capsid before being released by cell lysis. Because adenoviruses contain a small genome that encodes only about 30 different mRNA transcripts, replication relies upon commandeering cellular replication machinery. It is the role of the so-called early genes (E1–4) to prepare infected cells for viral DNA replication. Cellular entry into S-phase is regulated by viral E1A proteins (*see* Fig. 3). E1A is the first viral gene transcribed after infection, and its expression produces two related proteins, 243R and 289R. The 289R protein binds to and inactivates cellular Rb. E1A-mediated sequestration of Rb de-represses the transcriptional properties of E2F and allows for entry into S-phase and replication of the viral genome.

3.1.4. Engineering Δ 24: Exploiting the Link between E1A and Rb

Because viruses promote cellular proliferation by inactivating Rb through E1A, and because a *sine quo non* of tumor cells is dysregulation of the Rb pathway (p16/Rb/E2F), it is expected that mutating E1A so that it is unable to bind Rb would result in a virus that cannot replicate in normal cells (expressing functional Rb), but retains replicative competence in tumor cells that harbor inactive Rb and high levels of E2F (*see* Fig. 3).

Two segments of E1A are critical for binding Rb: one includes amino acids 30–60 in conserved region 1, and the other is amino acids 120–127 in conserved region 2. Whyte et al. showed that deletion of either region prevents the formation of detectable E1A/Rb complexes *(46)*. Consequently, Δ 24 was generated by deleting 24 base pairs (from nucleotides 919–943, coding for amino acids 122–129) from the conserved region 2 (CR2) of the E1A gene *(17)* (*see* Fig. 4). This mutation did not disrupt viral replication, as shown by the fact that Δ 24 can express the E1A protein. However, immunoprecipitation assays demonstrated that the mutant E1A protein of Δ 24 was unable to form complexes with the host cell Rb protein *(17)*.

3.2. Therapeutic Effects of Δ 24

3.2.1. Effects of Δ 24 on Glioma Cells

The anticancer effects of Delta 24 have been demonstrated in a large number of glioma cell lines. The lines tested have included cells that harbored a mutation in Rb itself, although the majority had disruption of the p16/Rb/E2F pathway (*see* Fig. 5). In vitro viability assays have shown a dose-dependent killing of glioma cell lines, with cytopathic effects occurring at titers as little as 0.5 to 1 viral particle/cell *(17)*. Lysis of glioma cells was observed within 10 to 14 d after infection with Δ 24 in vitro *(17)*. Moreover, these anticancer effects were shown to be caused by the replication of Δ 24, and studies analyzing the supernatant of Δ 24-infected tumor cells for progeny virus have shown an increase in the viral titers of 60 to 400× the initial infection titer as early as 6 d after initial infection, with the amount increase depending on the cell line tested. These studies, as well as cell-cycle analyses, confirm that lysis is the primary mode of cell death, although a small amount of apoptosis also occurs.

In vivo studies have demonstrated that treatment with Δ 24 significantly reduces the growth of subcutaneously grown glioma xenografts compared with controls treated with ultraviolet (UV)-inactivated-Δ 24, *(17)*. Similarly, the survival time of animals harboring intracranially established glioma xenografts was significantly extended after treatment with Δ 24 relative to controls treated with UV-inactivated Δ 24 or saline *(18)*. Most importantly, detailed histological analysis of Δ 24-treated tumors identified three zones of viral expression that are best explained by a wave-like movement of the vector from the injection site toward the edge of the tumor (*see* Fig. 6). Thus, there is substantial evidence that Δ 24 is effective as an anticancer agent against gliomas. Evidence

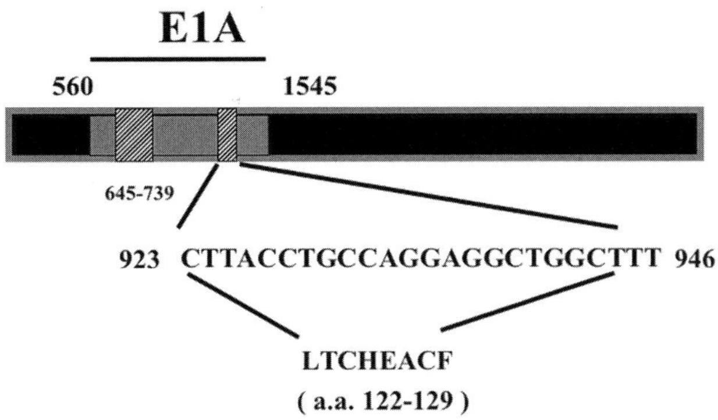

Fig. 4. The Δ 24 Construct. Δ 24 contains a deletion of 24 bp in the E1A region.

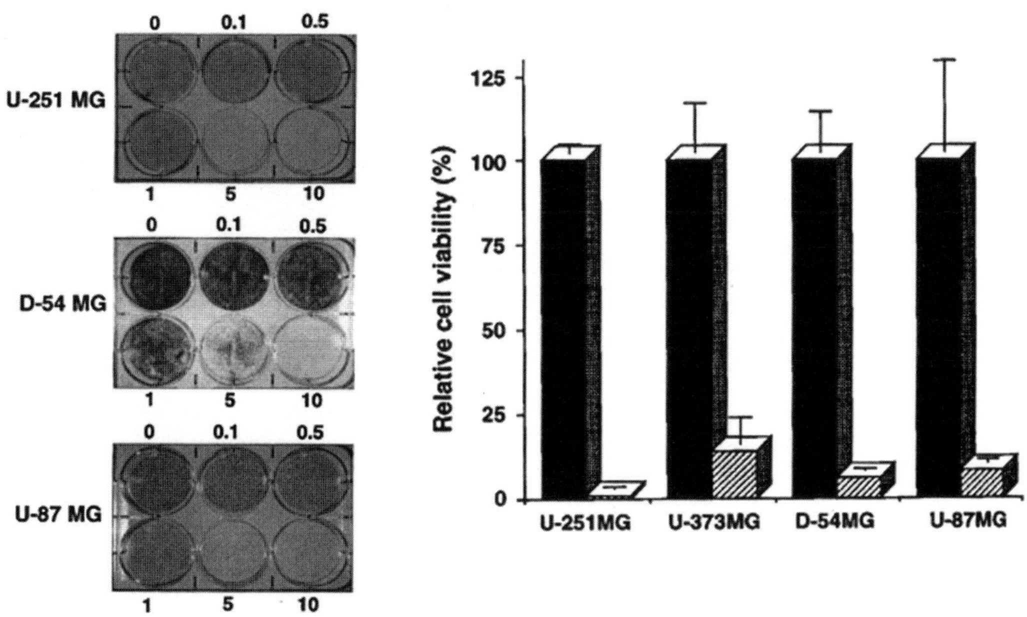

Fig. 5. Efficacy of Δ 24 against human gliomas. *(Left)* Dose-dependent assay. Cells of each cell line were plated and treated with increasing doses of Δ 24 (0-10 multiplicity of infection [MOI]). Cells were stained with crystal violet to assess viability. Δ 24 produced significant killing of tumor cells in a dose-dependent fashion with each cell line tested. *(Right)* Viability assay. Cells were plated and then infected with Δ 24 or UV-inactivated Δ 24 at 10 MOI. Cells were counted in triplicate 7 to 24 d after infection. The growth of cells treated with Δ 24 (hatched bars) compared with UV-inactivated Δ 24 (solid bars) is shown (Reproduced with permission from ref. *19*.)

is also accumulating that Δ 24 is effective against other tumor types, including sarcomas, lung cancer, ovarian cancer, and prostate cancer *(21–24)*. Δ 24 is expected to be a universal anticancer agent as inactivation of the Rb pathway is generally accepted to be an obligate alteration underlying the cancer cell phenotype.

3.2.2. Effects of Δ 24 on Normal Cells

Consistent with the hypothesis that mutation of E1A abrogates the capacity of normal cells to support adenoviral replication, Fueyo et al. initially showed that lung fibroblast cell lines are resistant to the cytotoxic effects of Δ 24 *(17)*. Important for

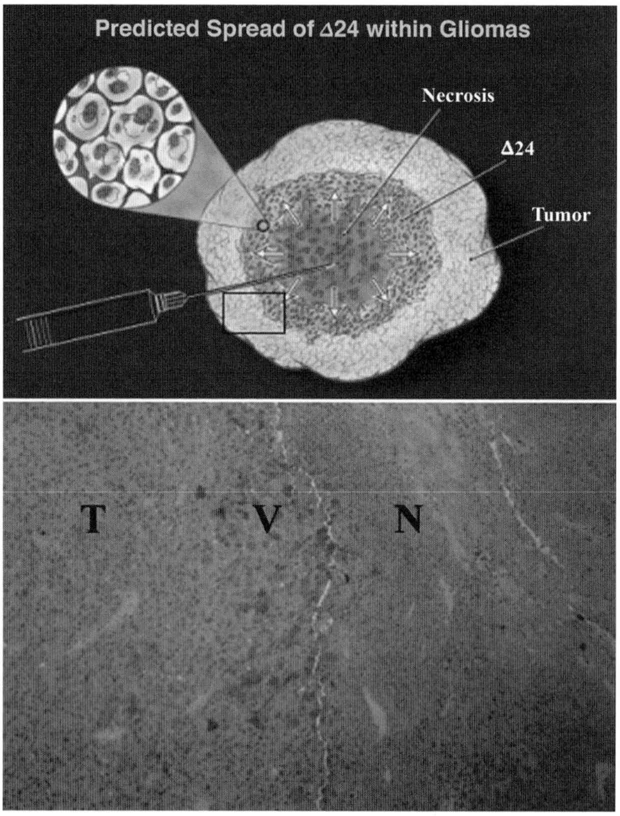

Fig. 6. Fueyo Dissemination of Δ 24 with glioma. *(Top)* Diagram showing predicted spreading of virus from point of injection. Three zones are evident: a central zone of necrotic cells that have been lysed by Δ 24, an intermediate zone of infected cells (inset shows viral inclusions in cells), and an outer zone of cells not yet infected. *(Bottom)* Photomicrograph of human xenograft taken from the brain of a mouse treated with Δ 24. The three zones are evident: T, uninfected tumor; V, cells infected with virus; N, necrotic lysed cells.

brain tumor therapy, similar studies performed on human astrocytes have confirmed the inability of Δ 24 to replicate in normal brain cells *(18)*. In contrast with tumor cells, treatment of these fibroblasts or astrocytes with Δ 24 resulted in no increase in progeny viral titer. These results did not result from the inability of the virus to infect the cells, but were specifically the result of the reduced capacity of the virus to replicate in these cells. The most convincing evidence for the capacity of Δ 24 to replicate only in Rb-inactivated cells comes from Rb-transfer studies. Specifically, using an Ad-Rb construct (replication incompetent adenoviral vector carrying the Rb gene) Fueyo et al. restored Rb function in Saos-2 cells (harbor an inactive Rb gene) *(17)*. They then showed that Δ 24 was only able to replicate in and kill the parental Saos-2 cell line (Rb inactive), but not the isogenetic Ad-Rb-infected Saos-2 cells (*see* Fig. 7). Thus, restoration of Rb was able to rescue the Saos-2 cells from the cytopathic effects of Δ 24, confirming the dependence of Δ 24 replication on the presence of an inactivated Rb pathway.

A caveat regarding Δ 24 is that *dividing* normal cells are potentially vulnerable to the cytopathic effects of the virus *(17–19)*. Because normal initiation of S-phase requires attenuating the activity of Rb (via cdk phosphorylation of Rb, see above) dividing cells

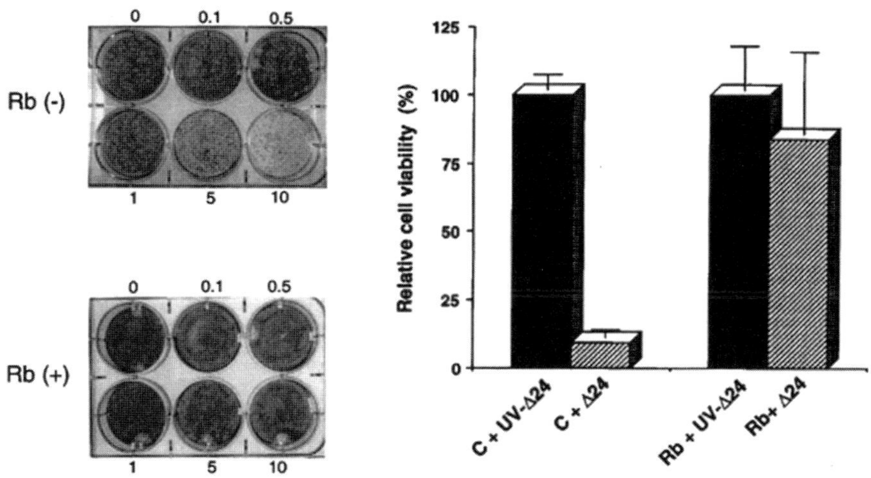

Fig. 7. Selectivity of Δ 24 for cells with inactive Rb. *(Left)* Saos-2 cells were infected with Ad-null (top) or Ad-Rb (bottom) and, 3 d later, with Δ 24 at the indicated dose (0–10 MOI). Cell viability was detected by staining with crystal violet. Cells containing Rb *(bottom)* are not killed by Δ 24, whereas Rb(-) cells *(top)* are killed. *(Right)* Saos-2 cells were infected with 100 MOI of Ad-null or Ad-Rb and, 3 d later, with 10 MOI of Δ 24 (solid bar) or UV-inactivated Δ 24 (hatched bar). Cell viability was assayed 5 d later. Cells containing normal Rb are not killed by Δ 24 (Reproduced with permission from ref. *19*.)

typically have low levels of active Rb (and high levels of E2F). Infection with Δ 24 during S-phase would thus result in viral replication and cellular lysis. For organs such as the brain in which the majority of functional normal cells do not divide (typically remaining in G0), the toxicity of Δ 24 would be anticipated to be low. Nevertheless, this shortcoming can also be addressed by further engineering Δ 24 to be more selective (*see* below).

4. SECOND GENERATION Δ 24 ADENOVIRUSES

Δ 24 can be viewed as a platform for the development of a selective oncolytic virus with increased infectivity *(18)*, reduced toxicity *(19)*, and augmented killing ability *(20)*. Although a variety of approaches to achieve these goals are conceivable, this section focus on alterations that to date have been reported and tested using Δ 24 as a backbone (Table 1).

4.1. Enhancing Infectivity by Exploiting Adenoviral Receptors: Δ 24-RGD

Elucidation of the mechanisms of viral entry into cells has led to the development of second-generation Δ 24 adenoviruses with improved infectivity in tumors. This development arose from knowledge of the mechanism underlying viral entry into cells.

4.1.1. Adenoviral Entry into Cells

Structurally, the adenovirus genome is contained in a capsid that consists of three major proteins: hexon (II), penton base (III), and a knobbed fiber (IV) *(44)*. An important function of these capsid proteins is to mediate viral entry into cells, which occurs by clathrin-dependent endocytosis and which is initiated by the interaction of the viral fiber knob protein with coxsackie-adenovirus receptors (CAR) located on cellular surfaces

Table 1
Δ 24 and Second Generation Δ 24 Viruses

Construct name	*Mutation*	*Molecular effect*	*Biological effect*	*Ref.*
Δ 24	24-bp deletion in E1A gene	Mutant E1A	Inability to replicate in Rb-positive cell	*(23)*
Δ 24-RGD	RGD-4C gene motif inserted into L4 region	Fiber knob with RGD insert	CAR-independent cell infection	*(18)*
CB1	24-bp deletion in E1A, deletion in E1B-55 kDa	Mutant E1A, nonfunctional E1B	Inability to replicate in Rb-positive cells and p53 positive cells	*(19)*
Δ 24-hyCD	Insertion of humanized yeast cytosine deaminase gene into E3 region	Expression of cytosine deaminase	Permits local conversion of 5FC to 5FU for enhanced cell kill	*(20)*
Δ 24-p53	Insert p53 gene into E3 region	Expression of wt-p53 protein during lytic phase	Enhanced cell lysis and viral progeny release	*(21)*

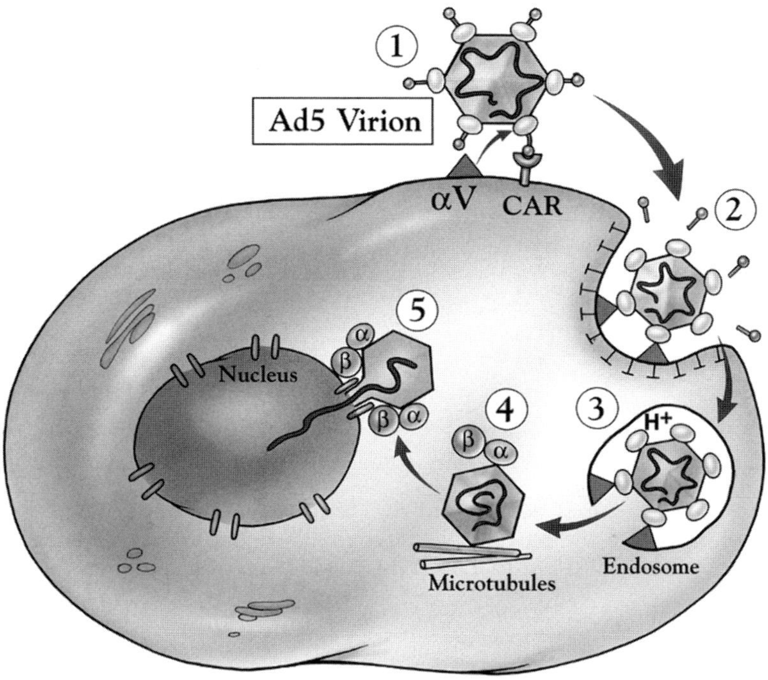

Fig. 8. Infection of cells by adenoviruses. Adenoviruses enter cells by initial binding of the fiber knob to CAR and subsequent interaction of the penton base with cell surface integrins. Clathrin-mediated endocytosis results in internalization of the virus and its subsequent movement into the nucleus.

(*see* Fig. 8) *(44,47,48)*. This interaction results in a conformational change in the fiber that allows the penton base protein, through its tripeptide amino acid sequence (arginine-glycine-aspartic acid [RGD] motif), to bind to α_v integrins, specifically $\alpha_v\beta3$ and $\alpha_v\beta5$ on the cell surface. This second interaction (penton base with integrins) results in a pH change (towards acidification) facilitating viral evasion of the endosome *(49,50)*. Once inside the cell, the viral core (containing the viral genome) moves into the nucleus through nuclear pores, and a viral DNA-cell histone complex is formed, initiating selective expression of early gene transcription.

4.1.2. CAR and Integrin Expression in Tumors

Examinations of CAR levels in neoplastic cells, revealed that CAR expression is typically low in tumors, including gliomas *(18)*. Indeed, in a study from our group, nearly 50% of glioma cell lines expressed very low levels of CAR *(18)*. Likewise, studies of paraffin-fixed brain tumor surgical specimens have documented the low CAR expression in gliomas *in situ*. This finding is important because a low-CAR level on tumor cells reduces viral infection and attenuates lateral spread of replication-competent viruses resulting from dependence on CAR for efficient viral infectivity. In addition, low-CAR expression on tumor cells can theoretically result in sequestration of virus by high-CAR expressing noncancerous normal cells, thereby limiting the infection of low-CAR expressing cancer cells. However, in contrast with their frequent low levels of CAR expression, tumor cells typically show high levels of $\alpha_v\beta3$ or $\alpha_v\beta5$. Indeed, in our study, glioma cell lines almost universally demonstrated high levels of $\alpha_v\beta3$ or $\alpha_v\beta5$, and many gliomas showed high expression of both integrins *(18)*.

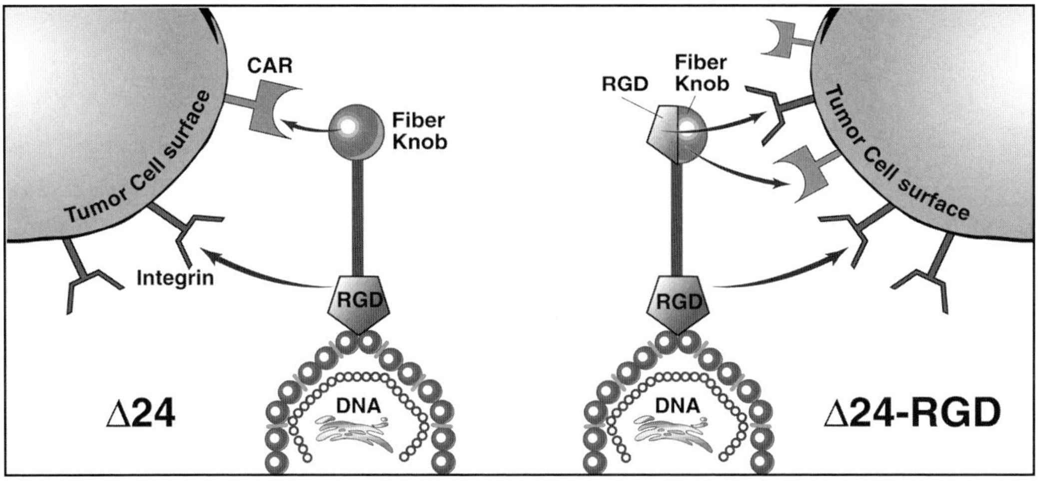

Fig. 9. Comparison between Δ 24 and Δ 24-RGD. The RGD motif in the penton base binds to integrins. Insertion of an RGD-motif into the fiber knob, permits Δ 24-RGD to infect cells irrespective of the presence of CAR. Note that Δ 24-RGD is still able to bind CAR.

4.1.3. Δ 24-RGD

Elucidation of the fiber knob/CAR and RGD/integrin interactions and the frequent low expression of CAR and high expression of integrins in tumors led to the development of second generation Δ 24 adenoviruses with improved infectivity in tumors. This development was fueled by the recognition that incorporation of an ACDCRGDCFCG peptide (RGD-4C) motif into the H1 loop of the fiber knob (H1 loop) is capable of facilitating adenoviral entry of tumor cells by bypassing the CAR interaction *(51)* (*see* Fig. 9). Curiel and coworkers were the first to demonstrate that this RGD motif could favorably augment the delivery of adenoviral vectors *(51)*. Subsequently, in order to improve the infectivity of Δ 24, Fueyo et al. reported a modified Δ 24 that included the RGD motif within the H1 loop, called Δ 24-RGD *(18)*. In vitro analyses have demonstrated that the presence of this RGD motif increases infection of glioma cells by as much as 6× more than infection with adenoviruses lacking RGD in the H1 loop. Blocking adenoviral infectivity mediated by CAR by incubating tumor cells with fiber knob protein did not significantly inhibit infection of RGD-containing adenovirus. In contrast, incubating them with RGD peptide to block integrin binding significantly reduced adenoviral infectivity. Thus, insertion of the RGD motif into the fiber knob allows for CAR-independent infection of gliomas.

The increased infectivity of Δ 24-RGD has been shown to translate into increased tumor cell killing *(18)*. Interestingly, in cells with low-CAR expression, Δ 24-RGD had higher cytopathic effects than Δ 24 or wild-type adenovirus. However, in cells with high-CAR expression, wild-type virus was more potent than Δ 24-RGD. Thus, the enhanced killing of Δ 24-RGD was most evident in tumor cells with low-CAR expression. This enhanced killing by Δ 24 RGD has been shown most convincingly in an intracranial glioma xenograft model of a low-CAR expressing glioma cell line (U87) (*see* Fig. 10). Intratumoral injection of Δ 24-RGD into established intracranial U87 xenografts was associated with a longer survival time (mean 131 d) than intratumoral injection of Δ 24 (mean 50 d). Furthermore, although long-term survivors were identified with both treatments, 60% of Δ 24-RGD treated mice, but only 15% of Δ 24-treated mice, survived for

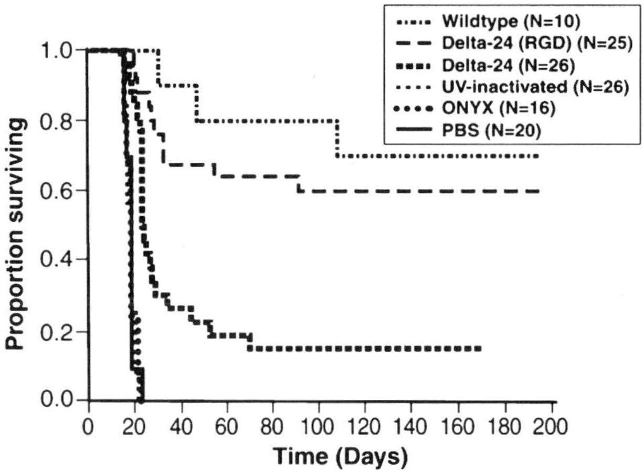

Fig. 10. Efficacy of Δ 24 and Δ 24-RGD in an intracranial glioma xenograft model. U87 glioma cells (low CAR expression) were implanted in the frontal lobes of nude mice, and after 3 d they were treated with the agents shown in the legend. Δ 24 treatment resulted in a significant increase in survival time relative to controls. Use of Δ 24-RGD further increased survival time in this model (60% of animals were cured). Treatment with Onyx-015 had no effect. Δ 24-RGD was as effective as wild-type adenovirus, indicating that its virulence was not significantly attenuated by the modifications.

more than 4 mo. Thus, there is substantial evidence that the addition of the RDG motif increased the capacity of Δ 24 to kill low CAR-expressing tumor cells.

Importantly, and in contrast to the case with tumor cells, the addition of the RGD motif to Δ 24 does not translate into increased killing of normal human astrocytes. Thus, the selectivity imposed by the mutant E1A is maintained in RGD modified Δ 24. Specifically, Δ 24-RGD was shown to be unable to replicate in serum-starved (non-dividing) normal human astrocytes, whereas wild-type adenovirus (not containing mutant E1A) was able to replicate. Indeed, Δ 24-RGD replication was 1000 to 10,000× greater in glioma cells than it was in normal human astrocytes. Thus, it is expected that Δ 24-RGD should have a high therapeutic index when used in the treatment of brain tumors. Moreover, recent reports have suggested that most normal cells in the brain have low levels of $\alpha_v\beta3$ or $\alpha_v\beta5$ integrins on their surface *in situ*, which would further extend the therapeutic index in glioma treatment.

4.2. Enhancing Tumor Selectivity and Decreasing Cellular Toxicity: CB1

As previously mentioned, a downside of the E1A-based oncolytic viruses, Δ 24 and Δ 24-RGD is their ability to replicate in *dividing* normal cells. Because normal cell division includes a period when Rb is inactivated, normal dividing cells are vulnerable to Δ 24 infection and replication. One approach that has been used to decrease toxicity in normal cells while maintaining efficacious replication and lysis of tumor cells has been to alter another early expressed protein, namely, the E1B protein. This double mutant adenovirus has been referred to as CB1 *(19)*.

4.2.1. Cellular p53 as Guardian of the Genome

Viral E1A expression inactivates Rb, resulting in the release and activation of E2F, inducing cell-cycle progression. Expression of E1A, increases in E2F, and unscheduled DNA synthesis are all capable of activating expression of one of the most critical cell-cycle check point genes, the p53 tumor suppressor *(52,53)*. p53 is a 393-amino-acid protein often referred to as the "guardian of the genome," as it is activated in response to genome-altering stresses including DNA damage, hypoxia, and oncogene expression. Both E2F and E1a are strong inducers of p53. Activation of p53 leads to increased expression of p21, a cdk inhibitor, and subsequent arrest of the cell in G1. This arrest allows cells to repair the DNA damage prior to proceeding to S-phase. However, if the damage is irreparable, activation of p53 leads to apoptosis, typically through p53-mediated transcriptional activation of apoptosis-related proteins (e.g., Bax, Fas, Puma, and Noxa). Importantly, p53 is negatively regulated by the mouse double minute-2 (mdm-2) protein, which binds to p53, thereby inhibiting its transactivating capacity *(54)* and targeting p53 for proteosome degradation *(55)*. Binding of mdm-2 to p53 is itself regulated by $p14^{ARF}$, which inhibits mdm-2 by sequestering it from p53 *(56)*. Thus, the expression of $p14^{ARF}$ activates p53 by releasing it from mdm-2. Increases in E1A and E2F activate p53 through this $p14^{ARF}$ pathway. Thus, the cell uses p53 to protect itself from the potential deleterious effects of viral infection.

4.2.2. The Role of Viral E1B in Replication

Because high levels of E2F are capable of activating $p14^{ARF}$ and leading to p53-mediated apoptosis, it is critical for adenoviruses to suppress the p53 apoptotic pathway in order to sustain replication. This is accomplished at last in part by the viral E1B-55kDa protein, which binds to and inactivates cellular p53. E1B-mediated inactivation of p53 prevents apoptosis and/or cell cycle arrest and permits viral replication and viral proliferation *(16)*.

4.2.3. CB1 (E1A-E1B Double Mutant)

In order to improve the safety, Gomez-Manzano et al. used this information to develop a double mutant adenovirus constructed on the backbone of the mutant-E1A Δ 24. Specifically, they deleted base pairs 2426 to 3328 in the E1B region, which prevents the expression of wild-type E1B-55kDa protein. This deletion was the same alteration incorporated into ONYX-015, first reported by Bischoff et al. *(31)*. Because p53 is inactivated in nearly all tumor cells (either by mutation of p53, increases in mdm-2 or loss of $p14^{ARF}$) *(25,57–60)*, abolishing the expression of viral E1B-55kDa does not attenuate viral replication in tumor cells. However, when E1B-mutant adenovirus infects normal cells, wild-type p53 is activated and viral replication is halted, either through cell-cycle arrest or apoptosis. The double mutant adenovirus (with E1A and E1B mutations), CB1, is unable to inactivate Rb and p53. Gomez-Manzano et al. showed that this virus replicates and lyses glioma cells as effectively as Δ 24 *(19)*. Furthermore, using a mouse intracranial glioma model, direct injection of CB1 significantly extended the survival time of mice compared with controls receiving ultraviolet-inactivated CB1, but their survival duration was not significantly different from mice receiving unmodified Δ 24. Important for reducing toxicity, the replication phenotype of CB1 was highly attenuated in both *nondividing* and *dividing* normal astrocytes. Although the effect of CB1 was no different from Δ 24 in nondividing astrocytes, in actively proliferating astrocyte cultures, CB1 produced significantly less toxicity than Δ 24. Thus, the inability of CB1 to inhibit cellular p53 acts as a secondary check on viral replication in dividing normal cells. In all, CB1 has improved selectivity, producing less toxicity on normal dividing cells than Δ 24 alone, while at the same time maintaining its replication efficiency and cytopathic effect on glioma cells.

4.3. Enhancing Cell Killing: Arming Δ 24

Given the potential of replication-competent viruses to spread throughout a tumor, a natural evolution of this therapeutic approach has been to "arm" replication-competent adenoviruses to deliver therapeutic transgenes. These genes are typically inserted into the E3 region, which modifies the host's immunological environment and can be deleted without interfering with viral replication. To date, Δ 24 has been used to deliver the cytosine deaminase gene (CD) *(20)* and the p53 gene *(61)*.

4.3.1. Δ 24-hyCD

In an effort to enhance tumor cell killing, Conrad et al. inserted a humanized version of the yeast cytosine deaminase gene driven by a CMV promoter into the E3 region of Δ 24 *(20)*. Activation of this gene results in expression of cytosine deaminase, an enzyme that converts the prodrug 5-fluorocytosine (5-FC) to the cytotoxic drug 5-fluorouracil (5-FU). This approach, called gene-dependent enzyme/prodrug therapy (GDEPT), is intended to enhance cell killing by increasing the local intratumoral concentration of 5-FU and thereby inducing a "bystander" effect on the surrounding tumor cells. Because 5-FU has a narrow therapeutic index and systemic dosing results in significant hematological and gastrointestinal toxicities, the GDEPT approach allows for systemic delivery of an inert nontoxic prodrug (5-FC) and subsequent local (intratumoral) conversion to the active drug (5-FC), thereby limiting systemic toxicity and enhancing cell kill by maximizing local intratumoral drug concentrations. However, in the context of replication-competent viruses, concern arose from the theoretical consideration that enhancing the killing of cells by 5-FU might attenuate viral replication by prematurely inducing apoptosis in both the infected cells and the surrounding cells.

Nevertheless, in vitro experimental studies have demonstrated that Δ 24-hyCD produces a catalytically active hyCD enzyme that efficiently converted 5FC to 5FU both in vitro and in vivo *(20)*. For glioma cell lines, the in vitro IC50 dose of FC required for complete cytopathic effect by the Δ 24-hyCD was 5-fold less than the dose required with Δ 24. Moreover, intratumoral treatment of mice bearing intracranial human gliomas with Δ 24-hyCD (delivered intratumorally) plus 5FC (delivered intraperitoneally) significantly improved survival time compared with the use of Δ 24 alone or Δ 24 plus 5FC. These studies indicate that the added bystander effect achieved by this prodrug approach enhances rather than limits tumor cell kill and thus represents an important improvement in the ultimate application of Δ 24.

4.3.2. Δ 24-p53

Cellular lysis at the end of the infection and replication cycle of the adenovirus is the critical step that determines the rate of viral progeny release. Whereas cellular lysis was initially thought to be a nonapoptotic process, it now appears that apoptosis is one mechanism used by adenoviruses to accomplish cell lysis *(62,63)*. Apoptosis is suppressed in the early stages of viral replication via the interaction of adenoviral proteins (encoded by E1 and E4 genes) with p53 such that p53 function is suppressed and its degradation is induced *(63)*. Inactivation of p53 prevents premature host cell death that would otherwise limit production of new viral progeny. However, at the end of the adenoviral cycle, cooperation with p53 to induce cell lysis is necessary for efficient viral replication *(63)*. Consequently, adenoviruses have the ability to lyse cells with functional p53 more efficiently than those that are p53-deficient *(62,63)*. Thus, many tumors that are p53-deficient, including malignant gliomas, may be resistant to the release of adenoviral progeny, thereby limiting intratumoral dissemination.

With the knowledge of the central role of p53 in coordinating the apoptotic response, van Beusechem et al. *(21)* recently engineered Δ 24 to carry a p53 transgene in the E3 region of the viral genome. *In vitro* studies demonstrated that Δ 24-p53 was more effective than Δ 24 at killing human cancer cells with various histologies (including gliomas) and p53 statuses. Thus, arming Δ 24 with apoptosis-enhancing genes such as p53 represents another therapeutic avenue that needs further testing.

5. CONCLUSIONS

The preclinical studies presented herein suggest that Δ 24 has significant promise as a therapeutic agent against human gliomas. Yet the true potential of this approach rests on the successful testing of these agents in clinical trials. Given the wealth of knowledge about the molecular function of Δ 24 and the second generation adenoviruses, it is paramount to properly design clinical trials so that the biological capacity of Δ 24 to lyse glioma cells, to spread to distant tumor cells, and to spare normal cells (in other words, to do what it was designed to do) is tested. Immediate success will require careful implementation of such trials. Ultimate success, however, will require continued understanding of the intersection between viral and tumor biology and the application of these findings to the refinement of ever more effective and safe Δ 24-based viral therapies.

ACKNOWLEDGMENT

The authors thank Sandra Flores for her excellent assistance with the preparation of this manuscript.

REFERENCES

1. Surawicz TS, Davis F, Freels S, Laws ER, Jr, Menck HR. Brain tumor survival: results from the National Cancer Data Base. J Neurooncol 1998;40(2):151–160.
2. Walker AE, Robins M, Weinfeld FD. Epidemiology of brain tumors: the national survey of intracranial neoplasms. Neurology 1985;35(2):219–226.
3. Alemany R, Balague C, Curiel DT. Replicative adenoviruses for cancer therapy. Nat Biotechnol 2000;18(7):723–727.
4. Biederer C, Ries S, Brandts CH, McCormick F. Replication-selective viruses for cancer therapy. J Mol Med 2002;80(3):163–175.
5. Shah AC, Benos D, Gillespie GY, Markert JM. Oncolytic viruses: clinical applications as vectors for the treatment of malignant gliomas. J Neurooncol 2003;65(3):203–226.
6. Martuza RL. Conditionally replicating herpes vectors for cancer therapy. J Clin Invest 2000; 105(7):841–846.
7. Bergmann M, Romirer I, Sachet M, et al. A genetically engineered influenza A virus with ras-dependent oncolytic properties. Cancer Res 2001;61(22):8188–8193.
8. Phuangsab A, Lorence RM, Reichard KW, Peeples ME, Walter RJ. Newcastle disease virus therapy of human tumor xenografts: antitumor effects of local or systemic administration. Cancer Lett 2001;172(1):27–36.
9. Gromeier M, Lachmann S, Rosenfeld MR, Gutin PH, Wimmer E. Intergeneric poliovirus recombinants for the treatment of malignant glioma. Proc Natl Acad Sci U S A 2000;97(12):6803–6808.
10. Strong JE, Coffey MC, Tang D, Sabinin P, Lee PW. The molecular basis of viral oncolysis: usurpation of the Ras signaling pathway by reovirus. EMBO J 1998;17(12):3351–3362.
11. Timiryasova TM, Li J, Chen B, et al. Antitumor effect of vaccinia virus in glioma model. Oncol Res 1999;11(3):133–144.
12. Stojdl DF, Lichty B, Knowles S, et al. Exploiting tumor-specific defects in the interferon pathway with a previously unknown oncolytic virus. Nat Med 2000;6(7):821–825.

13. Kruyt FA, Curiel DT. Toward a new generation of conditionally replicating adenoviruses: pairing tumor selectivity with maximal oncolysis. Hum Gene Ther 2002;13(4):485–495.
14. Lamfers ML, Grill J, Dirven CM, et al. Potential of the conditionally replicative adenovirus Ad5-Delta24RGD in the treatment of malignant gliomas and its enhanced effect with radiotherapy. Cancer Res 2002;62(20):5736–5742.
15. McCormick F. Cancer gene therapy: fringe or cutting edge? Nat Rev Cancer 2001;1(2):130–141.
16. McCormick F. Interactions between adenovirus proteins and the p53 pathway: the development of ONYX-015. Semin Cancer Biol 2000;10(6):453–459.
17. Fueyo J, Gomez-Manzano C, Alemany R, et al. A mutant oncolytic adenovirus targeting the Rb pathway produces anti-glioma effect in vivo. Oncogene 2000;19(1):2–12.
18. Fueyo J, Alemany R, Gomez-Manzano C, et al. Preclinical characterization of the antiglioma activity of a tropism-enhanced adenovirus targeted to the retinoblastoma pathway. J Natl Cancer Inst 2003;95(9):652–660.
19. Gomez-Manzano C, Balague C, Alemany R, et al. A novel E1A-E1B mutant adenovirus induces glioma regression in vivo. Oncogene 2004;23(10):1821–1828.
20. Conrad CA, Miller CR, Ji Y, et al. Delta-24-hyCD adenovirus suppresses glioma growth in vivo by combining oncolysis and chemosensitization. Cancer Gene Ther 2005;12(3):284–294.
21. van Beusechem VW, van den Doel PB, Grill J, Pinedo HM, Gerritsen WR. Conditionally replicative adenovirus expressing p53 exhibits enhanced oncolytic potency. Cancer Res 2002;62(21):6165–6171.
22. Cripe TP, Dunphy EJ, Holub AD, et al. Fiber knob modifications overcome low, heterogeneous expression of the coxsackievirus-adenovirus receptor that limits adenovirus gene transfer and oncolysis for human rhabdomyosarcoma cells. Cancer Res 2001;61(7):2953–2960.
23. Suzuki K, Fueyo J, Krasnykh V, Reynolds PN, Curiel DT, Alemany R. A conditionally replicative adenovirus with enhanced infectivity shows improved oncolytic potency. Clin Cancer Res 2001;7(1):120–126.
24. Bauerschmitz GJ, Lam JT, Kanerva A, et al. Treatment of ovarian cancer with a tropism modified oncolytic adenovirus. Cancer Res 2002;62(5):1266–1270.
25. Lang FF, Yung WK, Sawaya R, Tofilon PJ. Adenovirus-mediated p53 gene therapy for human gliomas. Neurosurgery 1999;45(5):1093–1104.
26. Lang FF, Bruner JM, Fuller GN, et al. Phase I trial of adenovirus-mediated p53 gene therapy for recurrent glioma: biological and clinical results. J Clin Oncol 2003;21(13):2508–2518.
27. Hentschel SJ, Lang FF. Current surgical management of glioblastoma. Cancer J 2003;9(2):113–125.
28. Sinkovics J, Horvath J. New developments in the virus therapy of cancer: a historical review. Intervirology 1993;36(4):193–214.
29. Huebner RJ, Rowe WP, Schatten WE, Smith RR, Thomas LB. Studies on the use of viruses in the treatment of carcinoma of the cervix. Cancer 1956;9(6):1211–1218.
30. Chiocca EA. Oncolytic viruses. Nat Rev Cancer 2002;2(12):938–950.
31. Bischoff JR, Kirn DH, Williams A, et al. An adenovirus mutant that replicates selectively in p53-deficient human tumor cells. Science 1996;274(5286):373–376.
32. Curiel DT. The development of conditionally replicative adenoviruses for cancer therapy. Clin Cancer Res 2000;6(9):3395–3399.
33. Dirks PB, Rutka JT. Current concepts in neuro-oncology: the cell cycle—a review. Neurosurgery 1997;40(5):1000–1013.
34. Ivanchuk SM, Rutka JT. The cell cycle: accelerators, brakes, and checkpoints. Neurosurgery 2004;54(3):692–699.
35. Weinberg RA. The retinoblastoma protein and cell cycle control. Cell 1995;81(3):323–330.
36. Ewen ME. The cell cycle and the retinoblastoma protein family. Cancer Metastasis Rev 1994;13(1):45–66.
37. Buchkovich K, Duffy LA, Harlow E. The retinoblastoma protein is phosphorylated during specific phases of the cell cycle. Cell 1989;58(6):1097–1105.
38. DeCaprio JA, Ludlow JW, Lynch D, et al. The product of the retinoblastoma susceptibility gene has properties of a cell cycle regulatory element. Cell 1989;58(6):1085–1095.
39. Farnham PJ, Slansky JE, Kollmar R. The role of E2F in the mammalian cell cycle. Biochim Biophys Acta 1993;1155(2):125–131.
40. Yamasaki L. Role of the RB tumor suppressor in cancer. Cancer Treat Res 2003;115:209–239.
41. Sherr CJ. The INK4a/ARF network in tumour suppression. Nat Rev Mol Cell Biol 2001;2(10):731–737.
42. Maher EA, Furnari FB, Bachoo RM, et al. Malignant glioma: genetics and biology of a grave matter. Genes Dev 2001;15(11):1311–1333.

43. Hanahan D, Weinberg RA. The hallmarks of cancer. Cell 2000;100(1):57–70.
44. Russell WC. Update on adenovirus and its vectors. J Gen Virol 2000;81(Pt 11):2573–2604.
45. Op De Beeck A, Caillet-Fauquet P. Viruses and the cell cycle. Prog Cell Cycle Res 1997;3:1–19.
46. Whyte P, Williamson NM, Harlow E. Cellular targets for transformation by the adenovirus E1A proteins. Cell 1989;56(1):67–75.
47. Bergelson JM, Cunningham JA, Droguett G, et al. Isolation of a common receptor for Coxsackie B viruses and adenoviruses 2 and 5. Science 1997;275(5304):1320–1323.
48. Meier O, Greber UF. Adenovirus endocytosis. J Gene Med 2003;5(6):451–462.
49. Wickham TJ, Mathias P, Cheresh DA, Nemerow GR. Integrins alpha v beta 3 and alpha v beta 5 promote adenovirus internalization but not virus attachment. Cell 1993;73(2):309–319.
50. Wang K, Huang S, Kapoor-Munshi A, Nemerow G. Adenovirus internalization and infection require dynamin. J Virol 1998;72(4):3455–3458.
51. Dmitriev I, Krasnykh V, Miller CR, et al. An adenovirus vector with genetically modified fibers demonstrates expanded tropism via utilization of a coxsackievirus and adenovirus receptor-independent cell entry mechanism. J Virol 1998;72(12):9706–9713.
52. Burns TF, El-Deiry WS. The p53 pathway and apoptosis. J Cell Physiol 1999;181(2):231–239.
53. Ryan KM, Phillips AC, Vousden KH. Regulation and function of the p53 tumor suppressor protein. Curr Opin Cell Biol 2001;13(3):332–337.
54. Haupt Y, Barak Y, Oren M. Cell type-specific inhibition of p53-mediated apoptosis by mdm2. Embo J 1996;15(7):1596–1606.
55. Haupt Y, Maya R, Kazaz A, Oren M. Mdm2 promotes the rapid degradation of p53. Nature 1997;387(6630):296–299.
56. Kamijo T, Weber JD, Zambetti G, Zindy F, Roussel MF, Sherr CJ. Functional and physical interactions of the ARF tumor suppressor with p53 and Mdm2. Proc Natl Acad Sci U S A 1998;95(14):8292–8297.
57. Bogler O, Huang HJ, Kleihues P, Cavenee WK. The p53 gene and its role in human brain tumors. Glia 1995;15(3):308–327.
58. Bruner JM, Saya H, Moser RP. Immunocytochemical detection of p53 in human gliomas. Mod Pathol 1991;4(5):671–674.
59. Frankel RH, Bayona W, Koslow M, Newcomb EW. p53 mutations in human malignant gliomas: comparison of loss of heterozygosity with mutation frequency. Cancer Res 1992;52(6):1427–1433.
60. Fults D, Brockmeyer D, Tullous MW, Pedone CA, Cawthon RM. p53 mutation and loss of heterozygosity on chromosomes 17 and 10 during human astrocytoma progression. Cancer Res 1992;52(3):674–679.
61. van Beusechem VW, Grill J, Mastenbroek DC, et al. Efficient and selective gene transfer into primary human brain tumors by using single-chain antibody-targeted adenoviral vectors with native tropism abolished. J Virol 2002;76(6):2753–2762.
62. Suzuki K, Alemany R, Yamamoto M, Curiel DT. The presence of the adenovirus E3 region improves the oncolytic potency of conditionally replicative adenoviruses. Clin Cancer Res 2002;8(11):3348–3359.
63. Hall AR, Dix BR, O'Carroll SJ, Braithwaite AW. p53-dependent cell death/apoptosis is required for a productive adenovirus infection. Nat Med 1998;4(9):1068–1072.
64. Vecil GG, Lang FF. Clinical trials of adenoviruses in brain tumors: a review of Ad-p53 and oncolytic adenoviruses. J Neurooncol 2003;65:237–246.

III Clinical Applications

20 Problems, Side Effects, and Disappointments in Clinical Cancer Gene Therapy

Ta-Chiang Liu, MD, PhD *and David H. Kirn,* MD

CONTENTS

Summary

Genetic therapeutic agents have been tested in cancer patients for over 10 yr. Five major approaches have been tested in clinical trials: tumor suppressor gene replacement, prodrug-activating enzyme delivery, oncolytic virotherapy, antisense oligonucleotide delivery, and cytokine immuno-gene therapy. Proof-of-principle demonstrations of transgene expression, as well as certain biological activities, have been shown; serious toxicity has been rare. However, the field faces several challenges, including limited efficacy, side effects, and lack of proper response indicators. Inefficient tumor delivery and/or transfection, and rapid clearance mediated by host immune responses result in inadequate transgene expression and limited efficacy. Major side effects include vector-/transgene-specific toxicities and disease-/host-specific idiosyncrasy. Discrepancies between certain biomarkers and imaging studies also increase the difficulties in interpretation. Future cancer gene therapy agents need to incorporate mechanisms that allow us to further understand the biodistribution, expression, and function of the vector/transgene. Immune responses toward vectors and transgenes should be reduced, whereas antitumoral immune responses should be enhanced. Vectors and transgenes that offer more than one mechanisms-of-action need to be explored and combined. Finally, our understanding of tumor biology, vectorology and immunology needs to be strengthened in order to improve efficacy and minimizing toxicity.

Key Words: Gene therapy; cancer; clinical trial; vector; genetics.

1. INTRODUCTION

The past decade has seen rapid development in cancer therapy. With the advantage of knowledge and technology advances in cancer biology, genetics, microbiology, and immunology, genetic therapy (a.k.a. "gene therapy") has entered clinical trials and provided useful information. The first human clinical cancer gene therapy trial was approved in 1989 for melanoma and renal cell carcinoma *(1)*. Hundreds of trials were subsequently carried out worldwide. The target tissues for these gene therapy studies can be divided into three categories. The first approach is to target cancer cells directly; this

From: *Cancer Drug Discovery and Development: Gene Therapy for Cancer*
Edited by: K. K. Hunt, S. A. Vorburger, and S. G. Swisher © Humana Press Inc., Totowa, NJ

includes, but is not limited to to, restoration of functional tumor suppressor genes (e.g., *p53*) *(2)*, "suicide" gene therapy followed by prodrug administration (e.g., herpes simplex virus tyrosine kinase [HSV-*tk*] followed by ganciclovir) *(3)*, transcriptional control of the vectors with the use of tumor-specific promoters to control the expression of vector genes or therapeutic transgenes (e.g., erbB-2 promoter-driven virus carrying suicide gene; prostate-specific antigen (PSA)-driven oncolytic adenovirus) *(4,5)*, and chemo- and radio-sensitization of tumor cells by the transgenes (e.g., adenovirus E1A) *(6)*.

Apart from cancer cells themselves, other host tissues are also targeted by cancer genetic therapy. Immunotherapy aims at restoring and/or enhancing the host antitumoral immune response. This includes the use of cytokines (e.g., interleukin [IL]-2, granulocyte macrophage colony-stimulating factor [GM-CSF]) *(7,8)*, costimulatory factors (e.g., B7) *(9)* and others (e.g., dendritic cells [DCs]) *(10)*. In some cases the therapeutic transgene products have direct antitumoral effect (e.g., IL-2), whereas in others the transgene products act through an indirect fashion (e.g., GM-CSF). Antiangiogenesis, initially proposed by J. Folkman, argues that the destruction of tumor angiogenesis can lead to tumor reduction *(11)*. This approach is exemplified by Avastin (bevacizumab; monoclonal vascular endothelial growth factor [VEGF] IgG), which has been approved by Food and Drug Administration (FDA) for the treatment of various cancers in conjunction with standard chemotherapy *(12,13)*. In terms of gene therapy, antiangiogenic factors can be delivered by vectors *(14)*. Finally, the third area of interest is to confer (chemotherapeutic) drug resistance on bone marrow stem cells, in order to avoid the bone marrow suppression which occurs frequently after high-dose chemotherapy *(15)*.

The gene delivery systems (vectors) can be divided into two broad categories: viral and nonviral vectors. Viral vectors, with the advantage of high transduction efficiency and sophisticated techniques for large scale clinical grade production, are frequently used vectors *(16–19)*. Examples include the use of adenovirus, retrovirus, herpes simplex virus (HSV), vaccinia virus, Newcastle Disease Virus, adeno-associated virus (AAV), measle virus, and others. Nonviral vectors have also been used in clinical trials. Examples include plasmids, liposomes, bacteriae, and cells *(20–24)*.

Although genetic therapy has been tested in cancer patients for more than 10 yr, no agent from this category has been approved to date. Tables 1–5 list results of a few major categories of cancer gene therapy approaches. Toxicity in most trials has been only transient and not severe. The expression levels of therapeutic genes or the replication of the vectors varied; higher doses tend to be associated with increased gene expression. Antitumoral immunity can be induced by immunostimulatory transgene products (e.g., GM-CSF, HLA-B7, IL-2) based on hematologic analysis. Immunity against viral vectors can also be demonstrated by neutralizing antibody levels. Although there are some promising results in these early trials, problems and limitations still exist which need to be tackled. The hurdles to be addressed include: (1) limited efficacy, (2) side effects, (3) lack of proper response indicators, and (4) lack of thorough understanding of mechanisms leading to therapeutic effects (Table 6).

2. HURDLES WITH CLINICAL CANCER GENE THERAPY

2.1. Limited Efficacy

Most clinical gene therapy trials reported to date consist of phase I and phase II trials. The overall response rate for cancer patients undergoing gene therapy as a single agent treatment has been less than 20% *(25–29)*. This has been largely attributed to

Table 1
Tumor Suppressor Gene Therapy (p53)

Route	*Cancer type/phase*	*Patient number*	*Vector*	*Doses*	*Schedule*	*AE (G3/G4 episodes; DLT; most freq. AE)*	*ORR*	*PD*	*TTP*	*Gene expression*	*Ref.*
IT (pre-op); cavity	Glioma I	15	Ad	3×10^{10}– 3×10^{12} vp	2 (1 pre-op, 1 post-op)	No DLT; headache, fatigue, fever	N/A	N/A	13 wk	13/13 p53 IHC + ;7/8 p21 IHC +(bx; within 8mm)	*84*
IT (pre-, intra-, post-op)	HNSCC I	15	Ad	1×10^{6}– 1×10^{11} pfu	3/wk × 2 (pre-); 3 d post-op (post-)	No DLT; fever, injection pain, headache	N/A	N/A	N/A	p53, p21 IHC + (bx)	*85*
IT (pre-/ post-op)	Laryngeal I	12	Ad	1×10^{10}– 1×10^{12} vp	2 × (qod × 5)	No DLT; fever	N/A	N/A	N/A	4 p53 IHC + (bx)	86
IT	Melanoma, breast I	6	Ad	2×10^{7}– 5×10^{8} pfu	single	No DLT; edema, fever, fatigue	0	2/6	N/A	5/6 p53 RT-PCR + (bx)	*87*
IT	NSCLC I	9	Retro	5×10^{8} cfu	qd × 5	No DLT	3/9	3/9	N/A	3/8 DNA PCR +(bx); 6/6 ISH + (bx)	*88*
IT	NSCLC I	15	Ad	1×10^{7}–1×10^{10} pfu	single	No DLT; fever, arthralgia, dyspnoea	0	13/15	N/A	6/15 RT-PCR + (bx; $\geq 10^{8}$ pfu)	*89*
IT	NSCLC I	28	Ad	1×10^{6}–1×10^{11} pfu	qm × (1–6)	No DLT; fever, inj site pain, nausea	2/28	10/28	N/A	18/21 PCR + (bx); 12 /26 RT-PCR + (bx)	*90*
IT or intra-vesicular (pre-op)	Bladder I	12	Ad	7.5×10^{11}– 7.5×10^{13} vp	single (3 .d prior op)	No DLT; GU burning sensation, abd pain,	N/A	N/A	N/A	0 PCR + (op) in IT arm; 7/9 RT-PCR + (op) in intra-vesicular arm	*91*

(*Continued*)

Table 1 (*Continued*)

Route	*Cancer type/phase*	*Patient number*	*Vector*	*Doses*	*Schedule*	*AE (G3/G4 episodes; DLT; most freq. AE)*	*ORR*	*PD*	*TTP*	*Gene expression*	*Ref.*
Intravesicular	Bladder I	13	Ad	1×10^{10}–1×10^{12} vp	days 1 and 4, days 1–4, or days 1–4 and 5–8	No DLT; bladder spasm	0	11/13	2m	2/7 RT-PCR + (bx)	*92*
IT (+C/T)	NSCLC I	24	Ad	1×10^{6}–1×10^{11} pfu	cisplatin 80 mg/m^2 on d1; virus 3 days post C/T × 6 courses	No DLT; fever, asthenia, dyspnea	2/24	5/24	N/A	6/14 RT-PCR +(bx; ≥3 × 10^9 pfu)	*93*
IT (+ C/T)	NSCLC II	25	Ad	7.5×10^{12} vp	d1/cycle, 1–3 cycles; + (1) carboplatin AUC = 6, taxol 175 mg/m^2 on days 1 or (2) cisplatin 100 mg/m2 on d1 + vinorelbine 25 mg/m^2 on days 1, 8,15, 22	13 G3/G4 AE; fever, flu-like, nausea	13/25	3/25	N/A	17/25 RT-PCR + (bx)	*29*

IT (+ R/T)	NSCLC II	19	Ad	3×10^{11}–3×10^{12} vp	days 1, 18, 32 + R/T 60 Gy/6w	14 G3/G4 AE; fever, pain, chills	6/19	11/19	9.2 m for mets	9/12 PCR + (bx); 10/12 RT-PCR (bx)	*94*
IT (+ R/T)	HNSCC II	42	Ad	1×10^{12} vp	qw × 8 + R/T 70 Gy/35f/7–8w	fever	16/17 (Combo); 22/27 (R/T alone)	0 (Combo); 0 (R/T alone)	N/A	N/A	*95*
IT (+ R/T)	NPC II	29	Ad	1×10^{12} vp	qw × 8 + R/T , 60–70 Gy/ 7–8 w	fever	100% (combo) 100% (R/T)	0	N/A	N/A	*96*
IP (± C/T)	Ovarian I/II	41	Ad	7.5×10^{10}–7.5×10^{13} vp	single; 2–3 doses + cisplatin 100 mg/m^2 on day 1, or carboplatin (AUC =6)/taxol (175 mg/m^2)	47 G3/G4 AE (1 possible DLT); fever, abd complaints, nausea	7/41 (CA125 _ with higher doses)	30/41	N/A	52/62 RT-PCR + (17/20 with multidosing) (bx)	*47*

Abbr: AE, adverse effect; DLT, dose-limiting toxicity; ORR, overall response rate; PD, progressive disease; TTP, time to tumor progression; HNSCC, head and neck squamous cell carcinoma; NPC, nasopharyngeal carcinoma; NSCLC, non-small cell lung cancer; IT: intratumoral, IP, intraperitoneal; pfu, plaque-forming units; vp, viral particles; R/T, radiotherapy; C/T, chemotherapy; N/A, non-available; bx, biopsy; IHC, immunohistochemistry; PCR, polymerase chain reaction; RT-PCR, reverse transcriptase-PCR; ISH, *in situ* hybridization; WB, western blotting; Ad, adenovirus; retro, retrovirus.

Table 2
Prodrug Activating Gene Therapy (HSV-*tk*)

Route	*Cancer type/ phase*	*Patient number*	*Vector*	*Doses*	*Schedule (incl. prodrug)*	*AE (G3/G4 episodes; DLT; most freq. AE)*	*ORR*	*PD*	*TTP*	*Gene expression*	*Ref.*
IT	Melanoma I/II	8	Retro-VPC	1×10^8–3×10^9 cells	Single or q5d × 3; GCV 5mg/kg q12h × 14 d from day7	No DLT; skin reaction, fever, pain	0	8/8	N/A	3/6 PCR + (bx)	*97*
IT	GBM I	5	Retro-VPC	1×10^8–1×10^9 cells	single; GCV 5mg/kg q12h × 14 d from d7	No DLT	N/A	N/A	N/A	N/A	*98*
IT	Brain I	13	Ad	2×10^9–2×10^{12} vp	single; GCV 5 mg/kg q12h × 14 d from d2	DLT at 2×10^{12} vp (CNS toxicity); hyponatremia, thrombocytopenia, increased hemiparesis	0	12/13	N/A	N/A	*99*
IT	Brain I	15	Retro-VPC	2.5×10^8–1×10^9 cells	single; GCV 5mg/kg q12h × 14 d	No DLT; seizure, hemorrhage	6/15	9/15	N/A	2/2 ISH + (resection)	*100*
IT	Refractory I	16	Retro	2×10^6 cfu	qd × 5; GCV 5mg/kg q12h × 14 d from d6	No DLT; inj. site pain	0	16/16	N/A	N/A	*101*
IT	Mesothelioma I	21	Ad	1×10^9–1×10^{12} pfu	single; GCV 5 mg/kg q12h × 14 d from day 5	No DLT; fever, anemia, bullae	0	15/21	N/A	10/20 PCR +, 3/14 RT-PCR +, 2/14 ISH + (bx)	*102*

IT (± steroid)	Mesothelioma I	10	Ad	1.5 × 10^{13} vp	single; GCV 5mg/kg q12h × 14 d ± methylpred 125mg q6h × 3 d	No DLT; fever, rash, anemia	0	10/10	N/A	PCR, RT-PCR, or ISH + (bx); no difference ± steroid	*71*
IT	CRC liver mets I	16	Ad	1 × 10^{10}– 1 × 10^{13} vp	single; GCV 5mg/kg q12h × 7 d	No DLT; pain, fever, transaminitis	0	5/16	8w	0/6 PCR + (bx)	*103*
IT	Prostate I/II	36	Ad	1 × 10^{8}– 1 × 10^{11} pfu	single (11 pts have a 2nd dose); GCV 5mg/kg q12 h or VCV 2g tid × 14 d	No DLT; fever, chills	N/A; 27/36 PSA	N/A	N/A	22/36 PCR + (bx)	*104*
IT	Prostate I	16	Ad	1 × 10^{10}– 1 × 10^{12} vp	single; GCV 5 mg/kg q12 h × 7 or 14 d; 5-FC 150mg/kg/d × 7 or 14 d	77/12; hematuria, lymphopenia, increased CPK	N/A; PSA ↓ > 25% (7/16)	N/A	N/A	12/16 PCR + (blood) 4/12 IHC + (bx)	*105*
IT	Prostate I	18	Ad	1 × 10^{8}– 1 × 10^{11} pfu	single; GCV 5mg/kg q12h × 14 d from d2	No DLT; fever, transaminitis	N/A; 3/18 PSA ↓ > 50%	N/A	N/A	10/18 PCR + (urine; vector DNA)	*106*
Intral-lesiona (+ bone)	Prostate I	11	Ad	2.5 × 10^{8}–2.5 × 10^{10} pfu	d1, 8; VCV 1g bid × 21 d	No DLT; flu-like; lymphopenia, neutropenia	N/A; PSA ↓ (2/11)	N/A	N/A	10/11 PCR + (bx)	*107*
cavity (post-op)	Glioma I/II	12	Retro-VPC	7.1–9.8 × 10^{6}	single; GCV 5mg/kg	No DLT; 11 G3/G4 AE	N/A	8/12	240 d (responder);	1/12 PCR + (blood)	*3*

(*Continued*)

Table 2 (*Continued*)

Route	*Cancer type/ phase*	*Patient number*	*Vector*	*Doses*	*Schedule (incl. prodrug)*	*AE (G3/G4 episodes; DLT; most freq. AE)*	*ORR*	*PD*	*TTP*	*Gene expression*	*Ref.*
				cells/cm^2	q12h × 14 d from day 8				75d (non-responders)		
cavity (post-op)	GBM I/II	30	Retro-VPC	1 × 10^9 cells	qw × 5; GCV 5mg/kg q12h × 14 d from day 21	22 SAE; seizure, meningitis, cerebral oedema	N/A	N/A	Time to KPS<60: 76 d	15/18 PCR + (brain; vector DNA)	*108*
cavity (post-op)	Glioma I	11	Ad	2.5 × 10^{11}–9 × 10^{11} vp	single; GCV 5mg/kg q12h × 14 d from d2	No DLT	2/11 (tumor control)	6/11	N/A	N/A	*109*
cavity (post-op)	GBM I/II	48	Retro-VPC	1 × 10^9 cells	single; GCV 5mg/kg q12h × 14 d from day 14	2 SAE	N/A	N/A	Time to KPS<60: 4.5 m	17/48 PCR + (blood); 4/10 PCR + (tumor; vector DNA)	*110*
cavity (post-op)	Glioma I	14	Ad	4.6 × 10^8–4.6 × 10^{11} vp	single; GCV 5mg/kg q12h × 14 d from d2	No DLT; transaminitis, UTI	0	14/14	2.3m	N/A	*111*
cavity (post-op)	Brain I	12	Retro-VPC	1 × 10^8 – 1 × 10^9 cells	single; GCV 5mg/kg q12h × 14 d from d15	No DLT	1/12	10/12	N/A	8/12 PCR + (PBL); 1/5 PCR + (bx; vector DNA)	*112*

cavity (post-op)	Glioma I	14	Retro-VPC; Ad	10^9 cells; 3×10^{10} pfu	single; GCV 5mg/kg q12h × 14 d	Fever	N/A	11/14	N/A	N/A	*113*
cavity (post-op)	Glioma II	17	Ad	3×10^{10} pfu	single; GCV 5mg/kg q12h × 14 d from d6	Transaminitis	N/A	8/17	Survival 70.6 wks (control 39 wks)	N/A	*114*
IP	ovarian I	14	Ad	1×10^9–1×10^{11} pfu	single; GCV 5mg/kg q12h × 14 d from d3	No DLT; fever, nausea, diarrhea	0	9/14	N/A	13/14 PCR + (ascites); 11/14 RT-PCR + (ascites)	*115*
IT (+ R/T, antiandrogen)	Prostate I/II	30	Ad	5×10^{11} vp	2–3 injections; VCV 2 g po tid × 14 d ± R/T 76Gy/35f ± antiandrogen	No DLT; fever, chills, fatigue	N/A	N/A	N/A	N/A	*116*
IT (+ R/T, antiandrogen)	Prostate I/II	59	Ad	5×10^{11} vp	2–3 injections; VCV 2 g po tid × 14 d ± R/T 76Gy/35f ± antiandrogen	N/A	N/A; PSA _ in low grade pts	N/A	N/A	N/A	*117*
IT (+ R/T)	Prostate I/II	85 (A: 36; B:	Ad	1×10^8 – 1×10^{12} pfu (A); 1×10^{10} –1×10^{11}	Single (A,B), 2 (C); GCV 5mg/kg q12h x 14d (A, B); VCV 2mg tid	N/A	N/A	N/A	N/A	(CD8_ in blood)	*118*

(*Continued*)

Table 2 (*Continued*)

Route	*Cancer type/ phase*	*Patient number*	*Vector*	*Doses*	*Schedule (incl. prodrug)*	*AE (G3/G4 episodes; DLT; most freq. AE)*	*ORR*	*PD*	*TTP*	*Gene expression*	*Ref.*
		22; C: 27)		pfu (B); 2.5×10^{10} pfu (C)	× 14 d + R/T 76 Gy/35 fr						
IT (+ R/T)	Prostate I	15	Ad	1×10^{12} vp	single; GCV 1800 mg/d × 1–4 wks; 5-FC 150 mg/kg/d × 1–4 wks + R/T 7000 –7400 cGy	No DLT; lymphopenia, urinary frequency, dysuria	N/A; PSA_ in all pts	N/A	N/A	4/9 IHC + (bx)	*119*
wall (post-op, R/T)	GBM III	248 (124 each group)	Retro-VPC	1×10^{9} cells	single; GCV 5 mg/kg q12h (days 14–27) + R/T 5–60 Gy, (days 14–21)	64 vs 53 G3/G4 AE; thrombo-embolism, seizure, hemiparesis	N/A	111/ 124 vs 103/ 124	180 d vs 183 d; 365 d vs 354 d (survival)	7/17 PCR + (tumor bx; vector DNA), 1/13 PCR + (normal brain); 9/121 PCR + (PB)	*120*
IP (+C/T)	ovarian I	10	Ad	2×10^{10}–2×10^{13} vp	single; ACV 15 mg/kg q8h × 14 d ; + topotecan 1 mg/m^2 iv qd × 5	No DLT; neutropenia, anemia, tranaminitis	N/A	N/A	4 m	4/10 PCR + (urine)	*121,122*

Abbr: AE, adverse effect; DLT, dose-limiting toxicity; ORR, overall response rate; PD, progressive disease; TTP, time to tumour progression; GBM, glioblastoma multiforme; HNSCC, head and neck squamous cell carcinoma; NPC, nasopharyngeal carcinoma; CRC, colorectal carcinoma; IT, intratumoral; IP, intraperitoneal; vp, virus particles; pfu, plaque-forming units; R/T, radiotherapy; C/T, chemotherapy; GCV, ganciclovir; VCV,valacyclovir; N/A, non-available; bx, biopsy; IHC, immunohistochemistry; PCR, polymerase chain reaction; RT-PCR, reverse transcriptase-PCR; ISH, *in situ* hybridization; Ad, adenovirus; retro, retrovirus; VPC, virus-producing cells; UTI, urinary tract infection.

Table 3
Oncolytic Virus (Ad-*dl*1520; Onyx-015)

Route	*Cancer type/ phase*	*Patient number*	*Doses*	*Schedule*	*AE (G3/G4 episodes; DLT; most freq. AE)*	*ORR*	*PD*	*TTP*	*Viral gene expression/ replication*	*Cytokine induction*	*Ref.*
IT	HNSCC I	22	1×10^7–1×10^{11} pfu	single; q4w if SD	No DLT; fever, nausea, chills	3/22	9/22	N/A	4/22 ISH + (Bx); - in plasma and oropharyngeal swab	N/A	*123*
IT	HNSCC II	37	1×10^{10} pfu	qd × 5/q 3 w; bid × 5/q 2 w	N/A	5/37	24/37	51 d	7/11 ISH, HE, EM (Bx)	N/A	*124*
IT	HNSCC II	40	2×10^{11} vp	qd × 5/q3w; bid × 5/ 2w	38 G3/G4 AE; inj site pain, asthenia, fever	5/40	19/40	22 (standard); 53 (hyper-fractioned)	12/29 PCR + (serum)	N/A	*125*
IT (pre-op)	Oral II	15	1×10^{10} pfu	Single; 1–14 days prior op	No DLT	N/A	N/A	N/A	10/15 (tumor),3/15 (normal) ISH, IHC + (bx); intensity greater in tumors than in normal tissues; 2/15 tumors receiving saline showed ISH +	N/A	*126*
IT	Pancreas I	23	1×10^8–1×10^{11} pfu	single/q4w	1 DLT at 1×10^{10} pfu (hyperbilirubinemia, transaminitis); fever, asthenia, pain	0	5/23	N/A	0 ISH + (Bx; day 22); 0 serum PCR + (> 1 d); 80% top 3 doses showed serum PCR + at 15 min post-injection	N/A	*127*

(*Continued*)

Table 3 (*Continued*)

Route	*Cancer type/ phase*	*Patient number*	*Doses*	*Schedule*	*AE (G3/G4 episodes; DLT; most freq. AE)*	*ORR*	*PD*	*TTP*	*Viral gene expression/ replication*	*Cytokine induction*	*Ref.*
Peritumoral (post-op)	Glioma I	24	10^7–10^{10} pfu	single	No DLT	0	23/24	46 d	N/A	N/A	*128*
IT (± IP for ascites)	Hepatobiliary II	19	6×10^9–3×10^{10} pfu	single	6 G3/G4 AE; fever, myalgia, abdominal pain	1/19 (AFP_8/16)	3/19	N/A	0 CPE (urine); 2/2 PCR + (bile stent); 4/4 ascites PCR + (days 1–9)	N/A	*129*
IP	Ovarian I	16	1×10^9–1×10^{11} pfu	qd × 5/q4w	No DLT; fever, flu-like, abdominal pain	0 (CA 125_1/16)	12/16	N/A	7/8 PCR + (peritoneal washing) on day 5, 5/5 + on day 15; 0/8 serum PCR +	N/A	*130*
IV then IT	HCC II	5	3×10^{11} pfu	IV (d1), IT (days 2,15, 16,29,30)	3 G3/G4 AE; fever, chills	1/5	4/5	N/A	HE, EM + (bx); serum PCR + (disappeared after 4 hrs)	N/A	*131*
IV	CRC II	18	2×10^{12} vp	day 1, 15/q28d × 6 cycles	3 G3/G4 AE; chills, fatigue, fever	0 (CEA _ 4/18)	10/18	N/A	5/18 PCR +(blood) at 72 h	N/A	*132*
IT (+ C/T)	HNSCC II	37	1×10^{10} pfu	qd × 5 + cisplatin 80 mg/m^2 day 1 i.v.b, 5-FU 800-1000 mg/m^2 days 1–5 c.i./q3w	42% pts G3/G4 AE; asthenia, fever, chills	19/37	N/A	150 d	4/7 ISH + (Bx)	Ab+	*81*

IT (+ C/T)	Pancreas I/II	21	2×10^{10}–2×10^{11} vp	days 1,5,8,15,36, 43,50,57; + gemcitabine 1000 mg/m^2 iv d 36,43,50,57	No DLT; fever, chills, myalgia	2/21	11/21	6 wks	0 ISH + (aspirate)	N/A	*133*
IT (+ C/T)	Sarcoma I/II	6	1×10^9–1×10^{11} pfu	d 1–5/m + mitomycin-C 8 mg/m^2 , doxorubicin 40 mg/m^2, cisplatin mg/m^2 qm; up to 6 cycles	No DLT; fever, fatigue, injection site pain	1/6	1/6	N/A	5/6 Q-PCR + (blood); 2/6 ISH + (bx)	N/A	*134*
IT, HAI, IV	Liver I, II	9 (I), 7 (II)	3×10^9–3×10^{11} pfu	days 1,2,15,16, 29,30 (IT); days1–5 (HAI, IV);+ 5-FU 300 mg/m^2qd × 3m, oxaleplatin 85 mg/m^2 q3w (extrahepatic cases)	No DLT; fever, chills	0 (CEA _ 3/7; phase II)	1/7 (phase II)	N/A	ISH, HE + (bx); EM: virus in sinusoids, endothelial cells, space of Disse, normal hepatocytes, tumor cells	N/A	*135*
HAI (+ IV C/T)	CRC liver mets I	11	2×10^8–2×10^{12} vp	days 1,8,22,50, 78 + 5-FU 425 mg/m^2/d iv days 22,50, 78	No DLT; fever, chills, liver enzymes _	N/A (1 PR at high doses)	N/A	N/A	Q-PCR + (blood) ≥ 6×10^{11} vp	N/A	*136*
HAI (+ IV C/T)	CRC liver mets II	27	2×10^{12} vp	days 1,8,22,50, 78 + 5-FU 425 mg/m^2/d iv	27 G3/G4 AE; fever, chills, ALP _	3/27	11/27	N/A	6/8 Q-PCR +(blood); 5/7 viremia (_ genome copies)	TNF, IFN-_, IL-1,	*59*

(*Continued*)

Table 3 (*Continued*)

Route	*Cancer type/ phase*	*Patient number*	*Doses*	*Schedule*	*AE (G3/G4 episodes; DLT; most freq. AE)*	*ORR*	*PD*	*TTP*	*Viral gene expression/ replication*	*Cytokine induction*	*Ref.*
				d22,50, 78					on d 4	IL-6, IL-10	
IV (+ C/T)	Refractory I	10	2×10^{10}–2×10^{13} vp	single/qw × 3 + carboplatin (AUC 2), taxol 425 mg/m^2 from cycle 3	No DLT; fever, chills, transaminitis	0	8/10	90 d	17/37 Q-PCR + (blood; d 7) 1 IHC, Q-PCR + (bx; d 5)	TNF, IL-6, IL-10	*137*
IV (+ C/T, IL-2)	Metastatic I	10	2×10^{11}, 2×10^{12} vp	single/qw × 6 ± CPT-11 125 mg/w, 5-FU 500mg/w iv single/qw × 4 or IL-2 iv single day 1	No DLT; fever, chills	0	6/10	120 d	2/10 Q- PCR + (blood) on d 7; Q-PCR + (tumor) on d 6	TNF, IFN-_, IL-6, IL-10	*138*

Abbr: AE, adverse effect; DLT, dose-limiting toxicity; ORR, overall response rate; PD, progressive disease; TTP, time to tumour progression; HNSCC, head and neck squamous cell carcinoma; HCC, hepatocellular carcinoma; CRC, colorectal carcinoma; IT, intratumoral; IP, intraperitoneal; HAI, hepatic arterial infusion; EUS, endoscopic ultrasound; R/T, radiotherapy; C/T, chemotherapy; N/A, non-available; bx, biopsy; IHC, immunohistochemistry; PCR, polymerase chain reaction; Q-PCR, quantitative PCR; RT-PCR, reverse transcriptase-PCR; ISH, *in situ* hybridization; ALP, alkine phosphate.

Table 4
Antisense Oligonucleotide (Bcl-2)

Route	*Cancer type/ phase*	*Patient number*	*Doses*	*Schedule*	*AE (G3/G4 episodes; DLT; most freq. AE)*	*ORR*	*PD*	*TTP*	*Gene expression*	*Ref.*
SC	NHL I	9	4.6–73.6 mg/m^2	Continuous × 14 d	No DLT; skin reaction, hyperglycaemia, lymphopenia	1/9 (LDH _ 4/9)	5/9	N/A	2/9 Bcl-2_ flow cytometry (PB, BM)	*139*
SC	NHL I	21	4.6–195.8 mg/m^2/d	Continuous × 14 d	DLT ≥ 147.2 mg/m^2/d (thrombocytopenia, fever, hypotension); skin reaction, lymphopenia	1/21	9/21	3.6 m	7/21 Bcl-2_ flow cytometry (PB, BM, LN)	*140*
IV	advanced I	35	0.6–6.9 mg/kg/d	Continuous × 14 or 21 d; 2 wk on/4 wk off × 3 cycles, or 2 wk on/2 wk off ×1 + 3 wk on/1 wk off × 2 cycles	No DLT; fatigue, transaminitis, anaemia	0	22/35	N/A	Bcl-2_ WB (PBMC)	*141*
IV (+C/T)	SCLC I	12	3mg/kg/d	Continuous × 7 d + paclitaxel 150 mg/m^2 on day 6	No DLT; fatigue, neutropenia, thrombocytopenia	0	8/12	N/A	1/12 Bcl-2_ WB (PBMNC)	*142*
IV (+C/T)	SCLC I	16	5–7 mg/kg/d	Days 1–8; 21 day cycle × 2 cycles +carboplatin (AUC =6) on day 6 +etoposide 80 mg/m^2/d on days 6–8	No DLT; fatigue, neutropenia, thrombocytopenia	12/16	0	162 d	0 Bcl-2_ WB (PBMNC)	*143*
IV (+C/T)	prostate I	26	0.6–5 mg/kg/d	Continuous × 14 d + mitoxantrone 4–12 mg/m^2/d ivb on day 8; 28-d cycles	No DLT; fatigue, nausea, lymphopenia	1/26; 2/26 PSA _	N/A	N/A	6/9 Bcl-2_ HPLC (plasma)	*144*

(*Continued*)

Table 4 (*Continued*)

Route	*Cancer type/ phase*	*Patient number*	*Doses*	*Schedule*	*AE (G3/G4 episodes; DLT; most freq. AE)*	*ORR*	*PD*	*TTP*	*Gene expression*	*Ref.*
IV (+C/T)	prostate II	20	5–7 mg/kg/d	Continuous × 6 d + docetaxel 60–100 mg/m^2 iv day 6/q3w	N/A; fever, fatigue	7/20 PSA _ (> 50%)		N/A	10/17 weak vs 5/19 strong + IHC (bx)	*145*
IV (+C/T)	prostate II	28	7 mg/kg/d	Continuous × 8 d + docetaxel 75 mg/m^2 iv day 6/q3w	Fever, transaminitis, hypophosphatemia	4/12 (with measurable disease); PSA _ 14/28	N/A	5.3 m (PSA progr-ession)	19/28 Bcl-2_ WB (PBMNC)	*146*
IV, SC (+C/T)	melanoma I/II	14	0.6–6.5 mg/kg/d	Continuous × 14 d + dacarbazine 200 mg/m^2/d on days 5–9; 28-d cycles	No DLT; transaminitis, lymphopenia, coagulopathy	3/14	6/14	N/A	10/14 Bcl-2_ WB (bx)	*147*
IV (+ C/T)	solid I	22	1–4 mg/kg/d (part I); 5–9 mg/kg/d (part II)	Continuous × 21 d + docetaxel 35 mg/m^2 on days 8,15,22 (part I); continuous days 1–5,12,13,19, 20 + docetaxel 35 mg/m^2 on days 6,14,21 (part II)	No DLT; fatigue, transaminitis	2/22	16/22	4.5 m	Variable Bcl-2 _flow cytometry (PB)	*148*
IV (+ C/T)	solid I	15	4.1–7 mg/kg/d	Continuous × 21 d + paclitaxel 100 mg/m^2 on days 1,8,15 or continuous × 5 d + docetaxel 75 mg/m^2 on day 5	No DLT; transaminitis	0/15; 2/15 PSA _ > 50%	N/A	N/A	Bcl-2_ WB (PB)	*149*
IV (+ C/T)	myeloma II	10	7 mg/kg/d	Continuous × 7 d + vincristine 0.4 mg qd + doxorubicin 9	10 G3/G4 AE; inj site pain, anemia, fatigue	4/10	3/10	6 m	Bcl-2_ flow cytometry (4/6 myeloma	*150*

				mg/m^2 on days 4–7 + decamethasone 40 mg; 2–6 cycles					cells, 9/9 B cells; PB)	
IV (+ C/T)	myeloma II	33	3–7 mg/kg/d	Continuous × 7 d (q3w) + thalidomide 100–400 mg qd (from d 4) + decamethasone 40 mg qd (days 4–7; q3w) ; total 3 cycles	Fever, creatinine_, hyperglycemia	18/33	7/33	12 m	6/9 Bcl-2_ RT-PCR (bx); 1/7 WB (bx)	*151*
IV , (+C/T G-CSF)	acute leukemia I	20	4–7 mg/kg/d	Continuous × 10 d; + fludarabine 15–30 $mg/m^2/d$, cytarabine 1–2 $mg/m^2/d$ on days 6–10; G-CSF 5 $\mu g/m^2/d$ on days 5–10	No DLT; diarrhea, fluid retention, hypocalcaemia, pancytopenia	9/20	11/20	N/A	10/14 Bcl-2_ RT-PCR (bx)	*152*
IV (+C/T, G-CSF)	AML I	29	4–7 mg/kg/d	Continuous ×10 d; + daunorubicin 45–60 $mg/m^2/d$ on days 4–6, cytarabine 100 $mg/m^2/d$ on days 4–10; G-CSF 5	No DLT	14/29	12/29	N/A	Responders showed significant Bcl-2_ than nonresponders (bx)	*153*

Abbr: AE, adverse effect; DLT, dose-limiting toxicity; ORR, overall response rate; PD, progressive disease; TTP, time to tumour progression; NHL, non-Hodgkin's lymphoma; SCLC, small cell lung cancer; IT, intratumoral; IV, intravenous; R/T, radiotherapy; SC, subcutaneous; C/T, chemotherapy; N/A, non-available; bx, biopsy; BM, bone marrow; IHC, immunohistochemistry; PCR, polymerase chain reaction; RT-PCR, reverse transcriptase-PCR; ISH, *in situ* hybridization; WB, western blotting; PB, peripheral blood; PBMNC, peripheral blood mononuclear cell; LN, lymph node.

Table 5
Immunotherapy (IL-2 gene therapy)

Route	Cancer type / phase	patient number	Vector	Doses	Schedule	AE (G3/G4 episodes; DLT; most freq. AE)	ORR	PD	TTP	Gene/ protein expression	Immune response	Ref.
SC	Neuroblastoma I	21	neuroblastoma cells (JF) and neuroblasts	10^7 cells/kg (JF; IL-2-secreting) + 10^4–10^7 cells/kg (lymphotactin-secreting)	qw × 2 – 2 w rest – qw × 2	No DLT; local inflammation	3/17	9/17	73 d	N/A	↑ IL-4, IL-5, WBC, CD4 +/CD8+ lymphocyte infil., NK cytotoxic activity	*154*
SC	CRC I	10	tumor cells (R/T), fibroblasts (-IL-2)	10^7 cells; IL-2: 100–800 U IL-2	q2w	No DLT; fatigue, flu-like	0	9/10	N/A	N/A	2/6 ↑ tumor-specific CTL	*155*
SC	Melanoma I	12	melanoma cells (R/T)	5×10^7–1.5 10^8 cells	days 1, 13, 26; qm	No DLT; erythema	0	8/12	N/A	N/A	↑ lymphocytes infiltration	*156*
SC	Melanoma I	12	melanoma cells (-IL-2)	5×10^6–7×10^7 cells (IL-2: 10 U/ 10^5 cells/48H)	1–3 injections	No DLT	0	9/12	9 wk	N/A	↑ CTL 4/12, DTH (1)	*157*
SC	Melanoma I/II	33	melanoma cells (-IL-2)	6×10^7–5.4×10^8 cells (IL-2: 120 ng/ 10^7 cells/24H)	qw × 3	No DLT; erythema	5/33	22/33	N/A	N/A	↑ CTL	158
SC	Melanoma I	6	melanoma cells (-IL-2)	1×10^5–9.6×10^6 cells (IL-2: 987 pg/ 10^6 cells/24H)	wk 1, 2, 3, 6	No DLT; erythemic reaction, fever	0	3	N/A	N/A	↑ CTL 2/6, DTH 2/6	*159*
SC	Myeloma I	8	plasma cells (-IL-2)	3.5–9 × 10^7 cells (IL-2: 2.95 ng/10^6 cells)	days 1, 14, then monthly	No DLT; erythema	6/6	0	N/A	no change; ELISA (serum)	↓ CD4+/CD8+ in high dose patients	*160*

SC	Breast, melanoma I	23	Ad	10^7–10^{10} pfu	qw × 1–5	No DLT; local inflammation, pain, myalgia	0	23/23	N/A	18/22 PCR+ (bx vector DNA); 4 RT-PCR + (bx IL-2)	↑ CD3 T-cell infiltration	*161*
ID, SC	Melanoma I	15	melanoma cells (-IL-2)	3 × 10^6–1 × 10^7 cells (IL-2:140-17060 U/ 10^6 cells/24H)	qw up to 8 cycles	No DLT; erythema, pain, fever	0	10/15	N/A	N/A	DTH 7/15, vitiligo, melanocyto-destruction, T-cell ↑ 2/15	*162*
SC ID	Mets I	15	tumor cells (R/T) + fibroblasts (-IL-2)	(tumor) 2 × 10^6 cells; (fibroblasts) 2 × 10^6 cells (IL-2: 5290 U/10^6 cells/ 24H	q 4–6 w	No DLT; fatigue, hemorrhage	1/15	13/15	N/A	PCR – (bx)	↑ CD4+ T-cells (bx), ↑ T-cell cytotoxicity, proliferation 4/15	*163*
IT	Prostate I	10	DNA-lipid complex	300–1500 μg DNA	qd × 8	No DLT; rectal spotting, perineal discomfort, myalgia	N/A; (PSA ↓ 16/ 24; ↑ 8/ 24)	N/A	N/A	N/A	↑ CD4+, CD8+ T-cells (bx), PBL proliferation	*164*
IT (pre-op)	Prostate I	12	Ad	10^9–10^{10} pfu	single	No DLT; neutropenia, flu-like, bleeding	N/A; (PSA ↓ 5/ 10)	N/A	N/A	0 RT-PCR (op; 1 m post-injection)	↑ IL-4, IFN-γ, CD8+ T-cells,	*165*
IT	Advanced solid tumors I, I/II	24 (I) 52 (I/II)	DNA/DMRIE/ DOPE lipid complex	10–1500 μg	qw 6	No DLT; injection site pain, malaise, fever	0	31/45	N/A	29/46 PCR + (bx); no difference ELISA (serum)	↑ CD8 infiltration	*23*
IT	SC metastatic solid tumors I	8	Vero cells (-IL-2)	5 × 10^5–5 × 10^7 cells (IL-2: 130 ng/ 10^6 cells/24H)	qw × 3	No DLT	0	6/8	N/A	ELISA- (serum)	↑ IL-4, IFN-γ 5/8	*7*

(*Continued*)

Table 5 (*Continued*)

Route	*Cancer type/ phase*	*patient number*	*Vector*	*Doses*	*Schedule*	*AE (G3/G4 episodes; DLT; most freq. AE)*	*ORR*	*PD*	*TTP*	*Gene / protein expression*	*Immune response*	*Ref.*
IT	Solid tumors I	14	Vero cells (-IL-2)	5×10^5–5×10^7 cells (IL-2: 229 ng/10^6 cells/24H)	days 1, 3, 5	N/A	1/13	7/13	N/A	RT-PCR - (bx)	↑ CTL, NK activity	*166*
IT	Mets. Solid I	9	Vero cells (-IL-2)	5×10^5–5×10^7 cells	days 1, 3, 5	No DLT; erythema, pain	1/8	3/8	N/A	↑ IL-2 ELISA at day 5 (serum); RT-PCR – (bx)	↑ IL-6, IL-10, IFN-γ 2/8	*167*
IT	MUC_1 +ve solid tumors I	13	VV	5×10^6–1×10^8 pfu	q 3–12 w	DLT; injection site pain, flu-like, myalgia	0	8/12	N/A	N/A	Ab to MUC_1 : (-); PBMC ↑ 2nd to MUC_1: 5/13	*168*
IV	CRC, RCC, lymphoma I	10	tumor cells (R/T)	2.19 × 107–9.21×10^9 cells (IL-2: 836 pg/106 cells/24H)	days 1–5; q3w	No DLT; fever	1/10	6/10	N/A	7 RT-PCR + (blood)	↑ IFN-γ (6/10), GM-CSF (2/10), ↑ PBL cytotoxicity, ↑ CD4+, CD8+ T-cells	*169*

Abbr: AE, adverse effect; DLT, dose-limiting toxicity; ORR, overall response rate; PD, progressive disease; TTP, time to tumor progression; CRC, colorectal carcinoma; RCC, renal cell carcinoma; bx, biopsy; IT, intratumoral; IP, intraperitoneal; SC, subcutaneous; ID, intradermal; R/T, radiotherapy; C/T, chemotherapy; N/A, non-available; bxIHC, immunohistochemistry; PCR, polymerase chain reaction; RT-PCR, reverse transcriptase-PCR; ISH. *in situ* hybridization; PB, peripheral blood; PBMC, peripheral blood mononuclear cells; V, vaccinia virus; DTH, delayed type hypersensitivity; CTL, cytotoxic T-lymphocyte; DTH, delayed type sensitivity.

Table 6
Issues to Address in the Genetic Therapy of Cancer

Issues to address	*Mechanisms*
Limited efficacy	Host immune response–transient expression Inefficient systemic delivery *in vivo* Low *in vivo* infection rate Inadequate patient selection for those likely to respond
Potential side effects	Insertional mutagenesis Vector- /transgene- specific toxicity Disease- /host- specific idiosyncratic toxicity Species-specificity: inadequate biodistribution and toxicity data with preclinical models Generation of replication-competent virus: recombination
Lack of proper response indicator	Discrepancy between tumor markers, imaging studies and true biological effects Lack of proper indicators for in vivo biological activities
Lack of thorough understanding of tumor biology, genetics and vectorology	Cancer cell signal transduction pathway redundancies (e.g., apoptotic blocks) Dominant-negative proteins in cancer cell block function of transgene product (e.g., p53) Inadequate biodistribution and toxicity data with preclinical models

host immune response to both vectors and transgenes *(30)*, which might lead to shorter vector persistence and/or inadequate transgene expression. Although the host immune system does not seem to block transgene expression after local injection *(31,32)*, long term (>6 mo) expression is still rare. In addition, tumor tissues are heterogeneous; stroma consists of fibrous and connective tissue that distribute throughout the tumor. Because of a lack of receptor to commonly utilized viral vectors, these areas are generally not easily infectable and do not efficiently support transgene expression/vector replication when infected. The central necrotic area in a tumor is another "dead space" which does not support transgene expression.

In addition, numerous studies have demonstrated that the more invasive the cancer is, the more likely it is to utilize multiple oncogenic pathways. Therefore, in any therapeutic targeting, including gene therapy, one or a limited number of these pathways might fail. For example, a phase III trial of Ad-p53 gene therapy in ovarian cancers did not show an adequate therapeutic benefit and was closed after the first interim analysis. It was proposed that the multiple genetic changes in cancer and epigenetic dysregulations led to aberrant silencing of genes *(33)*. Moreover, the recently identified dominant p53 mutants as well as p63 and p73 splice variants could also seriously hampered the effect of p53 gene therapy. This phenomenon can also be exemplified by the angiogenic profile of breast cancers in cancer development. Early breast cancers utilize solely vascular endothelial growth factor (VEGF) as angiogenic factor, but as the disease progressed it adapted to recruit/secrete up to six different angiogenic factors *(11)*. Thus, if a particular antiangiogenic factor is to be delivered to cancer patients by gene therapy, it is likely to receive a higher response rate in early stage patients, but might fail in late stage patients.

2.2. Potential Side Effects

Apart from the limited efficacy, cancer gene therapy also faces the concern of toxicity. Although no cases of treatment-related death have been reported in cancer patients under gene therapy trials, a few cases of treatment-related severe adverse effect (SAE) were documented. Moreover, death and SAE have been reported from gene therapy studies for other diseases. The first fatal case directly linked to gene therapy was of a patient with ornithine carbamyltransferase (OTC) deficiency, who received replication-deficient adenovirus-mediated OTC gene delivery via the hepatic artery. Investigation into this case pointed out an extremely high level of interleukin-6 (IL-6) postinjection in this patient and associated disseminated intravascular coagulation (DIC), which was not suppressed by a simultaneous rise in IL-10 *(34)*; whether IL-6 elevation was the cause or effect is unclear. Although it is uncertain whether this resulted from patient- or disease-specific idiosyncrasy to adenovirus, the tragedy has prompted investigators and patients to be more cautious in designing and participating in gene therapy trials *(35)*.

Another important report came from a X-linked severe combined immunodeficiency (SCID) trial in which patients without a matched bone marrow donor available underwent ex vivo retrovirus-mediated γ_C (common chain) gene delivery into autologous $CD34^+$ bone marrow cells *(36)*. Among more than 30 patients who entered the trial, 2 were found to develop acute leukemia after 2.5 to 3 yr *(37,38)*. Although gene integration is a hallmark of retrovirus based gene delivery, it has never been shown to promote insertional oncogenesis in rodent, dog, and nonhuman primate models, as well as in many other patients who previously received retrovirus-based gene therapy *(39,40)*. Moreover, the two patients who developed leukemia were both on the highest dose level, both among the youngest in the trial, but notably, they had the same locus of gene insertion *(37,38)*. A series of extensive investigations have been carried out, and several potential mechanisms were proposed to explain the SAE *(41–43)*. Some proposed that the activation of a yet poorly defined group of high risk proto-oncogenes (represented here by the gene LMO2 activated in both patients) was sufficient to induce premalignant transformation and further events (e.g., transgene expression and other signal alterations) would promote malignant progression. The other hypothesis suggested that non-physiologic transgene expression evoked a signal alteration that specifically cooperated with the activated oncogenes in the initiation of disease. Subsequent "hits" were also required in this model. However, it is unclear at this moment whether the transgene level at the local environment plays an equally critical role as proto-oncogene activation.

It is clear that current preclinical models are not ideal for predicting the type, frequency, and severity of toxicity, including insertional mutagenesis. Species difference between human and mouse or human and nonhuman primates is the major reason. For cancer gene therapy, animal models face another specific problem: most published preclinical models are human tumor-mouse xenograft systems and involved the use of athymic or even SCID mice. Thus, the results obtained from these studies may be misleading because one of the most crucial players in the cancer-vector-host interplay, the host immune system, is missing. In terms of the risk to humans, it is also unknown whether other patients who received retrovirus-based gene therapy developed leukemic disorders in the long term and whether the administration dosage, route, and duration have any impact on the development of these potential SAEs.

For studies involving the use of replication-deficient viruses, one potential concern is the recombination of replication-competent viruses. Similarly, for oncolytic viruses the risk of wild-type virus recombination (reversion) is another concern. Whereas herpesvirus can be eliminated by acyclovir, effective antibiotics are not readily available for other virus species, and the sequelae of circulating wild-type virus in patients are largely unknown, especially with HIV-based lentivirus. Although recombination has not been shown in preclinical and clinical studies, patients undergoing viral vector-mediated gene therapy should be closely monitored for replication-competent and wild-type virus recombination.

An equally important factor is the route of administration. Although systemic delivery is the ultimate goal for metastasing cancer cells, it is also likely to induce the highest immune reaction, and potential toxicity. To this end, "staged" clinical research and development approaches can ensure safety of the agent tested *(44)*. The goal of this approach is to increase systemic exposure to the test article sequentially only after safety with more localized delivery is demonstrated (*see* Fig. 1). Following demonstration of safety and biological activity by the intratumoral route, trials can sequentially be initiated to study intracavitary (e.g., intraperitoneal), intra-arterial (e.g., hepatic artery), and eventually intravenous administration. Finally, clinical trials of combinations with chemotherapy or radiotherapy will be initiated only after the safety of the test article as a single agent is demonstrated by the relevant route of administration.

In order to predict any potential toxicity to patients, proper preclinical toxicology testing is critical. However, the currently available preclinical models do not fully reflect clinical settings. In addition, because the latent period of the insertional mutagenesis in patients was more than 2 yr, long-term safety evaluation, which is not always practical for preclinical testing, needs to be improved. Furthermore, a large proportion of cancer patients have other comorbid diseases that might affect the biodistribution and toxicity of these gene therapy agents. Patients with liver function impairment (e.g., liver cirrhosis and/or chronic hepatitis) might have an impaired hepatic clearance of viral vectors; in contrast, pulmonary uptake might be increased in these patients, as shown in animal models *(45)*. It is also unknown whether patients with chronic viral infection (hepatitis B virus [HBV], Epstein-Barr virus [EBV], etc) will have acute exacerbation resulting from activation by viral genes and/or therapeutic transgenes. Indeed, age, comorbid index, and surgery were found to be risk factors for local delivery of low- and intermediate-dose adenovirus gene transfer vectors *(46)*. These need to be addressed in preclinical toxicity studies.

2.3. Lack of Proper Response Indicators

An equally important question that remains largely unresolved is the lack of a proper disease response monitoring index. Discrepancy between tumor-specific antigen (tumor marker) levels, imaging studies and efficacy has been shown in some trials *(47)*. Because tumor markers and imaging studies are the two main indices to monitor the disease status, the discrepancy leads to difficulty in interpretation. For prostate cancer, an ideal cancer model for gene therapy because of the ease of local access for vector administration, any local stimulation (including massaging and injection itself) will increase the serum PSA level, for example. This makes interpretation of the tumor markers difficult in these patients.

Furthermore, for biological activity determination, patients are required to have multiple invasive tissue samplings (biopsies). This adds to the inconvenience and potential risk to patients. In addition, significant sampling bias may be reflected from the data

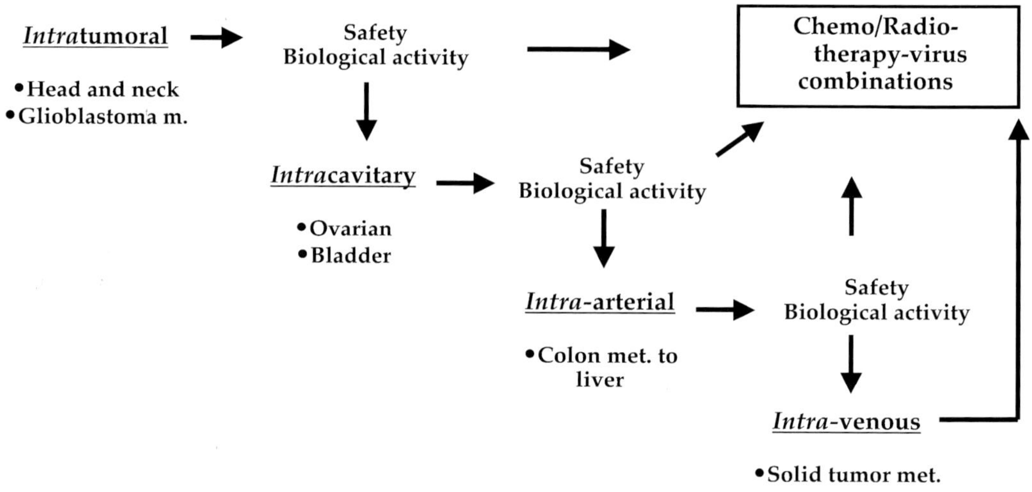

Fig. 1. Staged approach to cancer gene therapy trials.

obtained from biopsies, especially when the tumors are treated with local injections. Thus, a monitoring system for biological activity and disease status that can follow patients with minimal risks, convenience and cost while obtaining high-quality, real-time data is badly needed.

In cases where tumor suppressor gene(s) are delivered to restore the normal function of those genes, it is also worth reconsidering the current concept of gene delivery in the context of transgene expression level. Although transgene expression can be documented by various methods, one must bear in mind that successful gene delivery (as tested by polymerase chain reaction [PCR]) and/or transcription (mRNA expression) does not necessarily lead to functional protein expression. Hence, to monitor biological activities of this type of approach, more data must be obtained to realize the effect of gene restoration. In addition, the therapeutic level of transgene products that is high enough to induce significant antitumoral effect in patients must be determined.

2.4. Lack of Thorough Understanding of Biological Mechanisms

To date, the molecular and genetic targets selected for gene therapy has been largely based on our knowledge of tumor biology, genetics, and virology. However, little is known about the in vivo activities of these agents in humans. Whether the viruses and/or therapeutic transgenes behave in humans as predicted is unclear. For example, a functional gene product does not guarantee the restoration of any particular apoptosis induction pathway. A p53 pathway abnormality, for instance, can result from loss of p53 and/or its up- or downstream targets (i.e., p14, p21, MDM-2,). It remains to be determined in vivo whether p53 restoration can activate the downstream targets as shown in vitro. In addition, in patients who have evolved multiple blocks in the p53 pathway, simply restoring functional p53 might not be enough. As mentioned earlier, dominant- negative crosstalk between ectopic wild-type p53 and the dominant-negative p53 mutants could also limit the efficacy of the p53 gene therapy. In addition to the failed ovarian cancer Ad-p53 phase III trial, the early termination of retrovirus-BRCA1 trial in ovarian cancer patients also implies that a more thorough understanding of the mechanisms of the gene products and the interaction of these genes and vectors with the host is eagerly awaited *(28)*.

It is clear from the discussion above that there remains huge potential for improvement for clinical cancer gene therapy. Future directions in this field should include more efforts on improved understanding of the biological activities of the gene therapy agents in vivo in patients, enhancing efficacy, and reducing side effects (Table 7).

3. FUTURE DIRECTIONS

3.1. Improving the Understanding of Mechanisms and Monitoring of In Vivo Activities

As mentioned above, the lack of a thorough understanding of the biological activities of gene therapy agents in vivo has been a hurdle for cancer gene therapy. Several approaches can be taken to overcome this problem. First, the vectors can be designed to incorporate more sophisticated reporter genes to allow in vivo monitoring. For example, the use of radionucleotide imaging (e.g., positron emission tomography [PET] and single photon emission tomography [SPECT]) has been shown to improve the detection of regional/spatial distribution of vector/transgene expression in vivo *(48,49)*. With the use of Na/I symporter system, PET imaging can reveal biodistribution as well as quantification of gene expression *(50,51)*. SPECT can be used to image receptors, transporters, and other proteins expressed on cell surface. Similarly, vectors carrying bioluminescent activating enzymes (e.g., luciferases) can be monitored for their biodistribution and gene expression in vivo in real time *(52,53)*, although to date this approach is limited to animal models. Other examples of potential use in humans include magnetic resonance imaging (MRI) for gene expression through reporters/enzymes, fluorescence imaging with green fluorescent protein (GFP) introduced by the vector (for superficial tumors), as well as somatostatin receptor gene used in combination with radiolabeled octreotide *(54,55)*. These approaches offer detailed information on both distribution and quantitation of gene expression and they are expected to be incorporated into trials in the future. A detailed summary on molecular imaging of cancer gene therapy can be found in a recent review *(56)*.

In addition to imaging, the pharmacokinetics of the vectors as well as transgenes can also be monitored by incorporation of specific "marker" genes, such as the tumor-associated antigen carcinoembryonic antigen (CEA). An oncolytic measles virus encoding CEA has been tested in preclinical models *(57,58)*. As CEA is only expressed when the virus is replicating, the amount of virus replication/persistence of this virus can be easily followed by measuring the blood level of CEA. This strategy enables more frequent and rapid measurement of the replicating virus. In terms of replication-competent oncolytic viruses, pharmacokinetic monitoring can also be performed by obtaining the quantity of viral genomes in bloodstream following treatment. Mathematical models can be used to calculate the number of virus particles produced and shed into blood with each replication cycle *(59)*.

Treatment of highly accessible tumors for biopsy will definitely increase our knowledge of the in vivo activity of these genes. There is little technical difficulty in obtaining biopsies from superficial tumors, such as head and neck cancers, as well as melanoma. For tumors which post-treatment biopsy is prevented by technical and ethical reasons (e.g., brain tumors), applying gene therapy as a neoadjuvant therapy (i.e., given before operation) will allow us to analyze the biological endpoints from the resected tumors.

Table 7
Future Directions for Genetic Therapy Improvement

Directions	*Solutions*	*Examples*
Revealing the in vivo activities/mechanisms of gene therapy agents	Improving the design of new vectors to allow *in vivo* monitoring	Bioluminescence FIAU or Na/I symporter-based PET imaging Somatostatin receptor based imaging Viruses encoding CEA
	Proper patient selection/trial design	accessible tumors for biopsies Preoperative treatment to allow sampling
Enhancing efficacy	Transgene-armed, replication-selective oncolytic viruses	Oncolytic adenovirus armed with HSV-TK Oncolytic vaccinia virus armed with GM-CSF
	Reducing antivector and/or antitransgene immune response; enhancing antitumoral immune response	Steroid administration prior treatment Pseudotyping viruses Combining vectors with more than one serotypes Complexing with polycationic polymers Less immunogenic vectors Enhancing MHC I presentation Priming dendritic cell
	Targeting tumor stroma/ connective tissue to improve transfection efficiency	Use of matrix metalloproteinases?
	Expanding/manipulating viral tropism	Pseudotyping viruses with ligands to other cellular receptors
	Proper patient selection	Include early stage cancers Select cancers to include highly transfectable tumors
	Combination treatment with existing modalities	
Reducing side effects	More thorough understanding of vectorology	
	Decrease vector binding by antibodies and/ or uptake into reticuloendothelial (RE) cells	Complexing with polycationic polymers
	More sophisticated toxicology studies	Transgenic mice expressing human receptor homologue(s)
	Gene profile for patients receiving gene theraphy (tailored theraphy)	Tumor-necrosis factor promoter polymorphisms

3.2. Enhancing Efficacy

To enhance the antitumoral efficacy of the agents, a promising approach is to utilize replication-selective microorganisms as vectors for gene delivery. Indeed, replication-selective oncolytic viruses have emerged in recent years as powerful tools for cancer treatment *(44)*. These viruses are engineered to target cancer cells rather than normal cells. The self-perpetuating nature of these viruses leads to amplification of input dose in cancer cells, while reduced toxicity can be achieved by limiting the infection or replication of the viruses in normal cells. The past 5 yr have seen tremendous progress in this approach in both preclinical and clinical research *(60)*. New technology has been developed to improve the selectivity, viral spread, and transgene expression from oncolytic viruses, and it is expected to translate into improvement in clinical results in the next few years. Moreover, when "armed" with therapeutic transgenes, the effect is predicted to be greater than with replication-deficient viral vectors not only because of amplification of input dose, but also because of the different mechanisms employed by the armed oncolytic viruses to destroy tumors *(61)*. Apart from oncolytic viruses, certain bacteria have been tested for oncolytic activities. Attenuated Salmonella, Shigella, and other bacteria species have each been shown to be replication-selective *(22)*. Given the large capacity for transgene insertion, these engineered bacteria hold promise.

Because the limited efficacy seen in clinical trials can be at least partly attributed to efficient vector clearance by the host immune system, reducing the impact of host immunity may enhance the therapeutic efficacy. This has been achieved by several mechanisms. Examples include polyethylene glycol-coated (PEGylated) vectors that can avoid neutralizing antibodies and that have prolonged half-lives of the viruses *(62–64)* and plasmids *(65–67)*. Polycationic polymer-coated adenovirus has been shown to have extended systemic circulation, reduced toxicity and neutralizing antibody production *(68,69)*. The utilization of potentially less immunogenic vectors (e.g., recombinant adeno-associated viruses) may also reduce the immune-mediated clearance *(70)*. On the other hand, coinjection of viruses with immunosuppressive agents has been explored; although no significant antibody reduction or enhanced transgene expression was seen, the inflammation was largely reduced *(71)*. However, this approach was only tested in a limited number of patients and more studies are warranted.

Viral vectors can be engineered to boost the host antitumoral immune response or avoid antiviral immunity. Adenovirus, for example, has evolved several immunomodulatory genes (mostly in E3 region) to antagonize immune system-induced apoptosis signals *(72–74)*. The deletion of certain E3 gene regions, as in most adenoviral vectors, might thus contribute to the short in vivo vector persistence. On the other hand, with proper viral gene manipulation, the host antiviral immune response can be redirected to kill tumor cells. A good example is the adenoviral E3-gp 19kD gene, whose function is to downregulate the antigen-presenting cells (APCs) presentation of major histocompatability complex (MHC) I antigen. Adenoviral mutant with deletion in this gene has enhanced MHC I presentation, which correlates with enhanced cytotoxic T-lymphocyte (CTL) infiltration and enhanced antitumoral efficacy *(75)*. Similarly, the HSV viral ICP 47 gene product possesses a similar function, and HSV mutant with deletion in this gene also has enhanced CTL infiltration and antitumoral efficacy *(76)*. Therefore, this approach can be explored with other virus species.

For viral vectors that utilize specific cellular surface virus receptors, it is possible to alter the virus tropism so as to enhance tumor infectability *(77)*. Native viral proteins (e.g., adenovirus fiber) can be engineered to recognize tumor-specific surface protein to achieve tumor-selectivity. This approach redirects the viruses to desired target cells *(78)*. However, before translating this technique to clinical use, the tumor-specific receptor(s) must be thoroughly studied and confirmed, and safety and biodistribution must be obtained from tropism-modified viruses to exclude the possibility of infecting normal tissues *(44)*. Moreover, one must take into account the fact that tumor cells are heterogenous, and that these "tumor-specific" receptors might not be expressed in all tumor cells, and even in the cells that express the receptors, the intensity, and hence the infectibility, might be different from cell to cell. In addition, these vectors should be tested with primary tumor and normal tissues (e.g., from surgical specimens) whenever possible to closely mimic the clinical setting.

For oncolytic viruses, one possible way to enhance the potency is to engineer the virus for enhanced replication and/or viral spread in order to infect the maximum number of cells before being cleared by the immune system. For instance, overexpression of adenovirus death protein (ADP) can enhance the spread of oncolytic adenoviruses *(79)*. Similarly, the deletion of adenoviral E1B-19kD, which functions to balance the effect of ADP in a natural infection course, can also enhance viral replication and viral spread *(80)*. In addition, exploring other viral species that have a shorter viral replication cycle can potentially improve viral spread.

Targeting more than one critical regulator in oncogenic pathways may also enhance efficacy. Vectors can be engineered to carry multiple transgenes targeting different pathways. Similarly, combining gene therapy with existing treatment modalities not only may significantly increase efficacy, it may also reduce the likelihood of resistance *(81)*. It is likely that there will be multiple choices of gene therapy agents in the future, as is currently the case with chemotherapy. Finally, because oncogenesis takes multiple steps and requires a certain latent period, it is desirable to explore the role of gene therapy as a prevention medicine in premalignant lesions, in hope to block oncogenesis at an earlier stage *(82,83)*.

In terms of clinical trials, because end-stage cancers often develop multiple defects in apoptosis pathways, introducing single exogenous therapeutic genes is unlikely to affect the course of the disease. Therefore, patient inclusion criteria and protocol design should be modified to enroll more cancer patients in earlier stages of their disease once safety has been described. The design and enrollment of early stage cancer patients will enable us to potentially achieve optimal antitumoral effect of these agents in the clinic. In addition, for trials using viral vectors, it might be beneficial to include patients whose tumors express high levels of receptors for the particular virus to increase the infectibility.

3.3. Reducing Side Effects

To limit side effects, efforts should be made to enhance our understanding of both vectorology and immunology, particularly emphasizing the host immune reaction to the gene therapy vector and transgene products. As discussed above, vectors and transgenes that are less immunogenic will be of particular interest. Of note, the current preclinical toxicity models should be improved. Extra caution must be taken when interpreting data obtained from human tumor-mouse xenograft systems, whereas the development of immunocompetent syngeneic mouse tumor models or transgenic mouse models that allow for spontaneous tumor growth are useful for accessing the biological activities and efficacies of gene therapy. Of note, the FDA-recommended follow-up period for clinical trials has been extended to monitor any potential long-term side effects. Finally, studies should be initiated to analyze the gene profiles of patients undergoing gene therapy. Comparing the gene profiles before and after treatment with clinical outcome can help identify patients that are most likely to develop side effects (or conversely, clinical responses) after treatment.

A large amount of experience and knowledge has been gained from clinical gene therapy studies over the past 15 yr. Although hurdles have been identified, it is highly likely that genetic therapy will one day become part of the standard armamentarium against cancer.

REFERENCES

1. Gottesman MM. Cancer gene therapy: an awkward adolescence. Cancer Gene Ther 2003;10:501–508.
2. Nielsen LL, Maneval DC. P53 tumor suppressor gene therapy for cancer. Cancer Gene Ther 1998;5:52–63.
3. Klatzmann D, et al. A phase I/II study of herpes simplex virus type 1 thymidine kinase "suicide" gene therapy for recurrent glioblastoma. Study Group on Gene Therapy for Glioblastoma. Hum Gene Ther 1998;9:2595–2604.
4. Pandha HS, et al. Genetic prodrug activation therapy for breast cancer: A phase I clinical trial of erbB-2-directed suicide gene expression. J Clin Oncol 1999;17:2180–2189.
5. DeWeese TL, et al. A phase I trial of CV706, a replication-competent, PSA selective oncolytic adenovirus, for the treatment of locally recurrent prostate cancer following radiation therapy. Cancer Res 2001;61:7464–7472.
6. Hortobagyi GN, Hung M, Lopez-Berestein G. A Phase I multicenter study of E1A gene therapy for patients with metastatic breast cancer and epithelial ovarian cancer that overexpresses HER-2/neu or epithelial ovarian cancer. Hum Gene Ther 1998;9:1775–1798.
7. Tartour E, et al. Phase I clinical trial with IL-2-transfected xenogeneic cells administered in subcutaneous metastatic tumours: clinical and immunological findings. Br J Cancer 2000;83:1454–1461.
8. Mastrangelo MJ, et al. Intratumoral recombinant GM-CSF-encoding virus as gene therapy in patients with cutaneous melanoma. Cancer Gene Ther 1999;6:409–422.
9. Rubin J, et al. Phase I study of immunotherapy of hepatic metastases of colorectal carcinoma by direct gene transfer of an allogeneic histocompatibility antigen, HLA-B7. Gene Ther 1997;4:419–425.
10. Okada H, et al. Gene therapy of malignant gliomas: a pilot study of vaccination with irradiated autologous glioma and dendritic cells admixed with IL-4 transduced fibroblasts to elicit an immune response. Hum Gene Ther 2001;12:575–595.
11. Folkman J. Role of angiogenesis in tumor growth and metastasis. Semin Oncol 2002;29:15–18.
12. Yang JC, et al. A randomized trial of bevacizumab, an anti-vascular endothelial growth factor antibody, for metastatic renal cancer. N Engl J Med 2003;349:427–434.
13. Willett CG, et al. Direct evidence that the VEGF-specific antibody bevacizumab has antivascular effects in human rectal cancer. Nat Med 2004;10:145–147.
14. Kong HL, Crystal RG. Gene therapy strategies for tumor antiangiogenesis. J Natl Cancer Inst 1998;90:273–286.
15. Hesdorffer C, et al. Phase I trial of retroviral-mediated transfer of the human MDR1 gene as marrow chemoprotection in patients undergoing high-dose chemotherapy and autologous stem-cell transplantation. J Clin Oncol 1998;16:165–172.
16. Wu N, Ataai MM. Production of viral vectors for gene therapy applications. Curr Opin Biotechnol 2000;11:205–208.
17. Kay MA, Glorioso JC, Naldini L. Viral vectors for gene therapy: the art of turning infectious agents into vehicles of therapeutics. Nat Med 2001;7:33–40.
18. Kootstra NA, Verma IM. Gene therapy with viral vectors. Annu Rev Pharmacol Toxicol 2003;43:413–439.
19. Lundstrom K. Latest development in viral vectors for gene therapy. Trends Biotechnol 2003;21:117–122.
20. Nabel GJ, et al. Direct gene transfer with DNA-liposome complexes in melanoma: expression, biologic activity, and lack of toxicity in humans. Proc Natl Acad Sci U S A 1993;90:11,307–11,311.
21. Bermudes D, Low B, Pawelek J. Tumor-targeted Salmonella. Highly selective delivery vectors. Adv Exp Med Biol 2000;465:57–63.
22. Jain KK. Use of bacteria as anticancer agents. Expert Opin Biol Ther 2001;1:291–300.
23. Galanis E, et al. Immunotherapy of advanced malignancy by direct gene transfer of an interleukin-2 DNA/DMRIE/DOPE lipid complex: phase I/II experience. J Clin Oncol 1999;17:3313–3323.
24. Harrington K, et al. Cells as vehicles for cancer gene therapy: the missing link between targeted vectors and systemic delivery? Hum Gene Ther 2002;13:1263–1280.

25. Anklesaria P. Gene therapy: a molecular approach to cancer treatment. Curr Opin Mol Ther 2000;2:426–432.
26. Kirn D. Oncolytic virotherapy for cancer with the adenovirus dl1520 (Onyx-015): results of phase I and II trials. Expert Opin Biol Ther 2001;1:525–538.
27. Rainov NG, Ren H. Gene therapy for human malignant brain tumors. Cancer J 2003;9:180–188.
28. Tait DL, Obermiller PS, Hatmaker AR, Redlin-Frazier S, Holt JT. Ovarian cancer BRCA1 gene therapy: Phase I and II trial differences in immune response and vector stability. Clin Cancer Res 1999;5:1708–1714.
29. Schuler M, et al. Adenovirus-mediated wild-type p53 gene transfer in patients receiving chemotherapy for advanced non-small-cell lung cancer: results of a multicenter phase II study. J Clin Oncol 2001;19:1750–1758.
30. Harvey BG, et al. Variability of human systemic humoral immune responses to adenovirus gene transfer vectors administered to different organs. J Virol 1999;73:6729–6742
31. Gahery-Segard H, et al. Phase I trial of recombinant adenovirus gene transfer in lung cancer. Longitudinal study of the immune responses to transgene and viral products. J Clin Invest 1997;100:2218–2226.
32. Molnar-Kimber KL, et al. Impact of preexisting and induced humoral and cellular immune responses in an adenovirus-based gene therapy phase I clinical trial for localized mesothelioma. Hum Gene Ther 1998;9:2121–2133.
33. Zeimet AG, Marth C. Why did p53 gene therapy fail in ovarian cancer? Lancet Oncol 2003; 4:415–422.
34. Raper SE, et al. Fatal systemic inflammatory response syndrome in a ornithine transcarbamylase deficient patient following adenoviral gene transfer. Mol Genet Metab 2003;80:148–158.
35. Reid T, Warren R, Kirn D. Intravascular adenoviral agents in cancer patients: lessons from clinical trials. Cancer Gene Ther 2002;9:979–986.
36. Cavazzana-Calvo M, et al. Gene therapy of human severe combined immunodeficiency (SCID)-X1 disease. Science 2000;288:669–672.
37. Hacein-Bey-Abina S, et al. LMO2-associated clonal T cell proliferation in two patients after gene therapy for SCID-X1. Science 2003;302:415–419.
38. Kohn DB, Sadelain M, Glorioso JC. Occurrence of leukaemia following gene therapy of X-linked SCID. Nat Rev Cancer 2003;3:477–488.
39. Whitwam T, et al. Retroviral marking of canine bone marrow: long-term, high-level expression of human interleukin-2 receptor common gamma chain in canine lymphocytes. Blood 1998;92:1565–1575.
40. Hacein-Bey S, Basile GD, Lemerle J, Fischer A, Cavazzana-Calvo M. gammac gene transfer in the presence of stem cell factor, FLT-3L, interleukin-7 (IL-7), IL-1, and IL-15 cytokines restores T-cell differentiation from gammac(-) X-linked severe combined immunodeficiency hematopoietic progenitor cells in murine fetal thymic organ cultures. Blood 1998;92:4090–4097.
41. Insertional mutagenesis and oncogenesis: update from non-clinical and clinical studies. Gene Therapy Expert Group of the Committee for Proprietary Medical Products (CPMP), European Agency for the Evaluation of Medical Products - June 2003 meeting. J Gene Med 2004;6:127–129.
42. Baum C, et al. Chance or necessity? Insertional mutagenesis in gene therapy and its consequences. Mol Ther 2004;9:5–13.
43. Dave UP, Jenkins NA, Copeland NG. Gene therapy insertional mutagenesis insights. Science 2004;303:333.
44. Kirn D, Martuza RL, Zwiebel J. Replication-selective virotherapy for cancer: Biological principles, risk management and future directions. Nat Med 2001;7:781–787.
45. Smith JS, Tian J, Muller J, Byrnes AP. Unexpected pulmonary uptake of adenovirus vectors in animals with chronic liver disease. Gene Ther 2004;11:431–438.
46. Crystal RG, et al. Analysis of risk factors for local delivery of low- and intermediate-dose adenovirus gene transfer vectors to individuals with a spectrum of comorbid conditions. Hum Gene Ther 2002;13:65–100.
47. Buller R, et al. A phase I/II trial of rAd/p53 (SCH 58500) gene replacement in recurrent ovarian cancer. Cancer Gene Ther 2002;9:553–566.
48. Jacobs A, et al. Positron-emission tomography of vector-mediated gene expression in gene therapy for gliomas. Lancet 2001;358:727–729.
49. Vansteenkiste JF, Stroobants SG. Positron emission tomography in the management of non-small cell lung cancer. Hematol Oncol Clin North Am 2004;18:269–288.

50. Vassaux G, Groot-Wassink T. In Vivo Noninvasive Imaging for Gene Therapy. J Biomed Biotechnol 2003;2003:92–101.
51. Groot-Wassink T, et al. Quantitative imaging of Na/I symporter transgene expression using positron emission tomography in the living animal. Mol Ther 2004;9:436–442.
52. McCaffrey A, Kay MA, Contag CH. Advancing molecular therapies through in vivo bioluminescent imaging. Mol Imaging 2003;2:75–86.
53. Schellingerhout D, Bogdanov AA, Jr. Viral imaging in gene therapy noninvasive demonstration of gene delivery and expression. Neuroimaging Clin N Am 2002;12:571–581, vi–vii.
54. Zinn KR, et al. Noninvasive monitoring of gene transfer using a reporter receptor imaged with a high-affinity peptide radiolabeled with 99mTc or 188Re. J Nucl Med 2000;41:887–895.
55. Ray P, et al. Monitoring gene therapy with reporter gene imaging. Semin Nucl Med 2001; 31:312–320.
56. Shah K, Jacobs A, Breakefield XO, Weissleder R. Molecular imaging of gene therapy for cancer. Gene Ther 2004;11:1175–1187.
57. Peng KW, et al. Intraperitoneal therapy of ovarian cancer using an engineered measles virus. Cancer Res 2002;62:4656–4662.
58. Phuong LK, et al. Use of a vaccine strain of measles virus genetically engineered to produce carcinoembryonic antigen as a novel therapeutic agent against glioblastoma multiforme. Cancer Res 2003;63:2462–2469.
59. Reid T, et al. Hepatic arterial infusion of a replication-selective oncolytic adenovirus (dl1520): phase II viral, immunologic, and clinical endpoints. Cancer Res 2002;62:6070–6079.
60. Kirn D. Virotherapy for cancer: current status, hurdles, and future directions. Cancer Gene Ther 2002;9:959–960.
61. Hermiston TW, Kuhn I. Armed therapeutic viruses: strategies and challenges to arming oncolytic viruses with therapeutic genes. Cancer Gene Ther 2002;9:1022–1035.
62. Chillon M, Lee JH, Fasbender A, Welsh MJ. Adenovirus complexed with polyethylene glycol and cationic lipid is shielded from neutralizing antibodies in vitro. Gene Ther 1998;5:995–1002.
63. O'Riordan CR, et al. PEGylation of adenovirus with retention of infectivity and protection from neutralizing antibody in vitro and in vivo. Hum Gene Ther 1999;10:1349–1358.
64. Croyle MA, Chirmule N, Zhang Y, Wilson JM. PEGylation of E1-deleted adenovirus vectors allows significant gene expression on readministration to liver. Hum Gene Ther 2002;13:1887–1900.
65. Monck MA, et al. Stabilized plasmid-lipid particles: pharmacokinetics and plasmid delivery to distal tumors following intravenous injection. J Drug Target 2000;7:439–452.
66. Shi L, et al. Repeated intrathecal administration of plasmid DNA complexed with polyethylene glycol-grafted polyethylenimine led to prolonged transgene expression in the spinal cord. Gene Ther 2003;10:1179–1188.
67. Bruckheimer E, et al. In vivo efficacy of folate-targeted lipid-protamine-DNA (LPD-PEG-Folate) complexes in an immunocompetent syngeneic model for breast adenocarcinoma. Cancer Gene Ther 2004;11:128–134.
68. Fisher KD, et al. Polymer-coated adenovirus permits efficient retargeting and evades neutralising antibodies. Gene Ther 2001;8:341–348.
69. Green NK, et al. Extended plasma circulation time and decreased toxicity of polymer-coated adenovirus. Gene Ther 2004;11:1256–1263.
70. Sun JY, Chatterjee S, Wong KK, Jr. Immunogenic issues concerning recombinant adeno-associated virus vectors for gene therapy. Curr Gene Ther 2002;2:485–500.
71. Sterman DH, et al. A pilot study of systemic corticosteroid administration in conjunction with intrapleural adenoviral vector administration in patients with malignant pleural mesothelioma. Cancer Gene Ther 2000;7:1511–1518.
72. Burgert HG, et al. Subversion of host defense mechanisms by adenoviruses. Curr Top Microbiol Immunol 2002;269:273–318.
73. Fessler SP, Delgado-Lopez F, Horwitz MS. Mechanisms of E3 modulation of immune and inflammatory responses. Curr Top Microbiol Immunol 2004;273:113–135.
74. Windheim M, Hilgendorf A, Burgert HG. Immune evasion by adenovirus E3 proteins: exploitation of intracellular trafficking pathways. Curr Top Microbiol Immunol 2004;273:29–85.
75. Wang Y, et al. E3 gene manipulations affect oncolytic adenovirus activity in immunocompetent tumor models. Nat Biotechnol 2003;21:1328–1335.
76. Todo T, Martuza RL, Rabkin SD, Johnson PA. Oncolytic herpes simplex virus vector with enhanced MHC class I presentation and tumor cell killing. Proc Natl Acad Sci U S A 2001;98:6396–6401.

77. Nicklin SA, Baker AH. Tropism-modified adenoviral and adeno-associated viral vectors for gene therapy. Curr Gene Ther 2002;2:273–293.
78. Einfeld DA, Roelvink PW. Advances towards targetable adenovirus vectors for gene therapy. Curr Opin Mol Ther 4:444–451.
79. Doronin K, et al. Overexpression of the ADP (E3-11.6K) protein increases cell lysis and spread of adenovirus. Virology 2003;305:378–387.
80. Liu TC, et al. An E1B-19 kDa gene deletion mutant adenovirus demonstrates tumor necrosis factor-enhanced cancer selectivity and enhanced oncolytic potency. Mol Ther 2004;9:786–803.
81. Khuri FR, et al. a controlled trial of intratumoral ONYX-015, a selectively-replicating adenovirus, in combination with cisplatin and 5-fluorouracil in patients with recurrent head and neck cancer. Nat Med 2000;6:879–885.
82. Sandalon Z, Fusenig NE, McCutcheon J, Taichman LB, Garlick JA. Suicide gene therapy for pre-malignant disease: a new strategy for the treatment of intraepithelial neoplasia. Gene Ther 2001; 8:232–238.
83. Rudin CM, et al. An attenuated adenovirus, ONYX-015, as mouthwash therapy for premalignant oral dysplasia. J Clin Oncol 2003;21:4546–4552.
84. Lang FF, et al. Phase I trial of adenovirus-mediated p53 gene therapy for recurrent glioma: biological and clinical results. J Clin Oncol 2003;21:2508–2518.
85. Clayman GL, Frank DK, Bruso PA, Goepfert H. Adenovirus-mediated wild-type p53 gene transfer as a surgical adjuvant in advanced head and neck cancers. Clin Cancer Res 1999;5:1715–1722.
86. Han DM, et al. Effectiveness of recombinant adenovirus p53 injection on laryngeal cancer: phase I clinical trial and follow up. Zhonghua Yi Xue Za Zhi 2003;83:2029–2032.
87. Dummer R, et al. Biological activity and safety of adenoviral vector-expressed wild-type p53 after intratumoral injection in melanoma and breast cancer patients with p53-overexpressing tumors. Cancer Gene Ther 2000;7:1069–1076.
88. Roth JA, et al. Retrovirus-mediated wild-type p53 gene transfer to tumors of patients with lung cancer. Nat Med 1996;2:985–991.
89. Schuler M, et al. A phase I study of adenovirus-mediated wild-type p53 gene transfer in patients with advanced non-small cell lung cancer. Hum Gene Ther 1998;9:2075–2082.
90. Swisher SG, et al. Adenovirus-mediated p53 gene transfer in advanced non-small-cell lung cancer. J Natl Cancer Inst 1999;91:763–771.
91. Kuball J, et al. Successful adenovirus-mediated wild-type p53 gene transfer in patients with bladder cancer by intravesical vector instillation. J Clin Oncol 2002;20:957–965.
92. Pagliaro LC, et al. Repeated intravesical instillations of an adenoviral vector in patients with locally advanced bladder cancer: a phase I study of p53 gene therapy. J Clin Oncol 2003;21:2247–2253.
93. Nemunaitis J, et al. Adenovirus-mediated p53 gene transfer in sequence with cisplatin to tumors of patients with non-small-cell lung cancer. J Clin Oncol 2000;18:609–622.
94. Swisher SG, et al. Induction of p53-regulated genes and tumor regression in lung cancer patients after intratumoral delivery of adenoviral p53 (INGN 201) and radiation therapy. Clin Cancer Res 2003;9:93–101.
95. Zhang SW, et al. Treatment of head and neck squamous cell carcinoma by recombinant adenovirus-p53 combined with radiotherapy: a phase II clinical trial of 42 cases. Zhonghua Yi Xue Za Zhi 2003;83:2023–2028.
96. Chen CB, Pan JJ, Xu LY. Recombinant adenovirus p53 agent injection combined with radiotherapy in treatment of nasopharyngeal carcinoma: a phase II clinical trial. Zhonghua Yi Xue Za Zhi 2003;83:2033–2035.
97. Klatzmann D, et al. A phase I/II dose-escalation study of herpes simplex virus type 1 thymidine kinase "suicide" gene therapy for metastatic melanoma. Study Group on Gene Therapy of Metastatic Melanoma. Hum Gene Ther 1998;9:2585–2594.
98. Izquierdo M, et al. Human malignant brain tumor response to herpes simplex thymidine kinase (HSVtk)/ganciclovir gene therapy. Gene Ther 1996;3:491–495.
99. Trask TW, et al. Phase I study of adenoviral delivery of the HSV-tk gene and ganciclovir administration in patients with current malignant brain tumors. Mol Ther 2000;1:195–203.
100. Ram,Z, et al. Therapy of malignant brain tumors by intratumoral implantation of retroviral vector-producing cells. Nat Med 1997;3:1354–1361.
101. Singh S, Cunningham C, Buchanan A, Jolly DJ, Nemunaitis J. Toxicity assessment of intratumoral injection of the herpes simplex type I thymidine kinase gene delivered by retrovirus in patients with refractory cancer. Mol Ther 2001;4:157–160.

102. Sterman DH, et al. Adenovirus-mediated herpes simplex virus thymidine kinase/ganciclovir gene therapy in patients with localized malignancy: results of a phase I clinical trial in malignant mesothelioma. Hum Gene Ther 1998;9:1083–1092.
103. Sung MW, et al. Intratumoral adenovirus-mediated suicide gene transfer for hepatic metastases from colorectal adenocarcinoma: results of a phase I clinical trial. Mol Ther 2001;4:182–191.
104. Miles BJ, et al. Prostate-specific antigen response and systemic T cell activation after in situ gene therapy in prostate cancer patients failing radiotherapy. Hum Gene Ther 2001;12:1955–1967.
105. Freytag SO, et al. Phase I study of replication-competent adenovirus-mediated double suicide gene therapy for the treatment of locally recurrent prostate cancer. Cancer Res 2002;62:4968–4976.
106. Herman JR, et al. In situ gene therapy for adenocarcinoma of the prostate: a phase I clinical trial. Hum Gene Ther 1999;10:1239–1249.
107. Kubo H, et al. Phase I dose escalation clinical trial of adenovirus vector carrying osteocalcin promoter-driven herpes simplex virus thymidine kinase in localized and metastatic hormone-refractory prostate cancer. Hum Gene Ther 2003;14:227–241.
108. Prados MD, et al. Treatment of progressive or recurrent glioblastoma multiforme in adults with herpes simplex virus thymidine kinase gene vector-producer cells followed by intravenous ganciclovir administration: a phase I/II multi-institutional trial. J Neurooncol 2003;65:269–278.
109. Germano IM, Fable J, Gultekin SH, Silvers A. Adenovirus/herpes simplex-thymidine kinase/-ganciclovir complex: preliminary results of a phase I trial in patients with recurrent malignant gliomas. J Neurooncol 2003;65:279–289.
110. Shand N, et al. A phase 1-2 clinical trial of gene therapy for recurrent glioblastoma multiforme by tumor transduction with the herpes simplex thymidine kinase gene followed by ganciclovir. GLI328 European-Canadian Study Group. Hum Gene Ther 1999;10:2325–2335.
111. Smitt PS, Driesse M, Wolbers J, Kros M, Avezaat C. Treatment of relapsed malignant glioma with an adenoviral vector containing the herpes simplex thymidine kinase gene followed by ganciclovir. Mol Ther 2003;7:851–858.
112. Packer RJ, et al. Treatment of progressive or recurrent pediatric malignant supratentorial brain tumors with herpes simplex virus thymidine kinase gene vector-producer cells followed by intravenous ganciclovir administration. J Neurosurg 2000;92:249–254.
113. Sandmair AM, et al. Thymidine kinase gene therapy for human malignant glioma, using replication-deficient retroviruses or adenoviruses. Hum Gene Ther 2000;11:2197–2205.
114. Immonen A, et al. AdvHSV-tk gene therapy with intravenous ganciclovir improves survival in human malignant glioma: a randomised, controlled study. Mol Ther 2004;10:967–972.
115. Alvarez RD, et al. Adenoviral-mediated suicide gene therapy for ovarian cancer. Mol Ther 2000;2:524–530.
116. Teh BS, et al. Phase I/II trial evaluating combined radiotherapy and in situ gene therapy with or without hormonal therapy in the treatment of prostate cancer—a preliminary report. Int J Radiat Oncol Biol Phys 2001;51:605–613.
117. Teh BS, et al. Phase I-II trial evaluating combined intensity-modulated radiotherapy and in situ gene therapy with or without hormonal therapy in treatment of prostate cancer-interim report on PSA response and biopsy data. Int J Radiat Oncol Biol Phys 2004;58:1520–1529.
118. Satoh T, et al. Enhanced systemic T-cell activation after in situ gene therapy with radiotherapy in prostate cancer patients. Int J Radiat Oncol Biol Phys 2004;59:562–571.
119. Freytag SO, et al. Phase I study of replication-competent adenovirus-mediated double-suicide gene therapy in combination with conventional-dose three-dimensional conformal radiation therapy for the treatment of newly diagnosed, intermediate- to high-risk prostate cancer. Cancer Res 2003;63:7497–7506.
120. Rainov NG. A phase III clinical evaluation of herpes simplex virus type 1 thymidine kinase and ganciclovir gene therapy as an adjuvant to surgical resection and radiation in adults with previously untreated glioblastoma multiforme. Hum Gene Ther 2000;11:2389–2401.
121. Hasenburg A, et al. Thymidine kinase gene therapy with concomitant topotecan chemotherapy for recurrent ovarian cancer. Cancer Gene Ther 2000;7:839–844.
122. Hasenburg A, et al. Adenovirus-mediated thymidine kinase gene therapy in combination with topotecan for patients with recurrent ovarian cancer: 2.5-year follow-up. Gynecol Oncol 2001;83:549–554.
123. Ganly I, et al. A phase I study of Onyx-015, an E1B attenuated adenovirus, administered intratumorally to patients with recurrent head and neck cancer. Clin Cancer Res 2000;6:798–806.
124. Nemunaitis J, et al. Selective replication and oncolysis in p53 mutant tumors with ONYX-015, an E1B-55kD gene-deleted adenovirus, in patients with advanced head and neck cancer: a phase II trial. Cancer Res 2000;60:6359–6366.

125. Nemunaitis J, et al. Phase II trial of intratumoral administration of ONYX-015, a replication-selective adenovirus, in patients with refractory head and neck cancer. J Clin Oncol 2001;19:289–298.
126. Morley S, et al. The dl1520 virus is found preferentially in tumor tissue after direct intratumoral injection in oral carcinoma. Clin Cancer Res 2004;10:4357–4362.
127. Mulvihill S, et al. Safety and feasibility of injection with an E1B-55 kDa gene-deleted, replication-selective adenovirus (ONYX-015) into primary carcinomas of the pancreas: a phase I trial. Gene Ther 2001;8:308–315.
128. Chiocca EA, et al. A Phase I Open-Label, Dose-Escalation, Multi-Institutional Trial of Injection with an E1B-Attenuated Adenovirus, ONYX-015, into the Peritumoral Region of Recurrent Malignant Gliomas, in the Adjuvant Setting. Mol Ther 2004;10:958–966.
129. Makower D, et al. Phase II clinical trial of intralesional administration of the oncolytic adenovirus ONYX-015 in patients with hepatobiliary tumors with correlative p53 studies. Clin Cancer Res 2003;9:693–702.
130. Vasey PA, et al. Phase I trial of intraperitoneal injection of the E1B-55-kd-gene-deleted adenovirus ONYX-015 (dl1520) given on days 1 through 5 every 3 weeks in patients with recurrent/refractory epithelial ovarian cancer. J Clin Oncol 2002;20:1562–1569.
131. Habib N, et al. Clinical trial of E1B-deleted adenovirus (dl1520) gene therapy for hepatocellular carcinoma. Cancer Gene Ther 2002;9:254–259.
132. Hamid O, et al. Phase II trial of intravenous CI-1042 in patients with metastatic colorectal cancer. J Clin Oncol 2003;21:1498–1504.
133. Hecht JR, et al. A phase I/II trial of intratumoral endoscopic ultrasound injection of ONYX-015 with intravenous gemcitabine in unresectable pancreatic carcinoma. Clin Cancer Res 2003;9:555–561.
134. Galanis E, et al. Phase I-II trial of ONYX-015 in combination with MAP chemotherapy in patients with advanced sarcomas. Gene Ther 2005;12:437–445.
135. Habib NA, et al. E1B-deleted adenovirus (dl1520) gene therapy for patients with primary and secondary liver tumors. Hum Gene Ther 2001;12:219–226.
136. Reid T, et al. Intra-arterial administration of a replication-selective adenovirus (dl1520) in patients with colorectal carcinoma metastatic to the liver: a phase I trial. Gene Ther 2001;8:1618–1626.
137. Nemunaitis J, et al. Pilot trial of intravenous infusion of a replication-selective adenovirus (ONYX-015) in combination with chemotherapy or IL-2 treatment in refractory cancer patients. Cancer Gene Ther 2003;10:341–352.
138. Nemunaitis J, et al. Intravenous infusion of a replication-selective adenovirus (ONYX-015) in cancer patients: safety, feasibility and biological activity. Gene Ther 2001;8:746–759.
139. Webb A, et al. BCL-2 antisense therapy in patients with non-Hodgkin lymphoma. Lancet 1997;349:1137–1141.
140. Waters JS, et al. Phase I clinical and pharmacokinetic study of bcl-2 antisense oligonucleotide therapy in patients with non-Hodgkin's lymphoma. J Clin Oncol 2000;18:1812–1823.
141. Morris MJ, et al. Phase I trial of BCL-2 antisense oligonucleotide (G3139) administered by continuous intravenous infusion in patients with advanced cancer. Clin Cancer Res 2002;8:679–683.
142. Rudin CM, et al. A pilot trial of G3139, a bcl-2 antisense oligonucleotide, and paclitaxel in patients with chemorefractory small-cell lung cancer. Ann Oncol 2002;13:539–545.
143. Rudin CM, et al. Phase I study of G3139, a bcl-2 antisense oligonucleotide, combined with carboplatin and etoposide in patients with small-cell lung cancer. J Clin Oncol 2004;22:1110–1117.
144. Chi KN, et al. A phase I dose-finding study of combined treatment with an antisense Bcl-2 oligonucleotide (Genasense) and mitoxantrone in patients with metastatic hormone-refractory prostate cancer. Clin Cancer Res 2001;7:3920–3927.
145. Tolcher AW, et al. A Phase I pharmacokinetic and biological correlative study of oblimersen sodium (genasense, g3139), an antisense oligonucleotide to the bcl-2 mRNA, and of docetaxel in patients with hormone-refractory prostate cancer. Clin Cancer Res 2004;10:5048–5057.
146. Tolcher AW, et al. A phase II, pharmacokinetic, and biological correlative study of oblimersen sodium and docetaxel in patients with hormone-refractory prostate cancer. Clin Cancer Res 2005;11:3854–3861.
147. Jansen B, et al. Chemosensitisation of malignant melanoma by BCL2 antisense therapy. Lancet 2000;356:1728–1733.
148. Marshall J, et al. A phase I trial of a Bcl-2 antisense (G3139) and weekly docetaxel in patients with advanced breast cancer and other solid tumors. Ann Oncol 2004;15:1274–1283.
149. Morris MJ, et al. Safety and biologic activity of intravenous BCL-2 antisense oligonucleotide (G3139) and taxane chemotherapy in patients with advanced cancer. Appl Immunohistochem Mol Morphol 2005;13:6–13.

150. van de Donk NW, et al. G3139, a Bcl-2 antisense oligodeoxynucleotide, induces clinical responses in VAD refractory myeloma. Leukemia 2004;18:1078–1084.
151. Badros AZ, et al. Phase II study of G3139, a Bcl-2 antisense oligonucleotide, in combination with dexamethasone and thalidomide in relapsed multiple myeloma patients. J Clin Oncol 2005;23:4089–4099.
152. Marcucci G, et al. Phase 1 and pharmacodynamic studies of G3139, a Bcl-2 antisense oligonucleotide, in combination with chemotherapy in refractory or relapsed acute leukemia. Blood 2003;101:425–432.
153. Marcucci G, et al. Phase I study of oblimersen sodium, an antisense to Bcl-2, in untreated older patients with acute myeloid leukemia: pharmacokinetics, pharmacodynamics, and clinical activity. J Clin Oncol 2005;23:3404–3411.
154. Rousseau RF, et al. Local and systemic effects of an allogeneic tumor cell vaccine combining transgenic human lymphotactin with interleukin-2 in patients with advanced or refractory neuroblastoma. Blood 2003;101:1718–1726.
155. Sobol RE, et al. Interleukin 2 gene therapy of colorectal carcinoma with autologous irradiated tumor cells and genetically engineered fibroblasts: a Phase I study. Clin Cancer Res 1999;5:2359–2365.
156. Belli F, et al. Active immunization of metastatic melanoma patients with interleukin-2-transduced allogeneic melanoma cells: evaluation of efficacy and tolerability. Cancer Immunol Immunother 1997;44:197–203.
157. Palmer K, et al. Gene therapy with autologous, interleukin 2-secreting tumor cells in patients with malignant melanoma. Hum Gene Ther 1999;10:1261–1268.
158. Osanto S, et al. Vaccination of melanoma patients with an allogeneic, genetically modified interleukin 2-producing melanoma cell line. Hum Gene Ther 2000;11:739–750.
159. Sun Y, et al. Vaccination with IL-12 gene-modified autologous melanoma cells: preclinical results and a first clinical phase I study. Gene Ther 1998;5:481–490.
160. Trudel S, et al. Adenovector engineered interleukin-2 expressing autologous plasma cell vaccination after high-dose chemotherapy for multiple myeloma—a phase 1 study. Leukemia 2001;15:846–854.
161. Stewart AK. et al. Adenovector-mediated gene delivery of interleukin-2 in metastatic breast cancer and melanoma: results of a phase 1 clinical trial. Gene Ther 1999;6:350–363.
162. Schreiber S, et al. Immunotherapy of metastatic malignant melanoma by a vaccine consisting of autologous interleukin 2-transfected cancer cells: outcome of a phase I study. Hum Gene Ther 1999;10:983–993.
163. Veelken H, et al. A phase-I clinical study of autologous tumor cells plus interleukin-2-gene-transfected allogeneic fibroblasts as a vaccine in patients with cancer. Int J Cancer 1997;70:269–277.
164. Belldegrun A, et al. Interleukin 2 gene therapy for prostate cancer: phase I clinical trial and basic biology. Hum Gene Ther 2001;12:883–892.
165. Trudel S, et al. A phase I trial of adenovector-mediated delivery of interleukin-2 (AdIL-2) in high-risk localized prostate cancer. Cancer Gene Ther 2003;10:755–763.
166. Jantscheff P, et al. Gene therapy with cytokine-transfected xenogenic cells (Vero-IL-2) in patients with metastatic solid tumors: mechanism(s) of elimination of the transgene-carrying cells. Cancer Immunol Immunother 1999;48:321–330.
167. Rochlitz C, et al. Gene therapy study of cytokine-transfected xenogeneic cells (Vero-interleukin-2) in patients with metastatic solid tumors. Cancer Gene Ther 1999;6:271–281.
168. Rochlitz C, et al. Phase I immunotherapy with a modified vaccinia virus (MVA) expressing human MUC1 as antigen-specific immunotherapy in patients with MUC1-positive advanced cancer. J Gene Med 2003;5:690–699.
169. Schmidt-Wolf IG, et al. Phase I clinical study applying autologous immunological effector cells transfected with the interleukin-2 gene in patients with metastatic renal cancer, colorectal cancer and lymphoma. Br J Cancer 1999;81:1009–1016.

21 Trials and Tribulations in Developing Clinical Trials of Gene Therapy

E1A for Breast or Ovarian Cancer

Naoto T. Ueno, MD, PhD, *Judith K. Wolf,* MD,
David M. Gershenson, MD,
Gabriel N. Hortobagyi, MD,
and Mien-Chie Hung, PhD

CONTENTS

Summary

At The University of Texas M.D. Anderson Cancer Center, we have been investigating use of the adenovirus type 5 *E1A* gene as a cancer therapy for breast or ovarian cancer since 1995. *E1A* gene therapy is a nonimmunologic approach involving ectopic expression of a potentially therapeutic gene in cancer cells. During the late 1980s, *E1A* was shown to downregulate the overexpression of HER-2/*neu*, thus reversing the tumorigenic and metastatic phenotype of HER-2/*neu*-overexpressing breast and ovarian cancer cells. Since that time, *E1A* has also been shown to function as a tumor suppressor gene in several other types of tumor cells by inducing apoptosis and differentiation and by inhibiting metastasis regardless of HER2 expression level. This chapter highlights some of the issues and difficulties we encountered in designing clinical trials of *E1A* gene therapy for breast or ovarian cancer.

Key Words: Cationic liposome; breast cancer; ovarian cancer; adenovirus type 5 E1A; clinical trial.

From: *Cancer Drug Discovery and Development: Gene Therapy for Cancer*
Edited by: K. K. Hunt, S. A. Vorburger, and S. G. Swisher © Humana Press Inc., Totowa, NJ

1. ADENOVIRUS TYPE 5 *E1A*: AN ONCOGENE AND A TUMOR SUPPRESSOR GENE

Within the adenovirus genome, the *E1A* gene encodes proline-rich nuclear phosphoproteins that regulate the efficient replication of the adenovirus *(1)*. Because *E1A* proteins can transcriptionally transactivate proteins that can "immortalize" transformed cells, *E1A* was originally considered an "immortalization oncogene" *(2–4)*. Certain serotypes of *E1A* proteins, such as those of adenovirus type 12, are strongly oncogenic and induce tumors at high frequency *(1)*. Others, such as adenovirus type 5 and its closely related serotype adenovirus type 2, are nononcogenic *(5)*. We found that portions of *E1A* gene products inhibited HER2 overexpression in both rodent fibroblasts and human cancer cells, and they did so through transcriptional repression at the HER2 promoter *(6,7)*. This effect was thought to result from stimulation of transcription or repression of the activity of viral and cellular transcriptional enhancers.

These findings prompted us to investigate the possibility that *E1A* might function as a tumor suppressor gene in HER2-overexpressing cancer cells through repressing HER2 overexpression. First, to determine whether *E1A* could reverse the tumorigenicity of HER2-overexpressing human ovarian cancer cells, we transfected several such cell lines with the *E1A* gene and found that the transfected cells expressed less HER2 protein, produced fewer malignancies in immunosuppressed animal models, and were less able to induce tumors in immunocompetent mice *(8)*.

In addition to this tumor-suppressive activity in HER2-overexpressing cells, *E1A* has other suppressive activities independent of HER2 *(9,10)*. *E1A* has been shown to repress the transcription of various proteases involved in tumor cell invasion and metastasis, including type IV collagenase *(11,12)*, plasminogen activator *(13)*, stromelysin *(14)*, interstitial collagenase *(11)*, and urokinase *(11)*; *E1A* can also inhibit metastasis by elevating expression of the metastasis suppressor gene *Nm23 (15,16)*. *E1A* can also reduce the anchorage-independent growth and tumorigenesis of a variety of tumor cell lines, including human melanoma, fibrosarcoma *(17)*, rhabdomyosarcoma, Saos-2 osteosarcoma, non-small cell lung carcinoma, breast carcinoma *(18)*, and murine melanoma *(19)*, either by controlling cell proliferation through repression of growth factor-inducible genes *(14)* or by inducing differentiation *(20)*. *E1A* can also induce apoptosis in various cell types *(19,21–24)*. *E1A* was recently shown to suppress at least one other tyrosine kinase besides HER2—namely Axl, the prototype of a family of transmembrane receptors that also includes Sky and Eyk *(23,25)*, which may be involved in apoptosis or suppression of cell proliferation. *E1A* can also induce immune responses by sensitizing cells to apoptosis induced by tumor necrosis factor (TNF)-α *(26,27)* and cytolysis by activated natural killer (NK) cells and macrophages *(26,28,29)*.

In summary, *E1A* functions as a tumor suppressor gene through several mechanisms *(9,10)*: transcriptional repression of HER2, inhibition of metastasis-related genes, activation of metastasis suppressor genes, induction of differentiation or suppression of cell proliferation, induction of apoptosis, and induction of host immune responses.

2. SELECTING A GENE DELIVERY SYSTEM

Armed with these results, we then set out to choose a gene delivery system for our preclinical and clinical trials. Human gene delivery systems are of two types—viral or nonviral. Viral delivery of DNA plasmids is efficient, but the disadvantages include the inability of retroviral vectors to transfect nondividing cells and the strong immunogenicity of some adenoviral vectors *(30)*. Our initial choice for our preclinical animal studies was to use a replication-deficient adenoviral vector *(31)* to avoid potential problems with low-transfection efficiency. On the other hand, we reasoned that nonviral delivery systems might be more appropriate for clinical studies because they could be used repeatedly with minimal toxicity and immunogenicity; however, the transfection efficiency of such systems tends to be more limited than that of viral vectors *(32)*. One of the best-known nonviral delivery systems at that time was the cationic liposome, the first of which was developed for in vitro gene transfer in the late 1980s by Felgner and others *(33)*. The system was designed so that the overall charge remains positive after formation of the DNA/cationic liposome complex; this positive charge would promote the interaction of the complex with the negatively charged cell membranes and enhance transfection of the target cells. For our studies, we chose the 3-[*N*-(*N'*,*N'*-dimethyl-aminoethane)carbamoyl] cholesterol (DC-Chol) cationic liposome developed by Leaf and colleagues at the University of Pittsburgh. This system was shown to facilitate gene delivery into mammalian cells both in vitro and in vivo and was relatively nontoxic as well as being biodegradable, nonmutagenic, and nonimmunogenic *(34–38)*.

3. PRECLINICAL STUDIES

3.1. Safety and Efficacy of E1A *in Xenograft Mouse Models*

The first steps in the development of *E1A* as a therapeutic agent for human cancer involved establishing the antitumorigenic efficacy of *E1A* by using adenoviruses to transfect HER2-overexpressing ovarian or breast cancer cells and examining the behavior of those cells in vitro and upon their injection in mice *(31)*. The next steps involved using *E1A*, delivered by various means, to treat breast cancer or ovarian cancer in xenograft mouse models. In one such study, nude mice were injected in the mammary fat pads with the human HER2-overexpressing breast cancer cell line MDA-MB-361 and tumors were allowed to form. Then *E1A* genes complexed with DC-Chol cationic liposomes (*E1A*/DC-Chol complex) were injected into the tumors *(39)*,where they were shown to inhibit the growth of these breast cancer cells. Similar results were observed in an intraperitoneal (ip) model of ovarian cancer involving the HER2-overexpressing cell line SKOV-3; in that study, ip delivery of the *E1A*/DC-Chol complex inhibited the growth and dissemination of these ovarian cancer cells. About 70% of these mice survived for at least 365 d, whereas all untreated controls developed severe tumor-related symptoms and died within 160 d *(38)*.

3.2. Toxicity Studies

The final step before the phase I trial was to evaluate the toxicity (safety profile) of the *E1A*/DC-Chol complex after ip injection in normal mice. In the short term, cumulative doses of up to 40× those proposed for the phase I trial showed no adverse effects on renal, hepatic, or hematologic function in nude mice, nor were any major pathologic changes observed in any organs at necropsy. At 9 mo after discontinuation of treatment, no macroscopic or microscopic effects were noted in the genitals (uterus, fallopian tube, and ovary), liver, lung, heart, kidney, spleen, or brain. At 18 mo after treatment cessation, *E1A* DNA could still be detected in lung and kidney but not in liver, heart, spleen, brain, uterus, or ovary. Our conclusions from these tests were that the DC-Chol cationic liposome gene delivery system could allow repeated dosing of the *E1A*/DC-Chol complex without inducing any major toxicity but that long-term follow-up was needed to determine the ultimate effects of *E1A (36,37)*.

4. THE PHASE I TRIAL

On the basis of these results, an Investigational New Drug application was filed with the United States Food and Drug Administration and approved, and a phase I clinical trial of *E1A* gene therapy for metastatic breast or ovarian cancer was opened at MD Anderson Cancer Center in 1996 *(40)* (*see* Fig. 1). The goal of this study was to demonstrate the feasibility of the therapy and its effectiveness as assessed by downregulation of HER2 overexpression in tumor tissue. At first, only patients with tumors that overexpressed HER2 were eligible; the eligibility criteria were later expanded to include patients with tumors expressing low levels of HER2. Each patient was to receive a weekly injection of the *E1A*/DC-Chol cationic liposome complex through an indwelling Tenckhoff catheter placed in either the pleural cavity (for patients with breast cancer) or the peritoneal cavity (for patients with ovarian cancer). Each cycle consisted of three consecutive weekly injections followed by 1 wk off. The starting dose for the *E1A*/DC-Chol complex, 1.8 mg/m^2/injection, was derived from the effective dose established in the preclinical animal studies *(38,39)*. Three dose levels were tested: 1.8, 3.6, or 7.2 mg/m^2/injection.

4.1. Outcome

The median number of *E1A*/DC-Chol complex injections was 6 (range 1–8); the most common adverse event was development of fever 2 to 3 d after each injection regardless of dose. The appearance of grade 3–4 nausea/vomiting or pain in the 7.2 mg/m^2 dose group led us to reduce the MTD to 3.6 mg/m^2. Three patients experienced catheter-related infections requiring discontinuation of the treatment. No drug-related mortality was experienced. Several patients experienced stable disease with transient decreases in levels of the tumor markers CA-125 or carcinoembryonic antigen. Immunohistochemical staining of tumor tissue for HER2 expression showed downregulation of HER2 in all 6 patients so tested. Reverse transcriptase-polymerase chain reaction (RT-PCR) analysis of tissues from one patient at autopsy revealed *E1A* expression in lung, tumor, liver, and kidney but not in brain or ovary. *E1A* expression in tumor tissues was also confirmed by immunohistochemical staining, as was induction of apoptosis, after treatment with the *E1A*/DC-Chol complex. We concluded from these results that *E1A* delivery is feasible and that *E1A* expression could be detected in cancer cells after such treatment.

5. TRIBULATIONS IN DESIGNING CLINICAL TRIALS

5.1. Monitoring Gene Expression: Choice of End Point

One of the most difficult challenges in clinical gene therapy is planning how to monitor the presence and effects of the delivered therapeutic gene in vivo. The end points selected for our phase I trial were the maximum tolerated dose (MTD) and the maximum biologically active dose (MBAD) of the *E1A* plasmid. Because no toxicity had been detected during the preclinical toxicity study, we initially thought that we might not reach the MTD, and thus the dose of *E1A* plasmid was escalated in 100% increments rather than by the Fibonacci method. MBAD, the primary end point of the study, was defined as the dose of *E1A* plasmid (in mg/m^2) that would produce at least a 25% downregulation in HER2 expression in the tumor—the best-established end point at the time the trial was designed.

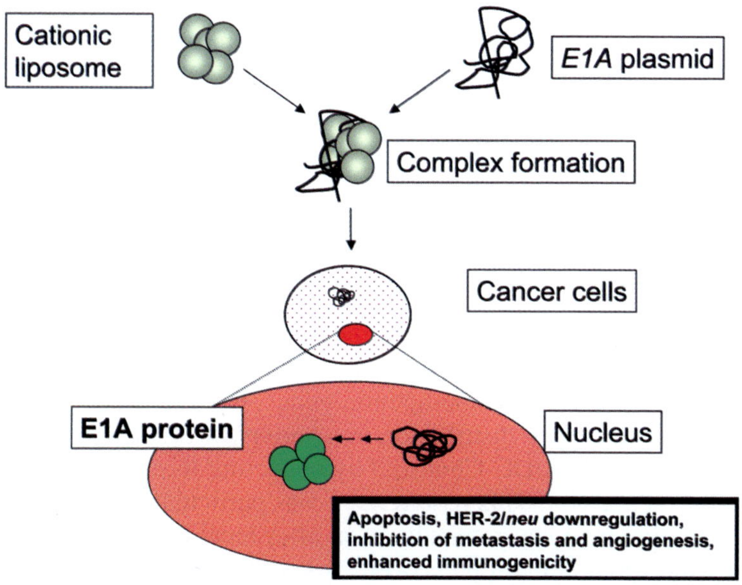

Fig. 1. Study concept of the phase I trial of *E1A* gene therapy in breast and ovarian cancer.

5.2. Choice of Measurement Techniques

Theoretically, the expression of a therapeutic gene in both targeted and nontargeted cells can be monitored at three levels: at delivery of the plasmid DNA into the cells (transfection), at mRNA synthesis from DNA (transcription), and at protein synthesis from mRNA (translation). Assays are available for monitoring gene expression at each of these levels (Table 1).

When designing a clinical trial, assay selection is critical for several reasons. First, the assays can be expensive and time-consuming. Second, the choice of assay is often affected by the type, source, and volume of tumor (or nontarget) tissue that can be collected for analysis. In our phase I trial, we chose immunohistochemical staining, which would reveal both the presence and the distribution of the *E1A* and HER2 protein products in tissue, and RT-PCR assays to detect *E1A* RNA. Western blotting was not considered feasible because it requires large amounts of *E1A*-transfected tissues.

5.3. Other Considerations: Efficiency, Distribution, and Duration of Gene Expression

Other issues to be considered before initiating our phase I trial were how to assess the efficiency, distribution, and duration of expression of the therapeutic gene. The optimal method for accurately determining the transfection efficiency of therapeutic genes in both tumor and nontumor cells in human subjects has yet to be established. In preclinical models, the efficiency of DNA transfection or protein expression is commonly described as a percentage of cells that stain positively for gene or protein expression among the entire cell population exposed to the transfecting agent. In intraperitoneal or intrapleural therapy, transfection of the *E1A*/DC-Chol complex into human cells is probably limited to those cells that were in direct proximity to or in contact with the complex, making measurement of gene expression difficult. Similar findings

Table 1
Assays for Monitoring Gene Expression

DNA	*RNA*	*Protein*
Southern blotting	Northern blotting	Immunohistochemical staining
Polymerase chain reaction	Reverse-transcriptase polymerase chain reaction	Western blotting
Fluorescence *in situ* hybridization		

have been reported from intratumoral gene therapy trials: expression of the gene tends to be strongest at the point at which the needle was inserted into the tumor.

Monitoring the distribution of therapeutic genes, even in local gene delivery systems, requires examining gene distribution in a variety of organ sites. We attempted to address this issue in our *E1A*/DC-Chol trial by collecting tissue samples from as many organs as possible at autopsy. This requirement was particularly acute because cationic liposomes can be distributed systemically even after local delivery. As for the duration of effect, many questions remain unanswered as to the transience or stability of gene expression in cancer gene therapy. Expression of genes delivered by cationic liposomes is transient in cells, and the DNA plasmid is degraded relatively quickly. However, we do not know how long the gene may be expressed in the cells, nor whether (or when) the transfected gene might become integrated into the host chromosomes. The potential for integration is a critical safety concern in gene therapy, as the integrated DNA could confer chronic adverse effects to normal host cells or even be passed on to the next generation if the transfected cells reside in the organs of fertility (e.g., the ovaries). Issues such as these are even more important for systemic (as opposed to local) gene delivery systems.

5.4. Accessibility of Tumor Tissue Samples

Another topic addressed in the design of this clinical study was the need to collect serial tumor specimens over time. Because intracavitary fluids are likely to contain tumor cells, we initially included only patients who had either ascites or pleural effusions, reasoning that insertion of a Tenckhoff (indwelling) catheter would allow repeated (weekly) fluid samples to be collected readily, with less risk and discomfort to the patient than other more invasive means of sampling tumors. We also considered that this approach might allow us to determine the ideal sampling intervals in terms of maximal transfection and protein synthesis after injection of the *E1A*/DC-Chol complex. Thus, our plan was to collect specimens before the first injection of *E1A*/DC-Chol complex and again 3 and 7 d thereafter. However, the wisdom of this approach remains controversial with regard to how aggressively one should attempt to collect tumor samples in light of the expense and the difficulty in obtaining samples in many clinical trials.

5.5. Monitoring Biological Effects

When we began designing the phase I study in 1995, we attempted to select an MBAD that would serve as the basis for establishing dosages for future phase II trials. Our reasoning was based on the assumption that the molecular effect (HER2 downregulation) triggered by the therapeutic gene (*E1A*) would be the dominant mechanism of antitumor activity. Our thought was that *E1A* may downregulate HER2 at dose A, but to induce rapid apoptosis, it may have to be given at a higher or lower dose. Alternatively, low *E1A* gene expression may induce strong antitumor activity by triggering a bystander effect, which could depend on the dose of the therapeutic gene or on a particular genetic abnormality in the cancer cells.

However, in the end, we abandoned the attempt to use MBAD to define the dosages for the phase II trial. Despite the confirmation that *E1A* had a biological effect at a dose lower than the MTD, the traditional MTD was used instead, for the following reasons. First, the possible therapeutic mechanisms suggested by the preclinical experiments do not always match the antitumor mechanism in clinical settings. Research by us and others suggested that *E1A* could reverse the malignant phenotype through more than one mechanism,(e.g., by triggering the host immune system), inducing apoptosis, inducing tumor lysis, and suppressing metastatic capability *(41)*. Even if antitumor activity could be detected in the treated patients, other activities associated with the *E1A*/DC-Chol complexes could have contributed to the antitumor effect in addition to the down-regulation of HER2. In attempts to clarify these issues, we studied several indices in several types of samples (i.e., tumor, intracavitary fluid, and serum) in the phase I trial. For example, we studied apoptosis and Ki-67 expression (an index of cellular proliferation) because *E1A* is known to induce apoptosis and suppress proliferation of certain cell types; we also measured cytokines (TNF-α and interferon [IFN]-γ) in the cavitary fluid because *E1A* is suspected of sensitizing cells to TNF-α.

Another problem was that assays to measure apoptosis, Ki-67, and cytokines had not been validated with clinical samples, and so any retrospective analyses of samples collected prospectively from phase I participants were limited by the possibility that the samples may not have been collected under the appropriate conditions or at appropriate times. Hence, the appearance of apparent associations among variables generated did not confirm the molecular mechanism of *E1A*; rather, they generated new hypotheses that needed to be tested in future trials.

By this reasoning, an accurate and useful MBAD for use in phase II trials would be difficult—if not impossible—to choose. In gene therapy trials for cancer, the threshold for triggering the molecular effect of a therapeutic gene is generally not known. This does not mean that one should not make an effort to determine these factors. Rather, a tremendous effort is needed to identify biological markers and at the same time come up with assays that can allow those markers to be monitored in a scientifically valid and reproducible manner.

6. PHASE II STUDY OF *E1A* MONOTHERAPY

As discussed above, the findings from our phase I trial actually led to additional hypotheses to test in both preclinical and clinical experiments. Our initial phase II study, which was to open in 2000, was designed to address some of these hypotheses, especially transfection efficiency. With this in mind, we restricted the study criteria to include only patients with ovarian cancer with relatively small tumors (i.e., 2 cm or less in largest diameter) and hence a generally better prognosis that those with metastatic disease. However, this restriction led to major difficulties in patient accrual, because several other potentially more attractive treatment options were open to such patients. In addition to the difficulties in competing for a relatively small pool of patients to participate in several clinical trials, encouraging patients to participate in gene therapy trials was particularly difficult after an 18-yr-old patient with an inherited enzyme deficiency died while participating in a clinical trial of human gene therapy in 1999. These difficulties led to premature closure of our phase II monotherapy study in 2002.

7. RATIONALE FOR A NEW AND IMPROVED TRIAL

After our experiences with the preclinical, phase I, and phase II studies recounted above, our next step was to open a phase II trial of *E1A* gene therapy used in combination with paclitaxel for ovarian cancer, with the hope that the addition of *E1A* would enhance the antitumor activity of paclitaxel and improve long-term outcome. Our initial hypothesis was that the ability of *E1A* to downregulate HER2 in HER2-overexpressing breast cancer cells could sensitize those cells to paclitaxel. Moreover, we showed that a paclitaxel-resistant phenotype in breast cancer cells was associated with enhanced p185 expression and that downregulation of p185 by *E1A* converted this resistant phenotype into a sensitive one *(42)*. These in vitro data led us to conduct a study in which *E1A* chemosensitization was tested in xenograft models of human HER2-overexpressing breast and ovarian cancer in which *E1A* gene therapy was combined with paclitaxel.

As noted earlier in this chapter, a major problem with gene therapy that remains to be resolved is how to deliver the therapeutic gene to distant target tissues. In our phase I trial of *E1A* gene therapy, delivery of the *E1A* gene into either the thoracic or the peritoneal cavity by means of DC-Chol cationic liposomes led to successful transfection of cancer cells. Use of the DC-Chol system is limited to intratumoral or intracavitary regional delivery, however, because of the vulnerability of the DNA/DC-Chol complex to serum. To overcome this limitation, another liposomal delivery system, the lipid-protamine-DNA or LPD system, was developed. In this formulation, the DNA is condensed, as it would be in natural vectors such as viruses, in a manner that makes it more resistant to degradation by serum. Injection of LPD complexes via the tail vein in nude mice has been shown to facilitate the delivery of the DNA to distant organ sites such as lung or liver *(43–45)*.

We used a version of this LPD system, LPDI, to deliver *E1A* gene therapy in combination with paclitaxel to mice implanted with human breast or ovarian cancer cells that overexpress HER2. Mice in the control groups (i.e., those given only *E1A* plasmid, only liposome, or a complex with a nonspecific gene) showed no suppression of tumor growth *(46,47)*. Mice treated with either the *E1A*/LPDI or paclitaxel showed some evidence of tumor suppression, but mice treated with the *E1A*/LPDI-plus-paclitaxel combination showed remarkable suppression of tumor growth. These findings led us to conclude that the *E1A* gene can enhance the sensitivity of HER2-overexpressing human breast cancer cells to paclitaxel and that intravenous (iv) delivery of *E1A* for gene therapy is in fact a feasible approach.

Another line of evidence indicates that the sensitization conferred by *E1A* is not limited to paclitaxel or to cancer cell lines that overexpress HER2. One group reported that *p53*-dependent apoptosis induced by *E1A* sensitized cells to the alkylating agent cisplatin *(21)*. Other groups have reported sensitization to cisplatin via a *p53*-independent mechanism *(48–50)*. Still another group has reported sensitization to cisplatin, etoposide, and gemcitabine by *E1A* in low-HER2-expressing cancer cell lines *(18,51,52)*. This chemosensitization by *E1A* was further confirmed in a xenograft model with the low-HER2-expressing breast cancer cell line MDA-MB-231 *(53)*.

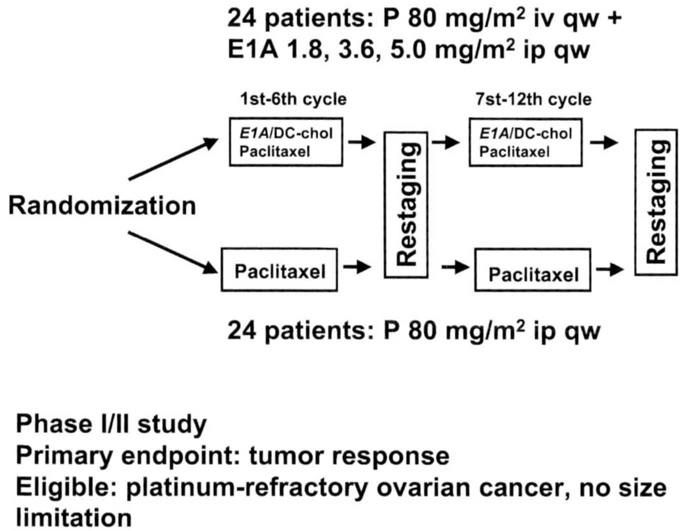

Fig. 2. Study design of the phase I/II trial of *E1A* gene therapy and paclitaxel.

8. NEW PHASE I/II RANDOMIZED TRIAL OF *E1A* GENE THERAPY WITH PACLITAXEL

On the basis of the findings described above, we are now planning a phase I/II trial targeting platinum-refractory ovarian cancer (*see* Fig. 2). The purpose of this randomized trial is to compare weekly paclitaxel vs weekly paclitaxel plus *E1A* gene therapy. The primary objectives are to evaluate the toxicity and establish the MTD of ip *E1A*/DC-Chol complex in combination with iv paclitaxel and to compare tumor response between treatment groups. Secondary objectives are to compare time with progression and overall survival and to examine the biological effects of the *E1A*/DC-Chol complex + paclitaxel combination on ovarian cancer cells through laboratory testing.

The study was designed to address whether the addition of *E1A* gene therapy is superior to weekly doses of paclitaxel, which is known to have antitumor activity in platinum-refractory disease. Our hope is that having attractive treatment options for both groups, and no limitations on tumor size, will improve accrual to the study.

Our plans for testing biological activity, derived in part from our phase I results, include measurements of apoptosis, HER2 downregulation, Ki-67, and cytokines (e.g., TNF-α) in ascites. This attempt to monitor potential biomarkers in a prospective manner is important for maintaining ongoing, bidirectional links between clinic and laboratory. Approaches that involve prospective study of molecular events that can trigger antitumor activity or side effects are crucial for improving the efficacy and safety of cancer gene therapy.

9. FINAL THOUGHTS

As is true for any other type of study, simply performing a clinical trial of cancer gene therapy is no guarantee of future success. Many attractive new therapeutic modalities that compete with gene therapy are available to patients. Mechanism-oriented monitoring strategies are needed that may allow the identification of new response prediction markers or improvements in the efficacy of therapeutic genes during the course of the trial. Results from phase I trials revealing some of the tumor suppression activities associated with *E1A* have already gone some way toward establishing this flexibility by laying the scientific groundwork for phase II clinical trials of *E1A* as an anticancer agent. In the end, however, any study, in addition to being ethical, must offer an attractive range of potential treatment options if it is to appeal to patients who might be persuaded to participate.

REFERENCES

1. Berk AJ. Functions of adenovirus E1A. Cancer Surv 1986;5(2):367–387.
2. Ruley HE. Adenovirus early region 1A enables viral and cellular transforming genes to transform primary cells in culture. Nature 1983;304(5927):602–606.
3. Byrd PJ, Grand RJ, Gallimore PH. Differential transformation of primary human embryo retinal cells by adenovirus E1 regions and combinations of E1A + Ras. Oncogene 1988;2(5):477–484.
4. Montell C, Courtois G, Eng C, Berk A. Complete transformation by adenovirus 2 requires both E1A proteins. Cell 1984;36(4):951–961.
5. Schrier PI, Bernards R, Vaessen RT, Houweling A, van der Eb AJ. Expression of class I major histocompatibility antigens switched off by highly oncogenic adenovirus 12 in transformed rat cells. Nature 1983;305(5937):771–775.
6. Yu D, Suen TC, Yan DH, Chang LS, Hung MC. Transcriptional repression of the neu protooncogene by the adenovirus 5 E1A gene products. Proc Natl Acad Sci U S A 1990;87(12):4499–4503.
7. Yan DH, Chang LS, Hung MC. Repressed expression of the HER-2/c-erbB-2 proto-oncogene by the adenovirus E1a gene products. Oncogene 1991;6(2):343–345.
8. Yu D, Wolf JK, Scanlon M, Price JE, Hung MC. Enhanced c-erbB-2/neu expression in human ovarian cancer cells correlates with more severe malignancy that can be suppressed by E1A. Cancer Res 1993;53(4):891–898.
9. Mymryk JS. Tumour suppressive properties of the adenovirus 5 E1A oncogene. Oncogene 1996;13 (8):1581–1589.
10. Frisch SM, Mymryk JS. Adenovirus-5 E1A: paradox and paradigm. Nat Rev Mol Cell Biol 2002; 3(6):441–452.
11. Frisch SM, Reich R, Collier IE, Genrich LT, Martin G, Goldberg GI. Adenovirus E1A represses protease gene expression and inhibits metastasis of human tumor cells. Oncogene 1990;5(1):75–83.
12. Yu D, Hamada J, Zhang H, Nicolson GL, Hung MC. Mechanisms of c-erbB2/neu oncogene-induced metastasis and repression of metastatic properties by adenovirus 5 E1A gene products. Oncogene 1992;7(11):2263–2270.
13. Young KS, Weigel R, Hiebert S, Nevins JR. Adenovirus E1A-mediated negative control of genes activated during F9 differentiation. Mol Cell Biol 1989;9(7):3109–3113.
14. van Dam H, Offringa R, Smits AM, Bos JL, Jones NC, van dEA. The repression of the growth factor-inducible genes JE, c-myc and stromelysin by adenovirus E1A is mediated by conserved region 1. Oncogene 1989;4(10):1207–1212.
15. Pozzatti R, McCormick M, Thompson MA, Khoury G. The *E1A* gene of adenovirus type 2 reduces the metastatic potential of ras-transformed rat embryo cells. Mol Cell Biol 1988;8:2984–2988.
16. Rosengard AM, Krutzsch HC, Shearn A, et al. Reduced Nm23/Awd protein in tumour metastasis and aberrant Drosophila development. Nature 1989;342(6246):177–180.
17. Frisch SM. Antioncogenic effect of adenovirus E1A in human tumor cells. Proc Natl Acad Sci U S A 1991;88(20):9077–9081.
18. Frisch SM, Dolter KE. Adenovirus E1A-mediated tumor suppression by a c-erbB-2/neu-independent mechanism. Cancer Research 1995;55(23):5551–5555.
19. Deng J, Xia W, Hung MC. Adenovirus 5 E1A-mediated tumor suppression associated with E1A-mediated apoptosis in vivo. Oncogene 1998;17(17):2167–2175.
20. Frisch SM. E1A induces the expression of epithelial characteristics. J Cell Biol 1994;127(4):1085–1096.
21. Lowe SW, Ruley HE. Stabilization of the p53 tumor suppressor is induced by adenovirus 5 E1A and accompanies apoptosis. Genes Dev 1993;7(4):535–545.
22. Debbas M, White E. Wild-type p53 mediates apoptosis by E1A, which is inhibited by E1B. Genes Dev 1993;7(4):546–554.
23. Lee WP, Wen Y, Varnum B, Hung MC. Akt is required for Axl-Gas6 signaling to protect cells from E1A-mediated apoptosis. Oncogene 2002;21(3):329–336.

24. Deng J, Zhang H, Kloosterboer F, et al. Ceramide does not act as a general second messenger for ultraviolet-induced apoptosis. Oncogene 2002;21(1):44–52.
25. Lee WP, Liao Y, Robinson D, Kung HJ, Liu ET, Hung MC. Axl-Gas6 interaction counteracts E1A-mediated cell growth suppression and proapoptotic activity. Mol Cell Biol 1999;19(12):8075–8082.
26. Chen MJ, Holskin B, Strickler J, et al. Induction by E1A oncogene expression of cellular susceptibility to lysis by TNF. Nature 1987;330(6148):581–583.
27. Shao R, Hu MC, Zhou BP, et al. E1A sensitizes cells to tumor necrosis factor-induced apoptosis through inhibition of IkappaB kinases and nuclear factor kappaB activities. J Biol Chem 1999;274 (31):21,495–21,498.
28. Duerksen HP, Wold WS, Gooding LR. Adenovirus E1A renders infected cells sensitive to cytolysis by tumor necrosis factor. J Immunol 1989;143(12):4193–4200.
29. Cook JL, May DL, Wilson BA, et al. Role of tumor necrosis factor-alpha in E1A oncogene-induced susceptibility of neoplastic cells to lysis by natural killer cells and activated macrophages. J Immunol 1989;142(12):4527–4534.
30. Friedmann T. Overcoming the obstacles to gene therapy. Sci Am 1997;276(6):96–101.
31. Zhang Y, Yu D, Xia W, Hung MC. HER-2/neu-targeting cancer therapy via adenovirus-mediated E1A delivery in an animal model. Oncogene 1995;10(10):1947–1954.
32. Felgner PL. Nonviral strategies for gene therapy. Sci Am 1997;276(6):102–106.
33. Felgner PL, Ringold GM. Cationic liposome-mediated transfection. Nature 1989;337(6205):387–388.
34. Nabel EG, Yang Z, Muller D, et al. Safety and toxicity of catheter gene delivery to the pulmonary vasculature in a patient with metastatic melanoma. Hum Gene Ther 1994;5(9):1089–1094.
35. Nabel GJ, Nabel EG, Yang ZY, et al. Direct gene transfer with DNA-liposome complexes in melanoma: expression, biologic activity, and lack of toxicity in humans. Proc Natl Acad Sci U S A 1993;90(23):11,307–11,311.
36. Xing X, Liu V, Xia W, et al. Safety studies of the intraperitoneal injection of E1A—liposome complex in mice. Gene Ther 1997;4(3):238–243.
37. Xing X, Zhang S, Chang JY, et al. Safety study and characterization of E1A-liposome complex gene delivery in an ovarian cancer model. Gene Ther 1998;5:1538–1544.
38. Yu D, Matin A, Xia W, Sorgi F, Huang L, Hung MC. Liposome-mediated in vivo E1A gene transfer suppressed dissemination of ovarian cancer cells that overexpress HER-2/neu. Oncogene 1995;11 (7):1383–1388.
39. Chang JY, Xia W, Shao R, et al. The tumor suppression activity of E1A in HER-2/neu-overexpressing breast cancer. Oncogene 1997;14(5):561–568.
40. Hortobagyi GN, Hung MC, Lopez-Berestein G. A Phase I multicenter study of E1A gene therapy for patients with metastatic breast cancer and epithelial ovarian cancer that overexpresses HER-2/neu or epithelial ovarian cancer. Hum Gene Ther 1998;9(12):1775–1798.
41. Mymryk JS. Tumor suppressive properties of the adenovirus 5 E1A oncogene. Oncogene 1996;13(8): 1581–1589.
42. Ueno NT, Yu D, Hung MC. Chemosensitization of HER-2/*neu*-overexpressing human breast cancer cells to paclitaxel (Taxol) by adenovirus type 5 *E1A*. Oncogene 1997;15:953–960.
43. Li S, Huang L. In vivo gene transfer via intravenous administration of cationic lipid-protamine-DNA (LPD) complexes. Gene Ther 1997;4(9):891–900.
44. Li S, Rizzo MA, Bhattacharya S, Huang L. Characterization of cationic lipid-protamine-DNA (LPD) complexes for intravenous gene delivery. Gene Ther 1998;5(7):930–937.
45. Li S, Wu SP, Whitmore M, et al. Effect of immune response on gene transfer to the lung via systemic administration of cationic lipidic vectors. Am J Physiol 1999;276(5 Pt 1):L796–L804.
46. Ueno NT, Bartholomeusz C, Herrmann JL, et al. E1A-mediated paclitaxel sensitization in HER-2/neu-overexpressing ovarian cancer SKOV3.ip1 through apoptosis involving the caspase-3 pathway. Clin Cancer Res 2000;6(1):250–259.
47. Ueno NT, Bartholomeusz C, Xia W, et al. Systemic gene therapy in human xenograft tumor models by liposomal delivery of the E1A gene. Cancer Res 2002;62(22):6712–6716.
48. Sanchez-Prieto R, Quintanilla M, Cano A, et al. Carcinoma cell lines become sensitive to DNA-damaging agents by the expression of the adenovirus E1A gene. Oncogene 1996;13(5):1083–1092.
49. Sanchez-Prieto R, Lleonart M, Ramon Y, Cajal SR. Lack of correlation between p53 protein level and sensitivity of DNA-damaging agents in keratinocytes carrying adenovirus E1a mutants. Oncogene 1995;11(4):675–682.
50. Sanchez-Prieto R, Vargas JA, Carnero A, et al. Modulation of cellular chemoresistance in keratinocytes by activation of different oncogenes. Int J Cancer 1995;60(2):235–243.

51. Zhou Z, Jia SF, Hung MC, Kleinerman ES. E1A sensitizes HER2/neu-overexpressing Ewing's sarcoma cells to topoisomerase II-targeting anticancer drugs. Cancer Research 2001;61(8):3394–3398.
52. Lee WP, Tai DI, Tsai SL, et al. Adenovirus type 5 E1A sensitizes hepatocellular carcinoma cells to gemcitabine. Cancer Res 2003;63(19):6229–6236.
53. Liao Y, Zou YY, Xia WY, Hung MC. Enhanced paclitaxel cytotoxicity and prolonged animal survival rate by a nonviral-mediated systemic delivery of E1A gene in orthotopic xenograft human breast cancer. Cancer Gene Ther 2004;11(9):564–602.

22 Phase I Clinical Experience with Intravenous Administration of PV701, an Oncolytic Virus

Andrew L. Pecora, MD
and Robert M. Lorence, MD, PhD

Contents

Summary

PV701 is a highly purified, replication-competent naturally attenuated strain of Newcastle disease virus, an avian paramyxovirus. PV701 directly lyses diverse human cancer cells in vitro (oncolytic) while being significantly less toxic toward normal human cells. In addition to its direct oncolytic properties, PV701 is capable of stimulating T-cell-mediated specific antitumor immunity and nonspecific activation of immune function, including interferon release and activation of tumoricidal macrophages. A high rate of complete tumor regression is observed in athymic mice implanted with human tumor cells following PV701 administered intravenously, or by intraperitonel or intratumoral routes. Objective responses have been observed in human phase I clinical trials of diverse tumor types. PV701 thus warrants further study as a novel therapeutic agent for cancer patients.

Key Words: Oncolytic; PV701; Newcastle disease virus; tumoricidal; paramyxovirus.

1. INTRODUCTION

Oncolytic viruses are an exciting new therapeutic modality being developed for cancer. The power of these novel agents reside in their ability to replicate within tumor cells, in effect creating more drug at the tumor site. A variety of oncolytic viruses are in various stages of preclinical testing or clinical development including Newcastle disease virus *(1–3)*, adenovirus *(4–6)*, herpes simplex virus (HSV) *(7)*, reovirus *(8)*, vaccinia virus *(9)*, myxoma virus *(10)*, vesicular stomatitis virus *(11–14)*, measles virus *(15)*, poliovirus *(16)*, coxsackievirus *(17)*, parvovirus *(18)*, and influenza virus *(19)*. Prior to the initiation of clinical testing, the ideal oncolytic virus for the broadest utility for cancer treatment would have the following properties:

From: *Cancer Drug Discovery and Development: Gene Therapy for Cancer*
Edited by: K. K. Hunt, S. A. Vorburger, and S. G. Swisher © Humana Press Inc., Totowa, NJ

- High selectivity for cytotoxicity toward human cancer cells compared with normal cells.
- High potency for killing of human cancer cells at low multiplicities of infection (MOI).
- Broad spectrum of antineoplastic activity.
- Systemic in vivo activity with a wide therapeutic index.
- Environmentally safe.
- High-titer growth sufficient for clinical and commercial manufacturing.
- Potential for genetic engineering.

Using such criteria, PV701, an attenuated, nonrecombinant, oncolytic strain of Newcastle disease virus (an avian paramyxovirus), was selected for clinical development by Wellstat Biologics Corporation. Additional attractive features of Newcastle disease virus include the lack of human pathogenicity, well-documented genetic stability of attenuated strains, the absence of genomic recombination or integration into the host genome, the lack of human-to-human transmission, and the very low incidence of pre-existing antibodies in the general human population *(3)*.

PV701 selectively kills human cancer cells versus normal cells in vitro by exploiting tumor-specific defects in the interferon (IFN)-mediated antiviral response of cancer cells *(20)*. These phenotypic defects in IFN response appear to be common among diverse malignancies, and are believed to confer a growth and/or survival advantage to cancer cells *(11,13)*. However, these same tumor defects disable important antiviral cellular defenses *(11,13)* resulting in significant vulnerability of cancer cells to infection and replication by oncolytic viruses such as PV701.

PV701 was the first oncolytic virus to enter phase I dose ranging studies by the intravenous (IV) route *(1)*. In the three phase I trials of PV701, key clinical variables of dose, dose frequency and the rate of intravenous (iv) administration were all systematically tested in a total of 113 patients (Table 1). These PV701 trials comprise the most extensive experience for any oncolytic virus using iv dosing and have resulted in a well-tolerated regimen for phase II studies with significant signs of anticancer activity and no signs of cumulative toxicity. This review provides an important up-to-date summary of these findings.

2. PRECLINICAL STUDIES WITH PV701

PV701 is a triple-plaque purified isolate of the attenuated Newcastle disease virus strain MK107 which demonstrates highly selective killing of human cancer cells compared with normal cells. PV701 was tested in cytotoxicity assays with 57 human cancer cells lines and eight normal cell strains *(20)*. In these 5-d assays, the median sensitivity (as measured by the concentration required to reduce the viability of the target cell population by 50%) of the 57 tumor cell lines was 1000 × higher than that of the eight normal cell strains. A high degree of potency for PV701 was also observed: For the majority of tumor cell lines tested, the multiplicity of infection (MOI) required to kill at least 50% of the cell monolayer was less than 10^{-5} (i.e, less than 10 plaque forming units [PFUs]/10^6 cells). PV701 displayed a broad spectrum of activity against tumor cells of multiple cellular origins, including carcinomas (such as breast, lung, prostate, and colon), melanomas, glioblastomas, and sarcomas *(20)*. In contrast, all normal cells tested were orders of magnitude more resistant to PV701 cytolysis than the tumor cells.

In human tumor xenograft models in mice, PV701 was highly active against a wide range of human tumor types by a variety of routes including intravenous, intratumoral, and intraperitoneal *(21–22)*. PV701 caused complete tumor regressions in animal

Table 1
Phase I Studies of Intravenous Administration of PV701

Study no.	*Ref.*	*No. of patients*	*Dosing regimens ($BPFU/m^2$)*	*Dose ranges*	*Dosing schedule*
1	Pecora et al. *(1)*	79	Single-Dose	5.9 to 24	1×, cycled every 4 wk
			Repeat-Dose	5.9 × 3; 12 × 3	3×/wk × 1wk, cycled every 4 wk
			1 wk desensitization	12, 24 × 2 to 12, 144 × 2	
			2 wk Desensitization	12, 96 × 5; 12, 120 × 5	3×/wk × 2wk, cycled every 3 wk
2	Laurie et al. *(25)*	16	Two-Step Desensitization[a]	1, 12, 24 × 4 to 1, 12, 120 × 4	
3	Hotte et al. *(26)*	18	Slow Infusion with Desensitization	12, 24 × 5 to 24, 120 × 5	
Total	—	**113**	—	—	—

[a]Two Step Desensitization refers to two increments in dose given to each patient (e.g., first dose of 1 BPFU/ m^2, second dose of 12 BPFU/ m^2, and third to sixth doses of up to 120 BPFU/ m^2). This is in contrast to all the other desensitization regimens which were "one-step" (e.g., first dose of 12 PFU/ m^2, followed by second and subsequent doses of up to 120 BPFU/ m^2).

models following iv administration of doses 100-fold below the maximum tolerated dose (MTD). In these tumor models, the response rate increased with higher doses or with more frequent dosing. For example, the incidence of tumor response in HT1080 fibrosarcoma xenografts in athymic mice increased from 55 to 100% by either raising the iv dose threefold or by increasing the number of doses from 1to 3 *(21)*.

Unlike many cancer chemotherapeutic compounds, the mechanisms effecting efficacy and acute toxicity for PV701 are distinct *(2)*. In these preclinical studies, PV701 antitumor effects resulted from virus replication within the tumor and required live virus, whereas acute toxicity was mediated by the induction of proinflammatory cytokines and was also seen with ultraviolet (UV)-killed virus. Also, in contrast to the traditional chemotherapeutic compounds, PV701 toxicity was principally associated with the first dose and was not cumulative. The term "desensitization" has been applied to describe the phenomenon whereby the first dose of PV701 reduces the toxicity of subsequent doses. Use of an initial "desensitizing dose" of PV701 allowed a 5- to 10-fold increase in the MTD for subsequent doses. Desensitization occurred as early as 24 h after the first PV701 dose and was also observed in severe combined immunodeficient (SCID) mice, indicating that this desensitization is not antibody mediated *(23)*.

The first dose of PV701 induces increased serum levels of proinflammatory cytokines such as interferon (IFN)-α, IFN-β, and tumor necrosis factor-α (TNF-α). In rodents, the transient release of these cytokines accounts for the acute toxicity and the reduction in their release into the serum after repeat dosing likely accounts for the desensitization seen on repeat PV701 doses. A similar desensitization phenomenon has also been observed following administration of individual cytokines. For example, a tolerance to acute toxicity has been reported for repeat doses of IFN *(24)*.

In addition to desensitization, PV701 toxicity was reduced in mice by slowing the rate of iv infusion. The same dose administered over 10 min vs 30 s was better tolerated in mice, whereas there was no loss in efficacy at the slower infusion rates. These preclinical findings indicated that a higher therapeutic index may be achievable by slowing the infusion rate.

3. CLINICAL EXPERIENCE WITH PV701

3.1. General

The clinical development of PV701 has focused on iv dosing, because systemic administration has the greatest utility for the treatment of metastatic disease. The preclinical conditions outlined above affecting efficacy and toxicity were incorporated into the phase I clinical studies and all have proven to be important translational observations. The primary objectives of these phase I studies were to characterize the safety and tolerability of intravenously administered PV701, to establish the MTD for single and repeat dose iv regimens, and to establish a regimen for phase II efficacy testing. Secondary objectives were to obtain antibody and viral shedding data as well as to document preliminary signs of efficacy in cancer patients.

In the first phase I trial involving 79 late-stage cancer patients *(1)*, bolus iv doses of PV701 were progressively escalated by cohort using several dosing regimens: single dose, repeat dose at the same dose level, and "desensitization" regimens with a lower first dose and subsequent higher doses escalated between cohorts (Table 1). Patients in the first cohort received a single dose of 5.9 BPUF/m^2, whereas those in the final cohort received a total of 612 BPFU/m^2/cycle (Table 1). In the most intensive regimen, patients were given six doses over 2 wk followed by 1 wk of rest with cycles repeated on a 3-wk basis. Two additional phase I trials *(25,26)* maintained that intensive schedule and evaluated either an additional desensitizing step or a slower infusion rate (Table 1). Advanced cancer patients with a variety of cancer types were enrolled in all of these studies after having failed all conventional therapies.

3.2. Single Dose Regimen

We started our clinical program by giving a single bolus injection of PV701 with dose escalation between cohorts from 5.9 to 12 to 24 billion PFU (BPFU)/m^2 *(1)*. Flu-like adverse events (AEs) were seen in all patients and most commonly consisted of fever, chills, nausea, vomiting, fatigue, and diarrhea. Patients were successfully managed with standard prophylactic measures (e.g., acetaminophen and ibuprofen for fever; antiemetics for nausea; loperamide to prevent diarrhea). Although not a dose-limiting toxicity (DLT), hypotension (grade 1 or 2) was the only dose-dependent toxicity noted and found to occur in four of five patients receiving 24 BPFU/m^2 *(1)*. With the goal of developing a safe outpatient regimen, we therefore selected 12 BPFU/m^2 as the first dose for continued testing of bolus administration.

The observed flu-like AEs, predicted from preclinical testing, were attributed to the induction of proinflammatory cytokines and their well documented symptoms *(1)*. At 6 h post dosing, increases in serum levels of proinflammatory cytokines were detectable and coincided with the occurrence of fever. All of these cytokines (IFN-α, interleukin [IL]-6, and TNF-α) consistently reached peak levels at 20 h post dosing and were approximately at baseline levels at the next time point tested (at three days after dosing).

3.3. Repeat Dosing and Desensitization Regimens

On repeat dosing with PV701, as predicted preclinically, there was a marked reduction in the incidence and severity of the flu-like AE that occurred following repeated dosing, even when subsequent doses were 8- to 10-fold higher than dose 1 (*see* Fig. 1). This phenomenon, termed "desensitization," also manifested as transient thrombocytopenia and leukopenia that recovered in spite of continued dosing. Desensitization allowed the MTD for the second and subsequent doses to be elevated to 120 BPFU/m^2 compared with the initial dose of 12 BPFU/m^2 *(1)*.

The reduction in side effects that occurred as a result of desensitization was coincident with a reduction in serum levels of two cytokines examined (IFN-α and TNF-α). The rapid onset of desensitization, within 2 d after the first dose, occurred before antibodies were undetectable *(1)* and is consistent with the preclinical observation that desensitization is an antibody-independent phenomenon. These findings are consistent with the tolerance to other inducers of proinflammatory cytokines that have been described in the literature *(27)*.

3.4. Successful Translation of Preclinical Regimens to Improve Patient Tolerability

Because the results of the 79 patient phase I trial using bolus dosing with PV701 were encouraging *(1,28)*, further dosing modifications to improve patient tolerability were warranted, especially for the first dose for which reversible grade 3 fatigue occurred in about one-third of patients. Because preclinical safety testing in rodents accurately predicted the toxicities observed clinically, we explored two alternative

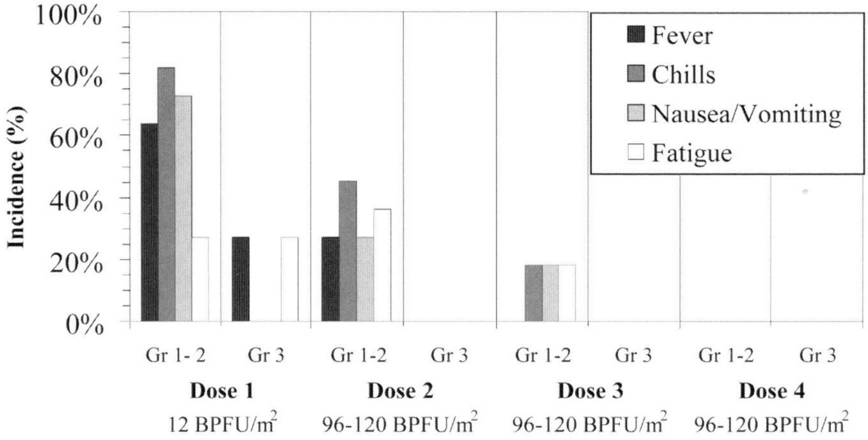

Fig. 1. An example of clinical desensitization using PV701: Decreased incidence and severity of the most common adverse events with repeat dosing. Data is from the 2-wk desensitization regimen using bolus dosing in which the first dose was 12 BPFU/m^2 and subsequent doses 8- to 10-fold higher. Severity is shown by grade (Gr).

dosing regimens in preclinical models first. One regimen tested an additional desensitizing step. In mice, a low first dose protected against the side effects of a moderate second dose, in turn protecting against higher subsequent doses. This approach, that we termed "two-step desensitization," was tested clinically in the second phase I trial of PV701. A first dose of 1 BPFU/m^2 was followed by a second dose of 12 BPFU/m^2 and then repeated higher doses escalated between patient cohorts from 24 to 120 BPFU/m^2 *(25)*. Adverse events observed in this 16 patient study still consisted of flu-like symptoms, but all were grade 2 or less (except for one patient noncompliant with prophylactic medications). No dose-limiting toxicities (DLTs) were observed in this study.

The second alternative dosing strategy examined the effects of infusion rate. In mice, we found that lengthening the infusion time to 10 min, as opposed to the original 30 s, dramatically reduced toxicity in mice while preserving the same degree of efficacy. Clinically, this concept was then tested in the third phase I trial with 18 patients (Table 1). As in the preclinical model, the rate of infusion of PV701 in patients was reduced approx 20-fold for the first dose (by means of a 3-h infusion instead of a 10-min bolus administration). All subsequent doses were administered over 1 h. Unlike the previous experience with bolus dosing, there were no grade 3 adverse events following a first dose of 12 BPFU/m^2 using the 3-hinfusion *(26)*. Escalation of the first-dose using slow-infusion established a first-dose MTD of 24 BPFU/m^2 for this regimen with moderate fever despite antipyretics and asymptomatic hypotension observed. Escalation of doses 2 to 6 continued up to the previously determined repeat dose MTD of 120 BPFU/m^2 with no DLTs reported.

3.5. Tumor Site Specific Adverse Events

An intriguing class of PV701-related AEs observed in the phase I studies were tumor site specific. Whereas flu-like symptoms appears to be common following administration of oncolytic viruses, tumor site specific AEs have not been reported with other viral agents. Tumor site specific AEs are associated with the specific location and size of tumor, were most commonly seen in the liver and the lung, and did not depend upon tumor type *(1)*. For example, reversible elevations in liver transaminases over 200 U/L occurred only in patients with liver metastases and not in patients without liver metastases *(1)*. In patients with pulmonary tumor masses, tumor site specific AEs were manifested as respiratory signs and symptoms *(1)*. Here, oxygen desaturation occurred only in patients with pulmonary or pleural tumors. Similarly, severe dyspnea was seen only in patients with lung/pleural involvement, particularly those with lung tumors larger than 5 cm. One such patient with pre-existing compromised lung function died of respiratory failure after his family refused additional therapy including intubation and mechanical ventilation. Findings in his autopsy included severe edema and inflammation confined solely to the tumor-bearing lobe along with thrombosis restricted to the tumor vessels and associated tumor necrosis. Based on these observations, two key changes in entry criteria were made. Patients with large lung tumors (≥5 cm in size) and baseline dyspnea were excluded and any other patients with lung tumors were required to have adequate pulmonary function as measured by FEV_1 and pulse oximetry. In subsequent patients who were enrolled after having met these revised entry criteria, there were no cases of treatment-related grade 3 dyspnea in the 11 patients with lung tumors nor in the other 23 patients.

Other tumor-site specific AEs included an enterocutaneous fistula at the tumor site in a patient with tumor extending from the bowel to the skin surface *(1)* and signs of bile duct obstruction in a patient that had a tumor encroaching the common bile duct (which was partially reversed upon administration of corticosteroid). Intestinal obstruction was also observed in a small percentage of patients with abdominal tumors, particularly those with large masses that had previously caused obstruction. In general, the time of onset of these tumor site specific AEs, usually within the first few days following dosing, is consistent with inflammation and swelling of the tumor in response to PV701.

3.6. Tumor Inflammation

Inflammation and swelling restricted to tumor sites following PV701 administration has been documented. This was a common occurrence in the latest phase I trial *(26)* and included intriguing effects observed in a patient with numerous cutaneous melanoma metastases. In this case, inflammation extensively developed in the skin metastases (and not seen anywhere else) after PV701 dosing, leading to an apparent increase the tumor dimensions. This inflammatory reaction was noted to occur before marked tumor regression (75% overall tumor reduction). For internal masses, tumor inflammation, however, may be inappropriately characterized as tumor progression on computed tomography (CT) scan and therefore new criteria (e.g., as outline by Sze et al. *[29]* for adenovirus) or alternative forms of imaging may be needed for tumor evaluation and response assessment. Nonetheless, with traditional scanning methods, 4 major and 2 minor responses were documented in 18 patients treated in the last trial (*see* Section 3.11.).

Tumor inflammation may underlie the occurrence of the tumor site specific AEs discussed above. The ability of a short course of an antiinflammatory corticosteroid to ameliorate a tumor site specific AE is consistent with a role for inflammation in the occurrence of this class of AEs. Infection with a virus expressing antigens foreign to the host would be predicted to generate an immune inflammatory response and the natural selectivity of PV701, based on preclinical experiments, for growth in tumor cells over normal cells would serve to restrict the inflammation to tumor sites. Clinically, signs of tumor inflammation and edema in palpable tumors have now been observed in six patients. Histological examination of tumors from five other patients revealed numerous mononuclear inflammatory cells in the tumors but not in adjacent normal tissues. A sample of inflamed tumor tissue obtained from one of these patients after his eighth cycle displayed evidence of PV701 budding from tumor cell membranes (*see* Fig. 2). Additional studies including tumor biopsies will be required to more fully understand the nature of these inflammatory and/or immune reactions and to address any association of tumor inflammation with virus levels in the tumor and with tumor response.

3.7. Adverse Events During Infusion

The third class of AEs observed initially in the first PV701 trial occurred during infusion, and consisted mainly of back pain, noncardiac chest pressure, and, less commonly, abdominal pain and hypertension. These were particularly noted on repeat dosing at the higher dose levels (particularly ≥96 BPFU/m^2) and were managed effectively by slowing the infusion rate. Indeed, in second PV701 trial *(25)*, this class of AEs became rare when the infusion time beginning for cycle 3 was doubled: AEs during infusion occurred with 1 of 62 doses when 120 BPFU/m^2 was administered over 1 h vs 12 of 44 doses when 120 BPFU/m^2 was administered over 30 min. Likewise, in the third trial with PV701, all of the doses were administered slowly (over at least 1 h) throughout the trial and again AEs during infusion were rare (with only one mild case observed among the 18 patients treated).

3.8. Lack of Cumulative Toxicity

Sixty-nine patients received multiple cycles of PV701 with no evidence of cumulative toxicity *(1,25,26)*. This includes a patient with peritoneal mesothelioma who received 41 courses over 4 yr without adverse effects on any organ system noted *(1)*. Nevertheless, continued monitoring for any signs of cumulative toxicity will be important for future patients receiving PV701 treatment.

3.9. Virology

Transient and low-level viral shedding was noted during these phase I studies *(1)*. Recovery of virus from sputum was rare (0.7% of those samples tested), occurring in only 2 patients, and was of very low concentration (median of 26 PFU/gram of sputum). Recovery of virus from urine (median level of 820 PFU/mL) was more common (15% of samples tested), but again the shedding did not persist, being cleared within 3 wk. This level of shed virus was very low, at least two orders of magnitude below the standard vaccine dose required for an antibody response in chickens, the most sensitive species *(30,31)*. From an environmental safety perspective, this low and transient virus shedding may be part of the explanation for the lack of any observed human-to-human transmission seen with Newcastle disease virus *(3)*.

3.10. Antibody Response

To date, 66 patients have been tested for antibodies to PV701 using assays for anti-PV701 IgG antibody and/or neutralizing antibody. Almost all patients were negative for

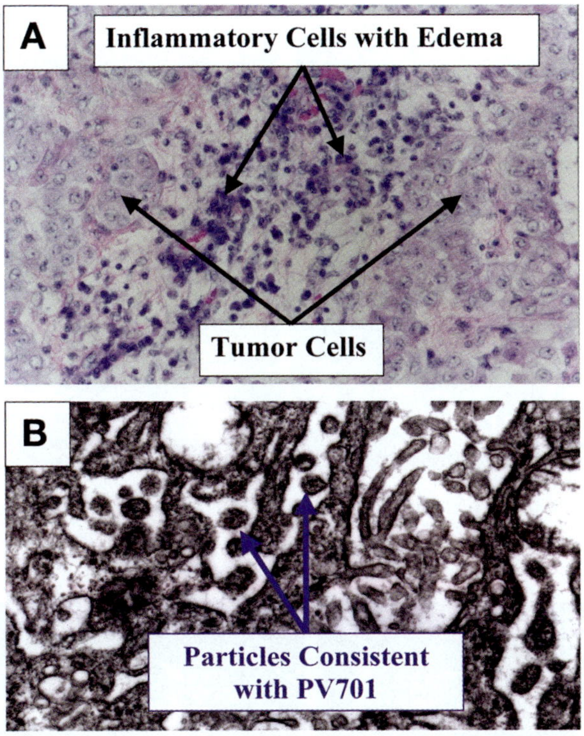

Fig. 2. Microscopic sections of tumor after eight PV701 cycles in a 46-yr-old man with advanced peritoneal mesothelioma (4 baseline tumor of 8 to 10 cm each) who went on to receive a total of 41 cycles of PV701 and who remained progression-free for 40 mo. (**A**) Tumor parenchyma demonstrating significant inflammation (H&E staining). (**B**) Electron micrograph displaying particles consistent with PV701 budding from the tumor cell membrane.

any detectable antibodies toward Newcastle disease virus at baseline *(1)*, consistent with previous reports that the general human population is seronegative to this virus *(32,33)*. In most of the patients tested post-dosing, neutralizing antibody titers was first detectable at 1 to 2 wk after their first dose. At 5 to 10 wk post-dosing, the median neutralizing antibody titer was 1:640, which is significantly less than the reported titers for patients treated with adenovirus vectors *(34–36)*. For those patients receiving several courses of PV701, a plateau in neutralizing antibody titer was seen at approx 1:2560 in all 7 cases analyzed thus far, including 1 patient who was followed for the first 18 mo of therapy *(1)*.

Understanding the effects that neutralizing antibodies have on PV701 therapy will require further studies. However, in spite of the presence of neutralizing antibodies, 19 patients receiving more than 1 cycle of PV701 had a second peak in viral shedding in the urine. Among the few patients enrolled with cutaneous metastases, visible signs of inflammation or tumor necrosis were seen in three patients after PV701 dosing during repeat cycles. Importantly, from a clinical perspective, the occurrence of tumor regressions was not restricted to the first two cycles, and included five patients noted to have regressions which developed in later cycles, long after the establishment of neutralizing antibody titers. Additional investigations that will shed further light on these issues will include studies on the immune response to PV701 and studies on viremia, viral clearance and virus levels in tumor biopsies during the initial cycle and during repeat cycles.

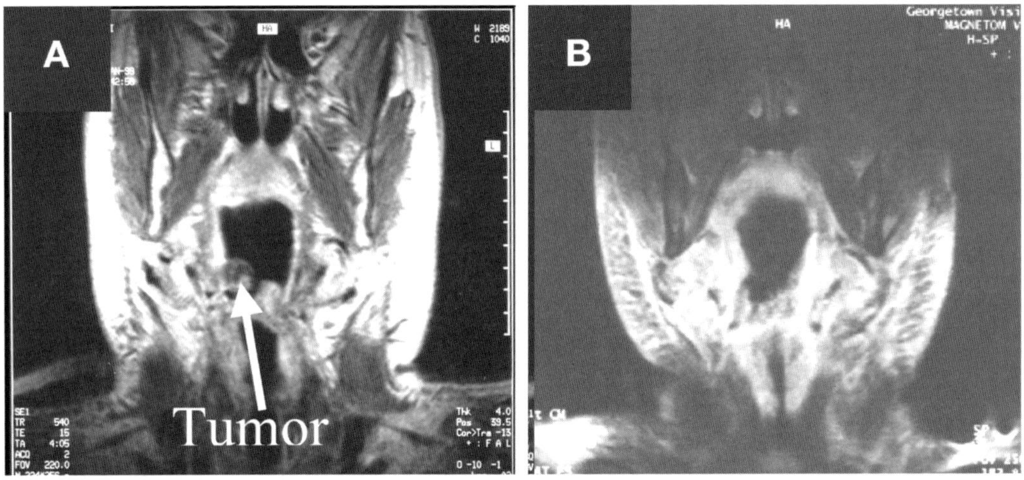

Fig. 3. Complete response in a 51-yr-old man with tonsillar carcinoma. (**A**) Baseline MRI scan showing a 1.5-cm tumor in the posterior pharynx. (**B**) MRI scan at 3 mo demonstrates complete regression of the tumor mass.

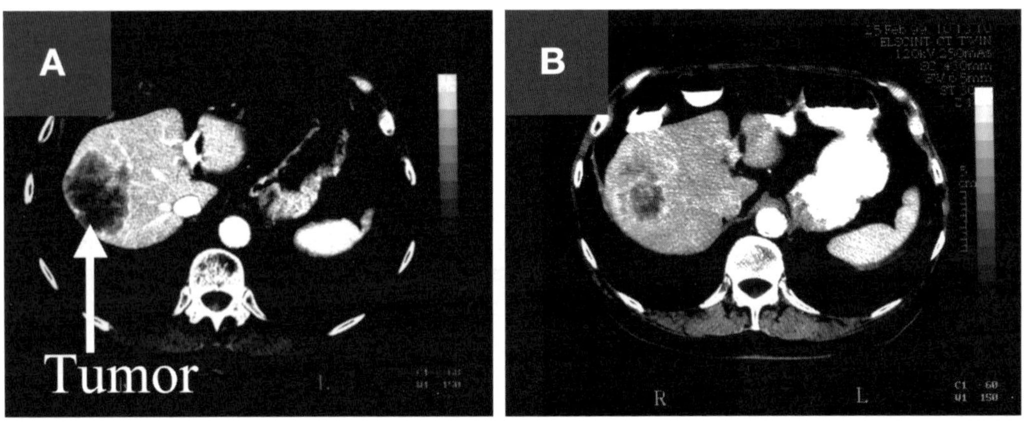

Fig. 4. Partial response in a 79-yr-old man with colorectal carcinoma. (**A**) Baseline CT scan showing a 10-cm liver metastasis. (**B**) CT scan at 1 m demonstrates a major response.

3.11. Tumor Responses

In the most recent trial using a slower infusion rate along with desensitization, there were 6 objective responses (33% rate of response) (1 complete response [CR] in cervical, 2 partial responses [PRs] in colorectal, 1 PR in melanoma, and 2 minor responses in carcinoid) among the 18 patients who had all failed all standard treatments *(26)*. Eleven patients (61%) had a progression-free survival (PFS) of at least 4 mo including 4 of 9 patients with colorectal carcinoma. Currently, one woman with advanced cervical carcinoma refractory to radiation and chemotherapy has clinically maintained a CR at 20 mon post-enrollment to the PV701 trial.

In the first 2 trials *(1,25)*, there were 8 other responses (1 CR in head and neck cancer [*see* Fig. 3]; 1 PR in colorectal cancer [*see* Fig. 4]; 1 PR in anal carcinoma, 2 minor responses [mesothelioma, pancreatic] and 3 mixed response [melanoma, colorectal and breast]). It is important to realize that all of these responses occurred in a heavily pretreated population that had failed a median of 2 prior chemotherapeutic regimens.

4. CONCLUSIONS

The three phase I trials of PV701 in 113 patients compromise the most extensive clinical testing by iv infusion of an oncolytic virus to date. These studies include systematic evaluation of dose levels, infusion rates, and various treatment schedules with a greater than 100-fold increase in dose intensity. In these studies, the safety and tolerability of intravenous administered PV701 has been characterized for phase II testing. The PV701 induced adverse events are manageable and can be categorized into 3 classes: (1) flu-like, (2) tumor site specific, and (3) those occurring during infusion. All patients experienced flu-like symptoms. Desensitization and slower infusion rates lessened the incidence and severity of flu like symptoms and allowed for a significant increase in dose intensity. Interestingly, all 11 major and minor responses were only noted at higher dose levels achievable with desensitization.

Collectively, the observations in the three phase I studies support the concept that systemic therapy with the replication competent virus, PV701, can provide a novel and potentially important therapy for patients with solid tumors including those unresponsive to standard therapy. The safety profile of PV701 is predicable, manageable with standard prophylactic measures such as antipyretics and antidiarrheals, and favorable compared with most chemotherapeutic agents. Repeated long-term iv PV701 administration seems feasible in humans and does not show any signs of cumulative toxicity to any organ system including the bone marrow, in contrast to many chemotherapies. Therapy with PV701 either alone or in combination with other agents may play an important role in the treatment of solid tumors. Additional clinical trials of PV701 will soon be underway.

ACKNOWLEDGMENTS

We thank the following other PV701 clinical investigators: Pierre P. Major and Sebastien Hotte (Hamilton Regional Cancer Centre), Scott A. Laurie and Harold L. Atkins (Ottawa Regional Cancer Centre), Naiyer Rizvi and John L. Marshall (Georgetown University Medical Center); Gary I. Cohen (The Cancer Center at Greater Baltimore Medical Center); Neal J. Meropol (Fox Chase Cancer Center); and Daniel Sterman (University of Pennsylvania Medical Center). We are grateful to John Bell at the Ottawa Regional Cancer Centre for general advice and assistance. At Wellstat Biologics Corporation, we thank Michael Bamat, Jim O'Neil, Scot Roberts, Scott Groene, Michael Myers, Jeff Miller, Steve Mueller, Pete Buasen, Tom Higgs, Jean Guyader, Joan Helton, Mari Toal, Bill Kusmik, Candice Duhon, Sandra Doveikis, Sharon Polidoro, Grace McDaniel, Bei Bei Li, Russell Jang, Mengdong Hu, and Chitra Sudarshan.

REFERENCES

1. Pecora AL, Rizvi N, Cohen GI, et al. Phase I trial of intravenous administration of PV701, an oncolytic virus, in patients with advanced solid cancers. J Clin Oncol 2002;20:2251–2266.
2. Lorence RM, Pecora AL, Major PP, et al. Overview of phase I studies of intravenous administration of PV701, an oncolytic virus. Curr Opin Mol Ther 2003;5:618–624.
3. Lorence RM, Roberts MS, Groene WS, Rabin H. Replication-competent, oncolytic Newcastle disease virus for cancer therapy. In: Replication-Competent Viruses for Cancer Therapy, Hernaiz Driever P, Rabkin SD, eds., Monographs in Virology. Basel, Switzerland: Karger 2001;22: pp. 160–182.
4. Hallden G, Thorne SH, Yang J, Kirn DH. Replication-selective oncolytic adenoviruses. Methods Mol Med 2004;90:71–90.

5. DeWeese TL, van der Poel H, Li S, et al. A phase I trial of CV706, a replication-competent, PSA selective oncolytic adenovirus, for the treatment of locally recurrent prostate cancer following radiation therapy. Cancer Res 2001;61:7464–7472.
6. Kanevera A, Bauerachmitz GJ, Yamamoto M, et al. A cyclooxygenase-2 promoter-based conditionally replicating adenovirus with enhanced infectivity for treatment of ovarian adenocarcinoma. Gene Ther 2004;11(6):552–559.
7. Markert JM, Medlock MD, Rapkin ST, et al. Conditionally replicating herpes simplex virus mutant G207 for the treatment of malignant gliomas: Results of a Phase I trial. Gene Ther 2000;7:867–874.
8. Yang WQ, Senger DL, Lun XQ, et al. Reovirus as an experimental therapeutic for brain and leptomeningeal metastases from breast cancer. Gene Ther 2004;11:1579–1589.
9. Thorne SH, Kirn DH. Future directions for the field of oncolytic virotherapy: a perspective on the use of vaccinia virus. Expert Opin Biol Ther 2004;4:1307–1321.
10. Sypula J, Wang F, Ma Y, et al. Myxoma virus tropism in human tumor cells. Gene Ther Mol Biol 2004;18:103–114.
11. Stojdl DF, Lichty BD, tenOever BR, et al. VSV strains with defects in their ability to shutdown innate immunity are potent systemic anti-cancer agents. Cancer Cell. 2003;4:263–275.
12. Lichty BD, Stojdl DF, Taylor RA, et al. Vesicular stomatitis virus: a potential therapeutic virus for the treatment of hematologic malignancy. Hum Gene Ther 2004;15:821–831.
13. Stojdl DF, Lichty B, Knowles S, et al. Exploiting tumor specific defects in the interferon pathway with a previously unknown oncolytic virus. Nat Med 2000;6:821–825.
14. Obuchi M, Fernandez M, Barber GN. Development of recombinant vesicular stomatitis viruses that exploit defects in host defense to augment specific oncolytic activity. J Virol 2003;77:8843–8856.
15. Dingli D, Peng KW, Harvey ME, et al. Image-guided radiotherapy for multiple myeloma using a recombinant measles virus expressing the thyroidal sodium iodide symporter. Blood 2004;103:1641–1646.
16. Ochiai H, Moore SA, Archer GE, et al. Treatment of intracerebral neoplasia and neoplastic meningitis with regional delivery of oncolytic recombinant poliovirus. Clin Cancer Res 2004;10:4831–4838.
17. Shafren DR, Au GG, Nguyen T, et al. Systemic therapy of malignant human melanoma tumors by a common cold-producing enterovirus, coxsackievirus A21. Clin Cancer Res 2004;10:53–60.
18. Raykov Z, Balboni G, Aprahamian M, Rommelaere J. Carrier cell-mediated delivery of oncolytic parvoviruses for targeting metastases. Int J Cancer 2004;109:742–749.
19. Mustar T, Rajtarova J, Sachet M, et al. Interferon resistance promotes oncolysis by influenza virus NS1-deletion. Int J Cancer 2004;110:15–21.
20. Welch AR, McDaniel GP, Sudarshan C, et al. The broad spectrum oncolytic activity of Newcastle disease virus PV701 is a result of a functional defect in the antiviral interferon response in tumor cells. Eur J Cancer 2001;37(1):S69.
21. Lorence RM, Roberts S, Groene WS, et al. Regression of human tumor xenografts following intravenous treatment using PV701, a naturally attenuated oncolytic strain of Newcastle disease virus. Proc Am Assoc Cancer Res 2001;42:454 (abst # 2442).
22. Roberts MS, Buasen PT, Incao BA, et al. PV701, a naturally attenuated strain of Newcastle disease virus, has a broad spectrum of oncolytic activity against human tumor xenografts. Proc Amer Assoc Cancer Res 2001;42:454 (abst # 2441).
23. Savage PD and Muss HB. Renal Cell Cancer. In: Biologic Therapy of Cancer. Devita VT, Hellman S, Rosenberg SA, eds., Philadelphia, PA: JB Lippincott 1995;pp.373–387.
24. Laurie SA, Atkins HL, Bell JC, et al. Novel 2-step desensitization dosing regimen of intravenous PV701, an oncolytic virus, results in improved tolerability: A phase I study of patients with advanced solid tumours. Eur J Cancer 2002;38(7): Abs 516.
25. Hotte SJ, Major PP, Hirte HW, et al. Slow intravenous infusion of PV701, an oncolytic virus: Final results of a phase I study. J Clin Oncol 2004; 22:204s (Abstr #3037).
26. Zeisberger E, Roth J. Tolerance to pyrogens. Ann N Y Acad Sci 1998;856:116–131.
27. Bergsland EK, Venook AP. Shedding old paradigms: Developing viruses to treat cancer. J Clin Oncol 2002;20:2220–2222.
28. Sze DY, Freman SM, Slonin SM, et al. Dr. Gary J. Becker Young Investigator Award: Intraarterial adenovirus for metastatic gastrointestinal cancer: Activity, radiographic response, and survival. J Vasc Interv Radiol 2003;14:279–290.
29. Newcastle disease virus vaccine. United States Code of Federal Regulations. 1999; Title 9, Part 1213, Section 329.
30. Thorton DH. Quality control of vaccines. In: Newcastle Disease. Alexander DJ, ed., Boston, MA: Kluwer Academic Publishers 1988;pp.347–365.

31. Miller LT, Yates VJ. Reactions of human sera to avian adenoviruses and Newcastle disease virus. Avian Dis 1971;15:781–788
32. Charan S, Mahajan VM, Agarwal L. Newcastle disease virus antibodies in human sera. Indian J Med Res 1981;73:303–307.
33. Nemunaitis J, Cunningham C, Tong AW, et al. Pilot study of intravenous infusion of a replication-selective adenovirus (ONYX-015) in combination with chemotherapy or IL-2 treatment in refractory cancer patients. Cancer Gene Ther 2003;10:341–352.
34. Hamid O, Varterasian ML, Wadler S, et al. Phase II trial of intravenous CI-1042 in patients with metastatic colorectal cancer. J Clin Oncol 2003;21:1498–1504.
35. Reid T, Galanis E, Abbruzzese J, et al. Intra-arterial administration of a replication-selective adenovirus (dl1520) in patients with colorectal carcinoma metastatic to the liver: A phase I trial. Gene Ther 2001;8:1618–1626.
36. Reid T, Galanis E, Abbruzzese J, et al. Hepatic artery infusion of a replication-selective oncolytic adenovirus (dl1520): Phase II Viral, immunologic, and clinical endpoints. Cancer Res 2002;62: 6070–6079.

23 MDA-7/IL-24 as a Multi-Modality Therapy for Cancer

Sunil Chada, PhD, *Dora Bocangel,* PhD,
Abujiang Pataer, MD, PhD,
Abner M. Mhashilkar, PhD, *Satoshi Inoue,* MD,
Ryo Miyahara, MD, *Jack A. Roth,* MD,
Elizabeth A. Grimm, PhD, *Stephen G. Swisher,* MD,
Kelly K. Hunt, MD, *and Rajagopal Ramesh,* PhD

CONTENTS

Summary

The protein encoded by the melanoma differentiation-association gene 7 (MDA-7/IL-24) is a novel interleukin (IL)-10 family cytokine with unique tumor-specific apoptotic and antiangiogenic properties that make it especially attractive for use in cancer gene therapy applications. *Mda-7* gene transfer with a replication incompetent adenoviral vector (Ad-mda7) induces apoptosis in a tumor specific manner, an effect that is independent of the status of other tumor suppressor genes, such as p53, Rb, or $p16^{INK4}$. In addition to its direct cytotoxic effects, Ad-mda7 transduction causes secretion of a processed, glycosylated form of MDA-7 protein. MDA-7 is a novel interleukin (IL-24) with unique apoptotic functions. Studies on the secreted MDA-7/IL-24 protein have shown that it can act as a pro-Th1 cytokine, and induces secretion of interferon-gamma, tumor necrosis factor-α, IL-6, IL-12, and granulocyte macrophage colony-stimulating factor in human peripheral blood mononuclear cells . Additional studies in syngeneic mice indicate that MDA-7 can function as an immune adjuvant and enhance immune reactivity against tumors. More recently, our group demonstrated that MDA-7 protein functions as a potent antiangiogenic factor in vitro and in vivo that is 50-fold more active than angiostatin or endostatin. In phase I clinical trials intratumoral delivery of Ad-mda7 showed tumor regression in patients with advanced carcinomas who failed conventional therapies. This chapter provides a comprehensive perspective on MDA-7/IL-24 research, highlighting its proapoptotic, antimetastatic, and antiangiogenic properties. The combination of these potent effector mechanisms makes mda-7/IL-24 a promising and novel approach for the treatment of cancer.

Key Words: Mda-7; IL-24; apoptosis; cancer; cytokine; antiangiogenesis.

From: *Cancer Drug Discovery and Development: Gene Therapy for Cancer*
Edited by: K. K. Hunt, S. A. Vorburger, and S. G. Swisher © Humana Press Inc., Totowa, NJ

1. INTRODUCTION

Tumor cells are characterized by mutations in critical tumor suppressor and proto-oncogenes. These genomic alterations result in apparently distinct, but mechanistically overlapping phenotypes: resistance to apoptosis and the ability to detach from normal tissue architecture and migrate to new environments. Multiple overlapping and redundant signaling pathways are involved in control of cell fate. In order to develop new targeted therapies to treat and ultimately prevent cancer, we must be able to integrate the burgeoning dataset of intracellular molecular interactions with an understanding of the pharmacologic modulation of these pathways. By developing a comprehensive understanding of these complex signals, we can recognize and validate tumor-specific molecular targets, and exploit the pleiotropic activities of overlapping signaling pathways to identify molecules that may interfere with multiple cancer specific phenotypes. One such interesting candidate that we have explored is a multifunctional gene called *mda-7*. This chapter summarizes preclinical findings showing the potent proapoptotic, antiangiogenic, and antimetastatic activities of mda-7/IL-24 and its implications in cancer therapy.

2. OVERVIEW OF MDA-7/IL-24 BIOLOGY

2.1. Initial Identification and Characterization

The melanoma differentiation associated gene-7 (*mda-7*) was identified in HO-1 melanoma cells induced to terminally differentiate by treatment with fibroblast interferon (IFN-β), and the protein kinase C activator mezerein (MEZ) *(1)*. The differentiated and growth arrested HO-1 melanoma cells mRNAs were used to generate a cDNA library; another library was generated from proliferating HO-1 cells. Differentiation induction subtraction hybridization (DISH) of these two yielded a temporally spaced subtracted cDNA library enriched for genes activated during HO-1 terminal differentiation *(2,3)*. The underlying hypothesis of the above approach was that cancer cells would stop or significantly reduce expression of genes regulating growth control or differentiation, and that treatment with IFN-β and MEZ would reactivate them. *mda-7* was identified as a gene with minimal or absent expression in proliferating melanoma cells, high expression in normal melanocytes, and inducible expression in terminally differentiated melanoma cells *(4–6)*. Studies on patient-derived specimens reported that MDA-7 protein expression inversely correlated with melanoma progression and that transfection of metastatic human melanoma cells with a vector encoding for *mda-7*/IL-24 reduced their colony formation capabilities *(6,7)*. The lack of MDA-7 protein expression in cancer cells did not result from mutations in the gene but rather from permanent defects in the signaling pathways or mRNA/protein stability *(8,9)*.

Subsequent studies on *mda-7* have shown that it encodes an evolutionarily conserved protein of 206 amino acids, with a predicted size of 23.8 kDa (*see* Fig. 1A) *(1,9,10)*. Two orthologs have been identified: the rat *c49a* and the mouse *mob5* genes. The rat *c49a* gene, with 78% nucleotide homology to human *mda-7*, was initially identified by differential display polymerase chain reaction (PCR) as a gene overexpressed in wound healing and was associated with proliferation of fibroblasts *(8)*; *mob5* was identified as a *ras*-induced gene involved in intestinal epithelia neoplasia *(11)*. The mouse *mda-7* ortholog was later identified as a Th2-specific cytokine, and named IL-4 induced secreted protein (FISP) *(12)*.

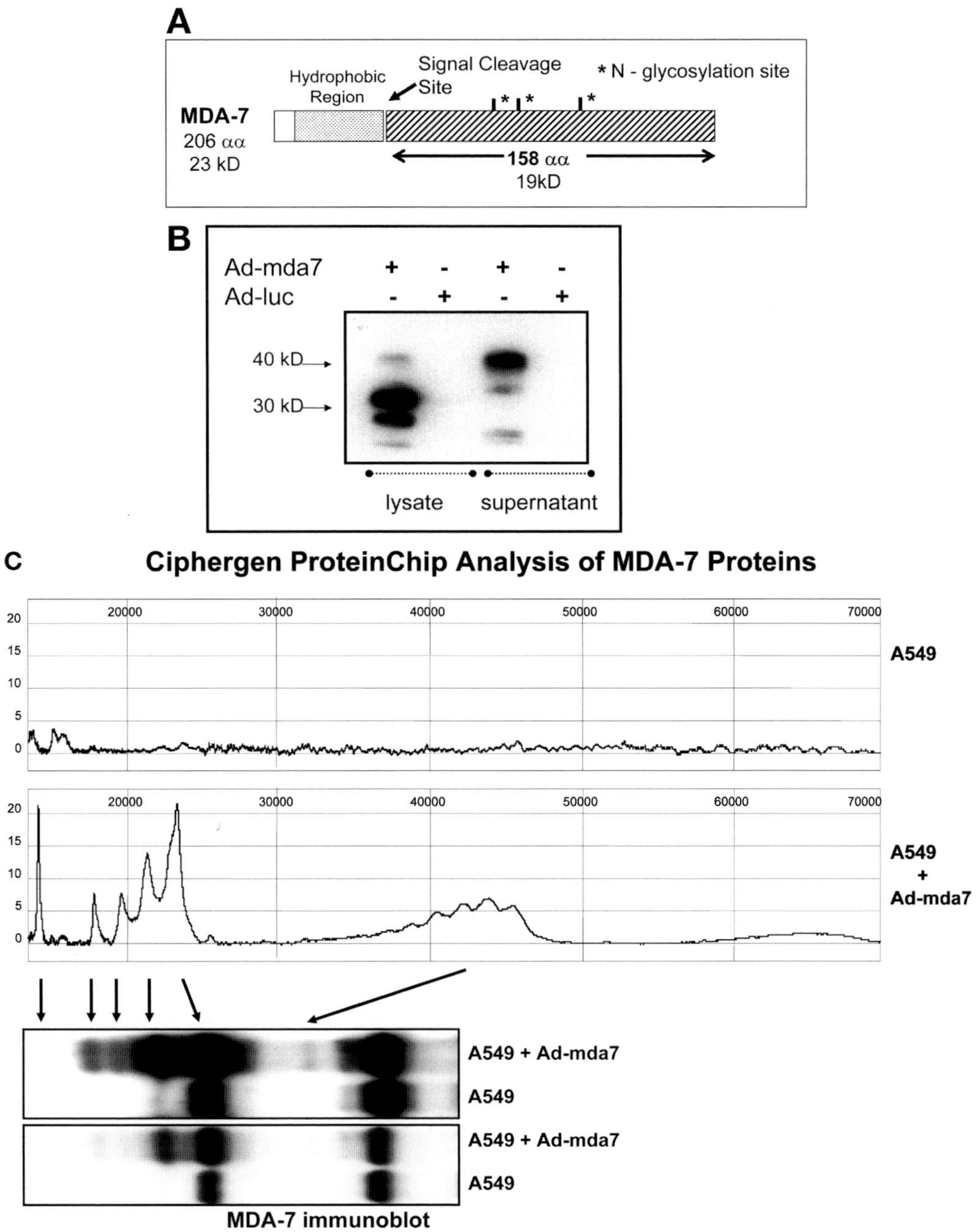

Fig. 1. Characterization MDA-7 protein after Ad-mda7 gene transfer. (**A**) Schematic of MDA-7 protein. The leader sequence is indicated by stippling and mature secreted protein is shown by hatched area. (**B**) Potential glycosylation sites are indicated. (**B**) Ad-mda7 transduction of H1299 NSCLC cells results in expression of protein intracellularly and glycosylated protein in supernatant. (**C**) Ciphergen proteomic analysis of intracellular MDA-7 protein. A549 NSCLC cells were untreated or treated with Ad-mda7 and lysates immunoprecipitated with anti-MDA-7 monoclonal antibody and evaluated using SELDI. Upper panels: SELDI traces of control A549 cells and Ad-mda7 treated cells. Molecular weights are indicated. *Lower panels*: western blot analyses of control A549 cells and Ad-mda7 treated samples. Note Ig heavy and light chains in control samples. Correlation of Western blot proteins with SELDI traces is indicated by arrows.

2.2. MDA-7 is an IL-10 Family Cytokine

The *mda-7* gene localizes to chromosome 1q32, a region within an IL-10 family cluster that also contains the genes for IL-10, IL-19, and IL-20 *(13)*. Although *mda-7* has little sequence homology with IL-10, the encoded protein has approx 19% amino acid identity with other IL-10 family members *(14,15)*. Based on its chromosomal location, the presence of an IL-10 signature motif, limited amino acid identity with other IL-10 cytokines, its translational regulation and predicted structural features, *mda7* has been renamed IL-24, and categorized as an IL-10 family cytokine *(16)*.

Chada S. et al. reported that exposure of melanoma cells to MDA-7/IL-24, induced secretion of interferon (IFN)-γ and IL-6, but not of IL-4 or IL-5; in contrast, Ad-luc treatment did not induce IFN-γ or IL-6, suggesting an MDA-7-specific effect *(15)*. Transduction of these cells with Ad-mda7 induced increases in mRNA that mirrored the cytokine induction observed with exposure to the MDA-7/IL-24 protein. The report suggested that the effect was also specific to some types of tumor cells, because similar treatment of lung and breast cancer cells did not induce release of cytokines. Microarray analysis of non-small-cell lung carcinoma (NSCLC) cells transduced with Ad-mda7 corroborated the cytokine-like activity of this gene, and confirmed that MDA-7 can activate IFN-γ and NF-κB signaling pathways. Given that IL-10 functions as an immunosupressive cytokine, and that it significantly inhibited MDA-7/IL-24 activity in human peripherral blood mononuclear cells (PBMCs), it is possible that *mda7*/IL-24 acts as an antagonist of IL-10 *(16)*.

Exposure of melanoma and PBMC cells to MDA-7/IL-24 protein also activated Stat3 pathways, which have previously been associated with cellular transformation. The specificity of STAT3 activation in these cells was demonstrated by addition of anti-MDA-7 antibodies, but was not affected by addition of anti-IL-6 antibodies. In this study, exposure of melanoma cells to bacterially expressed protein failed to induce similar results, and the authors hypothesized that post-translational modifications to the MDA-7 protein, in particular glycosylation, were important for its functional activity *(14)*.

Although the organization of the *mda-7* gene is better understood now in comparison with the other members of the IL-10 family cytokines, the crystal structure of the MDA-7 protein has not yet been solved. The IL-10 family of cytokines functions through the JAK/STAT signaling pathway and comprises six members: IL-10, IL-19, IL-20, IL-22, MDA-7/IL-24, and IL-26. In spite of the substantial degree of sharing of the receptor subunits, specificity of signaling is based on selective expression of either the receptors or of the cytokines themselves. Although the IL-10 family members share limited homology in some of their conserved domains, they are distinguished by their similar helical structure and IL-10 signature motif. There are three human IL-10 family proteins whose structures have been solved (IL-10, IL-19, and IL-22): all possess six α helices (A, B, C, D, E, and F) and at least one disulfide bond. The V-shaped complex is comprised of four helices (A through D) from one monomer and two helices (E and F) from the other. The classical four-helix bundle that is representative of all helical cytokines is formed by helices A, C, D, and F. Of the IL-10 family, *mda-7* seems to be the only member to posses an extensive (49 amino acids) leader sequence; but is otherwise organized into a similar consistent pattern of six predicted alpha helices (A through F) based on the structure of IL-10. Helix F is conserved in all the family members, whereas the NH_2-terminus is variable *(15)*. The regions in IL-10 corresponding to helix A, the A–B loop, and helix F are important in binding to its receptors. There are three potential glycosylation sites in MDA-7/IL-24; two are located on the top part of the V-shaped complex and seem to be readily accessible to modifications, the first is shared with IL-22 (Asn85-Ile-Thr), the second site maps to a unique loop between helices C and D. The third site maps to the base of helix B (aa99), but it is not likely to be used because glycosylation of this site would interfere with the structural integrity of the molecule. An in-depth review of the predicted structural features of IL-24 and how these relate to other IL-10 cytokines was recently presented *(15)*.

A combination of structural data, homology to known cytokines, chromosomal localization, a predicted N-terminus secretion signal peptide, and evidence of its regulation of cytokine secretion, all support classification of MDA-7/IL-24 as a IL-10 family cytokine *(4,9,16)*. A 49 amino acid leader sequence predicts it is a secreted protein; recent studies confirm this prediction and report that Ad-mda7 transduced cells release high levels of a 40-kDa form of the MDA-7 protein (*see* Fig. 1), which can bind to heterodimeric receptors IL-20R1/IL-20R2 and IL-22R2/IL-20R1 *(9,17,18)*. The intracellular form of the protein (23–30 kDa) is cleaved, and extensively modified (primarily by glycosylation) before its release into the extracellular compartment (*see* Fig. 1B,C) *(9,16,19)*. Expression of MDA-7 is rare in tumors, and correlates inversely with progressive stages of melanoma, as has also been shown of the expression of a novel mda-7 splice variant (*mda-7s*) *(6,7,20)*. Because its initial characterization as a differentiation factor in IFN-β and mezerein-treated human melanoma cells, MDA-7 has attracted interest because of its unique tumor-selective antiangiogenic and proapoptotic activities, which are reviewed below.

2.3. MDA-7 is a Tumor-Selective Apoptosis-Inducing Factor

The initial observation of *mda-7* loss of expression in melanomas and its correlation with progression of this type of tumors suggested growth suppressive properties in melanoma cells *(4–7)*. Ensuing studies investigated the effects of ectopic expression of *mda-7* in a wide variety of tumor cells (melanoma, carcinomas of the breast, colon, prostate, nasopharynx, high grade gliomas, and osteosarcoma) and proved that *mda-7* inhibits tumor cell growth regardless of the status of other genes (p53, Rb, Bax or p16) *(1,9,10)* (*see* Fig. 2 for a representative study of lung cancer cells). However, expression of the gene in normal human skin fibroblasts and mammary breast epithelial cells did not significantly affect their growth or trigger apoptosis *(9,10)*. Together, these reports indicate that MDA-7 is an IL-10 family cytokine with tumor cell apoptotic activity and that the cytotoxic effects it induces are specific to tumor cells *(5,10,22–24)*. Several studies have investigated the signal transduction pathways that mediate the apoptotic activity of *mda-7*. These appear to be multiple, cell-type specific, and include effects induced by the intracellular form of the protein, and by the secreted form (bystander effect) *(14)*.

Although activation of several apoptotic mediators (BAX, BAK, TRAIL, p53, Fas, and DR4), and signaling molecules (PKR, $p38^{MAPK}$, PI3K, JNK, GSK-3) have been reported, all these signaling molecules appear to converge on the common death effector mechanism mediated by caspase activation and mitochondrial destruction. In lung tumor cells, Ad-mda7-induced apoptosis is mediated by the release of cytochrome *c* (cyt *c*) and activation of a caspase 9/Apaf1/cyt *c* complex (apoptosome), which may involve cell death receptors *(14,19,28)*. Inhibition of caspase activation using ZVAD partially blocked apoptosis (*see* Fig. 3). Cytosolic cyt *c* is an essential part of the apoptosome, which activates caspase 9, which in turn activates other caspases (including caspase 3), triggering apoptosis. In lung cancer cells transduced with Ad-mda7, sharp increases in cytosolic cyt *c* levels were followed by induction of apoptosis, and occurred without changes in the mitochondrial membrane potential *(28)*. Staurosporine treatment

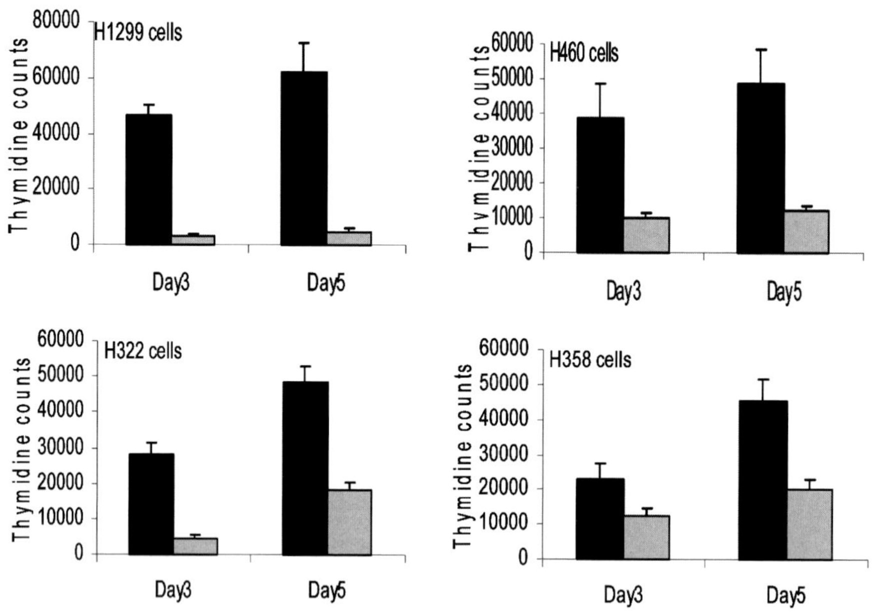

Fig. 2. Ad-mda7 kills lung tumor cells. Four NSCLC cell lines (H1299, H460, H322, and H358) were treated with Ad-luc (black bars) or Ad-mda7 (gray bars) at 2000 vp/cell and cell proliferation assayed at days 3 and 5 using tritiated thymidine assay. Data are shown as mean+SD.

was used as a positive control to induce cyt *c* release via mitochondrial permeability transition-dependent pores (MPTPs), and cyclosporine used to specifically inhibit MPTP. The authors report that Ad-mda7-induced cyt *c* release from the mitochondria was not blocked by cyclosporine, unlike that caused by treatment with staurosporine or Ad-p53. Western analysis of lysates from MDA-7 expressing cells showed no alterations in the levels of BAX, BAK, or Bcl-2, TNF-α, TNF-R1, or TNF-receptor associated death domain protein (TRADD), which are known to act via MPTPs; but pointed to a significant increase in FasL, which can activate caspase 8 and induce cleavage of Bid. This suggested that an MPTP-independent pathway is involved in the apoptotic effects induced by Ad-mda7. The effect, the authors hypothesized, could be mediated by an extrinsic death receptor pathway, involving activation of the IFN-inducible double-stranded RNA protein kinase (PKR), and other protein intermediaries. This hypothesis was in agreement with the results of a separate report by Pataer et al. which puts forward evidence for the key role of PKR in the apoptotic effects induced by MDA-7 expression *(29)*. In this study, infection with Ad-mda7 did not activate apoptosis when PKR function was inhibited by treatment with 2-AP (a specific serine and threonine kinase inhibitor). The need of a functional PKR pathway was further corroborated by Ad-mda7 transduction of PKR-null and PKR wild-type MEFs: apoptosis was absent in the PKR-null cells, but observed at high levels in their wild type PKR counterparts *(29)*.

In breast cancer cells, infection with Ad-mda7 results in a clear and dramatic increase of the proapoptotic protein BAX, as compared with normal human mammary epithelial cells (HMEC), and the ratio of BAX to antiapoptotic protein Bcl-2 becomes significantly higher *(9,24)*. The up-regulation of a proapoptotic member of the Bcl-2 family is of particular interest in breast cancer cells because estrogens regulate Bcl-2 gene expression in mammary epithelial cells and estrogen receptor (ER)-positive breast cancer lines *(24,30,31)*. Bcl-2 family members share four conserved motifs, Bcl-2

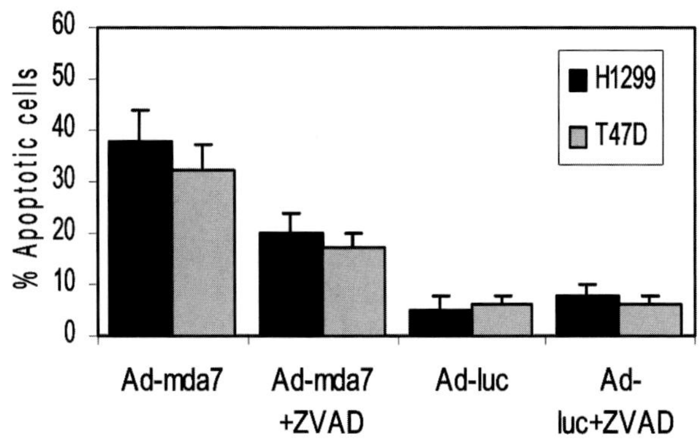

Fig. 3. Ad-mda7 induces apoptosis. H1299 NSCLC and T47D breast cancer cells were treated with Ad-luc or Ad-mda7 (2000 vp/cell) either alone or in presence of ZVAD (0.1 ug/mL). Apoptosis induction was assessed at day 3 using Annexin V assay. ZVAD significantly reduces apoptosis, but does not completely block it. Data are shown as mean+SD.

homology domains (BH-1 to BH-4); whereas antiapoptotic family members contain all four, proapoptotic members have only BH-3. The BH-3 domain is essential to one of their death-regulatory functions given that Bcl-2 proteins are known to homo- and hetero-dimerize with each other, and this domain acts as a peptide ligand that allows for the interaction *(32,33)*. Other death-related functions of this family of proteins are dimerization-independent: binding of the CED-4-like domain of Apaf-1, which prevents its association with pro-caspase 9, and its activation; and pore-forming capabilities that could induce alterations in mitochondrial permeability and thus the release of caspase-activating proteins like cyt *c (34–37)*. Bcl-2 family proteins act at the crossroads of several upstream pro- and antiapoptotic pathways. Thus, reports of *mda-7*-induced alterations in the level or activity of these proteins are in agreement with preliminary studies, and also with published studies by our group, showing that Ad-mda7 transduction significantly enhances the response of breast cancer cells to radiation therapy, and to a variety of chemotherapeutic agents (tamoxifen, docetaxel, adriamycin, and herceptin), in spite of their diverse mechanisms of action. Furthermore, the cancer growth inhibitory effects of Ad-mda7 expression were corroborated in vivo *(38,39)*.

3. SIGNALING PATHWAYS INVOLVED IN MDA-7 MEDIATED TUMOR CELL DEATH

There are numerous reports of MDA-7 growth-suppressor effects in tumors, and of its activation of various signaling pathways; including the β-catenin/PI3 kinase pathway in breast and lung cancer cells, general upregulation of BAX, p53, PKR, Fas, TNF-related apoptosis inducing ligand (TRAIL), DR4, and caspases, reduced levels of BCL-2 proteins, and down regulation of vascular endothelial growth factor (VEGF) and tumor growth factor (TGF)-β mRNA, among others. The inhibition of different kinases can have differential effects depending on the cell line used, and support the notion that MDA-7 can activate diverse signaling pathways and may activate signaling kinases in a tissue or cell line specific manner *(19,21)*. Indeed, Saeki et al. reported that *mda-7*-induced apoptosis and G2/M arrest correlates with an increase in p53 wild-type NSCLC cells, BAX and BAK proteins, established inducers of programmed cell death, and an increase in the ratio of BAX to BCL-2. In p53-null cells *mda-7* expression still induced apoptosis, although BAX and BAK were not upregulated. In all tumor cell lines tested, regardless of p53 status, the authors observed activation of caspases 3 and 9 and cleavage of PARP in tumor cells but not normal lung fibroblasts after Ad-mda7 treatment. Independent studies have also demonstrated up-regulation of p53, TRAIL, and DR4 after Ad-mda7 treatment. The antitumor effects were independent of the genomic status of p53, RB, p16, ras, bax, and caspase 3 in these cells *(9,10,40)*. Normal cell lines did not show inhibition of proliferation or apoptotic response to Ad-mda7. Although *mda-7* gene transfer induced cell-growth arrest and apoptosis in a broad-spectrum of cancer cells, the underlying signals mediating cell death varied and were reported to be cell-type dependent. MDA-7 markedly activated pc-Jun and pATF-2 transcription factors in ovarian cancer cells after Ad-mda7 treatment. The downstream targets NF = κB and AP-1 were both activated by Ad-mda7 at 24h. Activation of these molecules was not observed in normal cells. A key target of these proteins is the Fas-FasL protein family. Increased expression of both mRNA and proteins for Fas, FasL, FAF1, caspase 8 and FADD, but not TNF and TRADD, were observed at 24 h after Ad-mda7 treatment compared with PBS and Ad-luc treated cancer cells *(41)*. In ovarian cancer cells, Ad-mda7 increased Fas expression and Fas promoter activity in a p53-independent manner. Overexpression of FADD DN inhibited Ad-mda7 induced FADD activation and abrogated activation of caspases-9 and -8. Downregulation of Fas using Fas-specific siRNA resulted in the abrogation of Ad-mda7-mediated apoptosis compared with cells transfected with a scrambled siRNA. These results demonstrate the involvement of Fas-FasL signaling pathway in Ad-mda7-mediated apoptosis in ovarian cancer cells. Of the cell signaling pathways mentioned above, only $p38^{MAPK}$ in melanoma *(26)* and PKR in NSCLC *(29)* were reported to be essential for the apoptotic effects induced by expression of *mda-7* in tumor cells. Further confirmation for the role of PKR in NSCLC comes from the activation of downstream targets (eIF-2α, Tyk2, and Stats 1 and 3) of this IFN-induced kinase *(29)*.

A key gene involved in the genesis and pathological progression of many cancers is the adenomatous polyposis coli (APC) tumor suppressor gene, and the identification of direct interactions of APC with β-catenin has linked this type of neoplasia with the Wnt-signaling pathway, a highly conserved signal transduction pathway with functions in development, tissue homeostasis, and cancer. A major role of APC is the regulation of free β-catenin, a function that is carried out in part via a protein complex formed by APC, glycogen synthase kinase 3β (GSK-3β), and axin proteins. GSK-3β binds to β-catenin, and sequentially phosphorylates Thr 41, Ser 35, and Ser 33 of β-catenin, after β-catenin has been primed (phosphorylated at Ser 45) by (casein kinase 1 CK1). The β-catenin protein was first identified by its direct interaction with E-cadherin, which mediates its linkage to α-catenin, which in turn binds this complex to the cortical cytoskeleton. Activation of GSK-3β, results in degradation of β-catenin and inhibition of Wnt signaling. In gastrointestinal cancers lacking APC defects, mutations in GSK-3β phosphorylation sites near the β-catenin NH_2 terminus can render β-catenin resistant to regulation. The best studied part of the Wnt-pathway, called "The canonical Wnt pathway," involves the transcriptional activation of specific genes downstream active, membrane-bound, frizzled receptors. Frizzled receptors in turn activate, via phosphorylation, dishevelled, which binds to Axin and prevents phosphorylation of β-catenin by disruption of the APC/GSK-3β/Axin complex. Dishevelled functions to transduce wnt signals and activates the jun-N terminal kinase (JNK) pathway. Tight regulation of the free cytoplasmic pool of β-catenin seems to be a key switch of the Wnt-pathway, and three separate mechanisms can lead to accumulation of this protein: inactivation of the APC gene, axin mutations, and mutations of the β-catenin NH_2-terminus affecting its phosphorylation (residues S45–S33). Phosphorylated β-catenin binds to the F-box protein β-TRCP and undergoes ubiquitination and subsequent proteasomal degradation, whereas nonphosphorylated β-catenin translocates to the nucleus and binds to T-cell factor/lymphoid enhancer factor (Tcf/Lef) family, and activates transcription of the specific target genes (including c-Myc, cyclin D1, MMP7, gastrin, and ITF-2) *(42)*. Disruption of the PI3K and Wnt/β-catenin pathways are common in human tumors and appear to provide enhanced survival, antiapoptotic and metastatic phenotypes on tumor cells.

Ad-mda7 downregulates PI3K and Wnt/β-catenin pathways in breast, pancreatic, and lung cancer cells via the coordinate increase of tumor suppressor proteins: APC, GSK-3β, PTEN, and E-cadherin; thus, Ad-mda7 could indirectly regulate both, apoptosis and metastasis, in these tumor cells *(21)*. These changes, thought to be primarily post-transcriptional, induce reduced transcriptional activity (via TCF-LEF) and increase cell–cell adhesion in tumor cells, while sparing similar effects on their normal counterparts. Recent studies have shown that, although the more common ductal adenocarcinomas of the pancreas rarely harbor β-catenin or APC gene mutations, these alterations are common in other nonductal neoplasms and significantly correlate with the presence of lymph node and liver metastases *(43–46)*.

4. ANTIANGIOGENIC ACTIVITY OF MDA-7/IL-24

Angiogenesis, the formation of new blood vessels is important for the normal physiologic function of the body and is most commonly observed during the early stages of development *(47)*. Angiogenesis can also occur in the later stages of life, however, most frequently as a pathology-associated angiogenesis, such as tumor-related angiogenesis. Tumor-related angiogenesis is a multistep process that involves many cell types and is a finely orchestrated series of events that include endothelial cell proliferation, new capillary formation, attraction of pericytes and macrophages, disruption of existing extracellular matrix and deposition of new matrix *(48,49)*. A role for tumor-related angiogenesis is now well established, and recent studies support the concept that for tumors to grow and metastasize there is a need for blood supply that is provided by newly formed blood vessels adjacent to the tumor cells *(50)*. Importantly, extensive data exists demonstrating that solid tumors express genes coding for angiogenic mediators (e.g., VEGF, basic fibroblast growth factor [bFGF], platelet derived growth factor [PDGF], IL-8) in the local tumor milieu resulting in the production of new blood vessels *(51,52)*. Thus, metastasis from solid tumors is facilitated by angiogenesis of the primary tumor. Therefore inhibition of tumor angiogenesis is an effective means of inhibiting cancer growth and spread.

A number of angiogenesis inhibitors have evolved and can be used to block tumor growth *(53)*. These inhibitors can be broadly classified into four categories: (1) endothelial cell inhibitors such as thalidomide, TNP-70, angiostatin and endostatin *(54–56)*; (2) inhibitors of angiogenic factors, such as VEGF and VEGF receptor inhibitor *(51,57,58)*; (3) inhibitors of endothelial and smooth muscle migration, such as MMP inhibitor and integrin inhibition *(59,60)*; and (4) retinoids and cytokines such as IFN and IL-12 *(61–63)*. Although these antiangiogenic molecules have been shown to inhibit angiogenesis in preclinical studies, very few of them have demonstrated a therapeutic effect in clinical trials *(54)*. The failure to demonstrate activity and potency in clinical trials may result from the lack of understanding of the mechanism of angiogenic regulation by some of these inhibitors. Additionally, the optimal strategies for the use, monitoring, and validation of antiangiogenic agents in the clinic remain unclear. Angiogenesis is likely regulated on multiple levels; some inhibitors may function to block the formation of new blood vessels (antiangiogenic) whereas others may disrupt or modify the existing vessels (antivascular). A better understanding of the mechanism of action of vascular-targeted drugs will help in improving the treatment strategies that include combining with chemotherapy or radiotherapy.

Although antiangiogenic agents show great promise in preclinical models of cancer, their use may be limited in part by their delayed onset of inhibitory activity on tumor growth (e.g., tumors progressed as much as 400% in the first several days after initiation of antiangiogenic therapy) *(64,65)*. Given that the doubling time of murine tumors is several-fold higher than is observed in the presentation of human cancer, this delay in onset of activity could translate to several months in patients. For patients with metastatic and/or locally advanced cancer, this delay in onset of activity may make the use of these agents impractical. Another potential limitation with these agents is the high dose and prolonged treatment course that are required. Although recent work suggests that the delivery of antiangiogenic agents via continuous infusion or sustained release may allow for a reduction of the bolus dose, the amount of protein needed for widespread use will still be challenging *(56,65)*. Perhaps the most significant limit of current antiangiogenic therapy is the inability of these agents to completely eradicate the disease. Thus, there is an urgent to develop and test new and novel antiangiogenic agents that may overcome some of the limitations described above.

The concept to test the antiangiogenic properties of mda-7/IL-24 arises from several key observations made by us and several other investigators and are as follows: identification and demonstration of mda-7/IL-24 as a member of the IL-10 family with limited homology to IL-10 *(4)*, demonstration of IL-10-mediated antiangiogenic activity in vivo *(62,63)*, and reduced vascularization in tumors treated with an adenoviral vector expressing mda-7 (Ad-mda7) compared with tumors treated with control vectors *(61)*.

Initial in vitro studies demonstrated Ad-mda7 inhibited endothelial differentiation (ECD) and cell migration, assays that are routinely used to test the antiangiogenic activity of an agent *(23)*. Surprisingly, Ad-mda7 did not inhibit endothelial cell proliferation, an activity common to many antiangiogenic agents. The ability of Ad-mda7 to inhibit ECD and cell migration was similar to that observed with other antiangiogenic agents and suggested that mda-7/IL-24 may have antiangiogenic activity *(61)*. However, realizing the potential caveat that in vitro results do not always correlate with in vivo studies, a dorsal air-sac chamber assay was utilized to test the antiangiogenic activity of mda-7/IL-24 in vivo. In these experiments, human A549 lung tumor cells were used as the angiogenesis inducers. Tumor cells were treated with Ad-mda7 or Ad-luc (vector control) and loaded into chambers that were implanted into the dorsal side of nude mice. Seven to ten days later, the chambers were removed and observed for angiogenesis or neovascularization. A significant reduction in neovascularization was observed in chambers that contained Ad-mda7 treated tumor cells compared with chambers that contained Ad-luc treated tumor cells (*see* Fig. 4). That inhibition of tumor-vascularization was the result of tumor cell death was excluded by performing a viability assay and nuclear staining of cells inside the chamber (unpublished data). These results indicated that MDA-7/IL-24 possesses antiangiogenic activity.

An additional line of evidence supporting the antiangiogenic activity of MDA-7/IL-24 comprises the findings from in vitro tumor-endothelial cell mixing experiments that

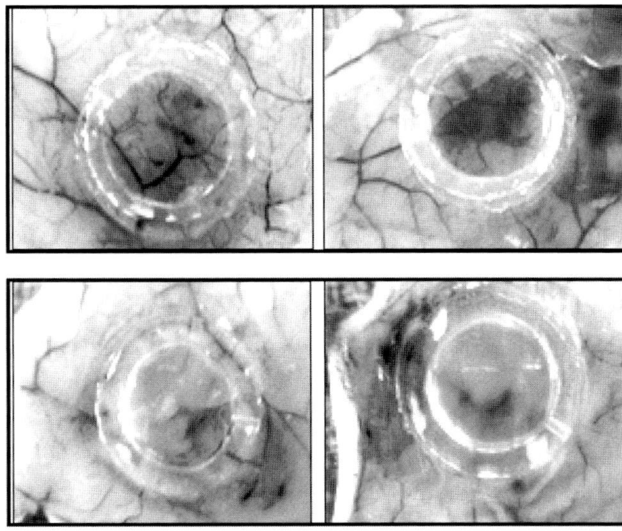

Fig. 4. Ad-mda7 inhibits angiogenesis in vivo. A549 tumor cells treated with Ad-luc or Ad-mda7 were plated on a semipermeable membrane (shown in circle) and implanted under the skin of a mouse. Five days later, the disc was isolated and neoangiogenesis evaluated by microscopy. Ad-luc treated cells demonstrate robust angiogenesis whereas Ad-mda7 treated cells shown significantly reduced vasculature.

mimic the in vivo conditions. Ad-mda7 infected A549 lung tumor cells when mixed with human umbilical vein endothelial cells (HUVEC) showed marked inhibition of ECD. In contrast, inhibition of ECD was not observed when Ad-luc (vector control) infected tumor cells were mixed with endothelial cells. These results demonstrated MDA-7/IL-24 expressing tumor cells when in close proximity to endothelial cells inhibited ECD.

Although the above findings support MDA-7-mediated antiangiogenic activity, several questions related to MDA-7-mediated antiangiogenic activity remain unanswered and are as follows: (1) is the antiangiogenic activity mediated by the intracellular MDA-7 protein or by the secreted MDA-7 protein, (2) can MDA-7/IL-24 directly affect the tumor vasculature or indirectly via inhibiting proangiogenic factors, and (3) what is the underlying mechanism for mda-7-mediated antiangiogenic activity?

4.1. Direct Inhibitory Effects on Angiogenesis

To test the direct inhibitory effects of MDA-7/IL-24 on angiogenesis, experiments were carried out using affinity purified human MDA-7/IL-24 protein *(16)*. In vitro, MDA-7/IL-24 protein selectively inhibited ECD in a dose-dependent manner with complete inhibition occurring at concentrations above 10 ng/mL (*see* Fig. 5). MDA-7/IL-24 had no effect on endothelial cell proliferation. Note that at the concentrations of MDA-7/IL-24 protein used, no significant cytotoxicity against lung tumor cells was observed, indicating selective activity against endothelial cells *(61)*. The specificity of the inhibitory effect of MDA-7/IL-24 on ECD was demonstrated by immunodepletion studies. Because MDA-7 belongs to the IL-10 family of cytokines and IL-10 has previously been reported to exhibit antiangiogenic activity studies, comparing the inhibitory effects of MDA-7 protein with those of recombinant IL-10 on ECD were also conducted. MDA-7, but not IL-10, inhibited ECD at the concentrations (5–50 ng/mL)

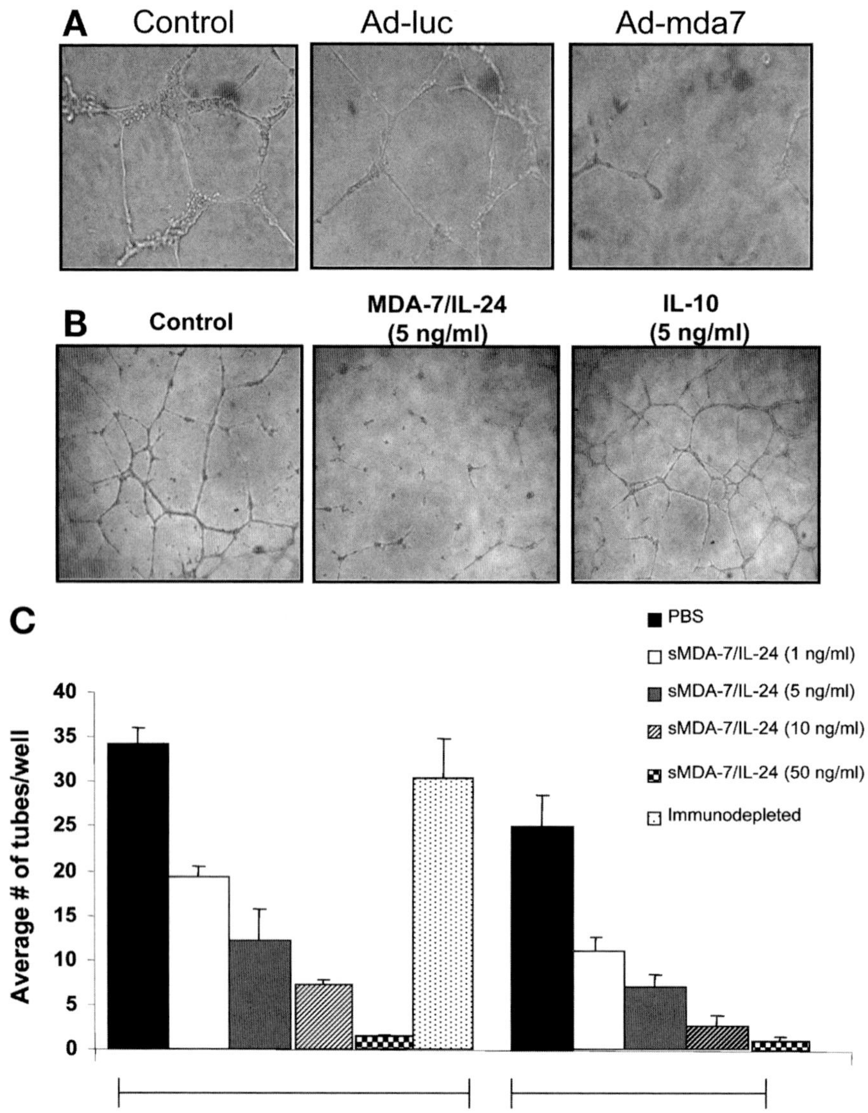

Fig. 5. Ad-mda7 and MDA-7/IL-24 inhibit endothelial cell differentiation. (**A**) HUVEC cells were treated with control media, Ad-luc or Ad-mda7 (5000 vp/cell), plated on matrigel and analyzed 24 h later for tube formation (in vitro angiogenesis assay). Ad-mda7 inhibits endothelial differentiation (tube formation) ut does not kill endothelial cells. (**B**) HUVEC cells were treated with control media, MDA-7 or IL-10, plated on matrigel and analyzed 24 h later for tube formation (in vitro angiogenesis assay). MDA-7 inhibits endothelial differentiation. (**C**) MDA-7 inhibits endothelial differentiation in a dose and ligand-dependent manner. Primary HUVEC and HMVEC endothelial cells were evaluated with PBS or increasing doses of MDA-7 (1; 5; 10; 50 ng/mL) or immunodepleted material.

tested (*see* Fig. 5). Similarly, comparison between the inhibitory effects of MDA-7/IL24 protein on ECD and equimolar concentrations of recombinant endostatin, IFN-γ, and IP10 agents that had previously shown to exhibit antiangiogenic activity *(65)* demonstrated MDA-7/IL-24 was 10 to 50× more potent than endostatin, IFN-γ, and IP10 in vitro *(61)*. The ability of MDA-7/IL-24 to inhibit ECD is similar to that seen with

IFN-γ *(66)*. Furthermore, IFN-γ production in MDA-7/IL-24 treated PBMCs has been reported *(16)*, raising the possibility that IFN-γ or IP-10 produced by mda-7/IL-24 treated endothelial cells could be responsible for the observed inhibitory effects. However, the possibility of MDA-7–mediated inhibitory effect resulting from IFN-γ or IP-10 was excluded by conducting antibody-blocking studies. Additionally, equimolar concentrations of recombinant IFN-γ or IP-10, when added to endothelial cells, showed less inhibition of ECD compared with MDA-7/IL-24 protein. These results showed that the in vitro antiangiogenic activity of MDA-7/IL-24 was more potent than IFN-γ or IP-10 and occurred via a novel mechanism.

Further evidence for MDA-7/IL-24-mediated antiangiogenic activity is its ability to potently inhibit VEGF-induced endothelial cell migration in a dose-dependent manner *(60)*. Inhibition of cell migration by MDA-7/IL-24 was also obtained when bFGF was used as an inducer (unpublished data). These results demonstrate the direct and specific antiangiogenic activity of MDA-7/IL-24 in vitro.

Evidence for direct effect of MDA-7-mediated antiangiogenic activity in vivo was next examined. Subcutaneous implantation of MDA-7 producing 293 cells (293-mda7) mixed with A549 lung tumor cells (1:1 ratio) in nude mice resulted in significant suppression of tumor growth compared with tumor growth in mice implanted with a mixture of parental 293 cells and tumor cells (*see* Fig. 6). That the tumor growth inhibitory effects resulted from exogenous MDA-7 was demonstrated by detecting MDA-7 protein in the tumors. Note that A549 tumor cells do not express detectable endogenous MDA-7 protein. Tumor growth inhibition was demonstrated to occur via apoptotic death of tumor endothelial cells. Associated with tumor growth inhibition was a marked reduction in tumor vascularization as demonstrated by the reduced hemoglobin content, and less $CD31^+$ endothelial cells *(61)*. These results demonstrated the direct antiangiogenic activity for MDA-7/IL-24 in vivo. Although these experiments established the "proof of concept" it is to be realized that most cancers such as cancer of the lung, breast, colon, and melanoma are often not localized but disseminated to distant sites in the body. Therefore for MDA-7/IL-24 to be an effective antiangiogenic agent it has to inhibit tumor growth at a distant site systemically. To test whether MDA-7 protein could exert its antiangiogenic effects systemically, two sets of experiments were performed. In the first set of experiment a mixture of 293 or 293-mda7 cells mixed with A549 tumor cells were implanted on the right lower flank of nude mice. On the contra lateral lower left flank of each mouse, tumor cells equivalent to that on the right flank were implanted. Animals were monitored daily for tumor growth on both the flanks. A significant delay in tumor growth was observed on both flanks of mice that were implanted with a mixture of tumor cells and 293-mda7 cells compared with animals that were implanted with a mixture of tumor cells and 293 cells (*see* Fig. 6). In the second set of experiments, lung tumor xenografts were established subcutaneously in the lower right flank of nude mice. Subsequently, when the tumors had grown to a size of 50 to 100 mm^3, matrigel containing parental 293 cells or matrigel containing 293-mda7 cells were implanted subcutaneously into the upper right flank of tumor-bearing animals and the effects of mda-7 on tumor growth were measured. A significant growth inhibition with 40 to 50% reduction in tumor size was observed in mice that were implanted with matrigel containing 293-mda7 cells compared with mice that were implanted with matrigel containing 293 cells (*see* Fig. 6B). That the observed tumor growth inhibition resulted from systemic inhibitory effects of MDA-7 protein on tumor angiogenesis was demonstrated by detecting the protein in the blood and a reduction in $CD31^+$ blood vessels *(61)*. Importantly, no gross pathological changes were observed in the animals

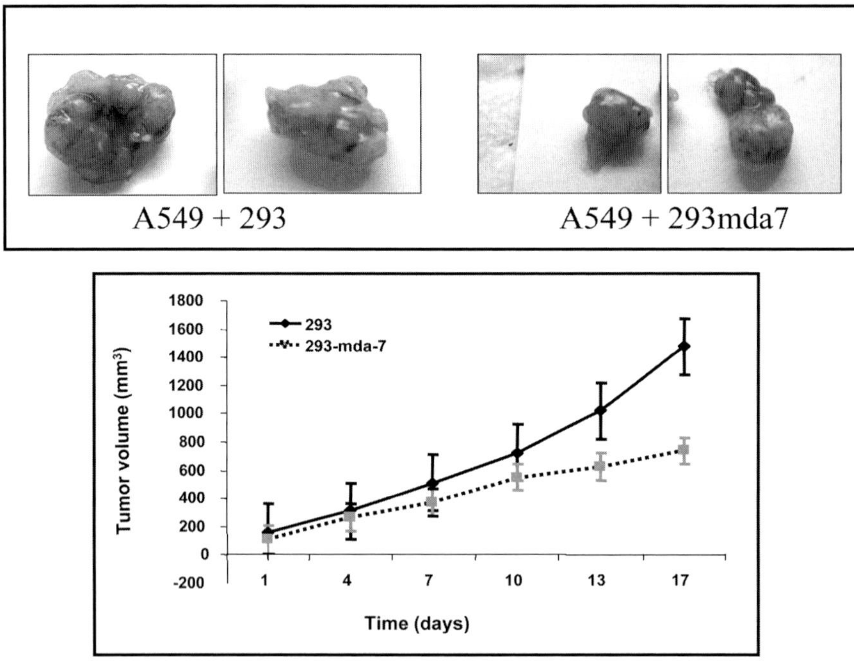

Fig. 6. Antiangiogenic activity of MDA-7/IL-24 in vivo. MDA-7/IL-24 systemically inhibits tumor growth and vascularization. Subcutaneous A549 lung tumor xenografts were established in nude mice in the lower right flank. When the tumors were measurable, Matrigel encapsulated 293 or 293-mda7 cells were implanted in the upper right flank. Tumor growth was monitored regularly for 3 wk. A significant inhibition of tumor growth was observed in animals implanted with Matrigel encapsulated 293-mda7 cells compared with animals implanted with Matrigel encapsulated 293 cells. Representative tumors are shown in upper panel and tumor growth kinetics are shown in *lower panel.*

implanted to 293-mda7 cells, suggesting that the protein had no toxic side effects. These results demonstrated MDA-7 protein systemically inhibited tumor growth by inhibiting tumor angiogenesis. Furthermore, our results establish a direct antiangiogenic activity for MDA-7/IL-24.

4.2. Indirect Inhibitory Effects on Angiogenesis

The possibility that MDA-7/IL24, like many other antiangiogenic agents can inhibit the expression of proangiogenic growth factors (IL-8, bFGF, VEGF) produced by the tumor cells existed *(67–70)*. Thus, inhibition of these tumor-derived growth factors by MDA-7/IL-24 will result in failure to support tumor vascularization thereby inhibiting angiogenesis. Preliminary cDNA array analysis demonstrated downregulation of VEGF, TGF-β, and IL-8 in human tumor cells treated with Ad-mda7 compared with tumor cells treated with Ad-luc (unpublished data). Subsequent in vitro studies demonstrated downregulation of VEGF protein expression in Ad-mda7 treated human prostate cancer (LNCaP) cells compared with Ad-luc treated control cells (*see* Fig. 7A). Correlating with our in vitro findings is the recent report by Nishikawa et al. *(68)* who showed Ad-mda7 inhibited VEGF, bFGF, and IL-8 expression in human lung tumor xenografts. In the same study, combining radiation therapy with Ad-mda7 demonstrated enhanced radiosensitization of lung tumor xenografts that was associated with a significant inhibition of VEGF,

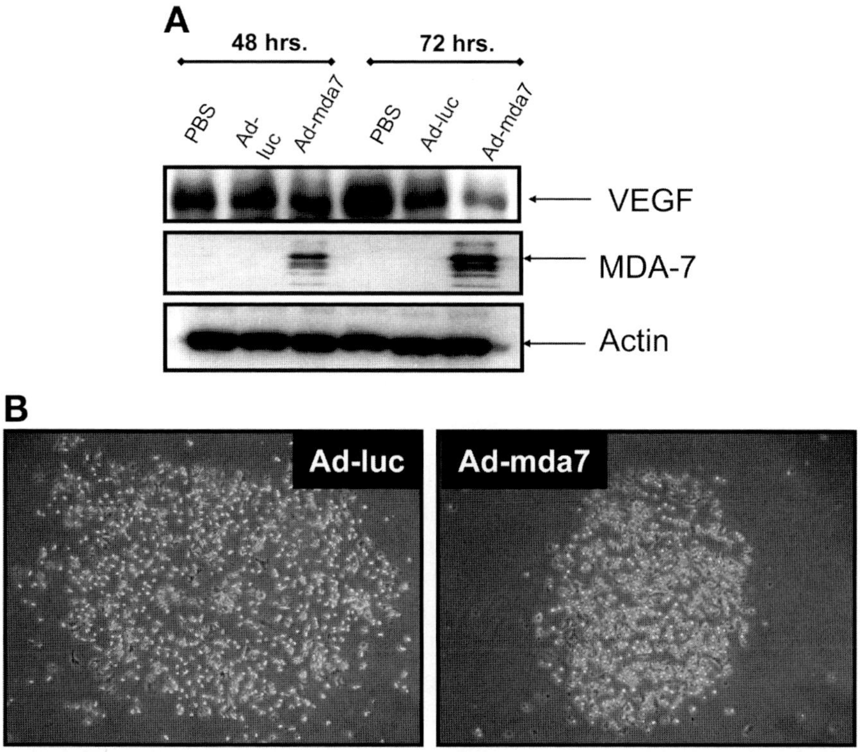

Fig. 7. MDA-7/IL-24 inhibits angiogenesis and tumor cell migration. (**A**) LNCap prostate tumor cells were treated with PBS, Ad-luc or Ad-mda7 (2000 vp/cell) and analyzed for MDA-7 and VEGF protein by western blot analysis. Ad-mda7 blocks VEGF expression. (**B**) H1299 NSCLC tumor cells were treated with 2000 vp/cell of Ad-luc or Ad-mda7 for 16 h and then replated. Cell migration was analyzed 24 h later. Control Ad-luc treated cells migrate whereas Ad-mda7 treated cells do not migrate.

bFGF, and IL-8 and tumor neovascularization. In fact, combination therapy showed higher inhibition of proangiogenic factors compared with radiation or Ad-mda7 treatment alone. These studies demonstrated that intracellularly expressed MDA-7 (Ad-mda7), albeit at supraphysiological levels, can inhibit tumor vascularization indirectly by down-regulating proangiogenic growth factor expression.

Based on our results it is clear that both extracellular and intracellular MDA-7 protein can inhibit angiogenesis. Thus we speculate that the antiangiogenic activity observed in vivo is the result of interplay of the direct and indirect antiangiogenic effects mediated by the intracellular and secreted form of the MDA-7/IL-24 protein. We are currently examining the expression of these proangiogenic (VEGF, IL-8, bFGF, CD31) markers in Ad-mda7 treated tumor specimens obtained from the recently concluded phase I clinical trial *(31,32)*.

4.3. Mechanism of MDA-7/IL-24-Mediated Antiangiogenic Activity

Recent studies have reported the identification of two heterodimeric receptors (IL-20R and IL-22R) for MDA-7/IL-24 *(72,73)*. In these studies binding of MDA-7/IL-24 to its cognate receptors and activation of STAT-3 as a measure of ligand-receptor interaction was demonstrated. Therefore, to test whether MDA-7-mediated antiangiogenic activity was receptor-mediated, activation of STAT-3 as a measure of receptor-ligand interaction and receptor blocking studies was performed. Prior to conducting these studies we determined the receptor expression for MDA-7/IL-24 in HUVEC. Reverse-transcription polymerase chain reaction (RT-PCR) and western blotting analysis showed expression of both IL-20R and IL-22R in HUVEC. Subsequent studies showed transient activation of STAT-3 in MDA-7 treated endothelial cells indicating receptor-ligand interaction *(61)*. However, in the presence of anti-IL-22R1 antibody, one of the two receptors for MDA-7/IL-24, MDA-7/IL-24-mediated inhibitory activity of ECD was abrogated that correlated with the loss of STAT-3 activation. These results demonstrated that MDA-7/IL24 exerts its antiangiogenic activity via the IL-22 receptor. Furthermore, the IL22R1 blocking antibody inhibited the antiangiogenic activity of mda-7 but not that of endostatin or IP-10, demonstrating its specificity *(61)*. Although we have demonstrated IL-22R-mediated antiangiogenic activity, the role of IL-20 receptor in MDA-7/IL-24-mediated antiangiogenic activity is yet to be elucidated. Furthermore, the role of STAT-3 activation other than receptor signaling in MDA-7/IL-24 mediated antiangiogenic activity remains unclear. Additionally, the downstream signaling mechanisms mediated by MDA-7/IL-24 in endothelial cells have not been studied. One possibility is the activation of STAT-1, a molecule that is associated with antiangiogenic phenotype *(75)*. Another possibility is the inhibition of the PI3K/AKT pathway that is associated with proangiogenic phenotype. In support of this is the recent demonstration of PI3K/AKT inhibition in lung and breast cancer cells ectopically expressing MDA-7/IL-24 *(21,72)*.

Although MDA-7 protein has demonstrated antiangiogenic activity in preclinical models, the idea to develop MDA-7 protein for cancer therapy is challenging and has to overcome some of the limitations that currently exist both in the fields of protein therapy and antiangiogenic therapy. For example, in order to develop MDA-7 for protein therapy it is important to know the biophysical and biochemical properties (i.e., stability, structure, glycosylation, half-life) of the protein. Similarly, lessons learned from the failures of previous antiangiogenic therapies suggest that an understanding of the mechanism of angiogenesis regulation is important. Additionally, the optimal strategies for the use, monitoring, and validation of antiangiogenic agents in the clinic remain unclear. Another potential limitation with antiangiogenic proteins is the high dose and prolonged treatment course that are required. Although recent works suggest that the delivery of antiangiogenic agents via continuous infusion or sustained release may allow for a reduction of the bolus dose, the amount of protein needed for widespread use will still be challenging *(75,76)*. Given these limitations, treatment of cancer using gene therapy vectors (adenovirus and non-viral vectors) is a promising approach and can overcome some of the obstacles described above.

The feasibility for systemic gene therapy using a nonviral (liposome) vector was tested in an experimental lung metastasis model. Treatment of lung-tumor bearing mice with mda-7/IL-24 plasmid DNA encapsulated in a cationic DOTAP: cholesterol (DOTAP:Chol) liposome resulted in significant inhibition of experimental metastasis *(77)*. Associated with the inhibition was a marked reduction in tumor angiogenesis. These results though preliminary indicate the feasibility of systemic gene therapeutic approach for treatment of cancer. Additional studies dissecting the antitumor versus antiangiogenic activities of mda-7 after systemic therapy are under investigation.

5. ANTIMETASTATIC ACTIVITY OF *MDA-7/IL-24*

Huang et al. showed that *mda-7* mRNA was stably expressed in the thymus spleen and peripheral blood leukocytes, and reported its *de novo* expression in human melanocytes, and *mda-7* induction in human hematopoietic cells after treatment with TPA. As mentioned above, *mda-7* was initially inversely correlated with melanoma progression *(10,22)*; which is consistent with our results demonstrating that MDA-7 protein expression localizes to superficial areas of primary cutaneous melanoma and decreases as one moves toward the deeper, more invasive, areas of the tumor *(6,7)*. Taken together, these results strongly suggest that MDA-7 expression is lost during melanoma progression and invasion. MDA-7 has reportedly high levels of expression in melanocytes, and in early stage melanomas. Immunohistochemical (IHC) analysis done by our group on a group of paired metastatic and primary melanomas from patients confirms MDA-7 expression at variable levels, in approx 70% of primary tumors. MDA-7 expression significantly decreased in both percent of positive cells and intensity of expression at the deep invasive front of the tumor as compared with its corresponding superficial areas *(6,7)*. The loss of MDA-7 expression in tumors indicates that this differentiation factor may act as a tumor suppressor, which would be consistent with its reported tumor-specific growth inhibitory, and antiangiogenic properties.

Studies to investigate the antimetastatic properties of MDA-7/IL-24 were based on the recent report by Ellerhorst et al. *(7)* who demonstrated a significant correlation between loss of MDA-7 protein expression and melanoma tumor invasion. In this study, the authors demonstrated the superficial layer of the tumor expressed MDA-7 and the MDA-7 protein expression was lost as the tumor invaded the surrounding tissue. The results from this study suggested that restoration of MDA-7 expression in tumor cells should inhibit tumor invasion and metastasis. Therefore we examined the effect of ectopic MDA-7 expression on migration and invasion of lung tumor cells in vitro and in vivo.

In vitro, MDA-7 expression resulted in significant inhibition of migration (*see* Fig. 7B) and invasion of tumor cells plated on Matrigel coated wells *(21,71)*. This inhibitory effect was independent of the previously established cytotoxic effects of MDA-7 on tumor cells and occurred by down regulating p85 PI3K, pFAK, MMP-2, and MMP-9 expression *(71)*. A role for these signaling molecules and proteolytic enzymes in tumor metastasis and angiogenesis has previously been reported *(62)*. For example, involvement of MMPs in invasion and angiogenesis in lung cancer has been demonstrated by the expression of MMP-2, -9 in several lung cancer cell lines and surgical specimens, their localization to the tumor neovasculature, and a correlation between MMP expression and prognosis. Inhibition of tumor metastasis by MDA-7/IL-24 was also demonstrated in vivo *(71,77)*. Intravenous injection of lung tumor cells treated with Ad-mda7 ex vivo into nude mice resulted in reduced number of lung tumor metastasis compared with mice injected with tumor cells treated with Ad-luc. Additionally, treatment of lung tumor bearing mice with DOTAP:Chol-mda-7 complex inhibited tumor metastasis as demonstrated by the reduced number of tumors in the lung compared with lungs from mice that were treated with PBS or DOTAP:Chol-luc (vector control) complex *(77)*. These results validate the antimetastatic activity of MDA-7/IL-24 and the underlying mechanism both in vitro and in vivo.

6. CONCLUSIONS

The preclinical data reviewed here clearly demonstrate the tumor-selective and potent proapoptotic, antiangiogenic, and antimetastatic activities of mda-7/IL-24 both, in vitro and in vivo. These effects of mda-7/IL-24, are induced by direct, indirect (bystander), and immune activation mechanisms, and appear to be independent of the status of other tumor suppressor pathways; offering a viable option for the treatment of cancers that resist current therapies. Taken together, the above findings demonstrate unique properties of mda-7/IL-24 make it a promising anticancer agent for the treatment of primary and disseminated cancers.

ACKNOWLEDGMENTS

The authors thank all the members of their respective laboratories and our collaborators who have contributed to this research. This work was supported by NCI grants CA89778, CA88421, and CA097598 (SC), 1RO1-CA102716, Texas Higher Education Coordinating Board ATP/ARP grant 003657-0078-2001, by an institutional research grant from The University of Texas MD Anderson Cancer Center, by WM Keck Gene Therapy Grant, by M.D. Anderson Cancer Center Support Grant CA16672, and a sponsored research agreement with Introgen Therapeutics, Inc. (RR).

REFERENCES

1. Jiang H, Lin JJ, Su Z-Z, et al. Subtraction hybridization identifies a novel melanoma differentiation associated gene, mda-7, modulated during human melanoma differentiation, growth and progression. Oncogene 1995;11:2477–2486.
2. Jiang H, Fisher PB. Use of a sensitive and efficient substraction hybridization protocol for the identification of genes differentially regulated during the induction of differentiation in human melanoma cells. Mol Cell Differ 1993;1:285–299.
3. Huang F, Adelman J, Jiang H, et al. Differentiation induction substraction hybridization (DISH): a strategy for cloning genes displaying differential expression during growth arrest and terminal differentiation. Gene 1999;236:125–131.
4. Huang EY, Madireddi MT, Gopalkrishnan RV, et al. Genomic structure, chromosomal localization and expression profile of a novel melanoma differentiation associated (mda-7) gene with cancer specific growth suppressing and apoptosis inducing properties. Oncogene 2001;20(48):7051-63.
5. Levedeva IV, Su ZZ, Chang Y, et al. The cancer growth suppressing gene mda-7 induces apoptosis selectively in human melanoma cells. Oncogene. 2002;21(5):708–718.
6. Ekmekcioglu S, Ellerhorst J, Mhashilkar AM, et al. Down-regulated melanoma differentiation associated gene (mda-7) expression in human melanomas. Int J Cancer 2001;94(1):54–59.
7. Ellerhorst JA, Prieto VG, Ekmekciouglu S, et al. Loss of MDA-7 expression with progression of melanoma. J Clin Oncol 2002;20(4):1069–1074.
8. Soo C, Shaw WW, Freymiller E, et al. Cutaneous rat wounds express c49a, a novel gene with homology to the human melanoma differentiation associated gene, mda-7. J Cell Biochem. 1999;74(1):1–10.
9. Mhashilkar AB, Schrock RD, Hindi M, et al. Melanoma differentiation associated gene-7 (mda-7): a novel anti-tumor gene for cancer gene therapy. Mol Med 2001;(4):271–282.
10. Jiang H, Su ZZ, Lin JJ, et al. The melanoma differentiation associated gene mda-7 suppresses cancer cell growth. Proc Natl Acad Sci U S A 1996;93(17):9160–9165.
11. Zhang R, Tan Z, Liang P. Identification of a novel ligand-receptor pair constitutively activated by ras oncogenes. J Biol Chem 2000;275(32):24,436–24,443.
12. Schaefer G, Venkataraman C, Schindler U. Cutting edge: FISP (IL-4-induced secreted protein), a novel cytokine-like molecule secreted by Th2 cells. J Immunol 2001;166(10):5859–5863.
13. Blumberg H, Conklin D, Xu WF, et al. Interleukin 20: discovery, receptor identification, and role in epidermal function. Cell 2001;104(1):9–19.
14. Chada S, Mhashilkar AM, Ramesh R, et al. Bystander activity of Ad-mda7: Human MDA-7 protein kills melanoma cells via and IL-20 receptor-dependent but STAT3-independent mechanism. Mol Ther 2004;10(6):1085–1095.
15. Chada S, Sutton RB, Ekmekcioglu S, et al. MDA-7/IL-24 is a unique cytokine-tumor suppressor in the IL-10 family. *Review*. Int Immunopharm 2004;4:649–667.
16. Caudell EG, Mumm JB, Poindexter N, et al. The protein product of the tumor suppressor gene, melanoma differentiation-associated gene 7, exhibits immunostimulatory activity and is designated IL-24. J Immunol 2002;168:6041–6046.

17. Dumoutier L, Leemans C, Lejeune D, et al. Cutting edge: STAT activation by IL-19, IL-20 and mda-7 through IL-20 receptor complexes of two types. J Immunol 2001;167:3545–3549.
18. Wang M, Tan Z, Zhang R, et al. Interleukin 24 (MDA-7/MOB-5) signals through two heterodimeric receptors, IL-22R1/IL-20R2 and IL-20R1/IL-20R2. J Biol Chem 2002;277:7341–7347.
19. Sieger KA, Mhashilkar AM, Stewart A, et al. The tumor suppressor activity of MDA-7/IL-24 is mediated by intracellular protein expression in NSCLC cells. Mol Ther 2004;9(3):355–367.
20. Allen M, Pratscher B, Roka F, et al. Loss of Novel mda-7 splice variant (mda-7s) Expression is Associated with metastatic melanoma. J Invest Dermatol 2004;123:583–588.
21. Mhashilkar AM, Stewart AL, Sieger K, et al. MDA-7 negatively regulates the β-catenin and PI3K signaling pathways in breast and lung tumor cells. Mol Ther 2003;8:207–219.
22. Madireddi MT, Dent P, Fisher PB. Regulation of mda-7 gene expression during human melanoma differentiation. Oncogene 2000a;19(10):1362–1368.
23. Saeki T, Mhashilkar A, Chada S, et al. Tumor-suppressive effects by adenovirus-mediated mda-7 gene transfer in non-small cell lung cancer cell in vitro. Gene Ther 2000;7(23):2051–2057.
24. Su ZZ, Madireddi MT, Lin JJ, et al. The cancer growth suppressor gene *mda-7* selectively induces apoptosis in human breast cancer cells and inhibits tumor growth in nude mice. Proc Natl Acad Sci U S A 1998;95:14,400–14,405.
25. Su ZZ, Lebedeva IV, Sarkar D, et al. Melanoma differentiation associated gene-7, mda-7/IL-24, selectively induces growth suppression, apoptosis and radiosensitization in malignant gliomas in a p53-independent manner. Oncogene 2003;22(8):1164–1180.
26. Sarkar D, Su ZZ, Lebedeva IV, et al. *mda-7* (IL-24) Mediates selective apoptosis in human melanoma cells by inducing the coordinated overexpression of the GADD family of genes by means of p38 MAPK. Proc Natl Acad Sci U S A 2002 (*Epub 2002 Jul 11*);99(15):10,054–10,059.
27. Lebedeva IV, Su ZZ, Sarkar D, et al. Melanoma differentiation associated gene-7, mda-7/interleukin-24, induces apoptosis in prostate cancer cells by promoting mitochondrial dysfunction and inducing reactive oxygen species. Cancer Res 2003;63(23):8138–8144.
28. Pataer A, Chada S, Hunt KK, et al. Adenoviral melanoma differentiation-associated gene 7 induces apoptosis in lung cancer cells through mitochondrial permeability transition-independent cytochrome c release. J Thorac Cardiovasc Surg 2003;125(6):1328–1335.
29. Pataer A, Vorburger SA, Barber GN, et al. Adenoviral transfer of the melanoma differentiation-associated gene 7 (*mda7*) induces apoptosis of lung cancer cells via up-regulation of the double-stranded RNA-dependent protein kinase (PKR).Cancer Res 2002;62(8):2239–2243.
30. Johnston SRD, MacLennan KA, Sacks NPM, et al. Modulation of Bcl-2 and Ki-67 expression in oestrogen receptor-positive human breast cancer by tamoxifen. Eur J of Cancer 1994;30A: 1663–1669.
31. Zapata JM, Krajewski S, Huang RP, et al. Expression of multiple apoptosis-regulatory genes in human breast cancer cell lines nad primary tumors. Breast Cancer Res. & Treatment 1998;47:129–140.
32. Oltvai Z, Milliman C, Korsmeyer S. Bcl-2 heterodimerizes *in vivo* with a conserved homolog, Bax, that accelerates programmed cell death. Cell 1993;74:609–619.
33. Zha H, Aime-Sempe C, Sato T, Reed JC. Pro-apoptotic protein Bax heterodimerizes with Bcl-2 and homodimerizes with Bax via a novel domain (BH3) distinct from BH1 and BH2. J Biol Chem 1996;271:7440–7444.
34. Zou H, Henzel WJ, Liu X, et al. Apaf-1, a human protein homologous to *C. elegans* CED-4, participates in cytochrome c-dependent activation of caspase-3. Cell 1997;90:405–413.
35. Hakem R, Hakem A, Duncan GS, et al. Differential requirement for caspase 9 in apoptotic pathways *in vivo*. Cell 1998;94:339–352.
36. Wolter KG, Hsu YT, Smith CL, et al. Movement of BAX from the cytosol to mitochondria during apoptosis. J Cell Biol 1997;139:1281–1292.
37. Reed JC. Double identity for proteins of the Bcl-2 family. Nature 1997;387:773–776.
38. Saeki T, Mhashilkar A, Swanson X, et al. Inhibition of human lung cancer growth following adenovirus-mediated mda-7 gene expression in vivo. Oncogene 2002;21(29):4558–4566.
39. McKenzie T, Liu Y, Fanale M, et al. Combination therapy of Ad-mda7 and trastuzumab increases cell death in Her-2/neu-overexpressing breast cancer cells. Surgery 2004;136(2):437–442.
40. Fisher PB, Gopalkrishnan RV, Chada S, et al. mda-7/IL-24, a novel cancer selective apoptosis inducing cytokine gene: from the laboratory into the clinic. Cancer Biol Ther 2003;2(4 Suppl 1):S23–S37.
41. Gopalan B, Litvak A, Sharma S, Mhashilkar AM, Chada S, Ramesh R. Activation of the Fas-FasL signaling pathway by MDA-7/IL-24 kills human ovarian cancer cells. Cancer Res 2005;65(8):3017–3024.

42. Van Noort M, Meeldijk J, Van der Zee R, et al. Wnt signaling controls the phosphorylation status of beta-catenin. J Biol Chem 2002:277(20):17,901–17,905.
43. Abraham SC, Wu TT, Klimstra DS, et al. Distinctive molecular genetic alterations in sporadic and familial adenomatous Polyposis-associated pancreatoblastomas: frequent alterations in the APC/beta-catenin pathway and chromosome 11p. Am J Pathol 2001;159(5):1619–1627.
44. Abraham SC, Klimstra DS, Wilentz RE, et al. Solid-pseudopapillary tumors of the pancreas are genetically distinct from pancreatic ductal adenocarcinomas and almost always harbor beta-catenin mutations. Am J Pathol 2002a;160(4):1361–1369.
45. Abraham SC, Wu TT, Hruban RH, et al. Genetic and immunohistochemical analysis of pancreatic acinar cell carcinoma: frequent allelic loss on chromosome 11p and alterations in the APC/beta-catenin pathway. Am J Pathol 2002b;160(3):953–962.
46. Li YJ, Ji XR. Relationship between expression of E-cadherin-catenin complex and clinicopathologic characteristics of pancreatic cancer. World J Gastroenterol 2003;9(2):368–372.
47. Wulff C, Weigand M, Kreienberg R, et al. Angiogenesis during primate placentation in health and disease. Reproduction 2003;126(5):569–577.
48. Folkman J. The role of angiogenesis in tumor growth. Sem. Cancer Biol 1992; 267:10,931–10,934.
49. Folkman J. Angiogenesis in cancer, vascular, rheumatoid and other diseases. Nat Med 1995.1:21–37.
50. Fidler IJ Ellis LM. The implications of angiogenesis for the biology ad therapy of cancer metastasis. Cell 1994;79:185–188.
51. Cristofanilli M, Charnsangavej C, Hortobagyi GN. Angiogenesis modulation in cancer research: Novel clinical apporoaches. Nat Rev 2002;1:415–426.
52. O'Reilly MS, Holmgren L, Shing Y, et al. Angiostatin: a novel angiogenesis inhibitor that mediates the suppression of metastases by a lewis lung carcinoma. Cell 1994;79:315–328.
53. O'Reilly MS, Boehm T, Shing Y, et al. Endostatin: an endogeneous inhibitor of angiogenesis and tumor growth. Cell 1997;8:277–285.
54. Shaheen RM, Davis DW, Liu W, et al. Antiangiogenic therapy targeting the tyrosinase kinase receptor for vascular endothelial growth factor receptor inhibits the growth of colon cancer liver metastasis and induces tumor and endothelial cell apoptosis. Cancer Res 1999;59:5412–5416.
55. Laird AD, Vajkoczy P, Shawver LK, et al. SU6668 is a potent antiangiogenic and antitumor agent that induces regression of established tumors. Cancer Res 2000;60:4152–4160.
56. Moses MA, Sudhalter J, Langer R. Identification of an inhibitor of neovascularization from cartilage. Science 1990;248:1408–1410.
57. Kumar CC, Malkowski M, Yin Z, et al. Inhibition of angiogenesis and tumor growth by SCH221153, a dual $\alpha_v\beta_3$ and $\alpha_v\beta_5$ integrin receptor antagonist. Cancer Res 2001;61:2232–2238.
58. Lingen MW, Polverini PJ, Bouck NP. Inhibition of squamous cell carcinoma angiogenesis by direct interaction of retinoic acid with endothelial cells. Lab Invest 1996;74:476–483.
59. Voest EE, Kenyon BM, O' Reilly MS, Truitt G, D'Amato RJ, Folkman J. Inhibition of angiogenesis in vivo by interleukin 12. J Natl Cancer Inst 1995;87:581–586.
60. Singh RK, Gutman M, Bucana CD, Sanchez R, Llansa N, Fidler IJ. Interferons alpha and beta down-regulate the expression of basic fibroblast growth factor in human carcinomas. Proc. Natl. Acad. Sci. U S A 1995;92:4562–4555.
61. Ramesh R, Mhashilkar AM, Tanaka F, et al. Melanoma differentiation-associated Gene 7/Interleukin (IL)-24 is a novel ligand that regulates angiogenesis via the IL-22 receptor. Cancer Res 2003;63: 5105–5113.
62. Stearns ME, Wang M. Antimestatic and antitumor activities of interleukin 10 in transfected human prostate PC-3 ML clones: Orthotopic growth in severe combined immunodeficient mice. Clin Cancer Res1998;4:2257–2263.
63. Huang S, Ullrich SE, Bar-Eli M. Regulation of tumor growth and metastasis by interleukin-10: the melanoma experience. J Interfer Cyto Res 1999;19:697–703.
64. Yamaguchi N, Anand-Apte B, Lee M, et al. Endostatin inhibits VEGF-induced endothelial cell migration and tumor growth independently of zinc binding. EMBO J 1999;18:4414–4423.
65. Zhang M, Volpert O, Shi YH, Bouck N. Maspin is an angiogenesis inhibitior. Nat Med 2000;6: 196–199.
66. Maheshwari RK, Srikantan V, Bhartiya D, Kleinman HK, Grant DS. Differential effects of interferon gamma and alpha on in vitro model of angiogenesis. J Cell Physiol 1991;146:164–169.
67. Tedjarati S, Baker CH, Apte S, et al. Synergistic therapy of human ovarian carcinoma implanted orthotopically in nude mice by optimal biological dose of pegylated interferon alpha combined with paclitaxel. Clin Cancer Res 2002;8:2413–2422.

68. Nishikawa T, Ramesh R, Chada S, Meyn RE. Suppression of tumor growth and angiogenesis by adenovirus-mediated mda-7/IL-24 gene transfer in combination with ionizing radiation. Mol Ther 2004;9(6):818–828.
69. Inoue K, Chikazawa M, Fukata S, Yoshikawa C, Shuin T. Frequent administration of angiogenesis inhibitor TNP-470 (AGM-1470) at an optimal biological dose inhibits tumor growth and metastasis of metastatic human transitional cell carcinoma in the urinary bladder. Clin Cancer Res 2002;8:2389–2398.
70. Hirata A, Ogawa S, Kometani T, et al. ZD1839 (Iressa) induces antiangiogenic effects through inhibition of epidermal growth factor receptor tyrosine kinase. Cancer Res 2002;62:2554–2560.
71. Ramesh R, Ito I, Gopalan B, Saito Y, Mhashilkar AM, Chada S. Ectopic production of MDA-7/IL-24 inhibits invasion and migration of human lung cancer cells. Mol Ther 2004;5:510–518.
72. Wang M, Tan Z, Zhang R, et al. Interleukin 24 (MDA-7/MOB-5) signals through two heterodimeric receptors, IL-22R1/IL-20R2 and IL-20R1/IL-20R2. J Biol Chem 2002;277:7341–7347.
73. Dumoutier L, Leemans C, Lejeune D, Kotenko SV, Renauld JC. Cutting edge: STAT activation by IL-19, IL-20 and mda-7 through IL-20 receptor complexes of two types. J Immunol 2001;167:3545–3549.
74. Hu H, Jove R. The STATs of cancer-new molecular targets come of age. Nat Rev Cancer 2004;4:97–105.
75. O'Reilly MS, Boehm T, Shing Y, et al. Endostatin: an endogenous inhibitor of angiogenesis and tumor growth. Cell 1997;8:277–285.
76. Drixlerm TA, Rinkes IH, Ritchie ED, et al. Continuous administration of angiostatin inhibits accelerated growth of colorectal liver metastasis after partial hepatectomy. Cancer Res 2000;60:1761–1765.
77. Ramesh R, et al. Local and Systemic Inhibition of Lung Tumor Growth After Liposome Mediated *mda-7/IL-24* Gene Delivery. DNA and Cell Biology 2004;23(12):850–857.

24 Development of Therapeutic Genes for Breast Cancer Treatment

Mien-Chie Hung, PhD
and Duen-Hwa Yan, PhD

CONTENTS

Summary

This chapter describes preclinical development of therapeutic genes in breast cancer treatment. Beginning from targeting HER-2/neu-overexpressing breast cancer cells by adenovirus E1A, we found E1A expression had profound effects on tumor cells including growth suppression, apoptosis, and sensitization to chemo-drugs and radiation. The mechanisms of the antitumor activities as well as the preliminary results obtained from multiple *E1A* clinical trials are discussed. Also identified are the antitumor activity of interferon inducible genes, *p202* and *IFIX*, and a proapoptotic gene, *bik*. The mechanism of action and the therapeutic potential of these genes in breast cancer models are also discussed.

Key Words: Gene therapy; E1A; p202; IFIX; Bik.

1. INTRODUCTION

It is estimated 216,000 new cases of breast cancer will be diagnosed and 40,000 deaths will be caused by the disease in the United States in 2004 (American Cancer Society statistics). Although conventional treatments on primary tumors by surgery, radiotherapy, and adjuvant/neoadjuvant chemotherapy have improved survival rates, the overall relapse rate remains high (10–40%) *(1)*. Therefore, novel treatment modalities are urgently needed for breast cancer. Given that cancer can be considered a genetic disease caused by the activation of cancer-promoting genes (oncogene) or the inactivation of cancer-suppressing genes (antioncogene), it is therefore possible to design strategies to compensate for these mutations in tumors by inhibiting the dominant oncogene function or by restoring the antioncogene function. This chapter discusses our experience in developing the adenovirus *E1A* (*E1A*) as a therapeutic gene that can inhibit a dominant breast cancer oncogene, *HER-2*. We will also describe the preclinical studies

From: *Cancer Drug Discovery and Development: Gene Therapy for Cancer*
Edited by: K. K. Hunt, S. A. Vorburger, and S. G. Swisher © Humana Press Inc., Totowa, NJ

on the development of HIN-200 (e.g., *p202* and *IFIX*) and *bik* as potential therapeutic genes in preclinical breast cancer treatment.

2. E1A

2.1. Tumor Suppressor Activity of E1A

E1A is the first transcriptional unit to be activated after the adenoviral genome reaches the nucleus. *E1A* encodes two major alternatively spliced proteins of 243 and 289 amino acids. Both proteins can activate or repress transcription of several viral and cellular genes *(2)* resulting in cell-cycle deregulation and virus replication. E1A accomplishes this by interacting with and modulating a host of cell-cycle regulatory proteins *(3)*. *E1A* was initially characterized as an oncogene by virtue of its ability to promote growth and immortalization of quiescent rodent cells *(4)* and to cooperate with *ras* oncogene to transform primary rodent cells *(5)*.

However, *E1A* was found to suppress experimental metastasis of rodent cells transformed by the *ras* oncogene *(6–8)*. We demonstrated that E1A could repress the promoter of rat *neu* oncogene *(9)* leading to both reversion of the *neu*-induced transformation and tumorigenicity *(10)* and experimental metastasis *(11,12)*. *E1A* was also shown to suppress human *HER-2* expression *(13)*, experimental metastasis *(14)*, and tumorigenicity *(15)* of certain human tumor cell lines. Together, these data strongly suggest that E1A can also function as a tumor suppressor.

2.2. Mechanisms of E1A-Mediated Tumor Suppressor Activity

The multifunctional E1A in tumor suppression is illustrated by its ability to sensitize tumor cells to chemotherapy and γ-irradiation, induce a bystander effect, suppress tumor growth, metastasis, and angiogenesis *(16)*. It is therefore not surprising that E1A targets multiple signal pathways to achieve these antitumor activities. Consistent with the antimetastasis activity, E1A activates metastasis-suppressor genes such as E-cadherins, NM23, TIMPs, and/or represses metastasis-promoting genes such as *HER-2*, *MMPs*, *uPA*, and *CD44s (16)*. E1A-induced growth inhibition has been linked to the upregulation of cell-cycle regulators such as the cyclin-dependent kinase inhibitor, *p21CIP1*, and the *p53* tumor suppressor gene *(17,18)*. In addition, the Axl tyrosine kinase receptor also plays a role in the E1A-mediated growth inhibition *(19)*. In particular, E1A represses the transcription of *Axl* gene and reduces cell growth-mediated by Axl and its ligand, Gas6 *(19)*. More importantly, E1A can target different signal pathways to sensitize tumor cells to apoptosis. For instance, E1A inactivates IKK resulting in NF-κB inactivation. Since NF-κB is an antiapoptotic molecule *(20–23)*, the inactivation of NF-κB by E1A renders the cells sensitive to apoptosis induced by tumor necrosis factor (TNF)-α or γ-irradiation *(24–26)*. More recently, we provided evidence to suggest that E1A targets a novel signaling pathway, the protein phosphatase 2A (PP2A)/AKT/p38 pathway, to sensitize tumor cells to chemotherapeutic drugs *(27,28)* (*see* Section 2.4.).

2.3. Tumor Suppressor Activity of E1A in Breast Cancer Experimental Models

The initial link between E1A and tumor suppression in breast cancer was based on the observations that E1A could suppress the transformation phenotype of the *neu*-transformed NIH mouse 3T3 cells *(10–12)* by transcriptionally repressing the promoter of rat *neu* oncogene *(9)*. *HER-2* is amplified and overexpressed in approximately 30% human breast cancer patients with poor prognosis *(29–31)*. Because the *neu* gene is a murine counterpart of the human HER-2 proto-oncogene, it was hypothesized that E1A could also repress HER-2 expression in human breast cancer. Indeed, both HER-2 protein and mRNA levels were reduced in HER-2-overexpressing breast cancer cell lines infected with an E1A-expressing adenovirus (Ad.E1A(+)) but not a mutant adenovirus (Ad.E1A(–)) in which E1A is deleted *(13)*.

To test whether the E1A-mediated HER-2 repression affects the cell growth in cell model systems, both the high-HER-2 (e.g., MDA-MB-361 and SKBR3) and the low-HER-2-expressing (e.g., MDA-MB-435 and MDA-MB-231) breast cancer cell lines were infected with either Ad.*E1A*(+) or Ad.*E1A*(–) followed by a growth assay. We showed that Ad.*E1A*(+), but not Ad.*E1A*(–), could specifically inhibit the growth of the high-HER-2 breast cancer cells as compared with those with the low-HER-2 expression *(32)*.

To demonstrate the efficacy of *E1A* in preclinical gene therapy settings, both Ad.*E1A*(+) and an E1A expression vector/liposome (3β-[*N*-(*N′*, *N′*dimethylaminoethyl) carbamoryl cholesterol [DCC]) complex (E1A/DCC) were used to assess the potential efficacy in an orthotopic, HER-2-overexpressing breast cancer model. MDA-MB-361 cells were transplanted into the mammary fat pads of female nu/nu mice. The mammary tumors become palpable usually about 45 d after implantation. Ad.*E1A*(+) or *E1A*/DCC was administered via intratumoral injection. Six months of *E1A* treatment (Ad.*E1A*(+) or *E1A*/DCC) resulted in suppression of tumor growth and prolonged survival (the mean survival was greater than 2 yr as opposed to less than 15 mo in the control groups). The Ad.*E1A*(+) treatment appeared slightly better than *E1A*/DCC treatment. Remarkably, no metastasis was found in intraperitoneal organs such as liver, intestine, spleen, and kidney *(32)*. These results suggested that E1A possesses antimetastasis activity, which is reminiscent of a previous finding that showed no detectable metastasis in the *E1A*-treated mice bearing HER-2-overexpressing ovarian tumors *(33)*. The suppression of mammary tumor by E1A correlated well with the expression of E1A and the reduced expression of HER-2 in these tumors *(32)*. Thus, these data suggest the feasibility of an *E1A*-based gene therapy against HER-2-overexpressing breast cancer in vivo. Importantly, the subsequent toxicity studies conducted in immuno-competent mice showed only minimum side effect associated with the *E1A* gene therapy *(34–36)*.

2.4. Chemosensitization of E1A

Previous studies have shown that E1A can sensitize both mouse embryo fibroblasts and human cancer cell lines to apoptosis induced by different anticancer agents *(37–39)*. Our rationale to study E1A-mediated chemosensitization was initially based on the hypothesis that E1A can sensitize cancer cells to anticancer agents by repressing HER-2 overexpression, which is a chemoresistance phenotype of breast cancer cells *(40–43)*. Combined treatment of Ad.*E1A*(+) infection and paclitaxel resulted in a synergistic suppression of growth and transformation phenotype of a high HER-2, paclitaxel-resistant MDA-MB-453 cell line *(44)*. Similarly, we showed an enhanced antitumor activity by a combined *E1A* and paclitaxel treatment in orthotopic breast cancer models derived from a high HER-2, MDA-MB-361 cell line *(45)*. Interestingly, E1A can also sensitize the low HER-2-expressing breast cancer cells (e.g., MDA-MB-231) to paclitaxel (10 n*M*)-induced killing *(46)*. This result indicates that a clinically relevant concentration (5~200 n*M*) of paclitaxel is able to synergize with *E1A* in cell killing. Although our earlier report indicated that E1A has minimum effect on paclitaxel sensitization in MDA-MB-435 cells, in light of our recent findings *(46)*, the synergistic effect by E1A is likely obscured by the high paclitaxel concentration (1 μ*M*) used in the study *(44)*. Together, these studies suggest that multiple mechanisms may be involved in the E1A-mediated sensitization by anticancer drugs. As such, *E1A*/anticancer drugs combined treatments may have a broad application in cancer therapy.

In the above studies, either a cationic lipid-protamine-DNA (LPD) (LPD-*E1A*) *(45)* or a SN cationic liposome *(47,48)* (SN-*E1A*) *(46)* was used as an *E1A* gene delivery system. These liposome formulations offer advantages that include the stability in serum and the high gene-transducing efficiency via intravenous (iv) administration *(47–50)*. These features are especially attractive because the treatment of metastatic breast cancer can only be effective by systemic administration of antitumor agents. Whereas injection of LPD-*E1A* (iv once/wk) and paclitaxel (intraperitoneal [ip] once every 3 wk) yielded additive efficacy as compared with LPD-*E1A* or paclitaxel treatment alone *(45)*, SN-*E1A*/paclitaxel combined treatment had a synergistic effect on tumor suppression and significantly prolonged survival *(46)*. As expected, E1A expression, reduced HER-2, and an increase of apoptotic cells were seen in the *E1A*-treated MDA-MB-361 tumor samples as determined by immunohistochemical assays *(45)*. These in vivo observations provided an important step forward to designing clinical trials using combinations of *E1A* and chemotherapeutic drugs for treating metastatic breast cancers.

2.5. Mechanisms of E1A-Mediated Chemosensitization

p53 was initially shown to be involved in E1A-mediated sensitization to anticancer drugs in mouse embryonic fibroblasts *(38,39)*. However, mounting evidence has indicated that E1A can also achieve such sensitization in human cancer cells that do not express wild type p53 *(25,27,28,37,44,46,51,52)*. Until recently, the mechanism underlying the E1A-mediated chemosensitization in cancer cells had been elusive. However, several findings uncovered a novel pathway by which E1A induces chemosensitization. We showed that E1A expression is associated with an increase of PP2A *(27)*, an enzyme that dephosphorylates and inactivates a key survival molecule, AKT *(53)*. The inactivation of AKT in E1A-expressing cells leads to activation of ASK1 and MEKK3 kinases, which, in turn, phosphorylate and activate a proapoptotic protein, p38 *(27,28)*. Importantly, the activation of p38 correlates with the E1A-mediated sensitization to apoptosis induced by commonly used anticancer drugs such as paclitaxel, adriamycin, cisplain, gemcitabine, and methotrexate. Specifically, treatment of E1A-expressing cells with p38 inhibitor or dominant negative p38 impaired the sensitization to paclitaxel-induced apoptosis *(28)*. These observations strongly suggest that E1A induces chemosensitization through the PP2A/AKT/(ASK, MEKK3)/p38 pathway.

2.6. E1A Clinical Trials

In 1995, the MD Anderson Cancer Center proposed to FDA and RAC of NIH a phase I clinical trial of *E1A* treatment targeting patients with advanced breast or ovarian cancer. At that time, our proposal represented the only gene therapy data that had a clear mechanism for antitumor activity. Four clinical trials using E1A gene therapy have been reported *(54–57)*. Currently, a phase I/II combined paclitaxel and E1A gene therapy for ovarian cancer is in progress at MD Anderson Cancer Center. Dr. Ueno will describe the details about the multiple clinical trials in a separate chapter.

3. HIN-200 GENES

The interferon (IFN)-inducible HIN-200 gene family encode a class of proteins that share a 200-amino acid signature motif of type *a* and/or type *b*. Previously, three human (*IFI16*, *MNDA*, and *AIM2*) and five mouse (*p202a*, *p202b*, *p203*, *p204*, and *p205* (or D3)) HIN-200 family proteins were identified *(58–60)*. HIN-200 genes are located at chromosome 1q21-23 as a gene cluster in mouse and human genomes *(60)*. The observations that HIN-200 proteins interact with several cellular regulators involved in cell cycle control, differentiation, and apoptosis strongly suggest the physiological roles of this family of proteins extend beyond the IFN system *(58–61)*. For example, with the availability of antibodies competent for *in situ* analysis, it is now clear IFI16 expression is not restricted to the hematopoietic compartment. IFI16 is found widely expressed in normal human tissues including endothelial and epithelial cells *(62–64)*.

3.1. p202

The antitumor activity of HIN-200 gene was first demonstrated by our study on *p202a* (*p202*). The p202 protein is encoded by one of the six or more murine IFN-inducible genes of the gene 200 cluster on chromosome 1q21-23 *(65)*. This family of proteins shares, close to their carboxyl termini, partially homologous 200 amino acid long segments. So far, p202 is the best-characterized murine member in this family *(65)*. The pathological relevance of *p202* was recently realized by the finding that *p202* is a candidate gene for systemic lupus erythematosus in a mouse model *(66)*.

p202 is primarily a nuclear, chromatin-associated 52-kD phosphoprotein involved in protein-protein interactions. Notably, several important transcriptional regulators such as retinoblastoma gene (Rb) *(67)*, E2F-1 *(68)*, E2F-4, p107 and p130 *(69)*, Fos/Jun (AP-1), a p53 binding protein (53BP-1) *(70)*, c-Myc *(71)*, NF-κB *(72–74)*, MyoD and myogenin *(75)*, are p202-interacting proteins. These observations strongly suggest a functional significance of p202 in cell cycle regulation, signal transduction, apoptosis, and differentiation. The p202 associated protein-protein interactions generally result in inhibition of transcription *(68,69,71,73–76)*. In most cases, a direct blocking of the transcriptional factor binding to its cognate DNA element by p202 is responsible for the transcription repression.

Similar to the IFN-induced growth inhibition, persistent expression of p202 was shown to be growth inhibitory in rodent cells *(68–70,73,77,78)* and in human cancer cells including breast cancer *(74,76,79,80)*. The p202-mediated growth inhibition was associated with attenuation at G1/S cell-cycle transition. It likely results from the interaction between p202 and E2F1, that in turn abrogates E2F-1-mediated transcriptional activation of certain S-phase genes such as *DHFR*, *b-Myb*, and *PCNA* resulting in attenuation of S-phase entry *(68)*. p202 also suppresses transformation as indicated by the reduced ability of p202-exprerssing breast cancer cells to grow in soft agar *(74)*. In addition, we recently showed that p202 expression also promotes apoptosis in breast cancer cells *(79)*. The p202-mediated apoptosis appears to be dependent on the activation of caspases. Based on the growth inhibitory and proapoptotic activities of p202, we subsequently performed the preclinical studies to evaluate the feasibility of using p202 as a therapeutic gene in treating experimental breast tumors.

3.2. Preclinical p202 Gene Therapy Studies

Our first attempt to test the therapeutic value of *p202* as an antitumor agent in breast cancer was conducted ex vivo. We showed that transfection of *p202*/PEI (polyethylenimine) complex into MCF-7 cells greatly inhibited tumor growth as compared with PEI alone in estrogen-supplemented nude mice *(74)*. Based on this encouraging result, we then developed a systemic delivery system that would allow delivery of *p202* gene through intravenous (iv) injection to the primary and metastasized tumor sites. To this end, we undertook two approaches and compared the efficacy of systemic p202 gene therapy treatment using either a p202-expressing recombinant adenovirus (Ad-*p202*) or CMV-*p202*/SN2 liposome complex in an orthotopic MDA-MB-468 breast cancer xenograft model. CMV-*p202* is a p202 expression vector driven by a cytomegalovirus (CMV) promoter. SN2 liposome formulation has been tested and shown to be an efficient gene delivery system in systemic gene therapy models *(47)*. The tumor growth was significantly reduced in both Ad-*p202* and CMV-*p202*/SN2 treatment groups *(79)*, (Wen and Hung, unpublished data). These results strongly suggest the feasibility of a systemic *p202*-based gene therapy treatment for breast cancer.

In addition, upon examining the tumor treated with Ad-*p202* or CMV-*p202*/SN2 by immunohistochemical assays, we found that the p202 protein levels correlates well with the extent of apoptosis in tumors in both models as determined by TUNEL (TdT [terminal deoxynucleotidyl transferase]-mediated dUTP nick end labeling) assay that stains the ends of DNA fragments. This observation is in agreement with our in vitro data that show Ad-*p202* infection induces apoptosis *(79)*. Thus, the p202-induced apoptosis contributes to the overall antitumor activities in vivo. Furthermore, we observed the levels of an angiogenic factor, vascular endothelial growth factor (VEGF), were significantly reduced in breast tumors treated with either CMV-*p202*/SN2 or Ad-*p202* as compared with that of the control treatments. This observation is also consistent to our previous finding that angiogenesis was reduced in *p202*-treated pancreatic tumors *(76)*. Together, our data strongly suggest *p202* is a potent therapeutic agent suitable for breast cancer therapy.

3.3. *IFIXα1*

Loss or reduced expression of human HIN-200 genes has been associated with several human malignancies: *IFI16* (breast cancer *[81]*), *AIM2* (melanoma, Li-Fraumeni syndrome, and colorectal cancer *[82–84]*), and *MNDA* (prostate cancer and adult myelodysplastic syndromes *[85–87]*). These observations support the hypothesis that HIN-200 genes function as putative tumor suppressors *(88)*.

We recently identified *IFIX* as a novel member of the human HIN-200 gene family. The *IFIX* transcriptional unit expresses at least six *IFIX* isoforms (α1, α2, β1, β2, γ1, and γ2) that show protein sequence homology to other human and mouse HIN-200 proteins. Importantly, we found the expression of IFIXα1, the longest IFIX isoform, is reduced in majority of breast tumors and breast cancer cell lines. These data suggest IFIXα1 may function as a tumor suppressor in breast cancer. Consistent with that notion, the IFIXα1 stable cell lines derived from MCF-7 and MDA-MB-468 exhibited reduced growth rates in both anchorage dependent and independent manner, suggesting a loss of transformation phenotype of these breast cancer cells. This observation was further substantiated by the suppressed tumorigenicity of IFIXα1 stable cell lines in nude mice. We further showed that the IFIXα1-mediated growth suppression is associated with an increase of the cyclin-dependent kinase inhibitor $p21^{CIP1}$ in a pRB- and p53 independent manner.

3.4. Preclinical *IFIXα1* Gene Therapy Study

To test the feasibility of using *IFIXα1* as an antitumor agent in breast cancer, we performed a preclinical gene therapy experiment using an orthotopic breast cancer xenograft model. Female nude mice were inoculated with MDA-MB-468 cells into the mammary fat pads (MFP). The mammary tumors were allowed to grow to 0.5 cm in diameter. Tumors were then injected with the liposome SN2 complexed with either an IFIXα1-expression vector (CMV-*IFIXα1*) or an empty vector (pCMV-Tag2B). We showed that the CMV-*IFIXα1*/SN2 treatment yielded significant antitumor activity as compared with the pCMV-Tag2B/SN2 treatment. This observation indicates that IFIXα1 possesses antitumor activity and shows a feasibility of using IFIXα1 gene therapy in breast cancer.

4. BIK

Another approach to target breast cancer is to induce programmed cell death by transducing proapoptotic genes into breast tumor cells *(90)*. The *bik* gene is a proapoptotic member of the Bcl-2 gene family *(91–93)*. It encodes an 18-kd BH3-only protein (914). It is now clear that these BH3-only proteins induce apoptosis by binding through a groove formed by the BH1 and BH2 domains on the surface of prosurvival Bcl-2 family members *(94)*. Interestingly, loss of chromosome 22q where *bik* gene resides is associated with breast tumorigenesis, suggesting *bik* gene may be a tumor suppressor *(95)*.

4.1. bik *Induces Apoptosis in Breast Cancer Cells*

In vitro, we showed that transfection of a *bik* expression vector and SN2 complex (SN-*bik*) into breast cancer cell lines such as MDA-MB-231, MDA-MB-468, and MCF-7 resulted in a drastic increase of apoptosis as measured by sub-G1 cell population *(47)*. As expected, the SN-*bik* transfected breast cancer cells exhibited drastic reduction of the number of colony in soft agar. These results suggest that *bik* is a potent proapoptotic agent and may be suitable for further development as a potential therapeutic gene in vivo.

4.2. Preclinical bik *Gene Therapy Study*

The initial indication that *bik* gene therapy might be feasible came from the result of an ex vivo experiment. Human breast cancer cell lines, MDA-MB-231 and MDA-MB-468, were transfected with SN-*bik* (or the control luciferase gene, SN-*luc*) prior to inoculation into MFP of female nude mice. The tumor size was monitored weekly post-inoculation. The growth of tumor transfected with SN-*bik* was significantly slower than those transfected with SN-*luc (47)*.

We then tested whether systemic delivery of SN-*bik* could yield antitumor activity in orthotopic breast cancer xenograft models. We treated the mice that bore tumors derived from either MDA-MB-231 or MDA-MB-468 with SN-*bik* (or SN-*luc*) via tail vein injection. This treatment protocol, i.e., 6 injections with 3 d between injections, resulted in a significant tumor suppression, an increase of apoptotic cells in tumors, and an increase of survival rate in mice treated with SN-*bik* as compared with those treated with SN-*luc*. More importantly, the SN-*bik*-treated mice had very few detectable metastatic nodules in the diaphragm and mesentery of these animals as compared with the control groups in which high incidence of metastasis was found *(47)*. Together, these results strongly support the notion that *bik* can be used as a potent therapeutic gene in breast cancer treatment.

4.3. Mutant bik *DD Enhances Apoptosis in Breast Cancer Cells*

Although *bik* gene therapy preclinical model yielded encouraging results *(47)*, complete tumor resolution remains the ultimate goal of this approach. As a step toward this objective, we attempted to modify the *bik* gene to make it more potent than the wild type *bik*. It has been implicated that phosphorylation of threonine 33 (T33) and serine 35 (S35) of bik protein are required for its maximum apoptotic activity *(96)*. We hypothesized that T33 and S35 substitutions with the negatively charged aspartic acids (D33 and D35) (i.e., *bik* DD) would be constitutively active and, thus, more potent. Indeed, we found that *bik* DD has higher binding affinity with the antiapoptotic molecules, Bcl-2 and Bcl-XL, than does the wild-type *bik*. Subsequently, transfection of *bik* DD led to higher apoptosis in breast cancer cells such as MCF-7 than did wild type *bik (97)*. These results suggest that *bik* DD is a more potent apoptotic agent than the wild type *bik*.

4.4. Preclinical Mutant bik *DD Gene Therapy Study*

To assess the antitumor activity of *bik* DD, we again performed an *ex vivo* experiment in which MCF-7 cells were transfected with *bik* DD and SN2 complex (SN-*bik* DD) or SN-*bik* before inoculation into the estrogen-supplemented female nude mice. Consistent with the in vitro data, SN-*bik* DD-transfected tumor cells grew significantly slower than those transfected with SN-*bik (97)*. Interestingly, the antitumor activity of single substitution mutants is also enhanced, but not to the same degree of potency as that of *bik* DD *(97)*. These encouraging ex vivo data set the stage for conducting a preclinical systemic gene therapy using MCF-7 orthotopic xenograft model. We showed that SN-*bik* DD intravenous injection (3×/wk with total 12 treatments) yielded greater tumor suppression activity and longer survival rates than SN-*bik* treatment *(97)*. Together, these observations suggest that *bik* DD is a better therapeutic agent than the wild type *bik*. The *bik* DD represents an improved version of a therapeutic agent that can be further developed to achieve the complete resolution of breast tumor.

5. FUTURE DIRECTIONS

In this chapter, we focused our discussion on the preclinical development of therapeutic genes in breast cancer treatment. Currently, *E1A* has been tested in multiple clinical trials and the preliminary data obtained so far are encouraging *(54–57)*. Both E1A and p202 could sensitize cancer cells to apoptosis induced by TNF-α or γ-irradiation *(24,25,74,79)*. These data provide a rationale to develop the combined therapy of *E1A* (or *p202*) and TNF-α (or γ-irradiation) that should yield better therapeutic effect than using single agent. Given that E1A and p202 inhibit NF-κB *(24,25,74,79)*, an antiapoptotic molecule, it is possible to achieve a better therapeutic effect with combined *E1A* (or *p202*) with chemotherapeutic agents *(98)*. Furthermore, because systemic treatment is imperative for treating metastatic tumors, the targeting specificity should be of concern to minimize the potential side effect. One way to overcome this drawback is to express these therapeutic genes under the control of tumor-specific promoter or to be delivered by a tumor-specific gene delivery system. To that end, we have successfully demonstrated that, using a p202 expression vector driven by a tissue-specific promoter, we were able to achieve a tissue-specific antitumor activity *(99)*. The similar approach should be applicable to *IFIXα1* and *bik* genes to achieve tumor-specific antitumor activity. With the availability of systemic gene delivery system that promises high efficiency of gene transfer (e.g., SN2 cationic liposome) it is possible that the tumor-specific expression of these therapeutic genes combined with appropriate chemotherapeutic agents would lead to a much effective killing of metastatic breast tumors.

REFERENCES

1. Miller BA, Feuer EJ, Hankey BF. Recent incidence trends for breast cancer in women and the relevance of early detection: an update. Ca: a Cancer J Clin 1993;43:27–41.
2. Berk AJ. Functions of adenovirus E1A. Cancer Surveys 1986;5:367–387.
3. Nevins JR. Adenovirus E1A: transcription regulation and alteration of cell growth control. Curr Topics Microbiol Immunol 1995;199:25–32.
4. Houweling A, van den Elsen PJ, van der Eb AJ. Partial transformation of primary rat cells by the leftmost 4.5% fragment of adenovirus 5 DNA. Virology 1980;105:537–550.
5. Ruley HE. Adenovirus early region 1A enables viral and cellular transforming genes to transform primary cells in culture. Nature 1983;304:602–606.
6. Pozzatti R, McCormick M, Thompson MA, Garbisa S, Liotta L, Khoury G. Regulation of the metastatic phenotype by the E1A gene of adenovirus-2. Adv Exp Med Biol 1988;233:293–301.
7. Pozzatti R, McCormick M, Thompson MA, Khoury G. The E1a gene of adenovirus type 2 reduces the metastatic potential of ras-transformed rat embryo cells. Mol Cell Biol 1988;8:2984–2988.
8. Steeg PS, Bevilacqua G, Pozzatti R, Liotta LA, Sobel ME. Altered expression of NM23, a gene associated with low tumor metastatic potential, during adenovirus 2 Ela inhibition of experimental metastasis. Cancer Res 1988;48:6550–6554.
9. Yu D, Suen TC, Yan DH, Chang LS, Hung MC. Transcriptional repression of the neu protooncogene by the adenovirus 5 E1A gene products. Proc Natl Acad Sci U S A 1990;87:4499–4503.
10. Yu DH, Scorsone K, Hung MC. Adenovirus type 5 E1A gene products act as transformation suppressors of the neu oncogene. Mol Cell Biol 1991;11:1745–1750.
11. Yu D, Hamada J, Zhang H, Nicolson GL, Hung MC. Mechanisms of c-erbB2/neu oncogene-induced metastasis and repression of metastatic properties by adenovirus 5 E1A gene products. Oncogene 1992;7:2263–2270.
12. Yu DH, Hung MC. Expression of activated rat neu oncogene is sufficient to induce experimental metastasis in 3T3 cells. Oncogene 1991;6:1991–1996.
13. Yan DH, Chang LS, Hung MC. Repressed expression of the HER-2/c-erbB-2 proto-oncogene by the adenovirus E1a gene products. Oncogene 1991;6:343–345.
14. Frisch SM, Reich R, Collier IE, Genrich LT, Martin G, Goldberg GI. Adenovirus E1A represses protease gene expression and inhibits metastasis of human tumor cells. Oncogene 1990;5:75–83.
15. Frisch SM. Antioncogenic effect of adenovirus E1A in human tumor cells. Proc Natl Acad Sci U S A 1991;88:9077–9081.
16. Yan DH, Shao R, Hung MC. E1A Cancer Gene Therapy. Gene Therapy of Cancer, Second ed. New York: Academic Press, 2002; pp. 465–477.
17. Li Z, Day C-P, Yang J-Y, et al. Adenoviral E1A targets Mdm4 to stabilize tumor suppressor p53. Cancer Res 2004;64:9080–9085.
18. Najafi SM, Li Z, Makino K, Shao R, Hung MC. The adenoviral E1A induces p21WAF1/CIP1 expression in cancer cells. Biochem Biophys Res Commun 2003;305:1099–1104.
19. Lee WP, Liao Y, Robinson D, Kung HJ, Liu ET, Hung MC. Axl-gas6 interaction counteracts E1A-mediated cell growth suppression and proapoptotic activity. Mol Cell Biol 1999;19:8075–8082.
20. Beg AA, Baltimore D. An essential role for NF-kappaB in preventing TNF-alpha-induced cell death. Science 1996;274:782–784.
21. Liu ZG, Hsu H, Goeddel DV, Karin M. Dissection of TNF receptor 1 effector functions: JNK activation is not linked to apoptosis while NF-kappaB activation prevents cell death. Cell 1996;87:565–576.
22. Van Antwerp DJ, Martin SJ, Kafri T, Green DR, Verma IM. Suppression of TNF-alpha-induced apoptosis by NF-kappaB. Science 1996;274:787–789.
23. Wang CY, Mayo MW, Baldwin AS, Jr. TNF- and cancer therapy-induced apoptosis: potentiation by inhibition of NF-kappaB. Science 1996;274:784–787.
24. Shao R, Hu MC, Zhou BP, et al. E1A sensitizes cells to tumor necrosis factor-induced apoptosis through inhibition of IkappaB kinases and nuclear factor kappaB activities. J Biol Chem 1999;274:21,495–21,498.
25. Shao R, Karunagaran D, Zhou BP, et al. Inhibition of nuclear factor-kappaB activity is involved in E1A-mediated sensitization of radiation-induced apoptosis. J Biol Chem 1997;272:32,739–32,742.
26. Shao R, Tsai EM, Wei K, et al. E1A inhibition of radiation-induced NF-kappaB activity through suppression of IKK activity and IkappaB degradation, independent of Akt activation. Cancer Res 2001;61:7413–7416.
27. Liao Y, Hung MC. A new role of protein phosphatase 2a in adenoviral E1A protein-mediated sensitization to anticancer drug-induced apoptosis in human breast cancer cells. Cancer Res 2004;64:5938–5942.

28. Liao Y, Hung MC. Regulation of the activity of p38 mitogen-activated protein kinase by Akt in cancer and adenoviral protein E1A-mediated sensitization to apoptosis. Mol Cell Biol 2003;23:6836–6848.
29. Gusterson BA, Gelber RD, Goldhirsch A, et al. Prognostic importance of c-erbB-2 expression in breast cancer. International (Ludwig) Breast Cancer Study Group. J Clin Oncol 1992;10:1049–1056.
30. Slamon DJ, Clark GM, Wong SG, Levin WJ, Ullrich A, McGuire WL. Human breast cancer: correlation of relapse and survival with amplification of the HER-2/neu oncogene. Science 1987;235: 177–182.
31. Slamon DJ, Godolphin W, Jones LA, et al. Studies of the HER-2/neu proto-oncogene in human breast and ovarian cancer. Science 1989;244:707–712.
32. Chang JY, Xia W, Shao R, et al. The tumor suppression activity of E1A in HER-2/neu-overexpressing breast cancer. Oncogene 1997;14:561–568.
33. Yu D, Matin A, Xia W, Sorgi F, Huang L, Hung MC. Liposome-mediated in vivo E1A gene transfer suppressed dissemination of ovarian cancer cells that overexpress HER-2/neu. Oncogene 1995;11:1383–1388.
34. Xing X, Liu V, Xia W, et al. Safety studies of the intraperitoneal injection of E1A—liposome complex in mice. Gene Ther 1997;4:238–243.
35. Xing X, Yujiao Chang J, Hung M. Preclinical and clinical study of HER-2/neu-targeting cancer gene therapy. Adv Drug Deliv Rev 1998;30:219–227.
36. Xing X, Zhang S, Chang JY, et al. Safety study and characterization of E1A-liposome complex gene-delivery protocol in an ovarian cancer model. Gene Ther 1998;5:1538–1544.
37. Frisch SM, Dolter KE. Adenovirus E1a-mediated tumor suppression by a c-erbB-2/neu-independent mechanism. Cancer Res 1995;55:5551–5555.
38. Lowe SW, Ruley HE, Jacks T, Housman DE. p53-dependent apoptosis modulates the cytotoxicity of anticancer agents. Cell 1993;74:957–967.
39. Nahle Z, Polakoff J, Davuluri RV, et al. Direct coupling of the cell cycle and cell death machinery by E2F. Nature Cell Biol 2002;4:859–864.
40. Yu D, Hung MC. Role of erbB2 in breast cancer chemosensitivity. Bioessays 2000;22:673–680.
41. Yu D, Jing T, Liu B, et al. Overexpression of ErbB2 blocks Taxol-induced apoptosis by upregulation of p21Cip1, which inhibits p34Cdc2 kinase. Mol Cell 1998;2:581–591.
42. Yu D, Liu B, Jing T, et al. Overexpression of both p185c-erbB2 and p170mdr-1 renders breast cancer cells highly resistant to taxol. Oncogene 1998;16:2087–2094.
43. Yu D, Liu B, Tan M, Li J, Wang SS, Hung MC. Overexpression of c-erbB-2/neu in breast cancer cells confers increased resistance to Taxol via mdr-1-independent mechanisms. Oncogene 1996;13: 1359–1365.
44. Ueno NT, Yu D, Hung MC. Chemosensitization of HER-2/neu-overexpressing human breast cancer cells to paclitaxel (Taxol) by adenovirus type 5 E1A. Oncogene 1997;15:953–960.
45. Ueno NT, Bartholomeusz C, Xia W, et al. Systemic gene therapy in human xenograft tumor models by liposomal delivery of the E1A gene. Cancer Res 2002;62:6712–6716.
46. Liao Y, Zhou Y, Xia W, Hung MC. Enhanced paclitaxel cytotoxicity and prolonged animal survival rate by a nonviral-mediated systemic delivery of E1A gene in orthotopic xenograft human breast cancer. Cancer Gene Ther 2004;11:594–602.
47. Zou Y, Peng H, Zhou B, et al. Systemic tumor suppression by the proapoptotic gene bik. Cancer Res 2002;62:8–12.
48. Zou Y, Peng H, Zhou BH, et al. Systemic tumor suppression by the pro-apoptotic gene, bik. (Correction). Cancer Res 2002;62:4167.
49. Li S, Huang L. In vivo gene transfer via intravenous administration of cationic lipid-protamine-DNA (LPD) complexes. Gene Therapy 1997;4:891–900.
50. Li S, Rizzo MA, Bhattacharya S, Huang L. Characterization of cationic lipid-protamine-DNA (LPD) complexes for intravenous gene delivery. Gene Ther 1998;5:930–937.
51. Brader KR, Wolf JK, Hung MC, et al. Adenovirus E1A expression enhances the sensitivity of an ovarian cancer cell line to multiple cytotoxic agents through an apoptotic mechanism. Clin. Cancer Res 1997;3:2017–2024.
52. Ueno NT, Bartholomeusz C, Herrmann JL, et al. E1A-mediated paclitaxel sensitization in HER-2/neu-overexpressing ovarian cancer SKOV3.ip1 through apoptosis involving the caspase-3 pathway. Clin. Cancer Res 2000;6:250–259.
53. Liu W, Akhand AA, Takeda K, et al. Protein phosphatase 2A-linked and -unlinked caspase-dependent pathways for downregulation of Akt kinase triggered by 4-hydroxynonenal. Cell Death Differ 2003; 10:772–781.

54. Hortobagyi GN, Ueno NT, Xia W, et al. Cationic liposome-mediated E1A gene transfer to human breast and ovarian cancer cells and its biologic effects: a phase I clinical trial. J Clin Oncol 2001;19:3422–3433.
55. Madhusudan S, Tamir A, Bates N, et al. A multicenter phase I gene therapy clinical trial involving intraperitoneal administration of E1A-lipid complex in patients with recurrent epithelial ovarian cancer overexpressing HER-2/neu oncogene. Clin. Cancer Res 2004;10:2986–2996.
56. Villaret D, Glisson B, Kenady D, et al. A multicenter phase II study of tgDCC-E1A for the intratumoral treatment of patients with recurrent head and neck squamous cell carcinoma. Head & Neck 2002;24:661–669.
57. Yoo GH, Hung MC, Lopez-Berestein G, et al. Phase I trial of intratumoral liposome E1A gene therapy in patients with recurrent breast and head and neck cancer. Clin Cancer Res 2001;7:1237–1245.
58. Asefa B, Klarmann KD, Copeland NG, Gilbert DJ, Jenkins NA, Keller JR. The interferon-inducible negative regulator of cell growth. Blood Cells Mol Dis 2004;32:155–167.
59. Choubey D. P202: an interferon-inducible negative regulator of cell growth. J Biol Regul Homeo Agents 2000;14:187–192.
60. Johnstone RW, Trapani JA. Transcription and growth regulatory functions of the HIN-200 family of proteins. Mol Cell Biol 1999;19:5833–5838.
61. Clarke CJ, Trapani JA, Johnstone RW. Mechanisms of interferon mediated anti-viral resistance. Current Drug Targets—Immune Endoc Metab Dis 2001;1:117–130.
62. Gariglio M, Azzimonti B, Pagano M, et al. Immunohistochemical expression analysis of the human interferon-inducible gene IFI16, a member of the HIN200 family, not restricted to hematopoietic cells. J Interferon Cytokine Res 2002;22:815–821.
63. Raffaella R, Gioia D, De Andrea M, et al. The interferon-inducible IFI16 gene inhibits tube morphogenesis and proliferation of primary, but not HPV16 E6/E7-immortalized human endothelial cells. Exper Cell Res 2004;293:331–345.
64. Wei W, Clarke CJ, Somers GR, et al. Expression of IFI 16 in epithelial cells and lymphoid tissues. Histochem. Cell Biol 2003;119:45–54.
65. Lengyel P, Choubey D, Li S-J, Datta B. The interferon-activatable gene 200 cluster: from structure toward function. Semin Virol 1995;6:203–213.
66. Rozzo SJ, Allard JD, Choubey D, et al. Evidence for an interferon-inducible gene, Ifi202, in the susceptibility to systemic lupus. Immunity 2001;15:435–443.
67. Choubey D, Lengyel P. Binding of an interferon-inducible protein (p202) to the retinoblastoma protein. J Biol Chem 1995;270:6134–6140.
68. Choubey D, Li SJ, Datta B, Gutterman JU, Lengyel P. Inhibition of E2F-mediated transcription by p202. EMBO J 1996;15:5668–5678.
69. Choubey D, Gutterman JU. Inhibition of E2F-4/DP-1-stimulated transcription by p202. Oncogene 1997;15:291–301.
70. Datta B, Li B, Choubey D, Nallur G, Lengyel P. p202, an interferon-inducible modulator of transcription, inhibits transcriptional activation by the p53 tumor suppressor protein, and a segment from the p53-binding protein 1 that binds to p202 overcomes this inhibition. J Biol Chem 1996;271:27,544–27,555.
71. Wang H, Liu C, Lu Y, et al. The interferon- and differentiation-inducible p202a protein inhibits the transcriptional activity of c-Myc by blocking its association with Max. J Biol Chem 2000;275:27,377–27,385.
72. Ma XY, Wang H, Ding B, Zhong H, Ghosh S, Lengyel P. The interferon-inducible p202a protein modulates NF-kappaB activity by inhibiting the binding to DNA of p50/p65 heterodimers and p65 homodimers while enhancing the binding of p50 homodimers. J Biol Chem 2003;278:23,008–23,019.
73. Min W, Ghosh S, Lengyel P. The interferon-inducible p202 protein as a modulator of transcription: inhibition of NF-kappa B, c-Fos, and c-Jun activities. Mol Cell Biol 1996;16:359–368.
74. Wen Y, Yan DH, Spohn B, Deng J, Lin SY, Hung MC. Tumor suppression and sensitization to tumor necrosis factor alpha-induced apoptosis by an interferon-inducible protein, p202, in breast cancer cells. Cancer Res 2000;60:42–46.
75. Datta B, Min W, Burma S, Lengyel P. Increase in p202 expression during skeletal muscle differentiation: inhibition of MyoD protein expression and activity by p202. Mol Cell Biol 1998;18:1074–1083.
76. Wen Y, Yan DH, Wang B, et al. p202, an interferon-inducible protein, mediates multiple antitumor activities in human pancreatic cancer xenograft models. Cancer Res 2001;61:7142–7147.
77. Choubey D, Gutterman JU. The interferon-inducible growth-inhibitory p202 protein: DNA binding properties and identification of a DNA binding domain. Biochem Biophy Res Commun 1996;221:396–401.
78. Gutterman JU, Choubey D. Retardation of cell proliferation after expression of p202 accompanies an increase in p21(WAF1/CIP1). Cell Growth Differ 1999;10:93–100.

79. Ding Y, Wen Y, Spohn B, et al. Proapoptotic and antitumor activities of adenovirus-mediated p202 gene transfer. Clin. Cancer Res 2002;8:3290–3297.
80. Yan DH, Wen Y, Spohn B, Choubey D, Gutterman JU, Hung MC. Reduced growth rate and transformation phenotype of the prostate cancer cells by an interferon-inducible protein, p202. Oncogene 1999;18:807–811.
81. Fujiuchi N, Aglipay JA, Ohtsuka T, et al. Requirement of IFI16 for the maximal activation of p53 induced by ionizing radiation. J Biol Chem 2004;279:20,339–20,344.
82. DeYoung KL, Ray ME, Su YA, et al. Cloning a novel member of the human interferon-inducible gene family associated with control of tumorigenicity in a model of human melanoma. Oncogene 1997;15:453–457.
83. Kulaeva OI, Draghici S, Tang L, Kraniak JM, Land SJ, Tainsky MA. Epigenetic silencing of multiple interferon pathway genes after cellular immortalization. Oncogene 2003;22:4118–4127.
84. Mori Y, Yin J, Rashid A, et al. Instabilotyping: comprehensive identification of frameshift mutations caused by coding region microsatellite instability. Cancer Res 2001;61:6046–6049.
85. Doggett KL, Briggs JA, Linton MF, et al. Retroviral mediated expression of the human myeloid nuclear antigen in a null cell line upregulates Dlk1 expression. J Cell Biochem 2002;86:56–66.
86. Pradhan A, Mijovic A, Mills K, et al. Differentially expressed genes in adult familial myelodysplastic syndromes. Leukemia 2004;18:449–459.
87. Varambally S, Dhanasekaran SM, Zhou M, et al. The polycomb group protein EZH2 is involved in progression of prostate cancer. Nature 2002;419:624–629.
88. Xin H, Geng Y, Pramanik R, Choubey D. Induction of p202, a modulator of apoptosis, during oncogenic transformation of NIH 3T3 cells by activated H-Ras (Q61L) contributes to cell survival. J Cell Biochem 2003;88:191–204.
89. Ding Y, Wang L, Su LK, et al. Antitumor activity of IFIX, a novel interferon-inducible HIN-200 gene, in breast cancer. Oncogene 2004;23:4556–4566.
90. Gomez-Navarro J, Arafat W, Xiang J. Gene therapy for carcinoma of the breast: Pro-apoptotic gene therapy. Breast Cancer Res 2000;2:32–44.
91. Boyd JM, Gallo GJ, Elangovan B, et al. Bik, a novel death-inducing protein shares a distinct sequence motif with Bcl-2 family proteins and interacts with viral and cellular survival-promoting proteins. Oncogene 1995;11:1921–1928.
92. Han J, Sabbatini P, White E. Induction of apoptosis by human Nbk/Bik, a BH3-containing protein that interacts with E1B 19K. Mol Cell Biol 1996;16:5857–5864.
93. Orth K, Dixit VM. Bik and Bak induce apoptosis downstream of CrmA but upstream of inhibitor of apoptosis. J Biol Chem 1997;272:8841–8844.
94. Huang DC, Strasser A. BH3-Only proteins-essential initiators of apoptotic cell death. Cell 103:839–842.
95. Castells A, Gusella JF, Ramesh V, Rustgi AK. A region of deletion on chromosome 22q13 is common to human breast and colorectal cancers. Cancer Res 2000;60:2836–2839.
96. Verma S, Zhao LJ, Chinnadurai G. Phosphorylation of the pro-apoptotic protein BIK: mapping of phosphorylation sites and effect on apoptosis. J Biol Chem 2001;276:4671–4676.
97. Li YM, Wen Y, Zhou BP, Kuo HP, Ding Q, Hung MC. Enhancement of Bik antitumor effect by Bik mutants. Cancer Res 2003;63:7630–7633.
98. Pahl HL. Activators and target genes of Rel/NF-kappaB transcription factors. Oncogene 1999;18: 6853–6866.
99. Wen Y, Giri D, Yan DH, et al. Prostate-specific antitumor activity by probasin promoter-directed p202 expression. Mol Carcinog 2003;37:130–137.

25 Steps in a Translational Cancer Gene Therapy Trial

Urs W. von Holzen, MD
and Stephen G. Swisher, MD

CONTENTS

Summary

This chapter reviews the requisite steps in a translational cancer gene therapy trial. As with all clinical trials, translational cancer gene therapy trials require clear concise objectives and endpoints. Several unique factors exist with gene therapy trials that must be considered prior to trial development, including the type of vector desired, the delivery mechanism and the different gene therapy strategies required for gene product expression. Progression of cancer gene therapy trials from the preclinical phase to the post approval phase IV stage require a careful strategy to meet the strict regulatory requirements at both the federal and local institutional level. Safety monitoring is especially important with gene therapy trials because of the high visibility of gene therapy trials and the impact on the trial, patient, and the gene therapy field in general if adverse events occur. Financial considerations should be addressed at the outset because of the increased costs associated with a translational gene therapy trial.

Key Words: Development of translational cancer gene therapy trial; gene therapy strategies; regulatory considerations; safety issues; financial considerations.

1. INTRODUCTION

Clinical gene therapy trials require a series of prerequisite steps that must be overcome prior to the initiation and completion of a successful translational trial. This chapter reviews some of the requisite steps in a translational cancer gene therapy trial. As with all clinical trials, translational cancer gene therapy trials require clear concise objectives and endpoints that depend in large part on the clinical experience and safety record

From: *Cancer Drug Discovery and Development: Gene Therapy for Cancer*
Edited by: K. K. Hunt, S. A. Vorburger, and S. G. Swisher © Humana Press Inc., Totowa, NJ

of the therapeutic agent and the principal investigator. Several unique factors exist with gene therapy trials that must be considered prior to trial development including the type of vector desired, the delivery mechanism, and the duration and amount of gene product expression required. In order to be successful, financial funding must be obtained but in the case of cancer gene therapy trials the amount of support is often much higher than conventional therapeutic agents because of the increased costs associated with the additional safety monitoring and regulation associated with human gene therapy trials. The strict regulatory requirements exist at both the federal and local institutional levels and require a careful planned strategy to fulfill. Finally, safety monitoring must be carefully considered because of the high visibility of gene therapy trials and the potential impact on the trial, patient and the gene therapy field in general if adverse events occur.

In 1989, Rosenberg et al. performed the first human gene therapy trial with a retrovirus construct that introduced the gene coding for resistance to neomycin into human tumor-infiltrating lymphocytes (TIL). These super-charged TILs were infused into five patients with advanced melanoma *(1)*. Since then the number of gene therapy trials has increased dramatically and as of January 31, 2004 there were 918 active clinical trials in 24 countries. The majority of these clinical trials are aimed at the treatment of various types of cancer (66%) and are designed to establish the feasibility and safety of the therapeutic agent and to demonstrate the expression of therapeutic proteins in vivo by transferred genes and in some cases to show therapeutic effect *(2)*.

2. STEP 1: GENE EXPRESSION—VECTOR SELECTION

The concept of gene therapy is based on the simple premise of transferring a gene into a cell or tissue with minimal toxicity and having the transduced cell express the transferred gene. The transferred gene product can then inhibit or stimulate a selected pathway to induce a desired biologic effect. Various techniques exist to transfer genes into cells and these can be broadly classified as viral or nonviral delivery systems. At the present time there is no perfect gene transfer technique. Each technique has its own inherent advantages and limitations that must be carefully considered in light of the patient population and the clinical objectives of the trial.

2.1. Viral Vectors

Viral vectors offer a higher efficiency of gene transfer compared with nonviral techniques. The most commonly studied vectors are replication-defective retroviruses, adenoviruses, and adeno-associated viruses (AAVs). Other viruses under study include herpes simplex, vaccinia, lentivirus, and baculovirus. Viral vectors have better transduction efficiencies than nonviral systems in vivo. Despite these advantages, problems with viral vectors include toxicity, transient protein production, limitations on the size of the transferred gene, lack of selective tissue targeting, expression of viral proteins, development of neutralizing antibodies, and inability to transduce all cell types. Viral vectors are used in about 70% of the clinical trials *(3,4)*. The most commonly used viral vectors are retroviruses and adenoviruses (28 and 26% of all trials respectively) *(2)*. Retroviruses have the ability to integrate into the genome leading to long lasting gene expression. Unfortunately, the ability to integrate into the genome has been associated with two cases of vector-induced leukemia. Retroviruses also have a relatively limited size capacity to carry therapeutic genes and are not able to target nonreplicating cells. Additionally, they are often difficult to produce to the large quantities necessary for clinical trials. Adenoviruses have a larger size capacity for therapeutic genes and are able to be produced in large quantities necessary for clinical trials. They have a higher transfer efficiency than retroviruses and are even able to transfect nondividing cells, but their gene expression is transient because they do not integrate into the genome. Another drawback is their tendency to induce immune and inflammatory responses that lead to mild clinical symptoms and the development of neutralizing antibody titers.

2.2. Nonviral Vectors

Limitations of the viral vectors have lead to the development of nonviral systems *(5)*. The most commonly used non-viral vector systems in clinical trials are the injection of naked DNA directly into certain tissues or the use of lipofection to improve transduction efficiencies of DNA. Nonviral vectors are normally nonimmunogenic. The transduction efficiencies, however, are much lower than with viral vectors making the ability to transduce adequate numbers of targets cells or tissues difficult especially in a clinical trial. The lack of neutralizing antibodies allows the possibility of systemic gene delivery but the low transduction efficiencies may limit this strategy in vivo.

3. STEP 2: GENE EXPRESSION—DELIVERY METHODS

One of the most difficult challenges to a successful clinical gene therapy trial is the selection of a gene delivery system. An effective delivery system that is able to transduce and express the transgene efficiently and safely to the target tissue has not yet been developed. The method of delivering genes in clinical trials may therefore need to be individualized to the objectives of the trial, the tissues targeted and the type of viral or nonviral vector selected *(6)*.

3.1. Viral Delivery Methods

Viral vectors are most commonly delivered to the target tissue by direct intratumoral injection through endoscopic or percutaneous means. This results in high levels of expression in the immediate area of injection but is limited because of diffusion in its ability to transduce large solid tumors. Selective tissue targeting also remains a limitation because all cells in the injected area are susceptible to transduction. Strategies to address these delivery limitations include the development of replication competent viruses that may enhance the amount of tissue transduced and the effective period of gene expression. Other targeting strategies under development include fusion proteins that are able to improve viral transduction efficiencies by selectively targeting specific extracellular receptors such as transferrin or endothelial growth factor receptor (EGFR) *(4)*. At the present time, systemic delivery of viral vectors has been limited by the rapid development of neutralizing antibodies that limit subsequent systemic delivery of the therapeutic vector. Although repeated systemic administration is limited by neutralizing antibodies, local intratumoral delivery can still lead to high levels of local gene expression perhaps because of the increased intratumoral tissue pressure in the injected site which limits systemic antibody accumulation *(7)*. Viral delivery limitations remain the largest obstacle to successful gene therapy trials in humans.

3.2. Nonviral Delivery Methods

The simplest technique of non-viral gene delivery involves injection of naked DNA. Depending on the type of cell, a small amount of the injected DNA will be taken up by the cell and expressed as its protein product *(5)*. Unfortunately, the rates of transduction are low and the periods of gene expression are short. Use in humans is also limited to areas where increased tissue pressures can be achieved to drive the plasmid DNA into the circulation and targeted tissue. Microinjection, electroporation, and calcium precipitation can all be used to increase efficiency, but these techniques are not usually applicable in vivo. Transduction efficiency can be improved by using a gene "gun" which blasts DNA into cells. At the present time, however, this technique is limited clinically to accessible sites such as the skin or mucous membranes. Deep-seated lesions in the lung or mediastinum cannot be targeted with the gene "gun." Liposomes are another alternative since they improve the efficiency of DNA transfer across the cell membrane and have been used in vivo to transfer various genes of interest. Unfortunately, liposomes are still not as efficient as viral delivery systems and are difficult to target or control in vivo. Liposomal transduction also results in transient expression because of lack of integration of the transferred DNA. In clinical trials systemic delivery is limited in part by interaction of the liposome–DNA complex with blood plasma proteins and the extracellular matrix. Novel liposomes are currently being developed with greater in vivo stability to improve clinical utility. Current research strategies to improve viral delivery included development of ligands and peptide sequences which aid receptor-mediated endocytosis and endosomal disruption *(5)*.

3.3. Cellular Delivery Methods

Another delivery method for both viral and non-viral vectors is ex vivo transduction of target cells that are then reintroduced into the patient *(6)*. This delivery mechanism was first used by Rosenberg et al. in the initial human gene therapy trial when human tumor infiltrating cells were transduced with retroviral constructs and reinfused in metastatic melanoma patients *(1)*. The advantage of this delivery method is that there is more control of the transduced cell and higher transduction efficiencies can be achieved in the target tissue. Disadvantages included difficulties in targeting the reinfused cells to specific anatomic locations as well as possible contamination with reintroduced biologic agents. Current research efforts are evaluating ex vivo transduction of stem and progenitor cells which may lead to more sustained gene expression and better tissue targeting.

4. STEP 3: SELECTION OF CANCER GENE THERAPY STRATEGY

The concept of gene therapy follows from the observation that certain diseases are caused by the inheritance of a single functionally defective gene. Replacement of this gene (i.e., in cystic fibrosis or in the severe combined immunodeficiency syndromes) can theoretically cure the disease *(3)*. In cancers, however, the situation may be more difficult because there are usually multiple genetic defects present, and the replacement of all these genes is not possible. To overcome these difficulties various gene therapy strategies have been proposed for the treatment of malignancies, including stimulation of the immune system, transfer of suicide genes, replacement or inhibition of critical genes such as oncogenes and tumor suppressor genes, induction of apoptosis or antiangiogenesis, and transfer of genes that enhance conventional treatments as radiotherapy or chemotherapy (Table 1).

4.1. Stimulating the Immune System

Different gene therapy approaches have been put forward to stimulate the immune system. The basic principle underlying immunotherapy in cancer is that tumors have

Table 1
Gene Therapy Strategies

Stimulating the immune system.
Transfer of suicide genes.
Replacement of tumor suppressor genes.
Inhibition of oncogenes.
Inhibition of angiogenesis.
Induction of apoptosis.
Enhancement of radiation therapy and/or chemotherapy.

antigens that are capable of provoking weak humoral or cellular reactions. By activating this immune response against tumor cells through gene transfer it is hoped that tumors can be eradicated either by the transferred gene product or activation of the patient's own immune system. In animal models, the administration of cytokines such as interleukin (IL)-2, IL-4, IL-6, IL-7, IL-12, tumor necrosis factor (TNF)-α, interferons and granulocyte macrophage colony-stimulating factor (GM-CSF) have resulted in tumor regression *(8)*. The systemic administration of cytokines in human trials though has been limited by the severe toxicity of these cytokines. Gene therapy strategies offer an opportunity to overcome these limitations because of the potential for local delivery to injected tumor with reduction in systemic toxicity *(9–11)*. Another approach to make tumor cells more immunogenic involves the cotransfer of stimulatory molecules such as B7.1 and B7.2. These molecules provide a key event in T-cell activation, and are often lacking on the surface of tumor cells. Zajac et al. used a nonreplicative vaccinia virus expressing HLA-A0201-restricted Melan-A/Mart-1_{27-35}, gp$100_{280-288}$, and tyrosinase$_{1-9}$ epitopes together with Human B7.1 and B7.2 costimulatory molecules in a phase I/II trial in metastatic melanoma patients *(12)*. In a large majority of patients, the reagent was able to induce specific CTL responses although major clinical responses were not seen *(12)*. The utilization of cytokine-based gene therapy strategies for the development of tumor cell vaccines through ex vivo delivery methods is another approach. Although these gene therapy strategies appear to stimulate the immune system and may ultimately produce long-term antitumor protection, problems with targeting the immune system include the heterogeneity of tumor antigen expression, which prevents a predictable response by the immune system to gene transfer.

4.2. Transfer of Suicide Genes

Another gene therapy strategy involves the transduction of tumor cells with a gene capable of converting a nontoxic compound into a toxic metabolite. The two most commonly used genes for this are the herpes simplex thymidine kinase gene (HSV-*tk*) and the cytosine deaminase gene. HSV-*tk* that convert non-toxic ganciclovir to a cytotoxic triphosphate metabolite, and cytosine deaminase converts 5-fluorocytosine to the cytotoxic antimetabolite 5-fluorouracil. This strategy could potentially lead not only to the killing of the transduced cells, but also to the killing of adjacent cells in a "bystander effect" so that only a fraction of the targeted cells are needed to be transduced for eradication of the tumor *(3)*. Potential limitations with the transfer of suicide genes include toxicity to normal cells that are transduced at the same time. These problems may be addressed by gene transfer strategies, that selectively target tumor tissue. One strategy to selectively target lung cancer cells involves the transfer of HSV-*tk* with a carcinoembryonic antigen (CEA) promoter because many lung cancer cells overexpress CEA. HSV-*tk* would then be selectively translated in CEA-overexpressing lung cancer cells.

4.3. Replacement or Inhibition of Critical Genes

Genes known to play a role in carcinogenesis include dominant oncogenes and mutated or deleted tumor suppressor genes. Gene therapy strategies that inactivate oncogenes or replace tumor suppressor genes may provide a target for tumor regression.

4.4. Oncogene Inhibition

Most oncogenes develop from proto-oncogenes that play an important role in fetal development but are later silenced to prevent abnormal cell growth. Point mutations, amplifications, translocations, or rearrangements in these protooncogenes can lead to a dominant transforming oncogene. Cancer cells often develop through activation and amplifications of these proto-oncogenes. Therefore, the disruption of tumor oncogenes may be one strategy of cancer gene therapy. Tumor oncogene expression may be disrupted through inhibition of the oncogene transcription into mRNA, or translation into protein, or interference with oncoprotein transport and function *(14)*. The transcription of oncogenes can be blocked by using DNA oligonucleotides, short single-stranded DNA sequences that bind to specific oncogene promotor regions. Another approach is to use antisense oligonucleotides which have been used to block bcl-2 oncogene translation in prostate and breast cancer cells *(15,16)*. Transduction of genes encoding for ribozymes (which directly cleave oncogene mRNA) has also been demonstrated in the laboratory to inhibit oncogene production and induce tumor regression.

4.5. Tumor Suppressor Gene Replacement

Tumor suppressor genes are a class of genes whose absence may contribute to tumor growth. In most situations tumor suppressor genes require both alleles of a gene to be deleted or inactivated to lead to tumor growth. The replacement of just one functional tumor suppressor gene may therefore be enough to restore normal growth regulation and induce tumor apoptosis. The tumor suppressor gene with the most clinical trial experience is the gene encoding for wild type (wt)-*p53*. The wt-*p53* gene may inhibit tumor development by either suppressing genes that contribute to uncontrolled cell growth and proliferation or activating genes that inhibit cell growth. Functional p53 is normally responsible for detecting damaged DNA and either directing repair of damaged cells or committing cells to apoptosis (programmed cell death) if the DNA is not able to be repaired. Several wt-*p53* gene replacement strategies are in clinical trials for head and neck cancer, melanoma, breast, brain, and lung cancer *(13,17,18)*. An additional advantage to tumor suppressor gene replacement is that normal cells are usually not affected by the tranduction of tumor suppressor genes whereas cancer cells often undergo irreversible apoptosis. This therapeutic index may allow the treatment of cancer cells with minimal toxicity to normal cells.

4.6. Induction of Apoptosis

The inhibition of apoptosis has also been implicated in tumorigenesis. Human papilloma viruses (HPV) have been implicated in the induction of cervical cancer through production of a protein (E6) that binds and inactivates the p53 gene promoter inhibiting apoptosis. Additionally, somatic mutations of the proapoptotic Bax gene have been implicated in the development of colon cancer. Because inhibition of apoptosis by cancer cells is a common trait, another cancer gene therapy strategy would be the tranduction of proapoptotic genes such as p53, Bax, Bak, TNF, or TNF-related apoptosis inducing ligand (TRAIL) *(19,20)*. Alternatively, strategies designed to inhibit antiapoptotic genes such Bcl-2 or Bcl-Xl with antisense nucleotides may be effective. It is important in this approach that the therapeutic index be carefully evaluated with each gene because some of these genes lack selectivity and induce apoptosis in normal cells as well (Bax and Bak) *(21)*. To improve selectivity, research efforts have developed viral constructs controlled by CEA or telomerase regulated promote that allow selective apoptosis induction of tumor cells with gene therapy delivery.

4.7. Inhibition of Angiogenesis

Angiogenesis is another critical component in tumor development regulating both the growth of the primary and metastatic deposits. The ability of a tumor to become vascularized allows rapid expansion of the primary tumor with increased metastatic potential. Multiple genes are involved in this process including vascular endothelial growth factor (VEGF). Gene therapy strategies to inhibit angiogenesis include inhibition of VEGF or its receptor with ribozymes or antisense nucleotides *(22)*. Alternatively, the induction of other genes involved in inhibiting angiogenesis such as p53 or angiostatin have been proposed. The transient nature of gene expression with current viral and nonviral vectors may limit this form of therapy for antiangiogenic strategies if prolonged expression of the gene is required to inhibit tumor growth.

4.8. Enhancement of Radiation Therapy or Chemotherapy

Chemotherapy and radiation therapy induce tumor cell death in large part by causing DNA damage that leads to apoptosis (programmed cell death). Toxicity to normal cells at higher doses with conventional agents often leads to the inability to completely eradicate tumor with conventional agents. Gene therapy strategies may therefore include transduction of genes that synergize with conventional agents without increasing toxicity to normal cells. One example of such a gene is wt-*p53* which is involved in monitoring DNA damage. Following DNA damage cellular p53 expression increases with tranduction of other genes such as p21 that induce G1 cell arrest and allow the cell to repair the damage. If the damage is not repaired, apoptosis may be induced. Cells with mutated p53 are more resistant to radiation therapy induced cell death than cells with wild type p53 leading to tumor resistance with conventional therapies *(23)*. In the laboratory, the administration of adenoviral p53 before chemotherapy and radiation therapy has demonstrated increased apoptosis both in vitro and in vivo without increased toxicity *(24)*. Preliminary trials in lung cancer with intratumoral Adp53 gene therapy and external beam radiation have also demonstrated high levels of tumor response and the induction of the proapototic Bak gene in the treated tumor *(7)*. Importantly, toxicity to normal cells did not appear to be increased. Combining gene therapy agents with conventional agents may therefore allow enhancement of antitumor activity without the increased toxicity seen with higher doses of conventional agents.

5. STEP 4: GENE THERAPY CLINICAL TRIAL DEVELOPMENT

In developing and conducting gene therapy clinical trials investigators must address biologic efficacy as well as regulatory requirements and safety and ethical issues. In this section we will focus on the endpoints that may need to be assessed in the different phases of gene therapy clinical trials (Table 2).

Table 2
Possible Endpoints in Clinical trials in Gene Therapy

Phase I	Maximum tolerated dose (MTD) Toxicity Safety Biological endpoints such as apoptosis Gene transfer efficacy
Phase II	Activity of strategy Tumor response Time to progression Tumor markers
Phase III	Disease-free survival Overall survival
Phase IV	Additional clinical indications Identification of genetic tests for sensitivity

5.1. Preclinical Phase

Preclinical studies in the laboratory are needed to support the clinical evaluation of gene therapeutics in human gene therapy trials. Preliminary in vitro studies must demonstrate "proof in principle" with efficacy and safety in laboratory and animal models *(25)*. The initial step usually involves demonstrating the potential of a proposed gene to address a clinical problem such as induction of the immune system to treat cancer. The second phase involves evaluating more closely a proposed vector construct that may be utilized in subsequent clinical trials. This phase involves animal models that more closely mimic the clinical situation and allow evaluation of both potential efficacy and safety in toxiciology and biodistribution studies. The data from these studies can then be put together in an application to the Food and Drug Administration (FDA) for an Investigational New Drug (IND) application *(26)*. It is therefore critical that the latter in vivo studies utilize the vector construct that will be utilized in the clinical trials and that combinations with proposed conventional agents such as radiation therapy or chemotherapy are also evaluated for efficacy and safety. The toxicology and biodistribution data that is required by the FDA will be dependent in part on the amount of information already available for that construct and the inherent potential for risk in a human gene therapy setting of the proposed gene therapy strategy *(27)*. The animal models utilized in these later preclinical studies are dependent in part on the vector and may often be performed in large part in mice although monkey studies with their increased costs may also be required for certain vectors. It is important that coordination with the FDA is established early to minimize potential cost over-runs from unforeseen problems. Final preclinical studies should use clinical-grade material produced in a Good Laboratory Practices (GLP) setting to satisfy safety and efficacy concerns of the FDA *(28)*.

5.2. Phase I Evaluation

In phase I trials the main focus is to monitor product safety in a small patient population. In these trials investigators traditionally look at the metabolic and pharmacological actions of a new agent in patients, the side effects and the maximum tolerated dose (MTD) of the new treatment agent, as well as the safety of the new approach. Clinical trials of gene therapy agents often follow nontraditional oncology trial design because phase I studies often do not achieve a MTD *(26)*. Dose escalation may also be limited by the cost and effort required to produce the gene therapy vector. Novel strategies and endpoints may therefore be required for gene therapy constructs. Phase I designs should address vector related toxicity, gene related toxicity and delivery related toxicity. Toxicity with biologic viral constructs may also be more related to the immune status of the patient than other traditional variables. In clinical stage III and IV patients, a compromised immune system may lead to greater toxicity than earlier stage immunocompetent patients. Novel endpoints may therefore need to be evaluated to demonstrate efficacy such as the number of apoptotic cells in a tissue sample after treatment *(29)*. Gene therapy trials must also address specific efficacy issues such as transduction efficiency and expression and effectiveness and safety of planned delivery methods such as repeated intratumoral injections. The assessment of vector transduction and gene expression may require quantitative reverse transcriptase-polymerase chain reaction (RT-PCR) of the target tissue for the therapeutic gene with vector specific primers or immunohistochemistry with careful evaluations of post-treatment tumor biopsies of tumor samples *(30)*. Incorporation of nontraditional endpoints such as surrogate tissue markers or functional imaging studies may allow a more effective demonstration of vector activity for subsequent phase II trials *(31)*.

5.3. Phase II Evaluation

Phase II studies are designed to assess potential efficacy and activity of the proposed gene therapy strategies in a larger patient population. These trials often evaluate the effectiveness and dose ranging of the new agent for a specific disease and patient population. Traditional endpoints of phase II trials with conventional agents often utilize tumor response (i.e., partial or complete response but many of the biologic agents may be cytostatic therapies that do not cause tumor shrinkage but still lead to antiangiogenic or immunomodulatory effects). Assessment of the true activity of these agents may therefore not be possible with these classic endpoints. Alternative endpoints such as time to progression, stable disease, or symptom improvement may therefore need to be considered *(32)*. Other potential endpoints may include decreases in tumor markers such as prostate-specific antigen (PSA) or CEA *(33)*. It is also critical to recognize that biologic agents may impact only a small subset of patients and studies may need to be designed to stratify patients according to biologic parameters. These correlative studies may be critical in identifying therapeutic subsets of patients. New federal regulations may impede this process by imposing strict criteria on the collection of tissue from patients and children with patients often choose not to participate in these critical steps *(34)*. The design of these trials should therefore take into account the need for biopsies to be limited in number to encourage active patient participation because the collection of tissue may allow future biologic information to be incorporated in sensitivity analyses that would not be possible if tissue collection had not occurred.

5.4. Phase III Evaluation

Phase III clinical trials are often expanded randomized studies in larger patient populations. These studies are designed to obtain further information about the effectiveness of the agent and safety. In these trials, the endpoint is a difference in disease free survival and overall survival as compared with the conventional treatment. Of all current gene therapy trials only 2.6% are clinical phase II/III or III trials *(3)*. Validation of gene therapy strategies will require more phase III trials to be performed yet the large number of potential gene therapeutics and the limited number of patients makes careful design of phase III studies critical. Additionally, the problem of limited numbers of patients may be reduced by properly designed phase II studies that utilize correlative studies to identify sensitive subsets so that large cohorts of patients do not have to be evaluated in phase III randomized setting to achieve statistical significance.

5.5. Phase IV (Post-Licensing) Evaluation

Following successful phase III studies which demonstrate benefit, most novel biologic agents receive FDA licensing for limited clinical use. A series of additional trials in a phase IV postlicensing stage than ensues. During these trials clinical studies are produced to extend claims or indications for the novel agent to different patients subsets, tumor types, or clinical situations *(28)*. These studies can also validate the surrogate endpoints allowing easier clinical use of the product in the market. Many of these trials allow fine tuning and marketing of the novel biologic agents to occur through presentations at national oncologic meetings and plenary discussions of clinical indications.

6. STEP 5: REGULATORY CONSIDERATIONS

Unlike other traditional therapeutics that are regulated by the FDA, gene therapy clinical trials are regulated by two federal agencies within the Department of Health and Human Services, the FDA, and the NIH (Table 3). Gene therapy clinical trials at the NIH are reviewed and discussed in a public forum by the RAC (Recombinant Advisory Committee) (Table 3). In contrast, the FDA review of gene therapeutics is confidential and conducted by the agency on an ongoing basis with the investigators. The roles of both groups are complementary and evaluate preclinical and clinical outcomes. The RAC, however, also focuses on ethical, legal and social implications of the research whereas the FDA is more concerned with review of product manufacturing as it relates to safety, purity, and efficacy *(28)*. After completing preclinical studies that focus on aspects such as toxicology, biodistribution, efficacy, and safety, investigators must file dual submissions to the FDA at CBER for an Investigational New Drug (IND) application and to the Office of Biologic Activity (OBA) to determine if full RAC review is required. The OBA submission is made prior to or at the same time as the IND submission to the CBER at the FDA. Full RAC review will be decided based on the novelty of the vector, gene-delivery system or application of the gene therapy. Because of timing and regulatory requirements, situations develop in which the FDA may approve a gene therapeutic prior to RAC discussion. The FDA therefore requests that sponsors agree to delay the clinical trial until the RAC has completed public discussion. Once the FDA and RAC have given approval for the clinical trial, Institutional Biosafety Committee (IBC) approval must be obtained from each institution at which recombinant DNA Material will be administered and Institutional Review Board (IRB) approval of the clinical protocol and informed consent documents must also be obtained prior to initiation of the clinical trial. Enrolment of patients can begin once the RAC review process has been completed and IBC and IRB approvals and FDA and all other applicable regulatory authorizations have been obtained *(35)*. Product development

Table 3
Regulatory Steps in Clinical Gene Therapy Trials

Preclinical studies on toxicology, biodistribution, potential efficacy and safety.
FDA Investigational New Drug (IND) Application.
NIH Office of Biologic Activities (OBA) Recombinant DNA Advisory Committee (RAC) Review.
Institutional Biosafety Committee (IBC) Approval.
Institutional Review Board (ICB) Approval of clinical protocol and informed consent documents.

then proceeds through IND stage (phase I–III) before product licensure occurs from the FDA. Phase IV post-licensing studies often continue during which further studies are peformed to expand product usage and define therapeutic subsets for therapeutic use. The FDA's primary role during this IND phase is to assure the safety of the gene therapy product and to validate the quality of the scientific data used to support the novel gene therapy product.

7. STEP 6: SAFETY CONSIDERATIONS

Safety of gene therapy clinical trials clearly is one of the key aspects. Two specific concerns unique to gene therapy include the use or development of replication competent viruses and the potential of inadvertent modifications of the patient's germline *(36)*. To date the safety profile in clinical gene therapy trials for cancer is excellent. In cancer gene therapy trials, hundreds of patients have been treated worldwide with a variety of vectors and gene therapy strategies without a death resulting from the vector. Most toxicity has been grade I or II related to inflammatory responses to the vector and has been much lower than toxicity associated conventional chemotherapeutics. Viral dissemination to people exposed to the patient has been limited and transient and there has been little evidence for germ line changes or development of replication competent viruses in patients. Because of this encouraging safety profile, most gene therapy trials have been able to move to outpatient settings allowing increased patient comfort and reduced cost. In 1999, however, the first major adverse effect was documented in a noncancer gene therapy trial at the University of Pennsylvania involving a patient undergoing gene transfer of the ornithine transcarboxylase gene *(37)*. The vector utilized was a replication deficient adenovirus type 5, deleted in E1 and E4 with a human ornithine transcarbamylase (OTC) gene insert. The vector was delivered by direct intrahepatic artery infusion and led to fulminant liver failure with death 4 d after administration from adult respiratory distress syndrome, multiple organ failure, and disseminated intravascular coagulation. An FDA investigation revealed several deficiencies in the trial. For example, researchers entered the patient into the trial as a substitute for another volunteer who had dropped out *(27)*. Additionally, the patient had a high ammonia level at the time of treatment that should have been an exclusion criteria. Further investigation revealed that two other serious side effects had not been immediately reported. These problems led to increased scrutiny of ongoing gene therapy trials although safety profiles for other cancer gene therapy trials continued to be good. The second major safety concern involved the trial with the first unequivocal gene therapy success which was the successful treatment of the X-linked form of SCID *(38,39)*. In this French gene therapy trial, two of nine patients successfully treated for X-SCID with a retroviral vector developed leukemia secondary to insertional mutagenesis. This report led to a temporary halt by the FDA of all gene therapy trials using retroviral vectors in blood stems cells.

The ability of certain viral vectors to integrate with the human genome, alter metabolic pathways and induce immunological responses to the virus and or its gene product emphasize the continued need for safety monitoring and development of novel strategies to ensure safe delivery. One safety mechanism that has been developed is the use of inducible promoters. In this case, the therapeutic gene can be turned on or off depending on the administration of another drug. Additionally the prompt reporting of adverse events reporting is critical. Currently, investigators are required to submit a written report on any serious unexpected adverse effect that is associated with the use of the gene transfer product and suggest a significant risk for human research participants to the NIH Office of Biotechnology Activities and to the local institutional Biosafety Committee. The high visibility of gene therapy trials mandates that extra caution be exercised for the safety of the patient, public and the gene therapy field in general.

8. STEP 7: FINANCIAL CONSIDERATIONS

The cost of developing therapeutics for cancer including novel chemotherapy agents is often quite high. Gene therapy products have additional costs associated with manufacturing, delivery, regulation, and monitoring of a novel biologic agent. There are increased public concerns with gene therapy agents because of ethical and safety issues. These concerns have led to additional regulatory and safety monitoring steps to safeguard these novel therapies. Regulatory approval requires both RAC and FDA submissions and adverse events are often scrutinized to a far greater degree by the government and press than conventional chemotherapy agents *(28)*. Additional costs are also encountered in manufacturing gene therapy agents for clinical trials because they must be produced in highly controlled conditions especially as they often cannot be sterilized *(32)*. Vectors must be manufactured under current GMP which requires that the facility, the raw materials, the training of personnel, and documentation of the process including the labeling and storage of the final product be approved. Increased local safety monitoring and approval is also required at each institution with not only IRB approval but also approval from specific biologic monitoring committees. Increased costs are also encountered in the method of delivery because the gene therapy vectors often have to be delivered intratumorally via interventional techniques and delivery of the agents often requires inpatient observation. Intratumoral delivery is usually performed in a negative pressure environment with monitoring of all exposed personnel. Additional costs can also be associated with intraoperative or intra-arterial administration.

The increased costs associated with regulation, safety monitoring, product development, and delivery make development of gene therapy products challenging especially in light of the often small population for targeted biologic agents *(40)*. Identification of sensitive patients through genetic testing may increase efficacy but may actually reduce the eligible patient population for therapy by eliminating nonresponders *(41)*. If this reduction in the patient population is not offset by higher drug prices commercial development may be impaired. Strategies to develop gene therapy products in the private sector include initial venture capital funding of "start-up" companies followed by association with more established pharmaceuticals. These funding strategies have become increasingly difficult with the lack of clear financial gene therapy successes. Governmental support of novel gene therapy strategies through NIH funding strategies are usually not able to support the large costs associated with phase II and III trials making clinical trial development beyond the phase I stage difficult. In the future, concerted collaborations with industry and government may need to occur to allow the development of gene therapy strategies for often fatal diseases without other conventional means of treatment. Investments in clinical trial development will need to occur in gene therapy because the increased costs of regulation, safety monitoring, product development and delivery will probably not disappear in the near future.

REFERENCES

1. Rosenberg SA, Aebersold P, Cornetta K, et al. Gene transfer into humans—immunotherapy of patients with advanced melanoma, using tumor-infiltrating lymphocytes modified by retroviral gene transduction. N Engl J Med 1990;323:570–578.
2. Edelstein ML, Abedi MR, Wixon J, et al. Gene therapy clinical trials worldwide 1989-2004-an overview. J Gene Med 2004;6:597–602.
3. Swisher SG, Roth JA. Gene therapy for human lung cancers. Surg Oncol Clin N Am 1998;7:603–616.
4. Jia W, Zhou Q. Viral vectors for cancer gene therapy: viral dissemination and tumor targeting. Curr Gene Ther 2005;5:133–142.
5. Glover DJ, Lipps HJ, Jans DA. Towards safe, non-viral therapeutic gene expression in humans. Nat Rev Genet 2005;6:299–310.
6. Trent RJ, Alexander IE. Gene therapy: applications and progress towards the clinic. Intern Med J 2004;34:621–625.
7. Swisher SG, Roth JA, Komaki R, et al. Induction of p53 regulated genes and tumor regression in lung cancer following intratumoral delivery of adenoviral p53 (RPR/INGN 201) and radiation therapy. Clin Cancer Res 2003;9:93–101.
8. Margolin KA, Rayner AA, Hawkins MJ, et al. Interleukin-2 and lymphokine-activated killer cell therapy of solid tumors: analysis of toxicity and management guidelines. J Clin Oncol 1989;7:486–498.
9. Sangro B, Mazzolini G, Ruiz J, et al. Phase I trial of intratumoral injection of an adenovirus encoding interleukin-12 for advanced digestive tumors. J Clin Oncol 2004;22:1389–1397.
10. Belldegrun A, Tso CL, Zisman A, et al. Interleukin 2 gene therapy for prostate cancer: phase I clinical trial and basic biology. Hum Gene Ther 2001;12:883–892.
11. Ren HBT, Soling A, Warnke PC, et al. Immunogene therapy of recurrent gliobastoma multiforme with a liposomally encapsulated replication-incompenent semliki forest virus vector carrying the human interleukin-12 gene - A pahe I/II clinical protocl. J Neuro-Oncol 2003;64:147–154.
12. Zajac P, Oertli D, Marti W, et al. Phase I/II clinical trial of a nonreplicative vaccinia virus expressing multiple HLA-A0201-restricted tumor-associated epitopes and costimulatory molecules in metastatic melanoma patients. Hum Gene Ther 2003;14:1497–1510.
13. Lang FF, Bruner JM, Fuller GN, et al. Phase I trail of adenovirus-mediated p53 gene therapy for recurrent giloma: biological and clinical results. J Clin Oncol 2003;21:2508–2518.
14. Hughes RM. Strategies for cancer gene therapy. J Surg Oncol 2004;85:28–35.
15. Tolcher AW. Preliminary phase I results of G3139 (bcl-2 antisense oligonucleotide) therapy in combination with docetaxel in hormone-refractory prostate cancer. Semin Oncol 2001;28:67–70.
16. Lopes de Menezes DE, Mayer LD. Pharmacokinetics of Bcl-2 antisense oligonucleotide (G3139) combined with doxorubicin in SCID mice bearing human breast cancer solid tumor xenografts. Cancer Chemother Pharmacol 2002;49:57–68.
17. Dummer R, Bergh J, Karlsson Y, et al. Biological activity and safety of adenoviral vector-expressed wild-type p53 after intratumoral injection in melanoma and breast cancer patients with p53-overexpressing tumors. Cancer Gene Ther 2000;7:1069–1076.
18. Roth JA, Cristiano RJ. Gene therapy for cancer: what have we done and where are we going? J Natl Cancer Inst 1997;89:21–39.
19. Pearson AS, Spitz FR, Swisher SG, et al. Up-regulation of the proapoptotic mediators Bax and Bak after adenovirus-mediated p53 gene transfer in lung cancer cells. Clin Cancer Res 2000;6:887–890.
20. Kagawa S, Gu J, Swisher SG, et al. Antitumor effect of adenovirus-mediated *Bax* gene transfer on *p53*-sensitive and *p53*-resistant cancer lines. Cancer Res 2000;60:1157–1161.

21. Pataer A, Fang B, Yu R, et al. Adenoviral bak overexpression mediates caspase-dependent tumor killing. Cancer Res 2000;60:788–792.
22. Kountouras J, Zavos C, and Chatzopoulos D. Apoptotic and anti-angiogenic strategies in liver and gastrointestinal malignancies. J Surg Oncol 2005;90:249–259.
23. Lowe SW, Ruley HE, Jacks T, et al. p53-dependent apoptosis modulates the cytotoxicity of anticancer agents. Cell 1993;74:957–967.
24. Nguyen DM, Spitz FR, Yen N, et al. Gene therapy for lung cancer: enhancement of tumor suppression by a combination of sequential systemic cisplatin and adenovirus-mediated p53 gene transfer. J Thorac Cardiovasc Surg 1996;112:1372–1377.
25. Pilaro AM, Serabian MA. Preclinical development strategies for novel gene therapeutic products. Toxicol Pathol 1999;27:4–7.
26. Aguilar LK, Aguilar-Cordova E. Evolution of a gene therapy clinical trial. From bench to bedside and back. J Neurooncol 2003;65:307–315.
27. Manilla P, Rebello T, Afable C, et al. Regulatory considerations for novel gene therapy products: a review of the process leading to the first clinical lentiviral vector. Hum Gene Ther 2005;16:17–25.
28. Miller AE, Simek SL. Regulatory aspects of gene therapy. 2005;371–382.
29. Amin S, Robins RA, Maxwell-Armstrong CA, et al. Vaccine-induced apoptosis: a novel clinical trial end point? Cancer Res 2000;60:3132–3136.
30. Schuler M, Herrmann R, De Greve JL, et al. Adenovirus-mediated wild-type p53 gene transfer in patients receiving chemotherapy for advanced non-small-cell lung cancer: results of a multicenter phase II study. J Clin Oncol 2001;19:1750–1758.
31. Parulekar WR, Eisenhauer EA. Phase I trial design for solid tumor studies of targeted, non-cytotoxic agents: theory and practice. Journal of the National Cancer Institute 2004;96:990–997.
32. Tan AR, Swain SM. Novel agents: clinical trial design. Semin Oncol 2001;28:148–153.
33. Teh BS, Ayala G, Aguilar L, et al. Phase I-II trial evaluating combined intensity-modulated radiotherapy and in situ gene therapy with or without hormonal therapy in treatment of prostate cancer-interim report on PSA response and biopsy data. Int J Rad Oncol Biol Phys 004;58:1520–1529.
34. Anderson BD, Adamson PC, Weiner SL, et al. Tissue collection for correlative studies in childhood cancer clinical trials: ethical considerations and special imperatives. J Clin Oncol 2004;22:4846–4850.
35. NIH Guidelines for research involving recombinant DNA molecules (NIH Guidelines). NIH 2002.
36. Lichtenstein DL, Wold WS Experimental infections of humans with wild-type adenoviruses and with replication-competent adenovirus vectors: replication, safety, and transmission. Cancer Gene Ther 2004;11:819–829.
37. Lehrman S. Virus treatment questioned after gene therapy death. Nature 1999;401:517–518.
38. Hacein-Bey-Abina S, Von Kalle C, Schmidt M, et al. LMO2-associated clonal T cell proliferation in two patients after gene therapy for SCID-X1. Science 2003;302:415–419.
39. Hacein-Bey-Abina S, Le Deist F, Carlier F, et al. Sustained correction of X-linked severe combined immunodeficiency by ex vivo gene therapy. N Engl J Med 2002;346:1185–1193.
40. Mehl B, Santell J. Projecting future drug expenditures—2001. Am J Health Syst Pharm 2001;58: 125–133.
41. Danzon P, Towse A. The economics of gene therapy and of pharmacogenetics. Value Health 2002;5:5–13.

Index

N

O

P

Q, R